NEUROLOGIC
EMERGENCIES

NEUROLOGIC EMERGENCIES

Edited by

Michael P. Earnest, M.D.

Associate Professor of Neurology and
Preventive Medicine
University of Colorado
Health Sciences Center
Director, Department of Neurology
Denver General Hospital
Denver, Colorado

With 20 Contributors

CHURCHILL LIVINGSTONE
New York, Edinburgh, London, Melbourne   1983

Distributed in the United Kingdom by Churchill Livingstone,
Robert Stevenson House, 1-3 Baxter's Place, Leith Walk,
Edinburgh EH1 3AF and by associated companies, branches
and representatives throughout the world.

First published 1983

Printed in U.S.A.

ISBN 0–443–08221–9

9 8 7 6 5 4 3 2 1

Library of Congress Cataloging in Publication Data

Main entry under title:

Neurologic emergencies.

    Bibliography: p.
    Includes index.
    1. Nervous system—Diseases.   2. Medical emergencies.
I. Earnest, Michael P.   [DNLM: 1. Nervous system
diseases.   2. Nervous system—Injuries.   3. Emergencies.
WL   100   N4942]
RC346.N384   1983   616.8′0425   83–2040
ISBN 0–443–08221–9

Contributors

H. Richard Beresford, M.D., J.D.
Professor of Neurology, Cornell University Medical College, New York, New York; Director of Neurology, North Shore University Hospital, Manhasset, New York

Jack S. Burks, M.D.
Associate Professor of Neurology, Microbiology and Immunology, Director, Rocky Mountain Multiple Sclerosis Center, University of Colorado Health Sciences Center, Denver, Colorado

John J. Caronna, M.D.
Professor of Clinical Neurology, Cornell University Medical College, Department of Neurology, The New York Hospital–Cornell Medical Center, New York, New York

Larry E. Davis, M.D.
Associate Professor of Neurology and Microbiology, Department of Neurology, University of New Mexico School of Medicine, Albuquerque, New Mexico

Michael P. Earnest, M.D.
Associate Professor of Neurology and Preventive Medicine, University of Colorado Health Sciences Center; Director, Department of Neurology, Denver General Hospital, Denver, Colorado

Paul A. Hwang, M.D.
Assistant Professor of Neurology, Director of the Electroencephalogram Laboratory, University of Colorado Health Sciences Center, Denver, Colorado

Joseph R. Lacy, M.D.
Assistant Professor of Neurology, University of Colorado Health Sciences Center, Department of Neurology, Denver General Hospital, Denver, Colorado

Michael Mestek, M.D.
Assistant Professor of Radiology (Neuroradiology), University of Colorado Health Sciences Center, Department of Radiology, Denver General Hospital, Denver, Colorado

Chester J. Minarcik, Jr., M.D.
Assistant Professor of Pediatrics and Neurology, University of Colorado Health Sciences Center, Department of Neurology, Children's Hospital of Denver, Denver, Colorado

Steven P. Ringel, M.D.
Associate Professor of Neurology and Immunology, Director of Neuromuscular Disease Clinic, University of Colorado Health Sciences Center, Denver, Colorado

Allan H. Ropper, M.D.
Instructor in Neurology, Harvard Medical School, Department of Neurology, Massachusetts General Hospital, Boston, Massachusetts

S. Clifford Schold, Jr., M.D.
Assistant Professor of Medicine (Neurology), Department of Neurology, Duke University Medical Center, Durham, North Carolina

John J. Sidtis, Ph.D.
Assistant Professor of Psychology in Neurology, Cornell University Medical College, Department of Neurology, The New York Hospital–Cornell Medical Center, New York, New York

David B. Simon, M.D.
Fellow in Neuromuscular Diseases, Department of Neurology, University of Colorado Health Sciences Center, Denver, Colorado

Russell D. Snyder, M.D.
Professor of Pediatrics and Neurology, Director of Pediatric Neurology, University of New Mexico School of Medicine, Albuquerque, New Mexico

John B. Sullivan, Jr., M.D.
Assistant Professor of Emergency Medicine and Pediatrics and Associate Director, Rocky Mountain Poison Control Center, University of Colorado Health Sciences Center, Denver, Colorado

David S. Thompson, M.D.
Assistant Professor of Neurology, Rocky Mountain Multiple Sclerosis Center, University of Colorado Health Sciences Center, Denver, Colorado

Jonathan D. Trobe, M.D.
Associate Professor of Ophthalmology, University of Florida Medical Center; Chief of Ophthalmology, J. Hillis Miller Hospital, Gainesville, Florida

Harold B. Vogel, M.D.
Associate Professor of Surgery (Neurosurgery), University of Colorado Health Sciences Center; Chief, Division of Neurosurgery, Denver General Hospital, Denver, Colorado

Bruce T. Volpe, M.D.
Assistant Professor of Neurology, Cornell University Medical College, Department of Neurology, The New York Hospital–Cornell Medical Center, New York, New York

K. M. A. Welch, M.D.C.H.B., M.R.C.P.
Clinical Professor of Neurology, University of Michigan; Chairman, Department of Neurology, Henry Ford Hospital, Detroit, Michigan

Preface

> Perhaps someone . . . will understand my illness, discover what a brain injury does to a man's mind, memory, and body, appreciate my effort, and help me avoid some of the problems I have in life. . . . Why doesn't my memory function, my sight return? Why does my head constantly ache and buzz? It's depressing, having to start all over and make sense out of a world you've lost because of injury and illness, to get those bits and pieces to add up to a coherent whole.*

This tragic plea of Lieutenant Zasetsky speaks for many patients. He received a bullet wound of the brain in World War II and for the next 25 years heroically struggled to piece together his shattered world. His journals were published and provide fascinating insights into the effects of brain injury upon an individual's life. He suffered a bullet wound, but patients with strokes, traumatic brain contusions, tumors, and those with anoxic brain damage have comparable stories to tell.

The human brain is the source of the human mind. Within the brain lie the structures and mechanisms that create human intelligence and personality (i.e., our humanity). When the brain is injured much more than a single organ suffers; the entire person is affected. The injury not only creates weakness, numbness, altered vision etc., but it also alters thinking, memory, perceptions of the world, insight, judgement, social interactions and emotions. Thus, the physician encountering the patient with an acute neurologic crisis must act swiftly and effectively to preserve the nervous system and the wholeness of the person.

Non-neurologists are often the first physicians called to manage patients with neurologic emergencies; the neurologist or neurosurgeon is consulted only later. However, the first few minutes to an hour is the critical period in which the process causing the emergency must be reversed, or at least

* Luria, A. R.: The Man with a Shattered World. Basic Books, Inc., New York, 1972.

halted, so that minimal brain injury will occur. Unfortunately, many physicians have had little training in neurology and so feel anxious and uncertain about the best steps toward a diagnosis and adequate treatment.

The purpose of this book is to provide several aids to the general physician, emergency room doctor or any other non-neurologist who wishes to learn more about managing neurologic emergencies. First, each chapter contains basic information on the anatomy and pathogenesis of the specific condition, information to expand the physician's understanding. Second, the chapter gives specific lists of differential diagnoses and management plans for the particular clinical syndrome. Third, key references are provided for further reading.

Each chapter is complete in itself, but it is recommended that the reader begin by reading Chapter 1, "Principles of Early Diagnosis and Management of Nervous System Emergencies." The concepts from that chapter apply to all neurologic crises and will provide a framework for a better understanding of later chapters.

The editor wishes to thank several persons who have given important advice and support. Dr. Stuart Schneck, whose suggestion was the origin of this project, generously advised the early development of the book. Drs. Robert Stone, Curtis Stine, Steven Ringel, and David Garr provided the editor with valuable suggestions about topics and how to present the important information. Drs. Schneck, Stine and Dr. Peter Rosen also reviewed and strengthened the draft for Chapter 1. The editor owes a special thanks to his office assistant, Ms. Clare Foster, who made scores of telephone calls, typed numerous letters, and in general, did everything necessary to keep the project going. Mrs. Colleen Epstein typed prodigious amounts of material and Ms. Marybelle Gotseff ran many important errands and made the reams of copies that are always necessary in any project of this sort.

Michael P. Earnest

Contents

1. **Principles of Early Diagnosis and Management of Nervous System Emergencies** 1
   Michael P. Earnest, M.D.

2. **Effective Use of Radiologic Tests in Neurologic Emergencies** 25
   Michael Mestek, M.D.

3. **Safe and Effective Use of the Lumbar Puncture** 47
   Michael P. Earnest, M.D.

4. **Acute Management of Increased Intracranial Pressure** 59
   Joseph R. Lacy, M.D.

5. **Coma in the Emergency Room** 79
   Allan H. Ropper, M.D.

6. **Emergency Management of Seizure Disorders** 103
   Paul A. Hwang, M.D., C.M., F.R.C.P.(C.)

7. **Emergency Diagnosis and Management of Brain Infarctions and Hemorrhages** 127
   Michael P. Earnest, M.D.

8. **Transient Neurologic Symptoms, Including Blackouts, Dizziness and Transient Ischemic Attacks** 161
   Michael P. Earnest, M.D.

9. **Trauma of the Head, Spine and Peripheral Nerves** 177
   Harold B. Vogel, M.D.

10. **Neuromuscular Emergencies**   219
    David B. Simon, M.D.
    Steven P. Ringel, M.D.
    Joseph R. Lacy, M.D.

11. **Drugs and Toxins Presenting as Neurological**   259
    Disorders
    John B. Sullivan, Jr., M.D.

12. **Acute Disorders of the Content of Consciousness**   275
    Bruce T. Volpe, M.D.
    John J. Sidtis, Ph.D.

13. **Diagnosis and Treatment of Spinal Cord Compres-**   311
    sion and Acute Myelopathy
    S. Clifford Schold, Jr., M.D.

14. **Neuro-Ophthalmologic Emergencies**   331
    Jonathan D. Trobe, M.D.

15. **Multiple Sclerosis**   361
    Jack S. Burks, M.D.
    David S. Thompson, M.D.

16. **Neurologic Emergencies of Children**   387
    Chester J. Minarcik, Jr., M.D.

17. **Acute Management of Severe Brain Anoxia**   413
    John J. Caronna, M.D.

18. **Evaluation and Management of Severe Headache**   439
    K.M.A. Welch, M.D.C.H.B., M.R.C.P.

19. **Early Diagnosis and Management of Acute Infec-**   465
    tions of the Nervous System
    Larry E. Davis, M.D.
    Russell D. Snyder, M.D.

20. **Legal Aspects of Neurological Emergency Care**   493
    H. Richard Beresford, M.D., J.D.

    INDEX   517

1

Principles of Early Diagnosis and Management of Nervous System Emergencies

Michael P. Earnest, M.D.

INTRODUCTION

The emergency room nurse is on the telephone, "Mr. Smith's family just brought him in. He has a bad headache, his right side is paralyzed and he has trouble talking. He really looks sick." The physician then must face one of the most challenging and one of the most serious health and life-threatening conditions in medicine. If the etiology of his symptoms is a subarachnoid or intracerebral hemorrhage Mr. Smith may die or suffer crippling, irreversible brain damage within minutes. However, he may also be having a neurologically complicated migraine attack or even an unusual transient ischemic attack, and so may recover normal function in a few hours. How can you determine what is actually happening? How can you treat the conditions you diagnose? How can you prevent progressive nervous system damage during the several hours of uncertainty before definitive diagnosis and treatment?

The general physician often faces such neurologic and neurosurgical emergencies with anxiety. The nervous system, especially the central nervous system, is an anatomically and functionally complicated organ complex, almost completely hidden from the eyes, ears and hands of the physician. He can't directly observe, palpate, percuss or auscultate it, so must infer the location and nature of the process by testing the functions of the system (i.e., by performing the neurologic examination). However, most general physicians have had limited training in neuroanatomy, neurophysiology and clinical neurology and neurosurgery, and so the anatomy, function, examination and differential diagnosis of the nervous system are not facile clinical tools for him. In addition, the nervous system is known to be extremely vulnerable to permanent injury and is widely believed to have little capacity for recovery, once damaged. This knowledge leads to an attitude of futility about the usefulness of treatment, especially concerning the older stroke patient. And finally, neurologists and neurosurgeons even themselves argue heatedly over how to work up and treat many acute illnesses. Anticoagulate the stroke patient or not? Do a carotid endarterectomy? Give steroids or mannitol? Do angiography or computerized tomography (CT scan)? These are difficult issues with no simple answers.

However, the general physician still must care for Mr. Smith. So he often must act out the clinician's art and "make adequate decisions based on inadequate data." In spite of the problems facing the clinician, adequate decisions are possible and the general physician can make them. Some basic principles can guide the physician in the diagnosis and management of acute neurologic disorders. Knowledge of these principles and their use as a framework within which to place clinical and laboratory observations can simplify and expedite the work-up and treatment.

THE CLINICAL METHOD IN NEUROLOGIC EMERGENCIES: GOALS, INITIAL MANAGEMENT AND DIFFERENTIAL DIAGNOSIS

The Primary Goals

The first goal of the physician in any emergency setting is to preserve the patient's life by maintaining his respiration and circulation. In the neurologic emergency setting the subsequent goal is to maintain the patient's brain and spinal cord or nerves and muscles in maximum possible health until the definitive diagnosis and treatment have been achieved. Effectively doing the latter requires knowledge of the ways the nervous system is vulnerable to injury and then responds to that injury.

The Pathophysiology Of Nervous System Injury

In spite of its complexity in detail, the nervous system can be understood in simple terms.[3,4] The basic working unit within the central nervous system (CNS) is the neuron, which is connected by its axon to other neurons. The axon is basically an electrical transmission cable. Surrounding the neurons are the glial cells giving mechanical and metabolic support. Wrapped around the axon is the myelin sheath, as insulation on the cable. The entire tissue is supplied with a luxurious blood system and is also bathed in cerebrospinal fluid.

The peripheral nervous system is composed of the effectors (muscles) and sensors (skin nerve endings) and the wiring (nerve roots and peripheral nerves) connecting them to the CNS.

These simple elements are arranged in a complex but balanced system.

The right side is balanced against the left at all levels. The more rostral structures are generally more complex and are functionally superimposed on and control the lower structures.[1]

So what happens when the nervous system is injured? Some of the neurons, axons and glial cells may die, but much more tissue is merely rendered dysfunctional. The first general principle for managing neurologic emergencies is then:

> ***PRINCIPLE 1:*** An injury of the nervous system does not cause instantaneous organ death. Viable tissue and function remain, and must be preserved.

In any type of injury to the nervous system, short of decapitation or some other event causing instantaneous total physical brain destruction, the process of injury is a dynamic and continuing one. There remain tissue and nervous system function that may be saved. The task for the clinician is to aggressively arrest the primary process, preserve the surviving but dysfunctional tissue and to prevent or reverse any secondary events that may cause further nervous system damage. Table 1.1 summarizes the mechanisms that are important in nervous system injury.

Table 1.1 Pathophysiology of Nervous System Damage in Neurologic Emergencies

Pathologic Events	Common Causes	Outcome
Primary Events		
Cell death	Anoxia	No recovery
	Intracranial hemorrhage	
	Ischemia	
	Trauma	
	Hypoglycemia	
Axonal or myelin disruption	Trauma	Partial recovery, if damage not severe
	Multiple sclerosis	
	Transverse myelitis	
	Tumors	
Interruption of transmission	Toxins	Full recovery, when primary lesion is treated
	Metabolic disorders	
	Spinal cord or nerve compression	
Secondary Events		
Edema		
Increased intracranial pressure		
Obstruction of CSF flow	Anoxia	
Vasospasm	Intracranial hemorrhage	Can be prevented or reversed with some recovery
Failure of cerebrovascular autoregulation	Ischemia	
	Trauma	
Failure of collateral vascular supply	Tumors	
Altered respiratory function		
Altered cardiac function		

The process of a simple ischemic infarct (bland stroke) or a traumatic contusion of the brain illustrates this concept. At the center of the damaged area there is dead or dying tissue, tissue where the neurons, axons and glia are irreversibly damaged. This portion of the lesion cannot, with current means, be saved or repaired. However, surrounding the central lesion is a zone of damaged but potentially salvageable tissue. In that zone are neurons, axons and glial cells that are alive but dysfunctional because of ischemia, local tissue acidosis, edema, toxic products from necrotic tissue, petechial hemorrhage or other local factors. If this marginal tissue can be maintained until the collateral blood supply develops or the local tissue factors resolve, then the tissue may function again.

However, within even a few minutes of nervous system injury other processes are initiated which may cause further tissue damage or even death. These are the secondary processes caused by the nervous system's own response to the initial injury (Table 1.1). Massive edema may follow a head injury and can occur in the hemisphere damaged by a large infarction. This produces increased intracranial pressure (ICP), thus further compromising brain function and altering cerebral blood perfusion. Herniation and death may follow. Arterial vasospasm, even severe enough to cause brain infarction, can follow head trauma or subarachnoid hemorrhage from an aneurysm. The normal flow of CSF can be obstructed by subarachnoid blood, causing hydrocephalus and increased ICP and further damage. Because of the nervous system injury the patient may develop changes in respirations and cardiac function, or shock in spinal injuries, which can further impair nervous system function and recovery. The clinician's task is to be aware of these secondary events and to reverse them as quickly and completely as possible. Quick action will preserve nervous system tissue and function; failure to act may be fatal for the patient.

Principles Of Basic Emergency Medicine In Neurologic Emergencies

Generally, what's good for the patient's whole body is good for the nervous system. The physician should initially focus on the standard "ABC's" taught by emergency medicine: Airway, Bleeding and Circulation. The first decision about treatment must focus on the Airway:

> **PRINCIPLE 2:** Always consider the need for intubation. If in doubt, intubate.

Patients with nervous system damage often have respiratory complications. Patients in coma often hypoventilate. With increased intracranial pressure and/or head injuries they often aspirate gastric contents. With status epilepticus they have post-ictal apnea, and with intracranial hemorrhages, may develop pulmonary edema. The abnormal ventilation may produce further nervous system damage by causing systemic hypoxia and acidosis and hypercarbia, which also aggravate increased ICP. Finally, the most common mode of death in brain-damaged patients is respiratory arrest, not primary cardiac arrest.

Early intubation gives the physician control of ventilation, access for ease of suctioning and allows immediate treatment for respiratory arrest. Intubation is also vital when brain herniation occurs. The first step in treatment is to forcibly hyperventilate the patient to reduce intracranial pressure.[10] (This will be discussed in Chapter 4.)

PRINCIPLE 3: Stop the bleeding.

Obviously, peripheral bleeding must be controlled, whenever present. Peripheral or internal bleeding is a common accompaniment in patients with multisystem trauma, including the head, in automobile or industrial accidents.

PRINCIPLE 4: Maintain systemic circulation.

Acute nervous system injury can be accompanied by life-threatening cardiovascular changes. Severe spinal injuries can produce peripheral vascular shock. Head injuries and non-traumatic intracranial hemorrhages can produce cardiac arrhythmias. Increased intracranial pressure, especially when due to hemorrhage, often causes marked systemic hypertension. The trauma that produces a head injury may also cause a ruptured spleen or other systemic injury, leading to shock. Such cardiovascular changes can produce further nervous system damage by causing further ischemia, edema or hemorrhage.

Thus each patient with an acute nervous system injury should be observed closely for changes in blood pressure and cardiac rhythm, and treatment begun as soon as serious changes occur.

Is It Structural Or Nonstructural?

Once the patient has been initially stabilized and the physician is free to focus on the diagnostic problem, the main question becomes:

PRINCIPLE 5: Is the disease structural or non-structural?

Structural lesions are those which are focal (i.e., localized to one area or one side of the nervous system). Often they produce focal mass effect, distorting surrounding brain and causing increased intracranial pressure. These lesions more than any other threaten the patient with death or permanent brain injury. They can usually be visualized by a radiologic procedure. Examples are brain tumors, abscesses, intracranial hematomas, and cerebral infarctions. Non-structural processes are those which usually affect the nervous system diffusely, produce little mass effect, and are usually diagnosed by blood or urine tests or lumbar puncture. Common diseases of this type are the metabolic comas, toxic disorders, meningitis, and multiple sclerosis.

Making this distinction early in the patient's course enables the physician to choose one of two quite different pathways (Fig. 1.1). If the tentative diagnosis is a structural one, the safest course is to promptly order a CT scan or other radiologic procedure, or transfer the patient to another institution where the test is available, and to observe the patient closely for brain herniation while preparing to treat it. Early consultation by a neurologist or neurosurgeon is important to aid in the decisions about tests and treatment. A *lumbar puncture is not done* because of the danger of precipitating brain herniation. (Chapter 3 will discuss the decision-making process and risks associated with lumbar puncture.)

If, on the other hand, the physician's initial impression is of a non-structural condition, he orders a broad range of blood and urine tests looking for a toxic or metabolic process. He also should consider a lumbar puncture early in the course. Examination of the spinal fluid can disclose an infectious process or unsuspected blood in the spinal fluid. If blood is found the possibil-

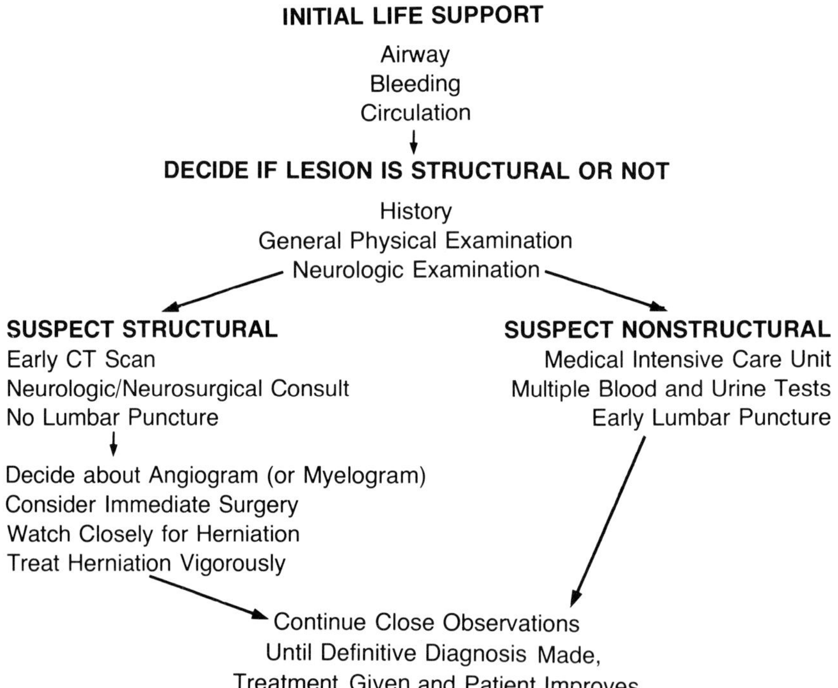

Fig. 1.1 The two decision pathways for structural and nonstructural neurologic lesions.

ity of a structural lesion (e.g., subdural hematoma or other intracranial hemorrhage) should be reconsidered.

The general bias of the physician should be to suspect a structural lesion and to prove one is *not* present by CT scan or another test, unless the diagnosis of a non-structural lesion is beyond reasonable doubt. The emphasis on structural lesions is necessary because undue delay in their diagnosis and treatment may allow progressive and permanent brain damage to occur. Delay in diagnosis of the non-structural process, other than hypoglycemia, continuing hypoxia, and bacterial meningitis, is generally not as immediately dangerous.

The use of the history and physical examination to distinguish structural from non-structural processes will be discussed. However, it may be helpful first to describe the thinking process a clinical neurologist uses to make a diagnosis.

The Clinical Neurologist's Analysis Of A Neurologic Emergency

In medical school and through later training the physician has been taught to gather all available data, form hypotheses and then, in a logical fashion, use further data to confirm or deny the diagnosis suspected. In neurology the mode taught required a full history, a detailed neurologic exam and then an exhaustive differential diagnosis followed by an outline of plans for the laboratory work-up. (I suspect that many general physicians have been frustrated because they have been trying to apply that process in their care of patients with neurologic emergencies.)

However, the actual behavior of the experienced clinical neurologist is quite different.[1,2] He begins with a minimal amount of data, quickly chooses a few most probable diagnoses, and then sharply focuses his history and neurologic examination to elicit data that confirms or excludes his hypotheses. Then, considering a short list of probable diagnoses, he chooses the test that will give the most information with the least risks.

The experienced clinician begins the process the minute he hears the syndrome the patient has presented with, and can clarify his diagnoses greatly by briefly observing the patient the moment he enters the examining room. For example, a 55-year-old man has been brought in by his family because today he developed trouble speaking and a right hemiparesis. The neurologist immediately suspects "stroke, left hemisphere, probably infarct, but rule out hemorrhage, tumor, abscess and subdural hematoma." Granted, it could be a transient ischemic attack, a post-ictal or migraine phenomenon, herpes encephalitis or some more rare condition, but the first diagnoses given are by far the most common and most immediately dangerous. Then the neurologist enters the room and sees the man is fully alert, has no fever, and has a limp, unmoving right arm. The diagnosis is almost certainly "left cerebral infarction" because a hemorrhage, tumor, abscess or subdural hematoma, by their mass, would almost invariably cause increased intracranial pressure and depression of consciousness if they were large enough to cause such profound focal signs (the paralyzed arm). This is not phenomenal clinical acumen or a mysteriously complex intuitive process. The process does take some training and experience in clinical neurology, but it is based on rather simple principles which also can be used by the general physician.

> ***PRINCIPLE 6:*** Keep the diagnosis simple, and don't initially worry about detailed localization of the lesion.

Immediately list only the few major types of lesions that often affect the nervous system, namely vascular disease, tumor, infection, trauma and seizures. You will refine, or change, the list as the work-up progresses. The principle and practice are: at first simply decide if the lesion is a focal, structural one or a diffuse, non-structural one. Then, if it's focal, decide if it is in the head, the spinal cord, or outside the spinal canal in the neuromuscular system. If it's in the head, is it on the right or left? Those judgements are about all that are immediately necessary in the emergency setting, and often those judgements are made before the detailed examination.

The keys to constructing the initial diagnostic list are easily available from the chief complaint, often given by the family, and the initial observation of the patient. They are: (1) the patient's state of consciousness; (2) the presence or absence of *gross focal signs;* and (3) the speed of onset of the symptoms (Table 1.2).

The state of consciousness (SOC) is the patient's degree of alertness. The SOC can be anything from fully alert (the patient has his eyes open, follows commands and talks spontaneously) to coma (eyes closed, no voluntary movements, and no verbal efforts), and any state in between. (Chapter 5 discusses the very important issue of defining the state of consciousness.) Focal signs are those findings on observation or on formal neurologic examination that show asymmetry of function of the nervous system. The most common and helpful ones in neurologic emergencies are hemiparesis, aphasia, paraparesis (weakness of both legs), deviation or abnormal movement of one or both eyes, asymmetric reflexes (corneal, deep tendon or toe reflexes), and asymmetric pupil size and/or reaction to light. "Gross focal signs" refers to those signs that the family reports or the physician sees with only a brief examination. The obvious arm weakness of the 55-year-old man with a stroke is an example. The speed of onset can be divided into acute (minutes or hours), subacute (1 day to a week) or chronic.

From the history alone or the history plus the brief initial observation of the patient several sets of diagnoses emerge (Table 1.2). If the patient is alert and has no gross focal signs then either he has no neurologic disorder, a symmetrical neuromuscular syndrome or has recovered from a transient neurologic syndrome. Such syndromes include transient ischemic attacks, seizures, migraine phenomena, anxiety symptoms, blackouts of cardiovascular origin and concussion. Depressed state of consciousness without focal

Table 1.2 Analysis of Neurologic Emergency Syndromes Based on Level of Consciousness, Presence of Focal Signs and Nature of Onset

Level of Consciousness	Focal Signs	Onset	Common Causes
Alert:	None	Acute	Resolved transient ischemic attack, seizure, migraine phenomenon or concussion Anxiety symptoms Cardiovascular events (e.g., syncope)
	Present	Acute	Strokes—ischemic Trauma with focal nervous system lesion (e.g., spinal or nerve injury)
	Present	Subacute	Multiple sclerosis Metastatic tumors
	Present	Chronic	Primary tumors (Glioma, meningioma)
Depressed:	None	Acute	Drug overdose Hypoglycemia Post-ictal state Meningitis Subarachnoid hemorrhage Cardiac arrest Trauma—concussion
	Ataxia Only	Subacute	Drugs
	Present	Acute	Intracerebral hemorrhage Cerebral contusion (traumatic) Large or bilateral cerebral infarcts Brainstem infarct Hypoglycemia
	Present	Subacute	Brain abscess Subdural hematoma Metastatic tumor Herpes encephalitis
	Present	Chronic	Primary tumor Subdural hematoma

signs usually results from metabolic or toxic depression of the nervous system or meningitis, or from a just completed grand mal convulsion. A patient who is fully alert but has prominent focal signs is more likely to have an ischemic infarct, multiple sclerosis or a spinal or peripheral nerve lesion, and unlikely to have an intracranial mass lesion. Finally, the patient with depressed SOC and obvious focal signs probably has one of the focal intracranial masses. However, a large cerebral infarction with severe edema or a brainstem infarction can produce similar findings. Hypoglycemia can sometimes produce depressed consciousness and focal neurologic signs and, although rare, should always be considered.

The nature of the onset of the condition then is used to add further precision to the diagnosis (Table 1.2). Only a few processes frequently cause serious neurologic dysfunction within a few hours. The most common are drug overdoses, hypoglycemia, anoxia associated with cardiac or respiratory arrest, seizures and related postictal states, trauma and vascular events, infarction or hemorrhage. Those commonly progressing in a subacute time course are brain abscess, meningitis, encephalitis, multiple sclerosis, most metabolic and toxic processes and metastatic tumors. The conditions to be considered in a chronically progressing syndrome are primary brain tumors and chronic subdural hematomas. Few other conditions cause chronic-onset dysfunction that presents as a neurologic emergency. (Chapter 12 discusses one important syndrome, the agitated patient with a known chronic organic brain syndrome.)

Given these three key pieces of data, the SOC, the presence or absence of focal signs and the nature of the onset, the physician often makes an accurate diagnosis, or compiles a very selective differential diagnosis to be explored. In the example above of the 55-year-old man, the acute onset, the patient's alertness and the paralyzed arm were all the physician needed to reach a reasonably secure primary diagnosis. Other clinical problems can be similarly analyzed, for example a patient with a depressed SOC and a hemiparesis. The patient has a focal exam and thus probably a structural lesion. He has a depressed state of consciousness as well, suggesting a mass-type structural lesion. If the onset had been acute the clinician would think of intracranial hemorrhage, but possibly trauma (the history usually makes this diagnosis) and far less likely a brainstem or massive edematous hemispheric infarction (both uncommon types of stroke). If the onset had been subacute, brain abscess, metastatic tumor or a subdural hematoma (especially if there were a history of recent trauma), or encephalitis would be most likely. A chronic onset would strongly suggest a primary brain tumor. Table 1.3 lists a number of syndromes commonly seen as neurologic emergencies and lists the most probable diagnoses, separated by mode of onset. A general principle should be stated here:

> **PRINCIPLE 7:** A patient with a depressed state of consciousness and focal signs probably has a mass-producing structural lesion of the brain.

Exceptions always exist to a rule. Exceptions to this principle are patients with two or more processes, for example an old stroke and diabetic ketoacidosis, patients following repeated focal motor seizures, and, rarely, patients following cardiac arrest or with hypoglycemia. However, the principle is strong enough that any patient with decreased SOC and focal signs should have a definitive radiologic test before another diagnosis is accepted and before a lumbar puncture is done.

Using The History, General Physical Examination And The Neurologic Examination Effectively

Further clarification of the diagnosis comes from the more detailed history, the general medical physical examination and then the focused neurologic examination. The emphasis in this step of the evaluation is to attempt to

Table 1.3 Differential Diagnosis and Suggested Tests for Some Common Emergency Neurologic Syndromes

Syndrome	Onset	Probable Diagnosis	Diagnoses to Exclude	Best Tests
Alert patient with hemiparesis, often with hemisensory deficit	Acute	Ischemic cerebral infarct or transient ischemic attack in progress	Small intracerebral hemorrhage Rare—Postictal after focal motor seizures Migraine with hemiparesis	CT scan or isotope brain scan plus lumbar puncture (LP)
Same focal signs but drowsy or comatose	Acute	Intracerebral or subarachnoid hemorrhage	Trauma with cerebral contusion or subdural hematoma Rare—Hypoglycemia	CT scan or isotope scan No LP
	Subacute or chronic	Brain tumor, abscess or subdural hematoma	Herpes simplex encephalitis	Same work-up
Alert patient with paraparesis	Subacute	Cord compression by tumor *must be* ruled out Multiple sclerosis	Cervical spine osteoarthritis Rare—Transverse myelitis Hydrocephalus Myopathy Neuropathy	Spine X-rays and/or myelogram (spinal CT scan helpful in some institutions)
Alert patient with ataxia	Acute	Cerebellar infarct or hemorrhage Vestibular disease	Multiple sclerosis Drugs (anti-convulsants) Rare—Spinal cord compression	CT scan—if negative, do LP, drug screen, otology consult
	Subacute	Drugs Cerebellar tumor In Child—parainfectious benign ataxia, meningitis	Multiple sclerosis Rare—Toxins (Mercury)	CT scan—if negative, same as above
Drowsy patient with ataxia only	Acute	Cerebellar hemorrhage or infarct	Brainstem stroke Drugs	CT scan—if negative, same as above
	Subacute	Drugs Cerebellar tumor	Toxins Hydrocephalus	CT scan—if negative, same as above
Alert patient with dizziness	Physician must first decide if it's vertigo (a sense of spinning or movement) or lightheadedness, fairtness, then for:			
Vertigo	Acute or Subacute	Vestibular disease	Brainstem stroke Multiple sclerosis	Otology or neurology consultation
Lightheadedness	Acute or Subacute	Anxiety	Systemic disease (e.g., anemia, postural hypotension) Vestibular disease	CBC, postural blood pressures, serum chemistry screen

establish whether the basic problem is a structural lesion or a non-structural process. The physician should always conduct a history and examination, focusing on the search for the nature of the lesion. A recent tendency among some physicians, especially junior house staff, has been to "get the CT scan and ask questions later." The clinician should *first* develop a differential diagnosis. Only then can he or she choose the proper test and interpret it intelligently. (See "Use of Laboratory Tests," later in this chapter.) The initial neurologic observations are the baseline with which to compare later observations while following the patient.

Once the patient has been stabilized and the clinician has developed his list of probable etiologies, he then can obtain more history. The patient, his family or friends who brought him in, the ambulance attendant, or even a telephone call to the patient's neighbors can be valuable sources of history. Obviously, the history will be focused on details that are relevant to the specific clinical problem. However, certain information should almost always be obtained to search for possible clues suggesting a structural lesion. If the clue is present it serves as a "red flag," alerting the physician's attention to consider a dangerous structural lesion. For example, a previously healthy 45-year-old woman was found at home in a coma. She was known to use sedative drugs. However, the added piece of history that she, in an ataxic drugged state, had fallen and struck her head would immediately raise the diagnosis of subdural hematoma, and require that it be ruled out before any other diagnosis would be accepted.

The "red flag" clues to be sought in most histories concerning neurologic emergencies are listed in Table 1.4. A very acute onset (within an hour) suggests cerebrovascular disease, either infarction or hemorrhage. A history of trauma suggests a subdural or other intracranial hematoma. A history of systemic bleeding or anticoagulant treatment suggests intracranial hemorrhage or subdural hematoma from minimal trauma. Prominent antecedent headache raises the specter of hemorrhage or tumor; known systemic tumor,

Table 1.4 Clues from the History Suggesting a Structural Lesion of the Nervous System

Clue	Diagnosis Suggested
Very acute onset	Cerebrovascular lesion
Trauma	Subdural hematoma (SDH)
Bleeding	Intracranial hemorrhage or SDH
Headache	Increased intracranial pressure (i.e., a mass)
Tumor elsewhere	Metastasis
Recent sepsis or bacterial infection of the face or sinuses	Brain abscess
Alcoholism	Subdural hematoma
Focal neurologic symptoms	Any structural lesion

metastases; prior focal symptoms (e.g., a weak arm or leg), a tumor or subdural hematoma; and known alcoholism, subdural hematoma, a disease endemic in that population. Recent sepsis, bacterial endocarditis, purulent sinusitis or mastoiditis suggest the possibility of a brain abscess.

The General Examination

The general physical examination is helpful in diagnosing the neurologic process in several ways (Table 1.5). First, the blood pressure, if markedly elevated, should alert the clinician to the possibility of increased intracranial pressure (ICP). In the author's experience high blood pressures (e.g., diastolic pressure above 120 mmHg) in a patient with depressed SOC and focal signs is often caused by a structural intracranial process, usually a hemorrhage, and is not often related to hypertensive encephalopathy. A pulse concomitantly slowed below 60 per minute is strong evidence for increased ICP. Arrhythmias without a known cardiac cause also suggest an intracranial mass or hemorrhage. One uncommon but dramatic (and often lethal) focal lesion that causes prominent cardiovascular abnormalities is a cerebellar mass. Either acute cerebellar hemorrhage, an infarction with edema or a tumor of the cerebellum can produce pressure on the cardiovascular regulating centers of the medulla and so cause marked hypertension and arrhythmias, even before causing prominent focal neurologic signs. Increased body temperature should raise the specter of possible nervous system infection.

Certain observations during the remainder of the general medical examination are also "red flags" suggesting a structural lesion. Signs of trauma suggest subdural hematoma. Even trauma distant from the head can be the only clue. Scalp contusions and abrasions must be sought, but are often hard to see because of the hair. Signs of excessive bleeding or bruising (associated with intracranial hemorrhage), systemic tumor (i.e., metastases),

Table 1.5 Clues from the General Examination Suggesting a Structural Lesion of the Nervous System

Clue	Diagnosis Suggested
Hypertension	Increased intracranial pressure (ICP) or cerebellar mass
Bradycardia	Same
Other arrhythmias without cardiac arrest	Same
Fever	Brain abscess
Purulent infection of the face or sinuses	Brain abscess
Trauma	Subdural hematoma (SDH)
Bleeding	Intracranial hemorrhage or SDH
Tumor	Metastasis

purulent sinusitis, or mastoiditis (i.e., brain abscess) and alcoholism (i.e., subdural hematoma) can also be important clues.

The Neurologic Examination

Next, the neurologic examination must be tailored to fit the clinical problem,
keeping clearly in mind the list of diagnoses developed in the first minutes
of the evaluation. For example, if the patient has presented with weakness
in both legs, progressive over 2 days and he is fully alert, the initial diagnostic
list includes spinal processes (e.g., metastatic tumor, multiple sclerosis or
transverse myelitis) and peripheral nerve disease (Guillain-Barré syndrome).
The examination is then focused on the legs and arms, with a cursory screening of mental status, cranial nerves and cerebellar function.

The formal neurologic examination can be helpful in several ways. With
it the clinician can confirm and clarify the focal signs he suspected from
his initial observation of the patient. The examination is also the best means
to localize the disease in the nervous system. Table 1.6 lists some common
neurologic exam findings that often help localize a lesion in the nervous
system. Localization of the process is important mainly to guide the choice
and interpretation of radiologic tests. If the lesion is in the head a CT scan
is by far the best tool, but an isotope brain scan may suffice. However,
those tests are not usually helpful to diagnose a spinal lesion, routine
X-ray films and/or a myelogram are the best test. The examination also
provides a valuable baseline of observations to follow. It is vitally important
in the emergency setting to observe if the patient is stable, improving or
deteriorating. Sequential observations of SOC and focal signs are necessary

Table 1.6 Some Common Syndromes of Focal Neurologic Signs and Their Anatomic Locations

Syndrome	Usual Localization
Hemiparesis, including face weakness, hemi-sensory loss, aphasia or hemianopia	Contralateral cerebral hemisphere
Hemiparesis without other findings	Usually small deep infarct (lacune) in contra-lateral cerebral hemisphere or pons
Hemiparesis with contralateral cranial nerve findings	Brainstem
Hemiparesis with contralateral trunk and limb sensory loss	Cervical spinal cord
Paraparesis	Thoracic or lower spinal cord or nerve roots
Monoparesis (most muscles or one arm or one leg)	Brachial or lumbar plexus lesion (Rule out small cerebral cortex lesion)
Weakness of isolated muscles of one limb	Peripheral nerve or spinal nerve root lesion
Bilateral distal limb numbness and/or weak-ness (legs usually worse)	Peripheral neuropathy
Bilateral proximal limb weakness without sen-sory symptoms	Muscle or neuromuscular junction

for that decision. Finally, the neurologic examination provides important clues toward answering the question "Is it structural or non-structural?".

The three types of neurologic observations that should be made in every case are the state of consciousness (SOC), the mental status and the "objective" observations of pupils, reflexes, etc.

The state of consciousness is the first thing that the physician observes, but is often not consciously noted as part of his examination. Even if the patient's SOC is normal and he is fully alert, that should be registered in the physician's mind and the chart. Next comes the mental status examination. A mental status that seems abnormal on first observation requires the physician to answer the next question: Is this a diffuse process (i.e., global confusion or dementia) or is it a speech problem (dysarthria from a brainstem lesion) or a language problem (aphasia from a left hemisphere lesion). The global confusional states are diffuse processes and are usually caused by metabolic or toxic processes. The other signs imply focal, structural lesions. (Chapter 12 discusses these issues more completely.)

The formal, "mechanical" part of the neurologic examination can take all day to perform and so intimidates many non-neurologists. However, in the emergency setting, when the exam is tailored to the few diagnoses entertained by the confident physician, it usually takes only a few minutes. The important part of the exam can be divided into three parts: the eyes, the motor function of the face and the limbs, and the reflexes. "The eyes" includes examination of the position of the eyes (Are they in midline position and conjugate?), the pupils (size, equality and light reaction), the extraocular movements (Are they full and conjugate?), the optic fundi (Is there blood or papilledema?) and the corneal reflexes (Are they symmetrical?). The face and limbs are observed for position (Is one side positioned grossly differently from the other?), tone, movement and strength. The key observation is to note any asymmetry of the motor signs (i.e., any inequality of the right versus the left side). Finally the reflexes are tested. Checking a few deep tendon reflexes often suffices, usually the biceps and knee jerks on both sides. Testing the toe reflexes following painful stimulation of the sole is essential, looking for the Babinski sign (the great toe moves upward). Again, a key observation is whether there is symmetry of the reflexes (i.e., whether the reflexes on the right and left are equal).

Other parts of the examination may be done, and must be done in some cases. If the physician suspects a stroke or other cerebrovascular disease the carotid arteries should be palpated and auscultated for bruits. If the patient is alert and cooperative and the exam seems non-focal, gait and station should be tested, looking for ataxia or unsuspected leg weakness. The sensory examination is the most variable, unreliable and least helpful part of the examination. It is also often the most difficult to do. However, in the alert, cooperative patient with a suspected spinal cord or peripheral nerve lesion it must be done to help localize the lesion.

Clues On Examination Suggesting A Structural Lesion

As previously stressed, an important early task in neurologic emergencies is to decide "Is it a focal, structural lesion or diffuse, non-structural one?" A structural, focal lesion is suggested by two different sets of observations (Table 1.7).

The first important set of observations suggests increased intracranial pressure. As mentioned before, unexplained hypertension, bradycardia and depressed SOC are the most common signs. However, a patient in coma with symmetrical but marked increase in muscle tone or hyperactive deep tendon reflexes should also be suspected of having increased intracranial pressure, if an antecedent cardiac arrest or other hypoxic event can be ruled out. Papilledema or hemorrhages in the retina also suggest possible increased intracranial pressure.

The second important set of clues suggesting a focal, structural lesion come from the "objective" part of the neurologic exam. Any consistent asymmetry of the signs of the eyes, limbs, reflexes or the presence of aphasia or other clearcut local sign usually means a structural, focal lesion of the nervous system (Table 1.7). Not all these clues have to be present. The unequivocal presence of any one of them, without another obvious explanation, is sufficient evidence to support a preliminary diagnosis of a structural lesion and to launch an aggressive plan to define and treat the lesion.

Table 1.7 Clues from the Neurologic Examination Suggesting a Structural Lesion of the Nervous System

Diffuse Signs—(Suggesting Increased Intracranial Pressure or Hemorrhage)		Focal Signs—(Significant Asymmetries)	
Eyes:	Papilledema or hemor-rhage in fundus	Eyes:	
		Position—	Deviation of both eyes to one side
Limbs:	Severely increased tone		Grossly disconjugate eyes
Reflexes:	Grossly increased deep tendon reflexes	Pupils—	Unequal size
			Unequal light reflex
		Movement—	Failure to move in one direction of gaze
			Disconjugate movements
		Corneal reflexes—	Asymmetric reflex
		Limbs:	
		Position—	Consistently asymmetric positions of arms or legs
		Tone—	Asymmetry, right vs. left
		Movement—	Hemi- or monoparesis
		Reflexes:	
		Deep tendon reflexes—	Consistently asymmetric, right vs. left
		Toes—	Unilateral Babinski sign

The Next Steps—Management Of The Suspected Lesion

If a structural lesion of the brain is suspected, especially if the patient has signs of increased intracranial pressure, the physician must begin to minimize the effects of the lesion on the brain and must prepare to treat complications. These steps should be instituted before the patient is sent for CT scan or transferred elsewhere. The first step is to slow the rate of infusion of any IV. Systemic fluid overload can aggravate an already increased intracranial pressure. The IV line should be kept open for infusion of drugs only. Secondly, if a focal mass is suspected (e.g., tumor abscess, hematoma), dexamethasone (Decadron, usually 10 mg) should be given intravenously. Then the physician should prepare to treat brain herniation. If the patient has not been intubated and is unconscious, he should be intubated. If he is conscious, the equipment for intubation should be kept at the bedside, ready for immediate use if his condition deteriorates. Osmotic diuretics should also be prepared for immediate administration if signs of brain herniation appear. (Chapter 4 discusses the detailed management of increased intracranial pressure.) The patient should be closely observed by the physician, nurses, and other attendants, as he is taken, as soon as possible, for the appropriate diagnostic test or prepared for transfer to an institution better equipped to make a definitive diagnosis. A *lumbar puncture should not be done* before the nature of the focal intracranial process is clarified.

If the physician's diagnosis is a non-structural, non-focal process, then appropriate management is to draw a broad spectrum of blood and urine tests to find the toxic, metabolic or infectious cause of the patient's problem. If the patient is in coma endotracheal intubation should be done. The patient is then best treated in a medical intensive care unit.

A lumbar puncture may also be performed, if there are no signs of increased intracranial pressure or a focal, structural lesion. Immediate examination of the spinal fluid is mandatory if the physician suspects bacterial meningitis.

SPECIAL CASES IN NEUROLOGIC EMERGENCIES: PITFALLS FOR THE UNWARY

Spinal Cord Compression

> **PRINCIPLE 8:** Any patient with progressing weakness in both legs has spinal cord compression until proved otherwise.

The spinal cord is a small (1–1½ cm diameter) structure enclosed in a rigid bony tube. The cord and its surrounding CSF meninges and spinal canal can compensate for slow growth of a tumor for weeks, or even years, as with a meningioma. However, once decompensation and clinical symptoms and signs begin, the process can advance very rapidly. A patient who comes in one evening with weakness in the legs may be totally and irreversibly paraplegic and incontinent the next morning. Clinical experience of neurologists and neurosurgeons has established that the sooner definitive treatment is begun, the better is the outcome. Even a few hours delay can make a significant difference, so the physician must make the clinical diagnosis, obtain the confirming tests and call for specialist consultations within hours of the patient's presentation.

The clinical syndrome is usually a distinct one to the alert physician. The patient has had some back pain, often in the thoracic region, and over a few days has had progressive weakness of his legs. He may also have noticed difficulty initiating urination or even urinary retention or incontinence. A past history of a primary neoplasm may be present, but is often absent. On examination the patient has weak legs and often has localized tenderness of the spine and Babinski signs. The knee and ankle jerk reflexes may be increased, normal or decreased. Careful sensory examination, best done with pinprick, may show a dermatomal sensory level on the trunk, thus localizing at least one level of spinal cord dysfunction.

The most helpful laboratory test is usually plain spine X-rays, with special attention to the area with localized tenderness or the region suggested by the level of sensory dysfunction. (Remember, the lesion in the spinal canal is often two or more vertebrae above the dermatome level found on the exam. Thus a sensory level at the tenth thoracic dermatome suggests a bony lesion and cord compression at the eighth thoracic vertebra.) A neurosurgical or neurological consultation should be obtained as soon as the diagnosis is suspected and a prompt decision should be made about myelography. No lumbar puncture should be done until the myelogram is performed or a decision is made not to do a myelogram.

Table 1.3 presents a more complete differential diagnosis of the syndrome of subacute onset paraparesis. However, spinal cord compression must always be considered and ruled out.

The Patient With Neurologic Signs And Fever

A patient with this syndrome presents the physician with a serious dilemma: Should he do a lumbar puncture to rule out meningitis, and risk brain herniation precipitated by the LP in the presence of a brain abscess, or should he do a CT scan or angiogram, and delay the LP several hours, risking progression of untreated meningitis? There is no simple, always correct answer, but a principle should be observed:

> **PRINCIPLE 9:** The patient with neurologic signs and fever should always be considered to have bacterial meningitis, until it is ruled out by lumbar puncture.

Fever, no matter how modest, and regardless of the presence of an obvious non-CNS infection, should raise the suspicion of purulent meningitis. If the patient has no signs of increased intracranial pressure and no prominent focal signs, an LP should be done to rule out meningitis. Delaying an LP for several hours could allow progression of the meningitis and more serious brain damage or death.

The more difficult case is the patient with signs of increased ICP or focal signs plus fever. An LP is contraindicated and yet meningitis must be ruled out. The safest course in this setting is to begin broad spectrum antibiotics and arrange a CT scan or angiogram as soon as possible. If a mass is then ruled out, the LP can be done and special microbiologic techniques used to attempt to isolate the organism.

Inadequate Observations

> *PRINCIPLE 10:* The patient with progressing symptoms is going to get much worse, and soon.

One of the most troubling events in a neurologist's career is to be called in to see a patient who arrived in the emergency room drowsy, confused and with a minimal hemiparesis, but who was later found by the nurse to be comatose and to have dilated, fixed pupils. This is an unfortunately too familiar course for a subdural hematoma, especially among alcoholic patients treated in busy emergency rooms.

Lesions of the nervous system can progress rapidly to cause severe, irreversible damage and death. The physician when he first sees the patient obtains some idea from the history about the rapidity of the patient's progression, but that does not tell him how fast the patient will progress over the next several minutes or hours. The brain and spinal cord are in closed bony containers, and once the space is filled enough by blood, pus or tumor to cause symptoms, the subsequent course is often a more rapid decline. Similarly rapid deterioration can occur when patients with neuromuscular disease or cervical spine injuries exhaust their ability to support adequate ventilation. They can progress to respiratory arrest within a few minutes. Physicians and nurses must make frequent, at least every 15 minutes, observations of vital signs, state of consciousness and focal signs for several hours, or until the patient is clearly improving. Any deterioration of the signs should prompt rapid decisions about intubation, immediate treatment (e.g., osmotic diuretics), rapid diagnostic work-up, neurosurgical consultation, etc.

The Diagnosis Of "Hysteria"

> *PRINCIPLE 11:* Patients with neurologic symptoms who are diagnosed as "hysterical" usually have organic neurologic disease.[7,8]

Patients with serious organic brain disease often "go crazy." Their behavior, their thinking, and their personality are changed because the brain is not functioning normally. The altered behavior and thinking are sometimes interpreted by the family and, all too often, by the physician as "hysterical." In addition, disorders of the nervous system often do present bizarre symptoms and signs that, especially early in the course, don't fit a coherent, organic pattern. So the physician often decides: "It doesn't fit any disease I know, so it must be hysterical." Finally, any patient with organic neurologic disease may also have a superimposed psychiatric disorder. One of the most difficult tasks in all of clinical medicine, even for an experienced neurologist or neurosurgeon, is to diagnose an organic neurologic disease behind the facade of an obvious psychogenic syndrome. But the general physician must try to do that, and should always have a bias toward diagnosing organic disease because it is the organic disease that, if not diagnosed, may progress to cause permanent nervous system damage or death.

The list of diseases that present in confusing, apparently "hysterical" patterns is long. Multiple sclerosis is the classic such disease, and often first presents in young women, the group often associated with "hysteria." Herpes simplex encephalitis, meningitis and drug toxicity often present as acute psychosis. Patients with the Guillain-Barré syndrome are seen early in their course by several physicians, and are often sent out from emergency rooms, because their vague sensory symptoms and complaints of weakness are not accompanied by clearcut signs. The young woman with known migraine headaches who comes to the emergency room with her "worst headache ever" may well have had a subarachnoid hemorrhage, so needs a lumbar puncture or CT scan. The man with a known seizure disorder who is brought in by his family because of strange behavior may be having multiple unrecognized partial complex (temporal lobe) seizures. The known schizophrenic patient with the bizarre tic or wry neck that suddenly began may not be "crazy" but may be having an idiosyncratic reaction to a new phenothiazine he recently began taking. The depressed middle-aged patient who "just can't get out of bed," and "has pain all over" may have spinal cord compression from metastatic carcinoma. (Each of these examples is based on one or more such actual cases seen by the author after an initial diagnosis of "hysteria.")

There are no easy solutions for this frequent problem. However, you can best protect your patient and yourself by: (1) always initially managing the problem as if it's organic; and (2) get help when you're not sure. A laboratory test (e.g., CT scan) or a consultation by a neurologist or neurosurgeon may prove very helpful.

Use Of Laboratory Tests

> **PRINCIPLE 12:** Always tell the radiologist or laboratory technician what diagnoses you suspect, tell the radiologist where you think the lesion is, and personally look at each important laboratory test.

The CT scan is a marvelous tool for diagnosis of central nervous system problems. However, it is quite fallible and can miss significant lesions. "Misses" occur mainly for two reasons: (1) an incomplete or technically inadequate study; and (2) the radiologist or physician interpreting the study does not look for, and so doesn't see the active process. An example of the former is a "normal" CT scan on a patient with a focal motor seizure, but the scan didn't include the most superior section over the cerebral hemispheres and so missed the small meningioma near the vertex. Failure to do contrast enhancement of CT scans is a common cause of failure to see lesions. Unenhanced scans often miss small tumors, recent strokes and small inflammatory lesions. The second problem usually results from the radiologist not knowing exactly where to look nor what to look for, so he may see and report the "left cerebral infarct, probably old" that was already known but may not see the subtle low density change of the early infarct in the right hemisphere, the current clinical problem. (Chapter 2 gives more examples of this problem.)

All other radiologic studies have similar limitations. The clinical physician must tell the radiologist the nature of the suspected lesion and direct his attention to the anatomic area of interest. This usually is best done by speaking directly to the radiologist before the test is done. The problem of the inadequate study can only be resolved by the physician reviewing the study himself to make sure the test shows the area of interest and was complete.

Interpretation of cerebrospinal fluid (CSF) findings presents a similar problem. Talcum powder crystals (from the sterile gloves used by the physician doing the lumbar puncture) or red blood cells may be interpreted as being white blood cells. Xanthochromia (yellowish discoloration of the CSF due to breakdown products from blood in the CSF) may be missed by the laboratory technician or may be reported when not present because of the presence of red blood cells in a poorly centrifuged CSF sample from a "traumatic tap." The physician should be aware of the level of expertise of his laboratory technicians and should himself examine the CSF whenever he has doubts.

Do No Harm

> **PRINCIPLE 13:** Do nothing that compromises the already injured nervous system.

One of the clinical tenets we all learn early in our medical career is "Do no harm!" This is true in neurologic and neurosurgical emergencies. Excessive intravenous fluids may cause a marked increase in intracranial pressure in a brain-injured patient. An LP in a patient with a brain abscess or large subdural hematoma can precipitate disastrous results by inducing brain herniation.

Several precautions should be considered in any patient with a neurologic or neurosurgical emergency:

1. If increased intracranial pressure or a focal mass-causing lesion (e.g., tumor, abscess, hematoma) is suspected, the rate of administration of intravenous fluids should be limited to "keep open."

2. Obviously, in the same clinical setting, lumbar puncture should not be done.

3. In any patient with a serious head injury or a patient with quadriparesis, suspect a neck injury and immobilize the neck until adequate cervical spine X-rays rule out a fracture.

4. In a patient with a stroke syndrome never anticoagulate until an intracranial hemorrhage has been ruled out by CT scan *and* lumbar puncture.

5. Don't give sedating drugs to a patient with a suspected intracranial mass or increased ICP. The exception to this rule is the combative, violently agitated patient who must be sedated for his own physical protection or who must be controlled to permit examination and tests (e.g., CT scan).

Don't Assume The Patient Is Lost

> *PRINCIPLE 14:* In the first hours following acute brain injury, the neurologic signs often suggest worse damage than actually exists.

In the early hours of a neurologic or neurosurgical emergency do not assume irreversible brain damage or brain death, no matter how ominous the clinical signs. Bilateral fully dilated, unreactive pupils may be drug induced. In the head-injured patient dilated, unreactive pupils may be due to brain hypoxia caused by systemic trauma and shock. Even dilated, unreactive pupils from brain herniation due to a large subdural or other hematoma may be occasionally reversed and the patient saved with aggressive medical and surgical treatment.[10]

Before the physician assumes the worst outcome, the patient should be vigorously supported and managed until the etiologic diagnosis is certain, other complicating factors are ruled out (e.g., drugs, hypothermia, hypoxia), and the early self-reversing effects of the acute brain injury have resolved (e.g., concussive, hypoxic, postictal effects). A reasonable period to wait is 6 hours. Diagnosing brain death or severe, irreversible brain damage in any less time should be reserved for very limited and well-defined cases. (see Chapters 5 and 20.)

CONCLUSION

The general physician is not expected to have the confidence nor the expertise of the experienced neurologist in managing neurologic and neurosurgical emergencies. However, conscientious use of the principles and practices that have been presented will enhance his ability to diagnose and effectively manage those emergencies. The subsequent chapters of this book give more detailed guidelines for the diagnosis and treatment of the most important emergencies of the nervous system. Reference 6 is excellent further reading on the neurologic examination, and read reference 9 on the differential diagnosis and management of neurologic syndromes.

REFERENCES

1. Adams, R.D., Victor, M.: Approach to the patient with neurologic disease. p. 1. In Adams, R.D., Victor, M., eds.: Principles of Neurology. 1st Ed., McGraw-Hill, New York, 1977.
2. Barrows, H.S., Bennett, K.: The diagnostic (problem solving) skill of the neurologist. Arch. Neurol., 26:273, 1972.
3. The Brain. Scientific American, Inc., W.H. Freeman and Company, San Francisco, 1979.
4. Eccles, J.C.: The Understanding of the Brain. McGraw-Hill Book Company, New York, 1973.
5. Luria, A.R.: The Man with a Shattered World. Basic Books, Inc., New York, 1972.
6. Mancall, E.L.: Essentials of the Neurologic Examination. 2nd Ed. F.A. Davis Company, Philadelphia, 1981.
7. Saravay, S.M., Koran, L.M.: Organic disease mistakenly diagnosed as psychiatric. Psychosomatics, XVIII:6, 1977.
8. Slater, E.: Diagnosis of "Hysteria." Brit. Med. J., 1:1395, 1965.
9. Weiner, H.L., Levitt, L.P.: Neurology for the House Officer. 2nd Ed. Williams & Wilkins, Baltimore, 1981.
10. Zervas, M.T., Hedley-Whyte, J.: Successful treatment of cerebral herniation in five patients. N. Engl. J. Med., 286:1075, 1972.

2

Effective Use of Radiologic Tests in Neurologic Emergencies

Michael Mestek, M.D.

INTRODUCTION

Before discussing the presently available radiologic methods for diagnosis of neurologic and neurosurgical emergencies several basic tenets should be emphasized.

First, patient problems often require multidisciplinary care, that is they necessitate the interaction of two or more physicians of different training and background. Often there must be verbal communication between the radiologist, the referring physician, and other physicians involved in the immediate care of the patient. In this way the clinical problem is clearly defined, the important questions to be answered are decided, and the available radiologic tests and their associated risks discussed.

Second, the radiologic work-up of any clinical problem depends a great deal upon the equipment available at a given hospital or facility as well as the expertise and interest of the available radiologic staff.

Third, technology is progressing at such a rate that today's procedure of choice will be obsolete and possibly inadequate tomorrow.[17] For example, several years ago the work-up of neurosensory hearing loss was plain films of the internal auditory canals followed by tomography. These studies often led to pantopaque posterior fossa myelography with angiography and/or pneumoencephalography as additional tests. Today a computerized tomographic scan (CT) with and without contrast for larger cerebellopontine masses or air-CT cisternography for smaller tumors are the key tests in the work-up of an acoustic neurinoma.

With these three remarks in mind, I will simply describe the current radiologic modalities available and then present more detailed discussion of the radiologic work-up of specific problems.

PLAIN FILMS

Plain skull and spine films are easy to perform and relatively inexpensive ($60–$100, depending on the number of views and the geographic region of the hospital). The radiation dosage (about 1 rad) for a full skull series is acceptable, while that for lumbar spine series (about 3 rads) represents a significant but small exposure to the gonads. Plain film techniques are based on an X-ray source, and film-screen-grid combination. X-rays produced via a generator and cathode ray tube are focused upon the desired part of the patient. Some X-rays pass through the patient, others are absorbed. Interaction of the X-rays with the intensifying screen results in the release of photons of light which interact with the film exposing the film in varying degrees to create the photographic picture. The resultant developed film has excellent spatial resolution (can distinguish between two objects close together) but less optimum contrast resolution (ability to distinguish between materials of similar density, i.e., CSF and brain). Spatial resolution problems such as fractures, foreign bodies, size and shape of the sella, position of the pineal, and bone destruction are well evaluated on the plain skull films. From a density standpoint calcium, water, fat, and air can be distinguished on plain films. Accordingly, processes having one of these densities can be evaluated (i.e., air-pneumocephalus, aeration of sinuses; calcium-meningioma, astrocytoma, aneurysm, infection; fat—some lipomas of the corpus callosum). Processes of near soft tissue density are not detected unless a calcified pineal is shifted (i.e., edema, hemorrhage, extracerebral blood or pus collections, hydrocephalus, infarction, neoplasm, abscess, arteriovenous malformation (AVM), and aneurysm). The sensitivity (number of false negatives) and specificity (number of false positives) of the plain skull film varies with the disease processes and will be covered in more detail in sections on specific disease processes.

Spine films are currently more useful than skull films because: (1) many emergency problems of spine involve bone, and (2) additional techniques such as CT of the spine are not as well suited to evaluation of the entire spine. Important information concerning fracture, subluxation, and size of the bony canal (particularly cervical) is obtained in trauma cases. In suspected infections, the integrity of the vertebral body is easily assessed. Absence of a pedicle, or destruction or sclerosis of a vertebral body aids the work-up of metastatic disease. Calcium in the spinal canal suggests a herniated disc or meningioma. Widening of an intervertebral foramen points to neurofibroma. Focal expansion of the canal suggests a spinal cord syrinx or other intramedullary process (e.g., tumor). On the other hand, spine films contribute little to the diagnoses of cord swelling or atrophy, spinal AVM, hematoma, discs, and most neoplasms.

Polytomography is an extension of plain film techniques in which the problem of superimposition of shadows or summation of densities is dealt with by blurring the tissues above and below the plane of interest by moving the X-ray tube and film simultaneously in opposite directions creating a fulcrum. Tomography is a particularly valuable tool in further evaluation of spine and facial fractures.

COMPUTERIZED TOMOGRAPHY (CT)

CT is the greatest advance in radiology since the discovery of the X-ray tube, especially for evaluating lesions of the brain. In this exciting technique the X-ray tube is combined with a computer to provide anatomic detail not previously seen. As stated before, plain films can resolve only four basic densities—water, fat, air, and calcium. In CT a tightly collimated X-ray beam (10 mm or less) is passed through an equal thickness of the part examined. The incident X-rays are absorbed in relationship to the linear attenuation coefficients (a measure of the ability of a given tissue to absorb X-rays) of the various brain constituents with the unabsorbed X-rays detected by xenon gas detectors. This information is processed by a computer according to an algorithm, a mathematical equation utilized to determine the locations of the attenuation coefficients in space. In this way a spatial representation of absorption coefficients or matrix is formed. The matrix consists of vertical or horizontal lines much like a regular television image. Each box of the matrix is called a pixel with dimensions of .8 mm × .8 mm or smaller. When the thickness of the slice is included one has a voxel. In this way an image of contiguous slices of the brain is formed composed of several hundred thousand voxels with each voxel being assigned a CT number from 0 to 1000. Using this digital information and converting it to analog information with a continuous gray scale, an image of the brain is obtained in which white matter can be differentiated from gray matter, and ventricles, fissures, and sulcal spaces seen. This image has excellent contrast resolution, but modest spatial resolution as compared to conventional X-rays. Iodinated contrast material is given intravenously to enhance or accentuate normal and pathologic anatomy.

The CT is relatively easy to perform with complications being essentially those of reactions to the contrast material. The cost is about $300 (varying from geographic region to region and depending on whether the study is done with or without contrast). The radiation dosage is about 2–5 rads, depending on certain technical factors and whether slices are contiguous. This technique is extremely sensitive for brain pathology involving structural abnormalities, approaching 100 percent in detecting abscesses, neoplasms, hemorrhage, and hydrocephalus.[15] It is somewhat less sensitive for brain infarction, AVM, and aneurysm, depending on size and location. The relationship of scanning to the ictus is also important with respect to infarcts. CT is not very sensitive for leptomeningeal processes. Specificity is not as great as sensitivity but combining the history and physical exam findings with CT details often permits a specific diagnosis. Infection, infarction, and neoplasm are often difficult to differentiate on the basis of the scan alone.[5,11] As technology improves limitations of CT will diminish, but these now include small lesions, lesions in regions of inherent artifact (e.g., acoustic neurinoma), patient motion, and poor detail of vascular structures.

NUCLIDE BRAIN SCAN

Before the advent of CT the nuclide brain scan was the radiologic screening procedure of choice. This study has two parts. The dynamic ("flow scan") portion consists of 16 images of the brain 2 seconds apart obtained immediately after the intravenous administration of the radionuclide. It is used to evaluate cerebral perfusion, brain death, and blood pool lesions such as AVM, aneurysm, and acute subdural hematoma. The static portion consists of frontal and lateral views of the brain obtained 1–3 hours after injection. This portion evaluates lesions affecting "blood-brain barrier" such as neoplasm, infarction, and infection. It is moderately expensive (about $200), easy to perform, and without significant complication. It is as sensitive as CT for most structural alterations of the brain but far less specific. However, there is a small percentage of cases in which CT is negative and nuclide scan positive (e.g., herpes encephalitis, superficial infarct, and metastatic disease). The nuclide scan depends on alterations in the blood brain barrier with accumulation of tracer, usually technetium pertechnetate. This is similar to but not the same as contrast enhancement in CT. Herniation of midline structures, brain edema, hydrocephalus and other secondary markers of brain abnormality easily seen in CT are not detected by nuclide scanning. Also not detected are processes in the midline and processes which minimally disturb the blood brain barrier. Nuclide tomographic scanning may help in these situations.

Considering the location and shape of the abnormality and correlating the static and dynamic portions of the exam one may obtain some specificity, although usually less than with CT.

In general nuclide scanning can be used when there is known allergy to CT contrast, an infarct superimposed on cerebral atrophy, suspected brain death, and occlusion of dural venous sinuses. In cases where the CT is normal but clinical suspicion of a brain lesion is high, a nuclide scan may disclose the lesion.

CEREBRAL ANGIOGRAMS

In the past cerebral angiography and pneumoencephalography were the definitive neuroradiologic processes. The role of PEG has almost become extinct while the role of cerebral angiography has changed considerably with CT. Diagnostic cerebral angiography is now reserved to clarify or add specificity to a CT diagnosis, to provide anatomic information for surgery (e.g., position and encasement of vascular structures by a tumor), and to evaluate vascular lesions such as AVM and aneurysm which are beyond the spatial resolution of CT. An angiogram involves the placement of a polyethylene catheter into the desired artery using a percutaneous approach and fluoroscopic localization. The test requires special equipment and training on the part of the radiologist and, even in the best of hands, can have serious although infrequent complications, among which is the production of a stroke. The cost is $600 and often more, while the radiation dosage is about 1.5 rads for each film run and 1.5–6.0 rads per minute of fluoroscopic time.

The specificity and sensitivity are similar to CT but require greater interpretive expertise. Diagnoses often are made by displacement of arteries or veins or alterations in caliber, or the number and type of vessels composing or supplying a lesion. There are also anatomically angiographic silent areas. In addition, small avascular lesions are difficult to detect and impossible to identify (i.e., whether tumor, blood clot or abscess).

MYELOGRAPHY

A myelogram is a procedure in which, via a spinal puncture, either air, pantopaque, or most recently metrizamide is instilled into the subarachnoid space allowing plain film visualization of spinal nerves, cord and subarachnoid space. In this way processes affecting the spinal axis can be localized and classified as extradural, intradural-extramedullary, and intramedullary. Air myelography is time consuming, necessitates polytomography, and is very uncomfortable for the patient. Pantopaque myelography involves the use of an oil based dye. It is easily manipulated and one can examine the whole spinal axis with good fluoroscopic control. It has the disadvantage of causing artifact on CT and in the presence of blood in the CSF may cause arachnoiditis. The standard of practice in the U.S. is to, as completely as possible, remove the pantopaque. It is best for assessing extradural processes.

Metrizamide (Amipaque) myelography involves the use of water soluble, non-ionic contrast which does not have to be removed and which can be combined with CT to show exquisite anatomic detail. It evaluates both cord and extradural spaces equally well, and has no reported incidence of arachnoiditis in humans. It has the disadvantage of being difficult to manipulate once in the spinal canal and it causes seizures if certain precautions are not taken.

In summary, the referring physician when ordering a test should be concerned with sensitivity and specificity of the test for the clinical problem, the radiation dose and cost incurred by the patient, as well as the potential complications of the procedure. (Table 2.1 summarizes the value, limitations,

Table 2.1 Value, Limitation, Risk, and Cost of Various Radiologic Tests

	Plain Skull	Computed Tomography	Nuclide Brain Scan	Cerebral Angiography	Plain Spine	Myelography
Main clinical value	Directs CT Air-fluid levels Depressed fracture Nature of intracranial Ca^{++}	Sensitive and often specific non-invasive screening test for variety of neurological problems	Adjunct to normal CT Brain death Patency of dural sinuses Occasionally more sensitive than CT in herpes encephalitis, superficial vascular processes	Adds specificity to CT Evaluate AVMs, aneurysms et al. vascular lesions Normal CT but pt. deteriorating, eg isodense SDH suspected	Inexpensive, easy to perform screen for bony pathology	Defines nature of process as extradural, intradural, intramedullary Information about cord, subarachnoid, and epidural space
Limitations	Does not give information about anatomy of brain or CSF spaces	Artifact common, particularly posterior fossa Small lesions, leptomeningeal processes missed Limited detail of vascular lesions and structures	Non-specific; Edema, mass shift, hydrocephalus, midline abnormalities not detected	Invasive Needs highly trained personnel	No information about cord, its coverings, and surrounding soft tissue	Misses lesions not impinging upon contrast filled sac; (this limitation may be overcome with use of CT)
Radiation dose	1 rad Depends on number of films and technical factors	3.5 rad Much variability with different machines	0.2 rad body 1 rad bladder	1.5 rads per vessel injected plus 1.5–6 rads/min for fluoroscopy	3 rads AP plus lateral	Variable, depending on part of spine and amount of fluoroscopy
Cost	$75	$325	$210	$600	$75	$250
Complications	None	Contrast reaction	None	Stroke Contrast reaction Femoral artery embolus or thrombosis	None	Headache Seizures with metrizamide Arachnoiditis with pantopaque

and risks of the tests discussed.) He should consider alternatives, especially in regard to invasive tests, and ask himself if the information sought will influence management of the patient.

SPECIFIC DISEASE PROCESSES

Cerebrovascular Disease—TIA, Ischemic Stroke

CT and radionuclide brain scanning can exclude processes such as neoplasm which may mimic a transient ischemic attack (TIA), but otherwise have no role in the evaluation of these events (see Chapter 8). Angiography at the present time is the main radiologic tool in the evaluation of TIAs (Table 2.2). If an angiogram is done within a day or two of the TIA, emboli can be demonstrated before they lyse. More importantly the status of the carotid bifurcation and vertebral basilar system can be assessed to aid in treatment planning. What vessels to study will vary with the symptoms of the individual patient and the management philosophy of the referring physician and radiologist. In the future the role of angiography may be altered by a new technique called digital subtraction angiography in which contrast is injected intravenously and, by means of a computer, processed images of arteries obtained.

In a suspected ischemic infarct, whether embolic or thrombotic, where anticoagulation might be used the role of CT is not to diagnose ischemic infarction but to exclude hemorrhage, and also to exclude processes such as subdural hematoma, brain abscess, or tumor which can mimic stroke. In this regard CT is unequaled because of its unique contrast resolution. The CT may be positive in stroke as early as 4 hours depending on the location and size of insult.[20] The earliest signs may be hemispheric mass effect with shift of midline structures or obliteration of sulci and/or a vague decreased density in the vascular territory affected (Fig. 2.1). Sensitivity of the CT is greatest at 3–5 days, usually showing reasonably well-marginated

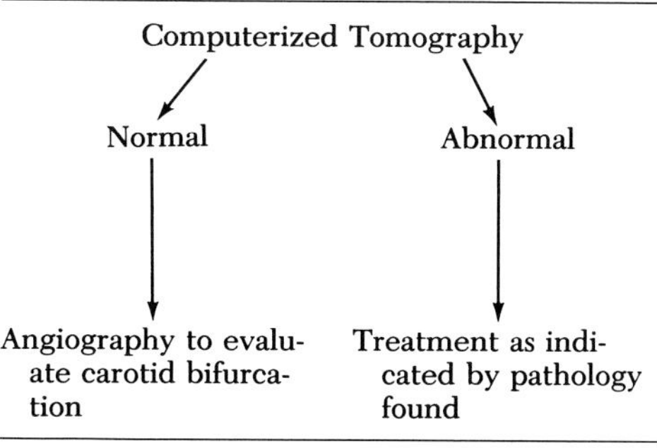

Table 2.2 Suggested Radiologic Workup for Carotid TIA

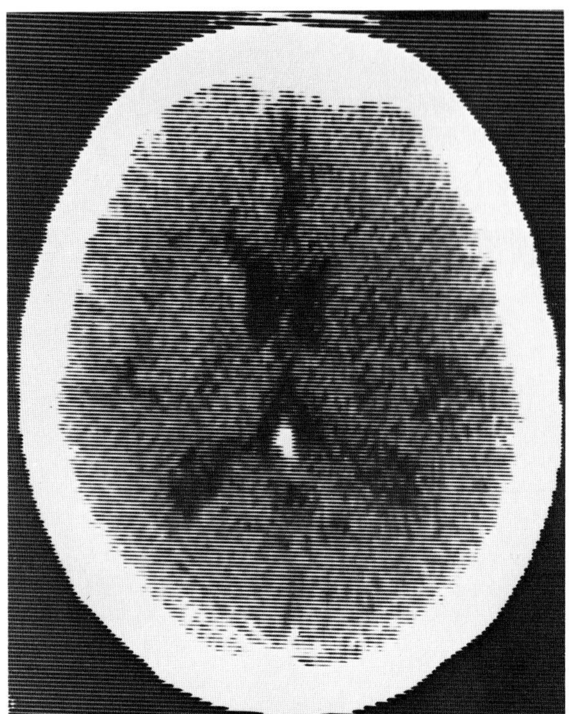

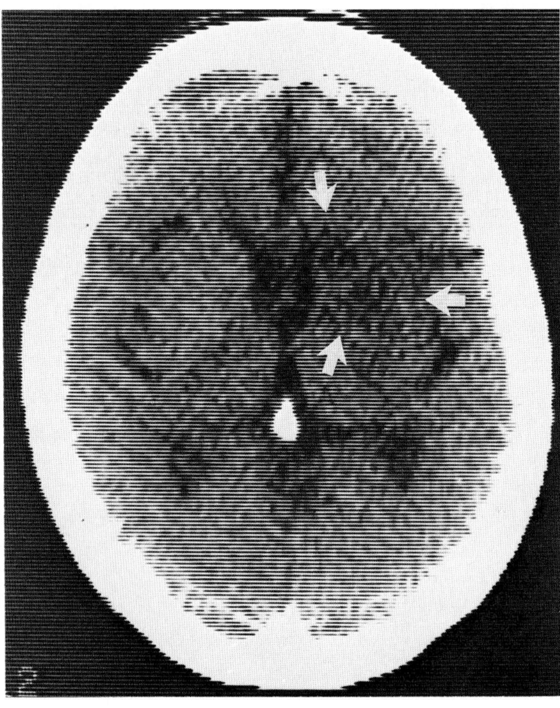

Fig. 2.1
(A) Recent cerebral infarct shown as a vague area of low density, right basal ganglia. (B) Eight days later the area of infarction is better marginated and lower in density (see Fig. 7.3).

decreased density in a vascular distribution (Fig. 2.2). Before 5 days, contrast infusion is not indicated unless tumor is a consideration. From 5–14 days an infarct may be isodense on the non-enhanced scan. Pathologic contrast enhancement of infarcted brain can occur from 3 days to 4 weeks, with a maximum incidence at 7–14 days. With maturation of the infarct, the density approaches CSF, the margins become well-defined, and mass effect and contrast enhancement are no longer evident. Lacunar infarcts as small as 0.1 ml in volume can be detected by CT, usually occuring in the internal capsule and thalamus.[10]

Radionuclide scanning is complimentary to CT. The dynamic part of the study can show differences in flow between the hemispheres. The static portion is seldom positive before 2 days, becomes increasingly positive, with a peak at 2 weeks, and fades at 2 months. Unlike CT, the nuclide brain scan gives no information about edema, ventricular shift or, most importantly, hemorrhage. However, it is often useful in patients with cerebral atrophy, previous infarction, or superficial lesions in which CT seems to be less sensitive.

Angiography should generally be reserved for those patients with mild clinical deficits in whom surgery on a correctable carotid lesion would be undertaken.

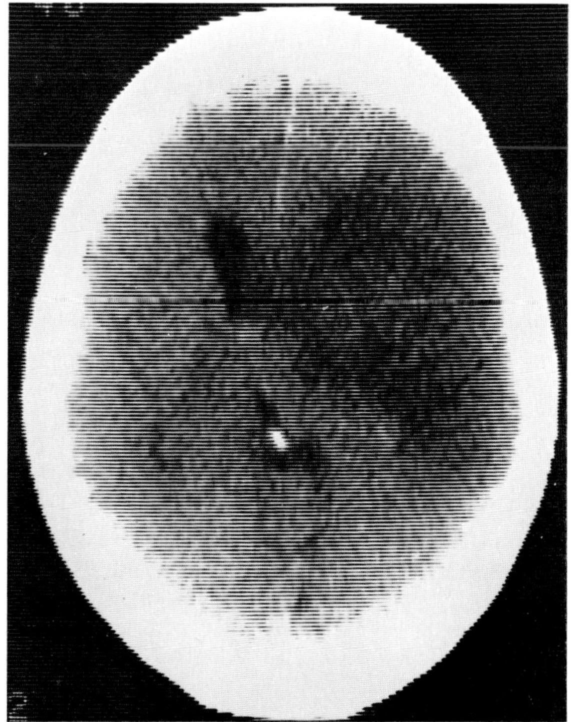

Fig. 2.2
Wedge shaped area of decreased density in the right cerebrum with shift of the septum pellucidum and compression of the lateral ventricle; a typical infarct.

Intracerebral Hematoma

In a suspected intracerebral hematoma it is important to define the size, location, surrounding edema, relationship to the ventricle, associated hydrocephalus, and etiology. CT definitively provides the answers to the first five questions and can often suggest the answer to the sixth.[7,21] Hematomas are usually well circumscribed, homogeneous in density, and often have halos of edema. History is often the most important factor in determining the etiology of a hematoma, but the location and whether there is contrast enhancement on CT can be very helpful. Hematomas in the basal ganglia, pons, cerebellum, and deep white matter raise the possibility of hypertension although AVMs, particularly in the brain stem and basal ganglia, are common (Fig. 2.3). Traumatic hematomas can occur anywhere but favor the frontal and temporal lobes. Hematomas secondary to blood dyscrasias or anticoagulants are usually supratentorial. Hemorrhagic infarcts are usually embolic or venous in nature and are located in the cerebral cortex. Those due to birth control pills seem to have a predilection for the temporal lobe. Hematomas secondary to neoplasm can be anywhere.

Contrast enhancement will often distinguish between spontaneous hematomas and those secondary to a structural lesion. Large AVMs and neoplasms usually enhance, although smaller lesions may be obliterated or compressed by the hematoma. Angiography adds specificity to the CT, providing further

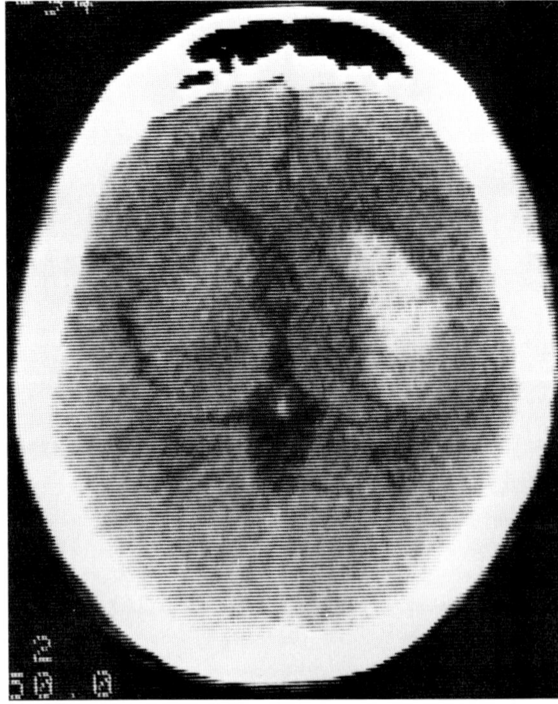

Fig. 2.3
Typical hypertensive hemorrhage in the putamen and globus pallidus.

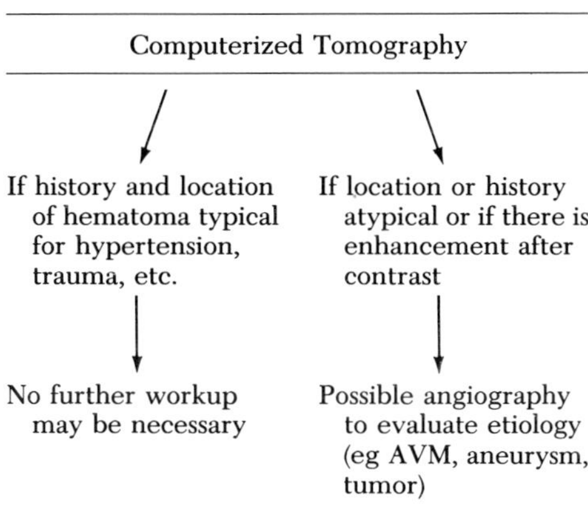

Table 2.3 Suggested Radiologic Workup for Intracerebral Hematoma

Computerized Tomography

If history and location of hematoma typical for hypertension, trauma, etc.

If location or history atypical or if there is enhancement after contrast

No further workup may be necessary

Possible angiography to evaluate etiology (eg AVM, aneurysm, tumor)

evaluation of the etiology. With its superior spatial resolution angiography can better delineate such entities as traumatically torn blood vessels or aneurysms. If there is no enhancement on CT the angiogram will usually be unrewarding and should be done only to define the etiology after the hematoma has resolved. The radionuclide scan has a limited role in the evaluation of intracerebral hemorrhage (Table 2.3).

Subarachnoid Hemorrhage (SAH)

In the context of severe headache SAH usually means aneurysm. The lumbar puncture is a more sensitive means of diagnosing SAH, although one can have a negative tap and positive CT. The CT will show blood as hyperdensity in the CSF spaces beneath or between the cerebral hemispheres. The primary role of CT is to evaluate hydrocephalus, hematoma, edema, and infarction.[3,4,19] With enhancement, aneurysms larger than 8 mm may be demonstrated as well as processes other than aneurysm which may cause SAH, such as AVM or tumor (Fig. 2.4). Because of the limited spatial resolution of CT, angiography is still needed to locate the aneurysm as well as to evaluate the neck and determine whether there is more than one aneurysm. CT can aid in the planning of the angiogram if an aneurysm is seen after contrast enhancement or if there is hematoma, or the SAH is in a specific limited location. However, the additional contrast may add an increased burden on the kidneys, especially if angiography is contemplated within 24 hours, and also may cause nausea and vomiting with a resultant increase in intracranial pressure. The skull film may show calcium in the wall of an aneurysm or AVM or an increase in vascular markings but provides little additional information beyond CT. Whether digital subtraction angiography can provide the detailed spatial information needed for aneurysm surgery remains to be seen.

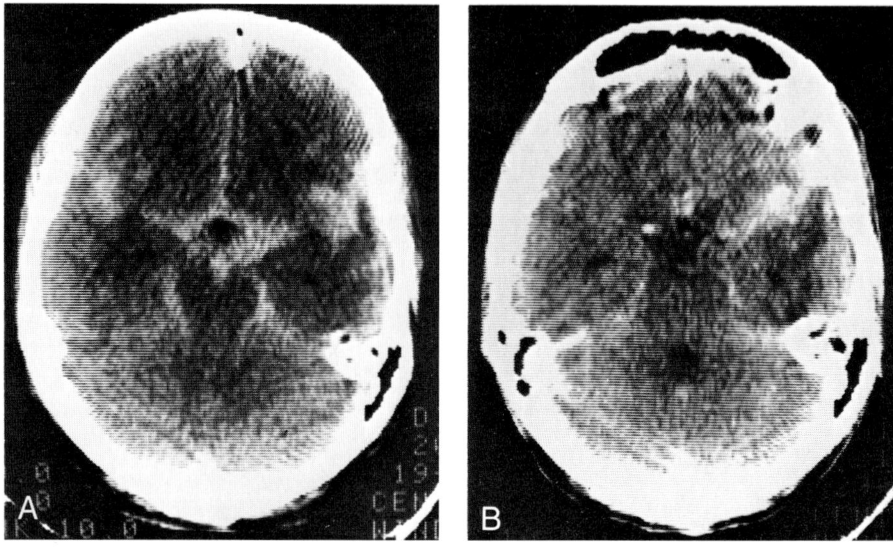

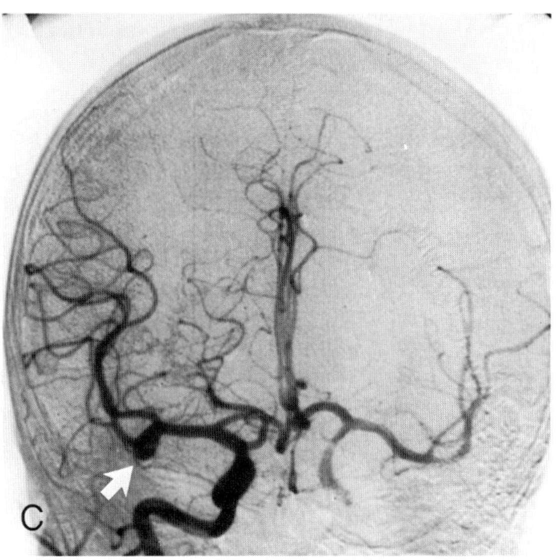

Fig. 2.4
(A) Subarachnoid hemorrhage in the typical "starfish" distribution in basal cisterns. (B) Contrast enhancement suggests an aneurysm of the right middle cerebral artery (RMCA). (C) Angiogram shows the aneurysm (arrow).

Trauma

Current radiologic techniques play a large role in the assessment of trauma. What studies are ordered depends on the clinical assessment of the state of consciousness, estimated intracranial pressure, and neurologic deficit. The role of skull X-rays is somewhat controversial. Skull films ordered on a routine basis have a low efficacy in the management of acute brain injury.[2] On the other hand, when ordered in the context of certain high yield criteria

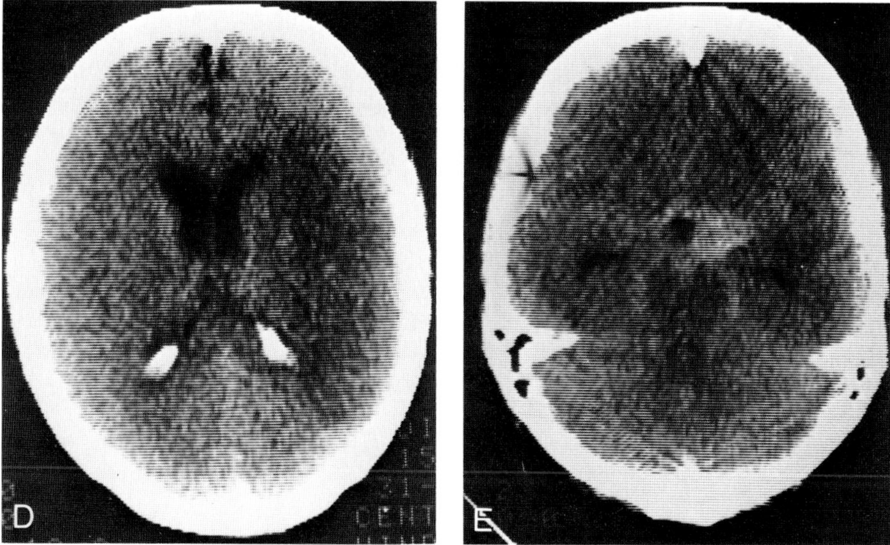

Fig. 2.4 *(continued)*   (D) Infarction in distribution of RMCA has developed (vague low density). (E) CT shows rebleeding three weeks after admission.

for skull fracture or brain injury, skull films can demonstrate significant findings and more importantly provide direction to the CT (Table 2.4).[9]

A linear skull fracture in itself may be unimportant but when related to a meningial artery groove or dural venous sinus it becomes quite significant. Such a plain film finding should direct the performance of the CT to exclude underlying epidural hematoma, contusion, and sinus thrombosis.

Table 2.4 High Yield Clinical Criteria for Predicting Skull Fracture and/or Significant Brain Injury*

Loss of consciousness more than 10 minutes by history
Altered level of consciousness on examination
Focal neurologic deficit
Seizure
Penetrating head wound
Palpable bony misalignment
Ear or nasal discharge (Blood or CSF)

* The author feels this list could also be used to determine the need for CT in trauma. (Adapted from Cummins, R.O.: Clinicians' reasons for overuse of skull radiographs. Am. J. Roentgenol., 135:549, 1980 and from Masters, S.J.: Evaluation of Head Trauma: Efficacy of skull films. Am. J. Roentgenol. 135:149, 1980; with permission).

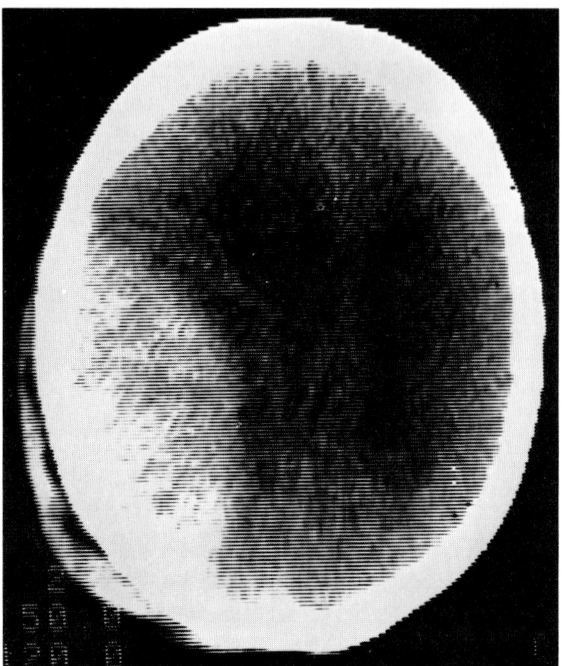

Fig. 2.5
CT shows a large left parietal epidural hematoma.

Depressed fractures, unless already suspected or diagnosed on plain films, may be missed or underevaluated on a CT without the proper window settings or proper angle of section. Basilar fractures are often difficult to demonstrate by any means, but if seen may require antibiotic therapy. Similarly, fluid levels in sinuses, especially the mastoids, are often first diagnosed on plain films.

Computed tomography can nicely demonstrate the mass effect of brain contusion and sometimes, if severe, show brain edema.[13] It is unsurpassed in showing small foci of contusional hemorrhage as well as intracerebral hematoma and intraventricular hemorrhage and SAH. Subdural and epidural hematomas can be diagnosed and their location, size and mass effect evaluated, thus guiding decisions as to immediate evacuation with a skull flap, delayed placement of a burr hole when liquification occurs, or nonoperative management (Fig. 2.5). If necessary, repeat studies are obtained easily and can be used to monitor resolution of the process, response to operation, evaluation of clinical worsening, and post traumatic atrophy or hydrocephalus. Angiography may be used to: (1) further assess abnormalities on CT (e.g., growing hematoma or possible isodense subdural hematoma (Fig. 2.6); (2) evaluate primary vascular injury, vascular spasm, carotid or intracranial artery stenosis; and (3) to clarify an abnormal clinical status (i.e., pulsating exopthalmus, unexpected neurologic course (Fig. 2.7)).[12]

Fig. 2.6
(A) CT equivocal; Possible left frontal mass compressing the ventricles. (B) Angiography reveals an extracerebral collection. Surgery showed a subdural hematoma.

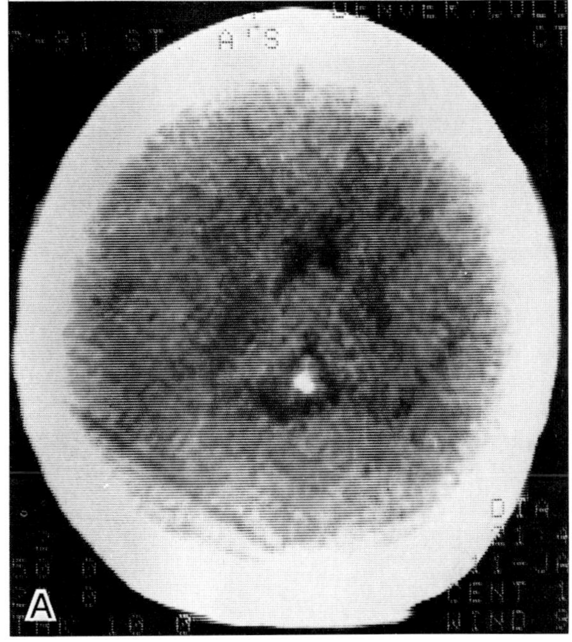

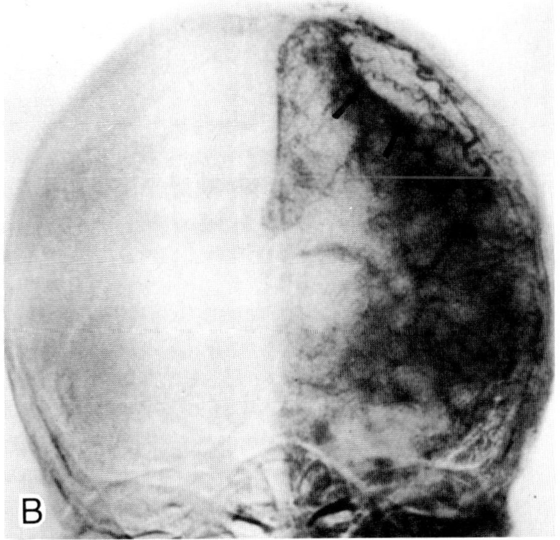

Infections

CT has dramatically changed the diagnosis and management of cerebral abscess. Size, number, location, thickness of capsule, and surrounding edema are accurately evaluated and guide the timing and method of treatment,

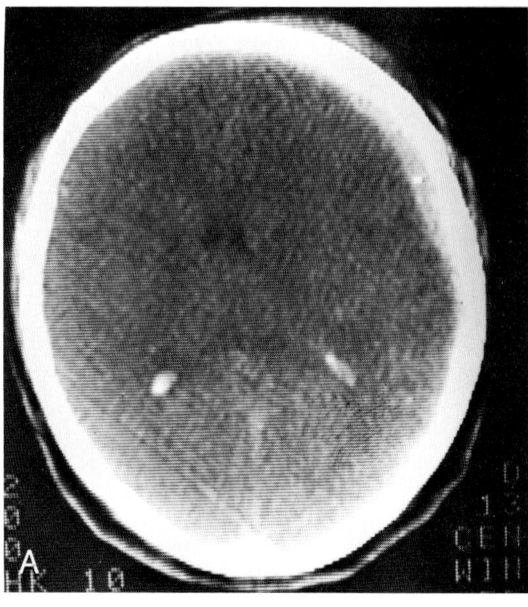

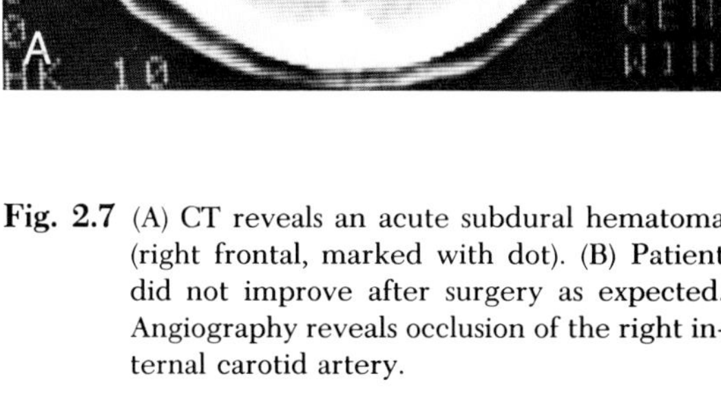

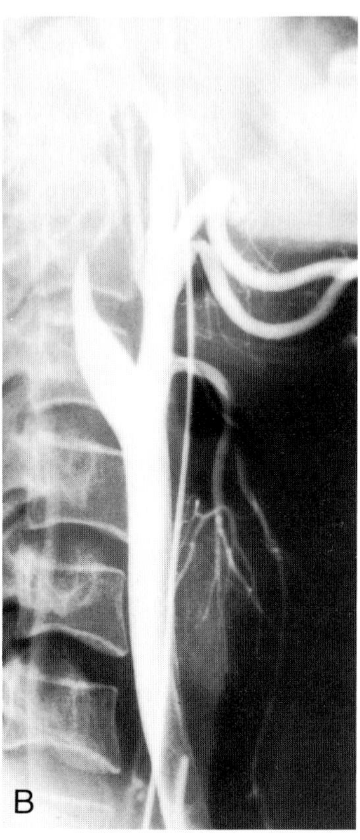

Fig. 2.7 (A) CT reveals an acute subdural hematoma (right frontal, marked with dot). (B) Patient did not improve after surgery as expected. Angiography reveals occlusion of the right internal carotid artery.

whether antibiotics, needle drainage, or open craniotomy (Fig. 2.8). In addition, response to treatment is easily obtained by follow-up CT scans.[16]

With regard to encephalitis and meningitis, CT plays a lesser but still important role. While a high degree of clinical suspicion is the most important factor instituting prompt therapy in herpes encephalitis, CT or nuclide scanning can support the clinical diagnosis by showing mass effect, edema, and enhancement in temporal or frontal lobes. It also can be used to assess response to treatment. In meningitis, CT is used to evaluate complications such as subdural effusion or empyema, hydrocephalus, and brain abscess. Angiography may be useful in excluding subdural empyema and, in difficult cases, angiography may be helpful in showing changes in caliber or occlusion of arteries at base of brain as well as more distally caused by the meningitis.

Seizures

In a patient with a first seizure, the role of radiology is to exclude a structural lesion (Fig. 2.9). If a high quality CT with and without contrast is normal, a major structural lesion is unlikely. Further work-up must be guided by the physician's clinical diagnosis of probable etiology of the seizure.

Fig. 2.8
Right occipital ring enhancing lesion, proven abscess.

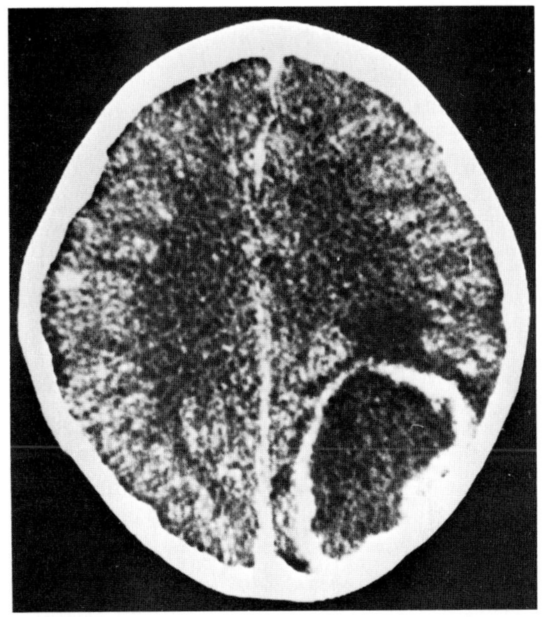

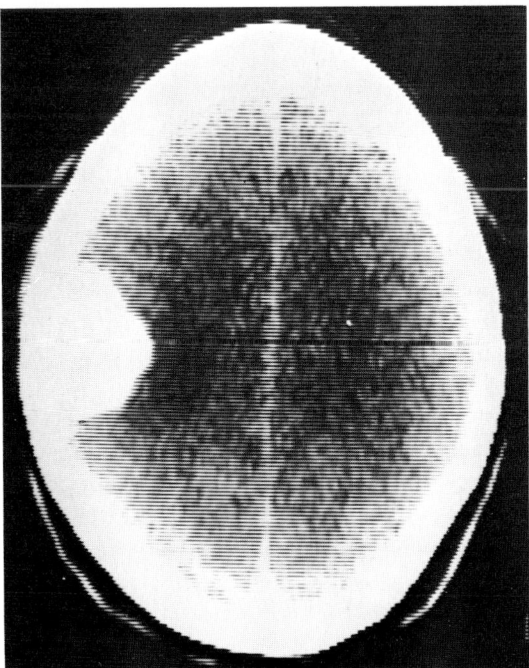

Fig. 2.9
59-year-old man with 1st seizure; CT shows left convexity meningioma.

Acute Disorders Of Mental Status

The primary role of radiology is to exclude a structural lesion and, in particular, a treatable lesion. In this light, CT would be the procedure of choice to evaluate possible subdural, hydrocephalus, or tumor (Fig. 2.10). Subdurals less than 4 mm or isodense subdurals may present diagnostic difficulties and in a few cases angiography may be necessary.

Sometimes the distinction between localized atrophy and a chronic subdural hematoma cannot be made by CT. Radionuclide scanning can distinguish between these two, as a subdural will show increased accumulation of the radionuclide.

Increased Intracranial Pressure (ICP)

ICP is a clinical diagnosis whose etiology can be accurately evaluated by radiologic techniques. The plain skull film may show changes in the sella or, if the patient is young, spreading of the sutures or increased digital markings. CT can demonstrate hydrocephalus as well as diagnose mass lesions.[14] With normal or small ventricles and an otherwise normal scan a diagnosis of pseudotumor cerebri can be made. Diagnosis of thrombosis of major sinuses sometimes can be made with a contrast enhanced CT scan, but angiography is more definitive.

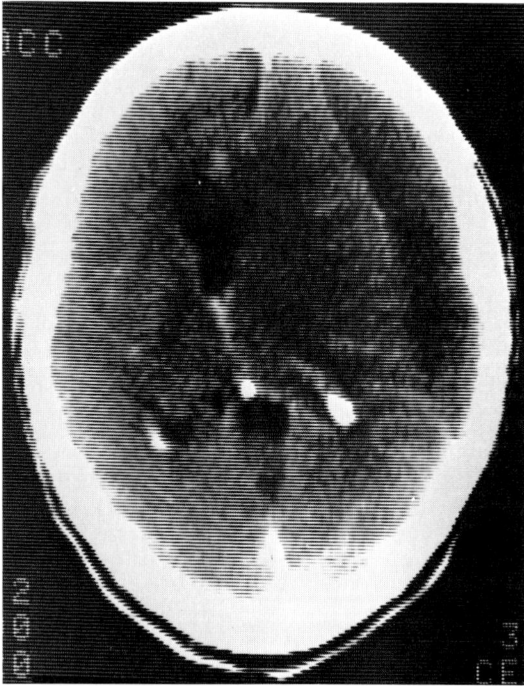

Fig. 2.10
78-year-old with suspected dementia; CT shows chronic subdural hematoma.

Coma

The role of radiology in coma is to exclude a structural lesion. This is most efficiently accomplished by CT, with radionuclide scanning and cerebral angiography playing secondary or complementary roles.

Anoxia

Diagnosis and causes of anoxia are heavily dependent on history and physical examination. CT can add additional information by demonstrating the location and extent of changes seen in anoxia (e.g., edema, demyelination, cortical infarction, and hemorrhage).[6,18] What changes are seen depend on the insulting agent, the degree of insult, and the time since the insult.

Multiple Sclerosis

CT can show enhancing white matter plaques as well as focal areas of decreased density within the white matter, thus supporting the diagnosis. However, often the CT in negative and its primary role lies in excluding mass lesions.

Toxins

Usually the diagnosis of exposure to cerebral toxins is made by history. Often, however, a patient is found unconscious and no history is available. In these cases CT can sometimes localize structural brain changes such as local brain necrosis and demyelination thereby suggesting an etiology as well as prognosis. Low attenuation areas bilaterally in the putamen are virtually diagnostic of methanol intoxication,[1] although sometimes seen after severe hypotensive shock. Exposure to carbon monoxide may result in areas of low attenuation in the occipital lobes or globus pallidus.

Spinal Disorders

Plain films of spine remain important for evaluating the bony changes of trauma, as well as the destructive lytic or blastic changes of metastatic disease. Processes such as syringomyelia and neurofibromatosis may also be diagnosed. In the case of metastatic disease or primary bone tumor of spine, the nuclide scan is often positive when plain films are normal. Occasionally both plain films and nuclide scans are negative in metastatic disease and a myelogram will show intraspinal involvement, especially in cases of lymphoma and lung carcinoma.

In trauma, polytomography diagnoses 20 percent more fractures than plain films and is used to further evaluate bony and ligamentous spinal injury.[8] Myelography may be indicated in progressing spinal cord deficit or a spinal cord deficit with some preserved function.

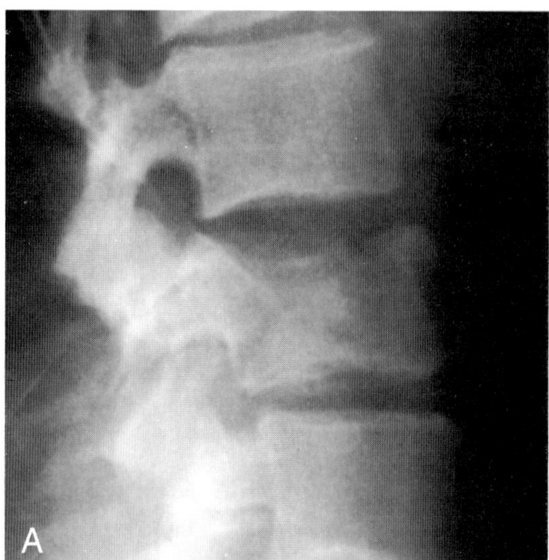

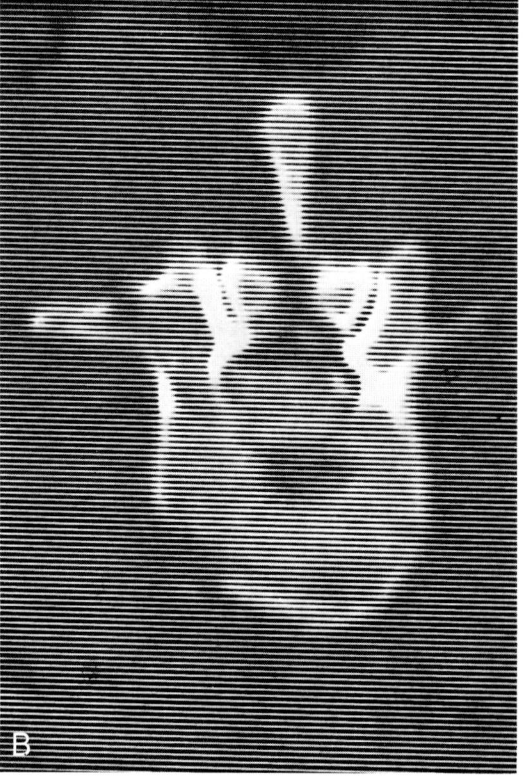

Fig. 2.11
(A) Plain lateral spine film shows compression of a lumbar vertebra and probable fragment in the spinal canal. (B) CT shows 50 percent stenosis of the canal from a herniated fragment of the vertebral body.

The role of CT in diseases of the spine is still being defined. Certainly it gives unequaled view of spinal stenosis (Fig. 2.11). With further refinements in spatial and contrast resolution increasing detail is being seen within the spinal canal and cord. In the future the diagnosis of disc disease, spinal tumors, AVM, cord hematomas, and cysts may be made by plain CT with no further work-up necessary.

CONCLUSION

Within the last 8–10 years there has been an explosion in non-invasive radiologic techniques. CT has made techniques such as cerebral angiography and nuclide brain scanning less important. Technical advancements are continuing and techniques such as intravenous digital subtraction angiography (IVDSA), Nuclear Magnetic Resonance (NMR), and positron emission tomography (PET) scanning may lessen the role of CT. It is imperative that the clinician have some knowledge of the tools available to him and that he work closely with the radiologist to better evaluate nervous system problems and thereby improve patient care.

REFERENCES

1. Aquilonius, S.M., Bergstrom, K., Enoksson, P., et al: Cerebral computed tomography in methanol intoxication. J. Comput. Assist. Tomogr., 4:425, 1980.
2. Cummins, R.O.: Clinicians' reasons for overuse of skull radiographs. Am. J. Roentgenol., 135:549, 1980.
3. David, K.R., New, P.F.J., Ojemann, K.G., et al.: Computed tomographic evaluation of hemorrhage secondary to intracranial aneurysm. Am. J. Roentgenol., 127:143, 1976.
4. Davis, J.M., Davis, K.R., Crowell, R.M.: Subarachnoid hemorrhage secondary to ruptured intracranial aneurysm, prognostic significance of cranial CT. Am. J. Neuroradiol., 1:17, 1980.
5. Davis, K.R., Taveras, J.M., Roberson, G.H., Ackerman, R.H.: Some limitations of computed tomography in the diagnosis of neurological diseases. Am. J. Roentgenol., 127:111, 1976.
6. Drayer, B.P., Rosenbaum, A.E.: Brain edema defined by cranial computed tomography. J. Comput. Assist. Tomogr., 3:317, 1979.
7. Hayward, R.A., O'Reilly, G.U.H.: Intracranial hemorrhage—Accuracy of CT in predicting underlying etiology. Lancet, 1:1, 1976.
8. Maravilla, K.R., Cooper, P.R., Sklar, F.H.: The influence of thin-section tomography on the treatment of cervical spine injuries. Radiology, 127:131, 1978.
9. Masters, S.J.: Evaluation of head trauma: Efficacy of skull films. Am. J. Roentgenol. 135:549, 1980.
10. Pullicino, P., Nelson, R.F., Kendall, B.E., Marshall, J.: Small deep infarcts diagnosed on computed tomography. Neurology, 30:1090, 1980.

11. Spetcler, R.F., Norman, D., Selman, W.R., et al: Computerized tomographic diagnosis: pitfalls for neurosurgeons. Neurosurgery, 5:231, 1979.
12. Tipper, M.H., Kishore, P.R.S., Girevendulis, A.K., et al: Delayed intracranial hematoma in patients with severe head injury. Radiology, 133:645, 1976.
13. Tsai, F.Y., Hyprich, J.E., Gardner, F.C., et al: Diagnostic and prognostic implications of computer tomography of head trauma. J. Comput. Assist. Tomogr., 2:323, 1978.
14. Weisberg, L., Nice, C.N.: Computed tomographic evaluation of increased intracranial pressure without localizing signs. Radiology, 122:133, 1977.
15. Weisberg, L.A., Nice, C., Katz, M.: Cerebral Computed Tomography: A Text-atlas. W.B. Saunders, Philadelphia, 1978.
16. Whelan, M.A., Hilal, S.K.: Computed tomography as a guide in the diagnosis and follow-up of brain abscesses. Radiology, 135:663, 1980.
17. Wolpert, S.M.: Central Nervous System: Approaches to Radiologic Diagnosis. Grune and Stratton, New York, 1979.
18. Yagnik, P., Gonzalez, C.: White matter involvement in anoxic encephalopathy in adults. J. Comput. Assist. Tomogr., 4:788, 1980.
19. York, D.H., Larson, D.A.: Computed tomography of hemorrhage from anterior communicating artery aneurysm with angiographic correlation. Radiology, 134:399, 1980.
20. York, D.A., Marshall, W.H.: Recent ischemic brain infarction and computed tomography. Radiology, 117:599, 1972.
21. Zimmerman, R.A., Bilaniak, L.T.: Computed tomography of acute intratumoral hemorrhage. Radiology, 135:355, 1980.

3

Safe and Effective Use of the Lumbar Puncture

Michael P. Earnest, M.D.

INTRODUCTION

For many physicians and patients the lumbar puncture (LP) has become synonymous with danger. The patient, and often his family, fears an LP because "My Aunt Minnie had one and she never walked again!" The physician, on the other hand, fears that his doing an LP will precipitate brain herniation, leading to progressive brain damage or even death. The physician usually is aware that the patient's fears are groundless: a lumbar puncture in the lower lumbar sac of the subarachnoid space will not cause a paraplegia. He knows that Aunt Minnie was probably paralyzed by the disease which prompted the LP. However, the physician's own fears are less easily assuaged. He wants to avoid harm to the patient. Nonetheless, in most neurologic emergencies, an LP can be safely done and should be done when the symptoms and signs give proper indications for the procedure.

INDICATIONS FOR AN LP (Table 3.1)

The general indication for an LP in the emergency setting is the physician's need to examine the cerebrospinal fluid (CSF) in order to establish or rule out a particular diagnosis. The LP is most urgent when infection of the central nervous system, other than brain abscess, is suspected. An immediate LP is indicated in a patient with suspected bacterial meningitis because delay in diagnosis and treatment, even delay for an hour to obtain a CT scan, can allow progression of the disease and serious brain damage.

The second common rationale for doing an LP is to look for blood in the CSF. An LP is an important part of the early work-up of a patient suspected to have a non-traumatic intracranial hemorrhage. The LP does

Table 3.1 Indications for Emergency Lumbar Puncture (LP)—Clinical Diagnoses Prompting an LP

Frequent Indications	Infrequent Indications
Bacterial meningitis	Multiple sclerosis exacerbation
Viral meningitis	Carcinomatous meningitis
Subarachnoid hemorrhage (nontraumatic)	Encephalitis
	Neurosyphilis

not have to be done if a CT scan shows subarachnoid blood or an intracranial parenchymal hemorrhage. However, in the clinical setting in which a non-traumatic intracranial hemorrhage is suspected and a CT scan shows no blood and no mass, the LP is the next step required in the work-up. A normal CT does not rule out subarachnoid blood; clinical experience indicates that over 20 percent of primary subarachnoid hemorrhages are not shown by the initial CT scan.[6] In some cases the LP may precede the CT scan. If a patient presents with a history strongly suggesting non-traumatic subarachnoid hemorrhage and, on exam, is not comatose and has no focal signs, the LP may be done as the first diagnostic test. If it shows blood in the CSF, then the patient should be admitted and the CT scan can be done later. However, if the lumbar CSF has no blood, the CT scan should be done soon to rule out intracranial blood that has not yet spread to the lumbar space. Sometimes as much as 2 hours may be required for intracranial subarachnoid blood to diffuse to the lumbar CSF.

In the emergency setting there are no other common indications for LP. In unusual cases the physician may do an LP primarily to measure the CSF pressure or to obtain CSF immunologic studies for multiple sclerosis or cytology to look for neoplastic meningitis.

CONTRAINDICATIONS FOR AN LP (Table 3.2)

Contraindications to an LP are all relative. They must be weighed against the value and urgency of the CSF examination. The physician should be aware of the various contraindications and their relative severity and should consider contraindications versus indications and then decide whether to do the LP.

Sometimes, in the author's consulting experience, the primary physician has been so concerned about the contraindications for LP that he has not done one and the patient has suffered harm. The most common situation is the comatose or confused patient with fever, in whom meningitis is suspected but in whom brain abscess has not been fully ruled out. The physician delays the LP and waits for a neurologic consultation or CT scan. If the patient does have meningitis, he is harmed by the delay in diagnosis and

Table 3.2 Contraindications for Lumbar Puncture (LP)—Clinical Syndromes in Which an LP May Be Dangerous

LP is Very Dangerous	LP has Some Danger	LP is Difficult, But Little Danger
Active brain herniation	Suspected increased intracranial pressure, but patient is stable	Prior spinal fusion
Suspected large, focal mass lesion of the brain	Small focal mass lesion with little shift of brain	Arachnoiditis
Cerebellar or brainstem mass	Skin infection near LP site	Severe spinal arthritis
Purulent skin or deep tissue infection at LP site	Prolonged prothrombin time, low platelet count, etc., without clinical bleeding disorder	
Clinical bleeding disorder or platelet count below 50,000	Spinal cord compression	

treatment. The LP should be done in spite of the concern about an abscess if the clinical history and examination do not disclose any strong contraindications to an LP.

The most nearly absolute contraindications against LP (i.e., the conditions in which an LP will have a high probability of doing harm) are:

1. A patient with a suspected focal mass lesion who is rapidly deteriorating or is having active brain herniation.[3,7,8]

2. Suspected mass lesion in the cerebellum or brain stem. The danger in this case, and in patients of the first category, is that the LP will draw off CSF from the lumbar space, and will create an imbalance of spinal CSF pressure with intracranial pressure, thus precipitating shift of the mass-pressured brain through the tentorial notch or the foramen magnum. The shifted brain then can suffer irreversible damage and the patient may die.

3. Severe local lumbar skin or subcutaneous infection.[14] The LP might introduce bacteria into the spinal canal and cause meningitis or an intraspinal abscess.

4. Severe bleeding disorder or platelet count below 50,000 platelets/mm.[3] The LP may produce an intraspinal hematoma that can cause paraplegia.[4]

Important, but less powerful, contraindications are:

1. Suspected increased intracranial pressure but the patient is not rapidly deteriorating, and is not believed to have a focal mass or posterior fossa lesion. An LP may be done even in the presence of papilledema in some

instances.[10,12] Patients with a diffuse increase in intracranial pressure are less likely to have progressive herniation after a lumbar puncture.[7]

2. Small focal mass lesion with little shift of the brain. In some cases a small mass seen on CT scan or angiogram might be an abscess, hemorrhage or tumor. An examination of the CSF is an important diagnostic tool. The LP may be done if the mass is not large and the brain is not badly shifted from its normal position or compressed by the mass.

3. Patients with skin infections near the proposed LP site (e.g., infected sacral decubitus or bacteremia) may have some increased risk of CSF contamination.[5] Careful technique will minimize that risk.

4. Patients with prolonged prothrombin times or moderately low platelets but no clinical bleeding disorder may have some increased risk of an intraspinal hemorrhage. However, gentle and accurate placement of the LP needle will minimize the risk of bleeding.

5. Suspected spinal cord compression.[14] An LP may precipitate rapid progression of the patient's course. In cases of suspected spinal cord compression it is safer to defer the LP until a neurology or neurosurgery consultation has been obtained and a decision made about doing a myelogram. If a myelogram is required, then obtain CSF for examination at the time of the myelography. If a myelogram is not required, but examination of the CSF is important, then an LP can be done.

An ill-advised LP in a patient with spinal cord compression can also create problems for the radiologist. The first LP may create a hole in the lumbar dura that leaks CSF. That leak may create an epidural CSF pocket which can make a subsequent LP for myelography impossible, or the epidural pocket may appear, on a successfully completed myelogram, to be an epidural spinal compression. The surgeon, the radiologist, the primary physician who did the LP and the patient all suffer when such an artefactual lesion is recognized only at the operating table.

6. Previous lumbar spine surgery. A spinal fusion can create a serious barrier to successfully passing the LP needle into the subarachnoid space. However, it is not a contraindication against attempting an LP when one is indicated. The major problems are the technical difficulty faced by the physician and the increased discomfort suffered by the patient. Known lumbar arachnoiditis presents similar technical and patient discomfort problems. A previous laminectomy and discectomy is not a contraindication.

The physician must be aware of all the above contraindications and must search for them in any neurologic emergency for which an LP is being considered. Any contraindications must be weighed against the urgency of need for an LP, and then the decision is made.

RECOMMENDED TECHNIQUE

Once the physician chooses to do the LP he must obtain a formal consent from the patient or the family. The physician's attitude of comfort about the safety and the indications for the procedure, and his confidence in his own ability to perform it, are important for reassuring the patient and obtaining his permission.

An LP is a simple procedure, and the technique uncomplicated. Figure 3.1 shows the most important step in doing a successful LP—correctly positioning the patient. The most common error made by inexperienced physicians is to attempt an LP when the patient is improperly positioned. The LP then is often unsuccessful.

The patient must be, for most LP's, in a lateral decubitus position on a firm bed with his head supported by a small pillow. The pillow allows the cervical spine and the thoracolumbar spine, to be straight and horizontal. The head is then flexed so the chin touches the chest and the legs are maximally flexed toward the head (Fig. 3.1). Maximal head and leg flexion produce maximal opening of the space between the vertebral spinous processes through which the LP needle must pass. The plane of the lumbosacral area should be maintained perpendicular to the table. Any rotation forward of the upper hip (usually the right hip) will produce rotation of the spine and so alter the relation of the internal open space between the vertebrae to the external landmarks. If the patient is uncooperative or unable to maintain the position, an assistant can hold the patient, and also can be helpful comforting and reassuring the patient as the procedure is done.

Most LPs are now performed using a pre-packaged sterile kit. The physician should position the kit in a place convenient for him while doing the LP and should scrub his hands and don sterile gloves. A large area of the lumbosacral skin is then scrubbed with an appropriate antiseptic and the area properly draped. The proper location for passing the LP needle is selected by the physician placing his hand on the iliac crest and then mentally marking a line perpendicularly downward to the spine.

At or near the intersection of the vertical line with the spine he should be able to feel with his thumb a space between two lumbar spinous processes. This is usually the L_4–L_5 interspace. This space, the next lower or the next higher one, may be selected. The highest space that should be considered is the L_2–L_3 interspace. A puncture above that space risks damaging the spinal cord, which usually ends at or just above the L_2 vertebra.[2]

Once the interspace is selected, an intradermal injection of local anesthetic numbs the skin and marks the desired spot for placing the LP needle. A deeper injection of local anesthetic may be given to numb deeper tissues. A 20 gauge needle is usually used. It should be used only with the stylet in place and should be initially passed through the skin and then angled to point cephalad toward the umbilicus. The initial skin puncture should be as exactly in the dorsal midline as possible. The bevel of the needle

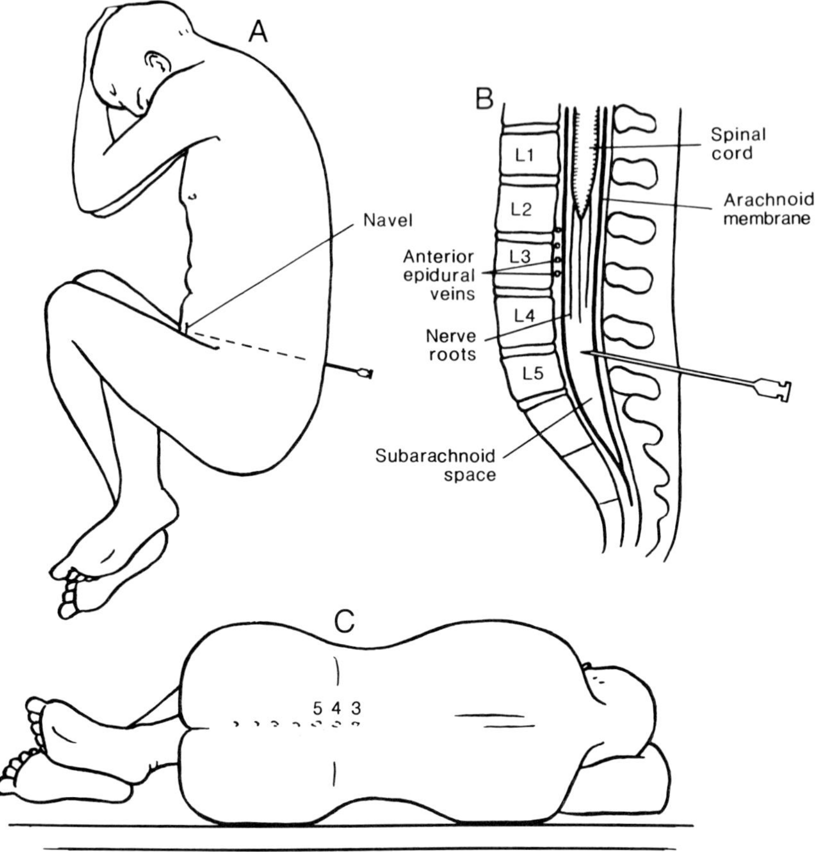

Fig. 3.1　Correct patient position and proper needle placement for successful lumbar puncture.

should be kept horizontal to produce separation, rather than transection, of the fibers of the dura. This, theoretically, reduces the chances of producing a prolonged CSF leak and post-LP headache.[1] Advancing the needle slowly will usually produce a soft "pop" as the needle penetrates the arachnoid membrane. The stylet should be withdrawn and the CSF should begin to drip from the needle, if the tap was successful. The referenced article by Posner gives a more detailed description of technique and what to do if the first attempt is unsuccessful. It also discusses proper handling of the CSF and treatment of the post-LP headache syndrome.[14]

COMMON PROBLEMS DURING THE LP (Table 3.3)

1. The unsuccessful tap—The most common cause is improper positioning of the patient and/or of the needle. The spine must be horizontal, unrotated and the lumbar spine in a kyphotic (bent dorsally) position.

Table 3.3 Common Problems and Their Management During the Lumbar Puncture

Problem	Solution
Patient moves too much	Have an assistant restrain patient Use more local anesthetic Sedate patient (a last resort)
Needle won't advance (hits bone or is deflected)	Correct patient's position Check for proper angle of needle towards umbilicus Make sure needle entry is midline If needle deflected by calcified ligament, use heavier gauge needle
Dry tap (needle in proper space and depth, but no CSF flow)	Twirl hub of needle Withdraw needle slightly Have patient cough Advance needle slightly (a last resort—risks hitting anterior veins) Try another space
Dry tap in spite of above measures	Do LP with patient sitting
Patient has nerve root pain	Don't advance the needle! Replace stylet Withdraw needle slightly & then advance at different angle
Traumatic tap	Withdraw needle slightly and let CSF drip until clear If CSF doesn't clear, retap at another spinal level
CSF pressure suspiciously high	Have patient relax Extend patient's legs & neck to neutral position Observe pressure for 5 minutes (it often drops as patient relaxes)
CSF pressure suspiciously low	Have patient cough Twirl hub of needle Withdraw needle slightly Advance needle slightly (risks hitting veins) Try another space

The plane of the hips and sacrum must be exactly vertical. The needle must then be exactly horizontal and directed toward the umbilicus. If all these criteria are met and several intervertebral spaces tried, and failed, then the LP can be done with the patient in a sitting, forward-flexed position. Very obese or muscular patients sometimes require this position.

2. The needle won't go in straight but is deflected by a tough or calcified midline interspinous ligament or scar tissue from prior surgery—Use of an 18 gauge needle often overcomes this problem.

3. The moving target—If a patient won't lie still, don't even try the LP, or, once begun, don't advance the needle until the patient can be completely restrained and positioned correctly. More local anesthetic, especially in deeper tissues, might help.

4. Poor CSF flow—Twirling the needle may improve flow. You may also slightly advance or retract the needle without the stylet while observing CSF flow.

5. A "traumatic" tap—This usually results when the needle has punctured epidural veins, usually ventral to the subarachnoid space (i.e., between the lumbar sac and the vertebral body). The needle was advanced too far. This can usually be avoided by slowly advancing the LP needle and feeling the distinctive "pop" as it enters the subarachnoid space, then not advancing further. Once bloody CSF is seen, the best procedure is to replace the stylet, withdraw the needle a few millimeters and then remove the stylet to observe the CSF. If it is still not clear, the physician should immediately withdraw the needle and perform an LP one or two interspaces higher using a clean needle.

When a traumatic tap is suspected immediate examination of the CSF can sometimes be helpful. A sample of CSF may be immediately centrifuged, carefully decanted to a clean tube and then examined for xanthochromia. If the fluid is distinctly xanthochromic (yellow-tinged because of products from red blood cell lysis), the blood, at least in part, is due to intracranial hemorrhage. If the CSF is colorless, no conclusion can be made about the LP being non-traumatic. Counting the red blood cells (RBCs) in the first CSF sample and in a later one, after several milliliters of fluid have been drained off, may show a large drop in the number of RBCs in the last versus the first sample. That difference suggests a traumatic tap. However, if the number of RBCs was equal, no conclusion can be made. The ratio of white blood cells to RBCs and the total protein in the CSF can also be helpful but are not as reliable.[7,14]

SPECIAL TECHNIQUES WHEN INCREASED INTRACRANIAL PRESSURE IS SUSPECTED

If the physician suspects increased ICP but must do the LP he should take several precautions. He should use a small gauge, number 22, needle. He should be especially careful to avoid multiple punctures, and so avoid a post-LP CSF leak through the dura. When he first enters the CSF space, he should take no samples but measure the pressure immediately. If it is elevated above 200 mmHg, he should remove only the minimum volume of CSF necessary for the essential laboratory tests. Following the LP the patient is kept horizontal at least 6 hours, probably best in the prone position, if possible. Continuous observation of the patient's level of consciousness and other neurologic signs should be begun. A neurologic or neurosurgical consultation should be called to help follow and manage the patient.

Care should be taken in documenting the CSF pressure. It should be measured only with the patient's legs and head extended in a comfortable position and when the patient is relaxed. Falsely elevated pressures are often produced by excessive muscle tension, flexion of the legs and head, pressure on the abdomen or an excessively obese abdomen.

The physician must be aware of falsely normal or low pressures as well. Such misleading values are usually produced by poor CSF flow through the LP needle. If poor flow is suspected the needle should be repositioned to obtain good flow or the LP repeated at another interspace. Good communication of the needle with the CSF space can be shown by brisk respiratory fluctuations of CSF in the manometer tube and by a prompt rise in the CSF pressure when pressure is applied to the patient's abdomen or when he performs a Valsava maneuver.

COMPLICATIONS FOLLOWING AN LP

The most life-threatening complication, herniation of the brain, has been discussed. However, it is a rare complication when the physician has taken proper care to rule out a focal, mass-producing intracranial lesion.

The most common residual of LP is probably lumbar spine aching pain and tenderness. Local heat, aspirin and rest will resolve those symptoms. A more vexing problem is post-LP headache.[1,9] Those headaches are thought to be caused by reduced intracranial pressure due to a continuing leak of CSF through a persistent hole in the dura from the LP needle. The frequency of post-LP headache is reduced by having the patient remain lying for several hours following the procedure. Best is probably the prone position, which, in theory, closes the hole in the dura.[1]

Once a post-LP headache has developed the patient should be instructed to lie down in the prone position whenever the headache starts. The headache classically occurs only or is most severe when the patient is sitting or standing. Occasionally, a few days of bed rest is required before the patient can be up without a headache. Having the patient drink copious liquids may help. Minor analgesics and anti-nausea medications are required in more severe cases.

INTERPRETATION OF CSF FINDINGS

Measurement of the pressure is the first step in examining the CSF; it's interpretation is discussed above. A CSF sample should then be examined for clarity. Is it cloudy or a normal, crystal-clear fluid? The color of the CSF should be next observed, after centrifugation if any RBCs are known or suspected to be present. The presence of xanthochromia indicates a prior intracranial or intraspinal hemorrhage. A specimen should be collected for stains and cultures appropriate for the clinician's diagnosis. However, CSF cultures are not mandatory if the differential diagnosis doesn't include infection. Specimens should routinely be sent to the laboratory for glucose and protein determination, and serologic testing for syphilis. In cases of suspected multiple sclerosis or fungal infections of the nervous system appropriate serologies should be collected, and for suspected cases of carcinomatous meningitis CSF cytology should be requested.

The author assumes that the physician is familiar with the CSF abnormalities in common diseases. Chapter 19 discusses CSF findings in various infectious conditions. However, the physician should be aware of several pitfalls that may lead to misdiagnosis:

1. Xanthochromia—Causes of CSF xanthochromia other than hemorrhage are a very high CSF protein (above 150mg/100ml CSF), high serum bilirubin, and lysis of RBCs not properly separated from the CSF by centrifugation immediately after the LP.[13] The latter imparts a more pink tint, however.

2. Excessive RBCs (Normal–0 RBC)—Talcum powder crystals or other debris in a CSF specimen may be mistaken for cells. The physician should know the level of expertise in his laboratory and should himself examine the CSF if there is any doubt about reported results.

3. Excessive white blood cells (Normal 0–5 WBC with 0 polymorphonuclear cells)—Increased WBCs are often a sign of infection. However, they are also increased in noninfectious inflammatory conditions. Within a few hours of an intracranial hemorrhage a marked inflammatory response occurs to increase both monocytes and polymorphonuclear cells (PMNs) in the CSF. Twelve or more hours after a cerebral infarction, WBCs may appear in the CSF. Convulsions alone rarely cause increased WBCs, so other causes must be sought in such cases. Large and irregularly shaped lymphocytes and other mononuclear cells may also be falsely identified as PMNs. Again, the physician should see the CSF himself, if in doubt.

4. Increased CSF protein (Normal 15–50 mg/100ml CSF) [7]—Increased CSF protein usually implies inflammation, hemorrhage or breakdown of the blood-brain barrier. However, diabetes mellitus may cause benign increases in CSF protein, up to about 100mg/100ml CSF maximum.[11] Other benign causes are hypothyroidism and advanced age.

5. Decreased CSF glucose (Normal 45–80mg/100ml CSF)—Low CSF glucose is usually caused by bacterial meningitis. However, some cases of subarachnoid hemorrhage, carcinomatous meningitis and aseptic meningitis also have low glucose.[7] Systemic hypoglycemia also causes low CSF glucose. The ratio of CSF to serum glucose is usually about 0.6. A CSF glucose severely below that ratio may suggest a pathologic process, however the ratio is not reliable when there is marked hyperglycemia.[7] Also, CSF glucose changes slowly in relation to blood glucose. Thus, a low ratio of CSF glucose in a patient with current hyperglycemia may merely reflect a lower blood sugar 2 hours before the LP. Two hours is the approximate time for equilibration of glucose between blood and CSF.

6. Fungus seen on India ink preparation—Again, an inexperienced lab technician and talcum powder crystals are often the culprits.

7. Bacteria not seen on Gram stain—When the physician suspects bacterial meningitis he must assure that the CSF specimen has been properly centrifuged, placed on the slide, fixed and stained by the laboratory. The CSF sediment can easily be washed off a slide. The physician should himself see WBCs present on the slide before he trusts the finding that there are no bacteria present. The absence of WBCs from a Gram stain of a centrifuged specimen implies an error in preparing the slide.

CONCLUSION

The LP is a valuable and safe clinical procedure in many neurologic emergencies. It should not be feared, but should be used when indicated. The physician should be familiar with the contraindications and the complications of an LP and the interpretation of the CSF findings. Such knowledge will enable him to safely use the LP for maximum clinical value.

REFERENCES

1. Brocker, R.J.: Technique to avoid spinal-tap headache. JAMA, 168:261, 1958.
2. Brodal, A.: Neurological Anatomy in Relation to Clinical Medicine. 2nd Ed. Oxford University Press, New York, 1979.
3. Duffy, G.P.: Lumbar puncture in the presence of raised intracranial pressure. Brit. Med. J., 1:407, 1969.
4. Edelson, R.N., Chernik, N.L., Posner, J.B.: Spinal subdural hematoma complicating lumbar puncture: occurrence in thrombocytopenic patients. Arch. Neurol., 31:134, 1974.
5. Eng, R.H.K., Seligman, S.J.: Lumbar puncture-induced meningitis. JAMA, 245:1456, 1981.
6. Findlay, G.F.G.: Computer-assisted (axial) tomography in the management of subarachnoid hemorrhage. Surg. Neurol., 13:125, 1980.
7. Fishman, R.A.: Cerebrospinal Fluid in Diseases of the Nervous System. W.B. Saunders, Philadelphia, 1980.
8. Garfield, J.: Management of supratentorial intracranial abscess: a review of 200 cases. Brit. Med. J., 2:7, 1969.
9. Glass, P.M., Kennedy, W.F.: Headache following subarachnoid puncture: treatment with epidural blood patch. JAMA, 219:203, 1972.
10. Korein, J., Cravioto, H., Leicach, M.: Re-evaluation of lumbar puncture: a study of 129 patients with papilledema or intracranial hypertension. Neurology, 9:290, 1959.
11. Kutt, H., Hurwitz, L.J., Ginsburg, S.M., McDowell, F.: Cerebrospinal fluid in diabetes mellitus. Arch. Neurol., 4:31, 1961.

12. Lubic, L.G., Marotta, J.T.: Brain tumor and lumbar puncture. Arch. Neurol. & Psychiat., 72:568, 1954.
13. Petito, F., Plum, F.: The lumbar puncture. N. Engl. J. Med., 290:225, 1974.
14. Posner, J.B.: Sure and careful lumbar puncture. Consultant, November, 1973, p. 17.

4

Acute Management of Increased Intracranial Pressure

Joseph R. Lacy, M.D.

ANATOMY AND PHYSIOLOGY

The skull encases the brain and protects it from everyday trauma. Within the skull, the brain is bathed by circulating cerebrospinal fluid and stabilized by two fibrous bands: the falx cerebri and the tentorium cerebelli (Fig. 4.1); these elements also serve to protect the brain from minor trauma. It should be recognized, however, that because of the rigid nature of the skull, there is very limited space for the brain to expand under conditions of significant increased intracranial pressure.

The tentorium cerebelli divides the intracranial cavity into two compartments (Fig. 4.2). The area above the tentorium, called the supratentorial compartment, contains the cerebral hemispheres and deep midline structures (basal ganglia, thalamus and hypothalamus). The area below the tentorium is called the subtentorial compartment (posterior fossa), and it contains the brainstem and cerebellum.

The brainstem, a critical structure, controls such reflex activities as respirations and houses the reticular activating system (the alerting center of the brain). It is also the origin of the cranial nerves. The brainstem connects with supratentorial structures through an opening in the tentorium called the tentorial notch. It is the midbrain portion of the brainstem with its exiting third cranial nerves which lies within the tentorial opening (Fig. 4.3). Here, the midbrain lies just mesial to the medial or uncal portions of the temporal lobes. Under conditions of increased intracranial pressure, the brainstem is especially susceptible to compression from the contents of the supratentorial compartment which may herniate either directly downward (central herniation) or medially and downward (uncal herniation). As will be discussed, compression of the brainstem has profound effects on the level of consciousness, brainstem reflexes, and tone and posturing of the extremities.

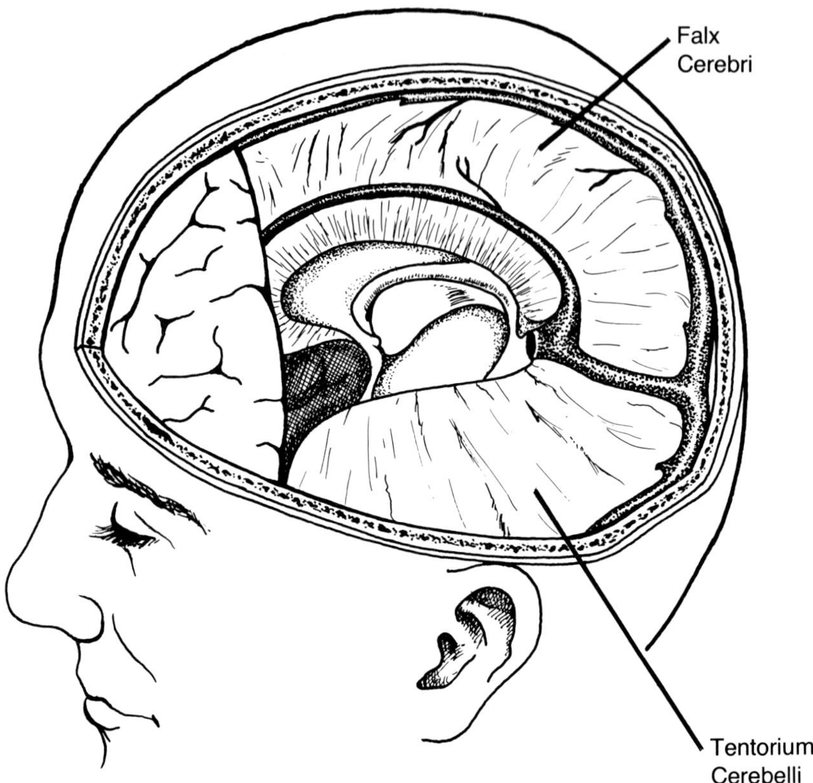

Fig. 4.1 Falx Cerebri and Tentorium Cerebelli. Falx cerebri is the fibrous band between the two cerebral hemispheres. Tentorium cerebelli is the fibrous band which separates the intracranial contents into supra- and subtentorial compartments.

As illustrated in Figure 4.4, the cerebrospinal fluid (CSF) is produced primarily by structures within the ventricular system of the brain called the choroid plexus. Once produced, the CSF travels within the lateral ventricles, the third ventricle and down through the acqueduct of Sylvius to the fourth ventricle. The fourth ventricle contains two lateral openings (foramina of Lushka) and one midline opening (foramen of Magendie) which allow the CSF to flow out into the subarachnoid space. The CSF circulates down into the spinal subarachnoid space and, eventually, circulates up and over the surface of the brain. There the CSF is absorbed into the dural venous sinuses by extrusions of the dural sinuses called arachnoid villi.

In summary, the cranial cavity contains the brain and circulating CSF. The brain is compartmentalized into supra- and subtentorial compartments by the tentorium cerebelli. The free space within the rigid skull is limited.

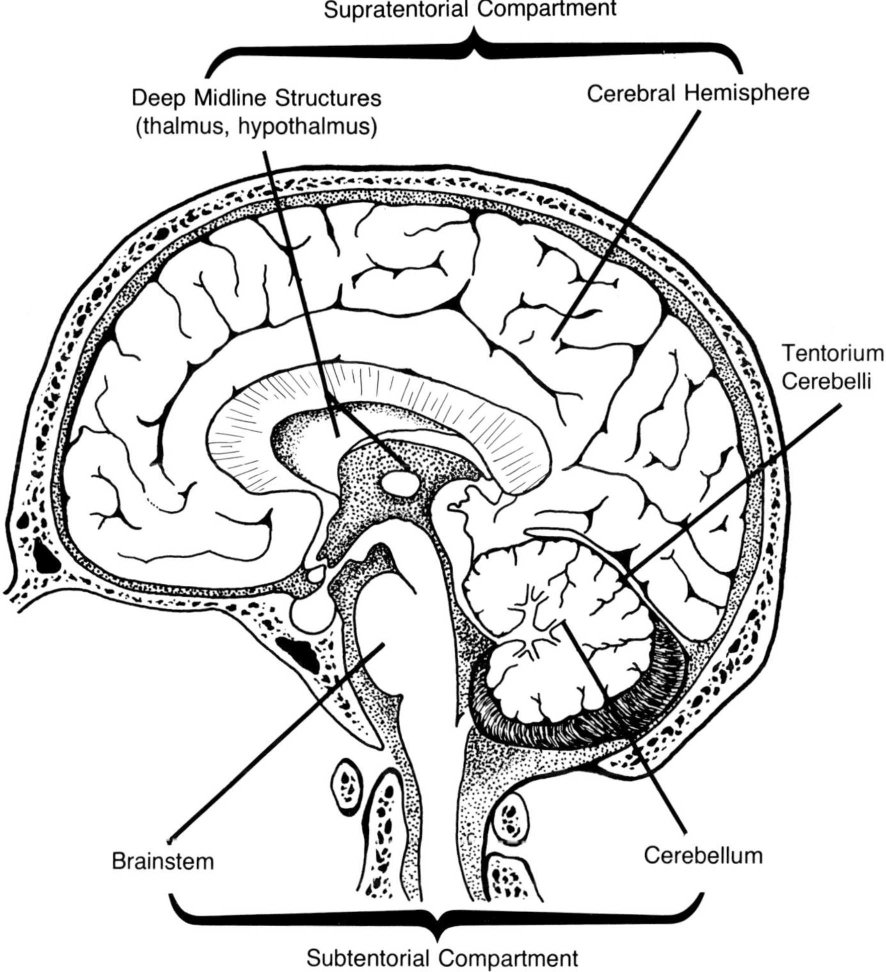

Fig. 4.2 Supratentorial and Subtentorial Compartments. Tentorium cerebelli divides the brain into supratentorial compartment (cerebral hemispheres and deep midline structures) and subtentorial compartment (brainstem and cerebellum).

Accordingly, disorders which cause the pressure within the brain or CSF to rise result in distortion and compression of various regions of the brain—most importantly, the brainstem. The mechanisms by which various processes produce increased pressure, the attendant neurologic signs and symptoms, and the treatment of intracranial hypertension are the principal issues of this chapter.

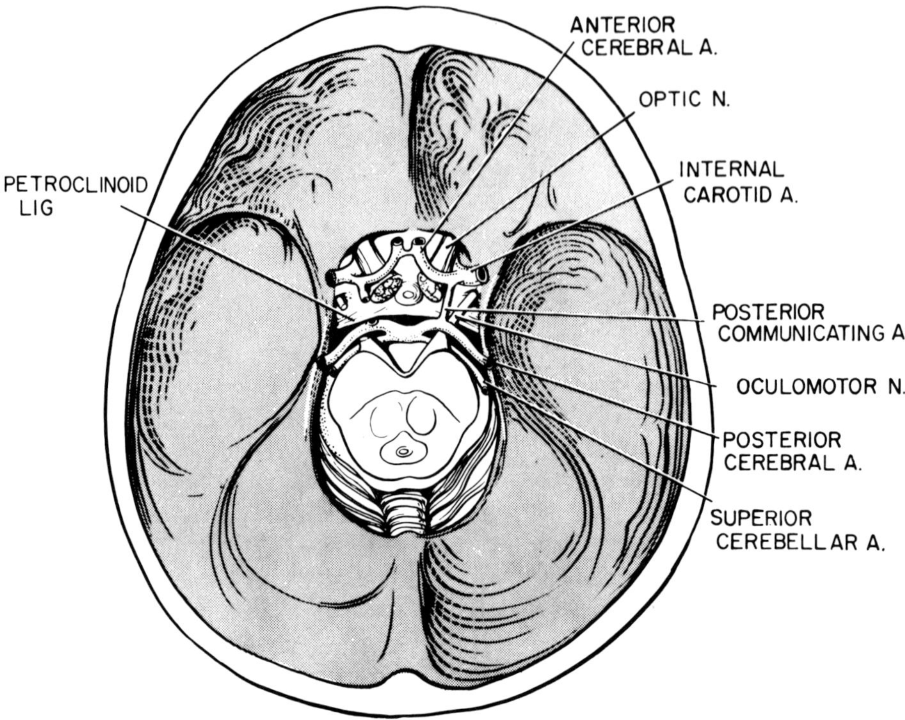

Fig. 4.3 Brainstem in the Tentorial Notch. Midbrain and third cranial nerves in the tentorial notch, and their relationship to the temporal lobes (not shown) which lie in the middle cranial fossa along medial edges of the tentorium (from Plum, F., Posner, J.B.: The Diagnosis of Stupor and Coma. 3rd Ed., F.A. Davis Co., Philadelphia, 1980; reprinted with permission).

MECHANISMS OF INCREASED INTRACRANIAL PRESSURE

There are three categories of pathological processes which cause critical increases in intracranial pressure: (1) disorders which cause diffuse edema or swelling of the brain; (2) expanding mass lesions of the supra- or subtentorial compartment; (3) hydrocephalus resulting from increased production of CSF or from obstruction of the flow or absorption of CSF.

Aside from its obvious place among disorders in the first category, significant brain swelling or edema may accompany disorders in the other two categories as well. There are three types of brain edema:

1. Cytotoxic edema refers to swelling of damaged nerve cells and other cellular elements as a result of the movement of extracellular fluid into the intracellular compartment.

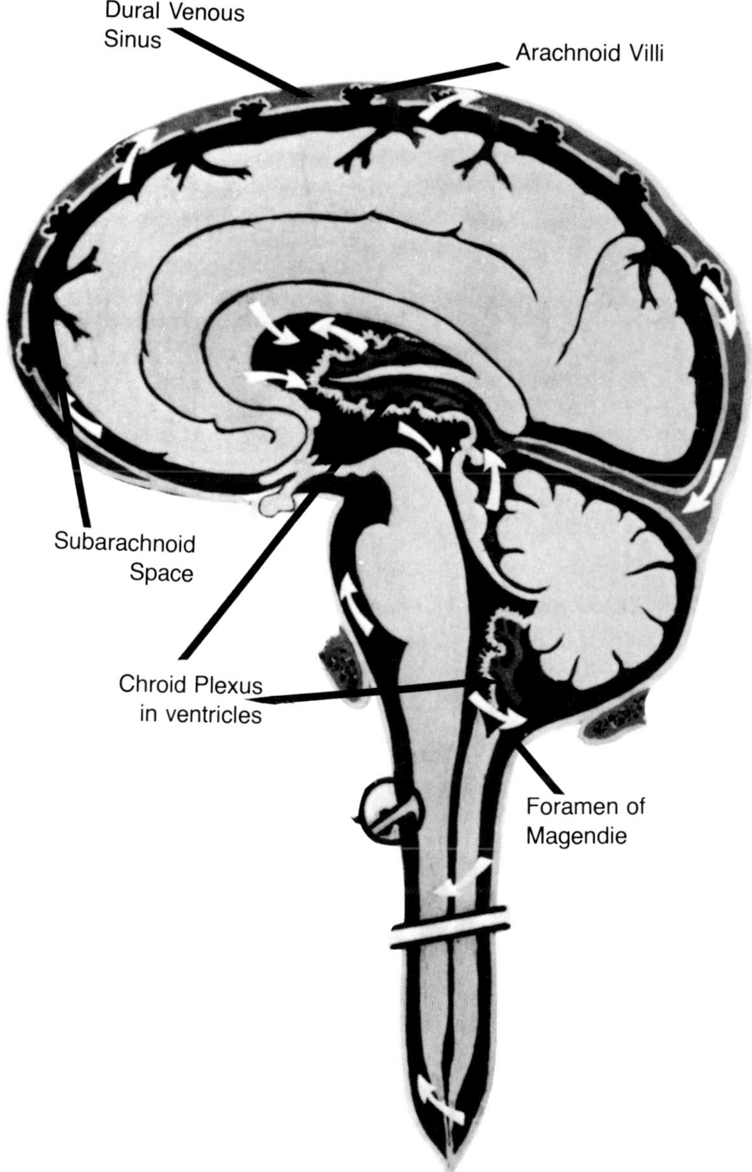

Fig. 4.4 Cerebrospinal Fluid Circulation. Sites of CSF production, circulation and absorption (from Fishman, R.A.: Cerebrospinal Fluid in Diseases of The Nervous System. W.B. Saunders Co., Philadelphia, 1980; reprinted with permission).

2. Vasogenic edema indicates a state in which brain swelling results from increased capillary permeability with leakage of albumin and other molecules into the interstitial spaces.

3. Hydrocephalic edema, which occurs with hydrocephalus, refers to the movement of CSF from the lateral ventricles into the adjacent white matter of the brain.

Many of the disorders which produce intracranial hypertension are discussed in detail elsewhere in this text. Accordingly, these will be reviewed only briefly here.

DISORDERS CAUSING DIFFUSELY INCREASED INTRACRANIAL PRESSURE

The disorders which cause a diffuse increase in intracranial pressure are listed in Table 4.1.

Hypoxic brain damage is a common sequela of sustained respiratory or cardiopulmonary arrest. Not only are the cerebral cortex, the deep midline structures, the brainstem, and the cerebellum immediately damaged, but also cerebral edema of the cytotoxic variety may develop with an attendant marked rise in intracranial pressure. The edema may begin within minutes. It tends to reach its peak intensity within several days and subsides within a week to 10 days.

Just as with hypoxic brain damage, significant cytotoxic edema and associated increased intracranial pressure may occur in patients with severe head injuries. The time course of the edema is quite similar to that seen with hypoxia. Patients with head trauma and hypoxic damage who develop cerebral edema are generally those who have suffered significant brain injuries and who have a depressed level of consciousness. The evolution of edema and raised intracranial pressure in such patients may signal a worsening of their already poor neurological status.

Subarachnoid hemorrhage usually results from a ruptured aneurysm bleeding into the subarachnoid space. Blood is an irritant which causes a marked rise in CSF pressure and, therefore, in intracranial pressure. When a large amount of bleeding occurs rapidly, a tremendous acute rise in pressure may occur which compresses vital brain structures; in such cases, the patient may either die or suffer irreversible brain damage.

The increased intracranial pressure associated with meningitis and encephalitis usually occurs several days after the onset of infection. It may

Table 4.1 Disorders Producing Diffusely Increased Intracranial Pressure

Hypoxia
Head trauma
Subarachnoid hemorrhage
Meningitis and encephalitis

be secondary to infection-induced vasogenic edema or it could be related to hydrocephalus which also develops as a direct consequence of the infection.

Other less common causes of diffuse increased intracranial pressure include lead encephalopathy, and dialysis and diabetic dysequilibrium syndromes. Because of their rarity, the general physician is not likely to encounter these disorders.

SUPRA- AND SUBTENTORIAL MASS LESIONS CAUSING INCREASED INTRACRANIAL PRESSURE

The common mass lesions of the brain which cause increased pressure within the intracranial cavity are listed in Tables 4.2 and 4.3.

Of the supratentorial mass lesions (Table 4.2), the increased pressure associated with epidural and intracerebral hematomas occurs rapidly while that associated with brain abscess and cerebral infarction develops subacutely. With regard to cerebral infarction, it should be noted that significant cerebral edema and increased pressure occur uncommonly, usually appearing in patients who have suffered large hemispheric infarctions involving an entire middle cerebral or internal carotid artery distribution.

The evolution of increased intracranial pressure in subdural hematomas and brain tumors is quite variable. With acute subdurals and rapidly growing primary or metastatic tumors, pressure rises rapidly. On the other hand, chronic subdurals and slowly growing tumors, such as meningiomas, may reach large proportions and produce significant distortions of the brain before signs of increased pressure occur.

As illustrated previously (Fig. 4.2), the subtentorial compartment or posterior fossa is small. Accordingly, the processes listed in Table 4.3 which develop in the posterior fossa tend to produce pressure changes which rapidly compromise brainstem function. An exception is certain brainstem tumors (gliomas) which tend to grow slowly and, therefore, produce insidiously evolving mass effect.

The mechanisms by which mass lesions cause intracranial hypertension include the actual mass effect of the lesion itself, associated vasogenic edema,

**Table 4.2 Supratentorial Mass Lesions Causing
Increased Intracranial Pressure**

Subdural hematoma
Epidural hematoma
Intracerebral hematoma
Brain tumor
Brain abscess
Cerebral infarction (massive)

**Table 4.3 Subtentorial Mass Lesions Causing
Increased Intracranial Pressure**

Brainstem tumor
Brainstem hemorrhage
Cerebellar hemorrhage
Cerebellar infarction
Cerebellar tumor
Cerebellar abscess (rare)

and obstruction of CSF flow with secondary hydrocephalus. For example, a large acutely evolving intracerebral hematoma or cerebeller hematoma causes increased pressure by virtue of sheer mass effect. In contrast, the rise in intracranial pressure associated with many brain tumors is in large part related to associated vasogenic edema or, less commonly, secondary to obstructive hydrocephalus.

ABNORMALITIES OF CSF FLOW CAUSING INCREASED INTRACRANIAL PRESSURE

As indicated in Table 4.4, several abberations of CSF circulation may result in raised intracranial pressure.

Obstructive hydrocephalus usually results from obstruction of CSF flow at the acqueduct of Sylvius or at the outlets from the fourth ventricle. Obstruction of this type may be congenital in nature, secondary to mass lesions including a variety of tumors, or a consequence of viral or bacterial infection. This increases pressure within the ventricular system with dilitation of the lateral and third ventricles, and sometimes of the fourth ventricle depending upon the level of obstruction.

The term communicating hydrocephalus indicates a state of hydrocephalus in which the openings or communications from the fourth ventricle to the subarachnoid space are open but the avenues of flow of CSF over the surface of the brain are blocked. This prevents absorption of the CSF and, as with obstructive hydrocephalus, results in increased CSF pressure and dilatation of the ventricular system. Figure 4.5 shows the head computerized tomographic (CT) scan of a patient with normal brain ventricles as compared to a patient with hydrocephalus who has markedly dilated ventricles.

**Table 4.4 Abnormalities of CSF Flow Causing
Increased Intracranial Pressure**

Obstructive hydrocephalus
Communicating hydrocephalus
Pseudotumor cerebri
Excessive production of CSF (rare)

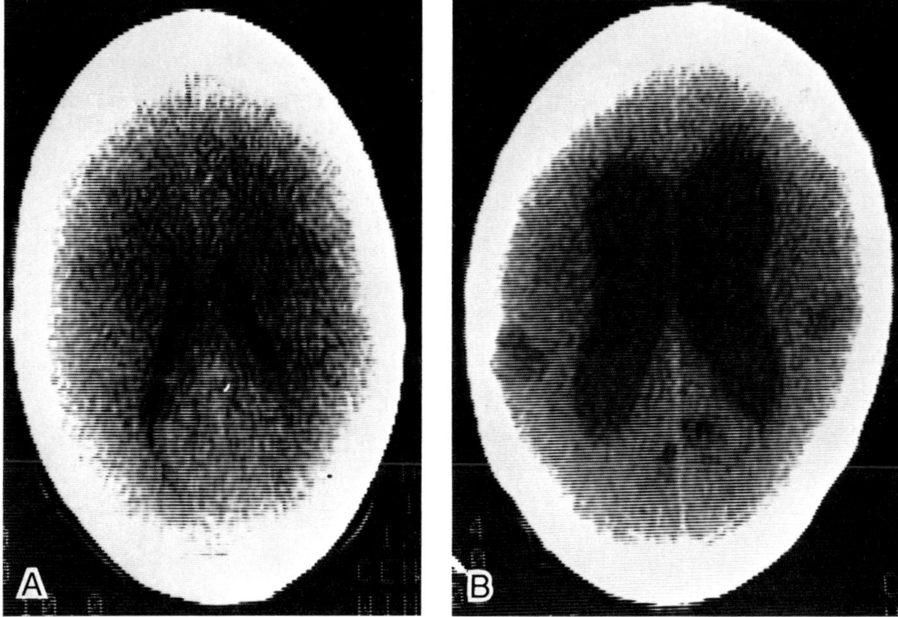

Fig. 4.5 Computerized Tomographic Scans of Lateral Ventricles. (A) Normal sized lateral ventricles. (B) Dilated lateral ventricles seen with obstructive hydrocephalus.

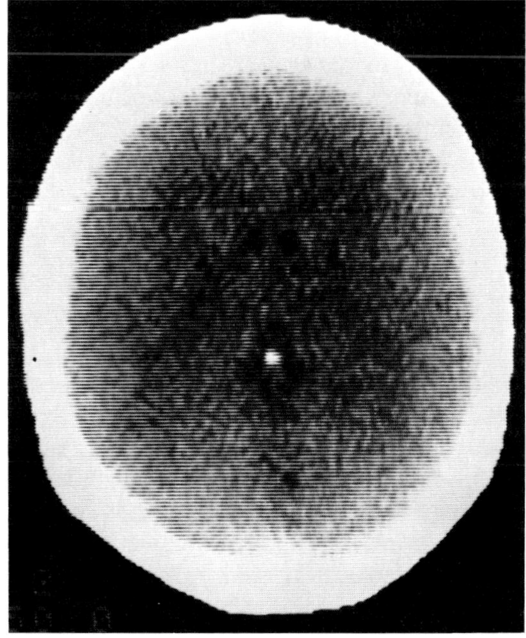

Fig. 4.6
Computerized Tomographic Scan in Pseudotumor Cerebri. Lateral ventricles are "slit-like," or nearly obliterated.

Another disorder which causes increased intracranial pressure and which appears to be related to an abnormality of CSF dynamics is pseudotumor cerebri or benign intracranial hypertension. This disorder typically occurs in young, obese women who present with a subacute course of headaches and papilledema. The lumbar CSF pressure is moderately to markedly elevated. The CT scan may be entirely normal or, as illustrated in Figure 4.6, may show slit-like lateral ventricles suggestive of a diffuse increase in brain volume and intracranial pressure. There is evidence that pseudotumor cerebri is related to a disturbance of CSF absorption. This disorder may require medical treatment but tends to run a benign course.

The least common mechanism of hydrocephalus is overproduction of CSF. This may occur with a rare brain tumor called choroid plexus papilloma.

SYMPTOMS AND SIGNS OF INCREASED INTRACRANIAL PRESSURE

Before discussing specific symptoms and signs of intracranial hypertension, certain basic facts should be reviewed:

1. Pain sensitive structures within the skull include the cerebral arteries, dural veins, and meninges or coverings of the brain. Increased pressure may cause pain when traction or distortion of these structures ensues. Pain and stiffness of the neck may occur when the meninges of the cervical spinal cord are irritated as in subarachnoid hemorrhage or stretched by increased pressure from above.

2. The alerting mechanism of the brain is known as the reticular activating system (RAS). The RAS is housed within the upper brainstem and has projections to the deep midline structures, the thalamus and hypothalamus (see Fig. 5.1). Compromise of these deep midline structures causes the patient to become drowsy while pressure upon the brainstem results in further depression of consciousness and, eventually, coma.

3. Damage to the frontal lobes or deep midline structure may result in Cheyne-Stokes respiration. Pressure upon the midbrain may cause hyperventilation (central neurogenic hyperventilation), while compromise of the lower portions of the brainstem (the pons and medulla) causes breathing to become irregular and, eventually, results in cessation of respiration altogether.

4. Pressure at the level of the deep midline cerebral structures may produce decorticate posturing (flexion of the arms with extension of the legs), while compromise at an upper brainstem level results in decerebrate posturing (extension of both arms and legs).

5. Pupillary reactivity is controlled by both parasympathetic (pupillary constriction) and sympathetic (pupillary dilitation) fibers. Both fiber types

travel down through the midbrain but at that point parasympathetic fibers exit to travel with the third cranial nerve (oculomotor nerve) to the eye. Sympathetic fibers continue through the brainstem and cervical spinal cord, and reach the eye by ascending along the carotid artery. Disorders which exert direct pressure upon the midbrain may disrupt both parasympathetic and sympathetic fibers such that the pupils become midposition and unreactive (fixed) to light. As illustrated in Figure 4.3, the third nerve may be compressed by herniation of the medial aspect by the temporal lobe; this produces disruption of parasympathetic fibers only, resulting in a fixed and widely dilated pupil on that side.

6. The sixth cranial nerves (abducens nerves) are susceptible to indirect pressure during intracranial hypertension. Accordingly, double vision because of inability to move one or both eyes laterally may occur as a non-specific or non-localizing effect of increased intracranial pressure.

7. The brainstem is responsible for a variety of other reflexes including oculocephalic (doll's eyes), oculovestibular (caloric), corneal, gag, and vomiting reflexes. These may be disturbed if increased intracranial pressure causes distortion or direct damage to the brainstem.

The symptoms and signs associated with intracranial hypertension vary and depend upon both the nature of the underlying process and the rapidity with which the rise in pressure develops. In slowly developing mass lesions, such as meningiomas, or with more diffuse processes, such as insidiously progressive hydrocephalus or pseudotumor cerebri, symptoms and signs tend to evolve slowly. In such cases, headache is often an early complaint. The headache is usually non-specific, being intermittent and generalized in nature. Less commonly, the headache is localized over a certain area of the head or is brought on by changes in posture as the responsible mass lesion causes variable distortions of pain sensitive structures or intermittent obstruction of CSF flow. Patients may appear less attentive and more drowsy than usual as pressure is exerted on deep midline structures. Intermittent vomiting because of indirect pressure upon the lower brainstem may occur as may diplopia (double vision) because of indirect pressure upon the sixth cranial nerves.

Examination of such patients may reveal some degree of inattentiveness, papilledema, abnormal lateral eye movements (sixth nerve palsies) and mild nuchal rigidity. These may be the only neurologic abnormalities in patients with increased intracranial pressure secondary to a diffuse process such as hydrocephalus. But when a slowly growing mass lesion is present, focal signs may also be found (e.g., mild hemiparesis, hemisensory deficit, increase in tone or reflexes, or a Babinski sign on the side opposite the mass).

In processes which produce rapid rises in intracranial pressure, accompanying signs and symptoms appear acutely and tend to have more dire consequences. As described earlier, the types of processes which may cause rapid increases in intracranial pressure include supratentorial mass lesions such as intracerebral hemorrhage, subtentorial mass lesions such as cerebellar hemorrhage, and diffuse disorders such as acute hydrocephalus. Symptoms associated with such rapidly evolving disorders may be the sudden onset of headache, nausea, vomiting, neck stiffness and depression or loss of consciousness.

Examination may reveal a patient with mild alteration of consciousness and minimal nuchal rigidity but with normal vital signs. Focal signs (i.e., unilateral facial weakness, hemiparesis, hemisensory deficit) are usually present where a supra- and subtentorial mass lesion is responsible. If the rise in pressure is limited, the patient may stabilize at this level.

Patients who experience acute and progressive rise in intracranial pressure will develop further signs of compression of deep midline structures and, eventually, of critical brainstem centers. The earliest signs of ongoing compression are subtle and non-specific (Fig. 4.7). These may include progressive depression of consciousness, appearance of small reactive pupils, worsening of focal signs and changing vital signs. The initial change in vital signs is often an increase in both pulse and blood pressure. With dramatic rises in intracranial pressures, the classical Cushing reflex may be observed: a vasopressor reflex manifested by a marked rise in blood pressure and significant slowing of the pulse and respirations.

Be aware of the early signs of ongoing compression, for it is at this juncture that treatment for intracranial hypertension should be instituted. All too often these early signs are not recognized, and the patient's condition is allowed to deteriorate to the point where brainstem compression or herniation occur. If the seriousness of his condition is not appreciated and if brainstem compression becomes fully developed, treatment may be only partially successful or, worse, entirely unsuccessful.

Once the early stage of compression has been passed, progressive supratentorial mass lesions will distort or compress the brainstem in one of two ways. Pressure upon the brainstem may occur in a central fashion (central herniation) or asymmetrically from displacement of the medial portion of the temporal lobe into the tentorial notch (uncal herniation).

Central herniation (Fig. 4.8) involves a progressive alteration of consciousness; a patient who is drowsy or inattentive because of pressure effects upon deep midline structures will become progressively more depressed and, eventually, comatose as pressure is exerted upon the midbrain and upper pons. Also, with compression of the upper brainstem, an alteration in respirations may occur. Respirations which were initially normal or Cheyne-Stokes in nature may change to central hyperventilation. Decorticate then decerebrate posturing of the extremities appears. The pupils become midposition and fixed to light as both parasympathetic and sympathetic fibers become disrupted. As compression progresses down the brainstem, other brainstem reflexes are lost including oculocephalic, corneal, oculovestibular and gag reflexes. Respirations, too, progressively change

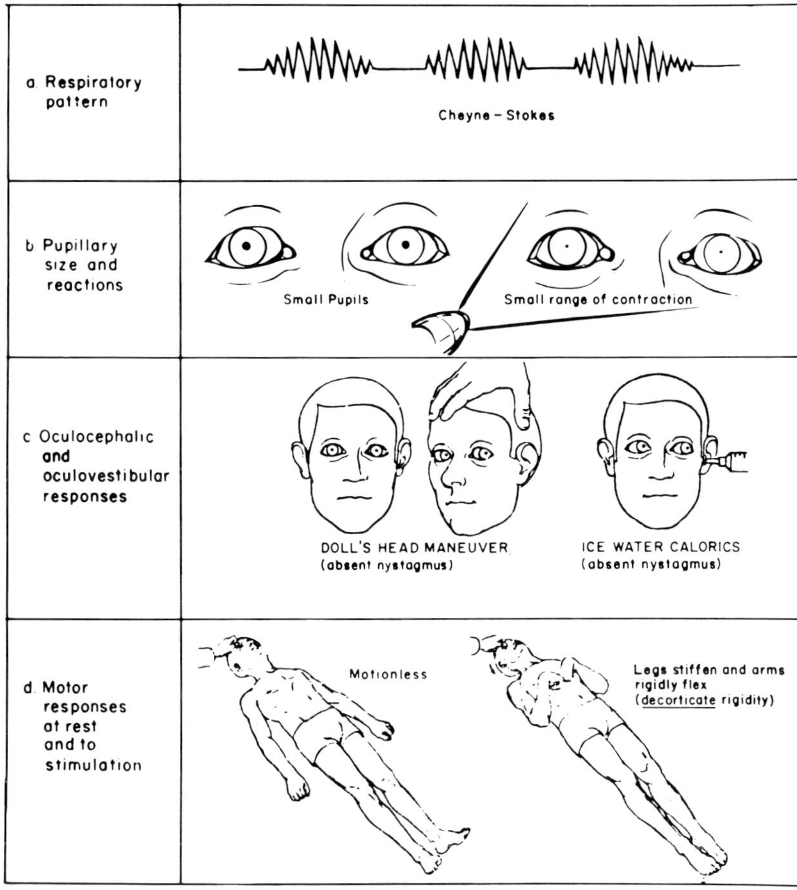

Fig. 4.7 Early Signs of Herniation. Signs which may appear with compression of thalamic and hypothalamic regions of the brain (from Plum F., Posner, J.B.: The Diagnosis of Stupor and Coma. 3rd Ed., F.A. Davis Co., Philadelphia, 1980; reprinted with permission).

from hyperventilation to irregular patterns of breathing; ultimately, respiratory arrest occurs.

In uncal herniation (Fig. 4.9) progression may be very rapid. The patient may appear to be relatively stable when the medial temporal lobe herniates, compressing the third cranial nerve on one side and distorting the midbrain. With compression of the third nerve, parasympathetic fibers are disrupted so that the pupil on that side becomes widely dilated and fixed to light. The appearance of a fixed and dilated pupil is of localizing significance as the mass lesion and herniating tissue are always on the same side as the abnormal pupil. Together with alteration of the pupil, coma and central hyperventilation rapidly ensue as the midbrain is compressed. So too a hemi-

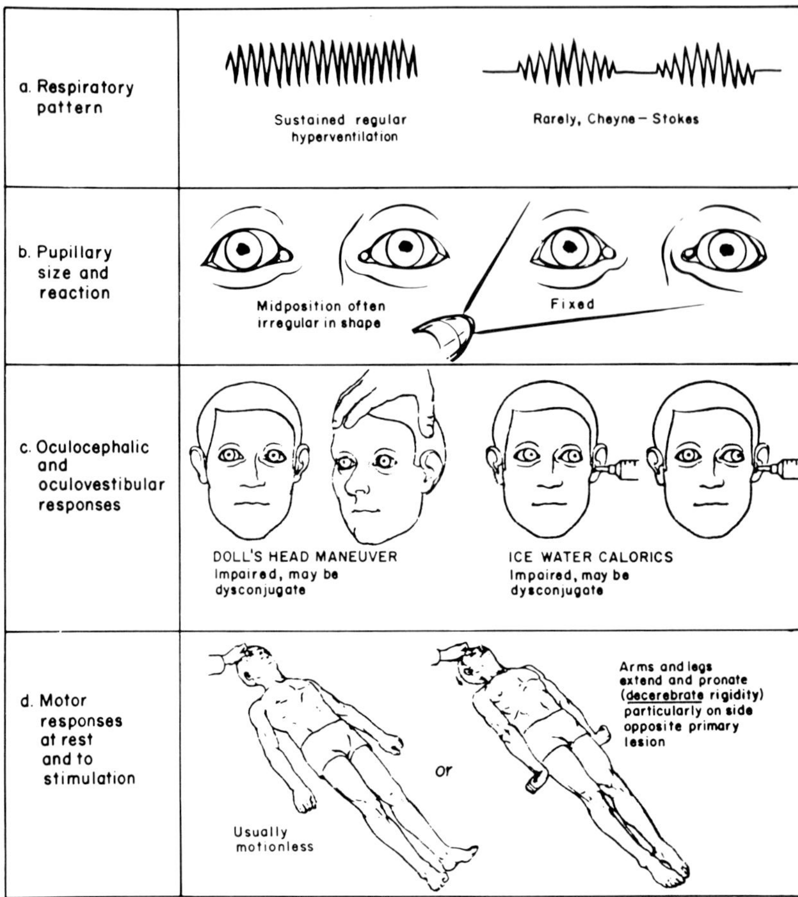

Fig. 4.8 Signs of Central Herniation. Signs which appear with compression of the midbrain (from Plum, F., Posner, J.B.: The Diagnosis of Stupor and Coma. 3rd Ed., F.A. Davis Co., Philadelphia, 1980; reprinted with permission).

paresis with decorticate or decerebrate posturing may appear, this also on the side opposite the herniating mass and abnormal pupil. With sustained compression, both pupils may become fixed and dilated and posturing may appear bilaterally. From this point, continued pressure results with much the same signs as in central herniation with progressive loss of brainstem reflexes and failure of respiration.

In summary, supratentorial mass lesion may result in either central or uncal herniation depending upon where the lesion is located and in which direction it exerts its maximal force. The orderly progression of signs of herniation may occur over the course of minutes to hours in acutely advancing processes, or over the course of a few days in subacutely progressing lesions. However, regardless of whether the underlying disorder is an acute,

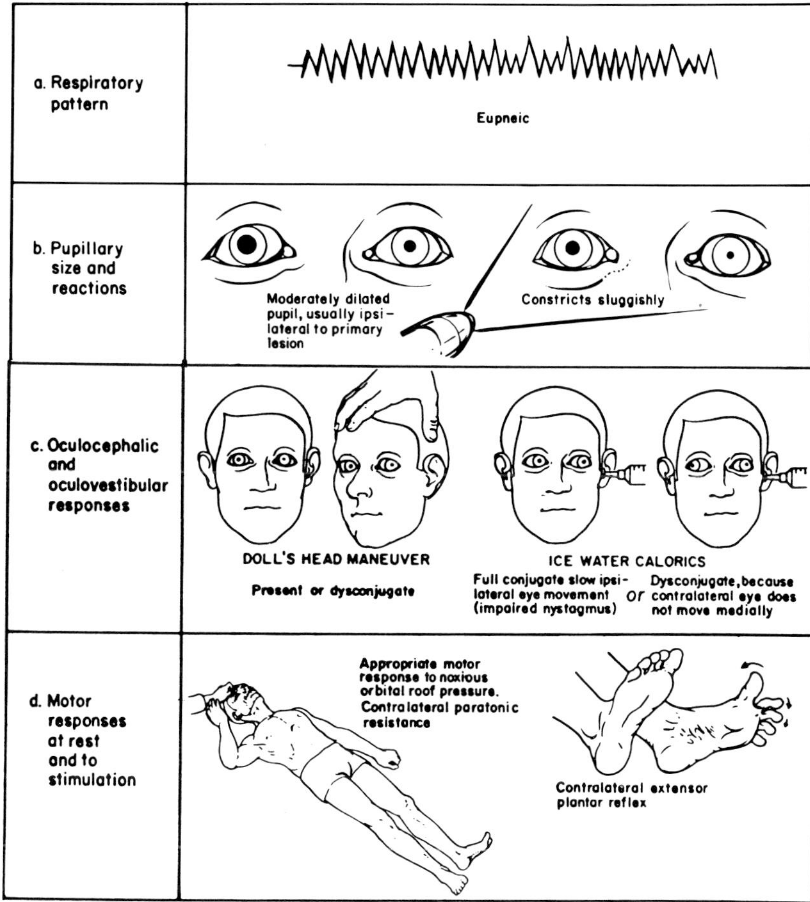

Fig. 4.9 Signs of Uncal Herniation. Early signs which appear with compression of the third cranial nerve and midbrain by the medial portion of the temporal lobe (from Plum, F., Posner, J B · The Diagnosis of Stupor and Coma. 3rd Ed., F.A. Davis Co., Philadelphia, 1980: reprinted with permission).

subacute, or chronic process which has reached a critical level of pressure, once signs of upper brainstem (midbrain) or third nerve dysfunction appear, progression tends to be relatively rapid. Again, it is critical to recognize the early signs of compression of the deep midline structures and of the upper brainstem because appropriate treatment must be instituted as these signs are evolving; otherwise, the brainstem will be irreversibly damaged.

Because of the limited space within the posterior fossa, subtentorial mass lesions tend to compromise brainstem functions quickly and with relatively little mass effect. Initially, consciousness may or may not be altered. Brainstem signs are variable and tend not to appear in the orderly sequence seen with central or uncal herniation. With posterior fossa lesions, alterations in pulse, blood pressure, and respirations often occur early and may be extreme.

Cerebellar hemorrhage may be taken as an example. Patients with cerebellar hemorrhage frequently complain of the sudden onset of occipital headache, vertigo, vomiting and difficulty walking or even standing. Examination may reveal a patient who is quite alert but whose blood pressure is markedly increased and whose pulse may be either abnormally increased or decreased. Signs often include unilateral facial weakness, nystagmus, gaze paresis (inability to move the eyes conjugately to one side), and arm/leg ataxia as well as marked difficulty with sitting, standing or walking. If cerebellar hemorrhage is suspected clinically and confirmed by CT scan, surgical evacuation of the clot may be lifesaving. However, if left untreated, rapid decompensation because of brainstem compression typically occurs with a fatal outcome.

EVALUATION OF PATIENTS WITH SUSPECTED INCREASED INTRACRANIAL PRESSURE

A sequence of evaluation of patients with suspected intracranial hypertension is proposed in Table 4.5.

A complete but brief history of events preceding the patient's presentation to the emergency room should be obtained either from the patient or, if the patient is unable to give a history, from relatives, friends, or ambulance attendants. Based upon the history, it should be possible for the physician to begin to decide whether the patient is suffering from a chronic, relatively stable disorder or has suffered a sudden intracranial event which is producing an acute increase in intracranial pressure.

A brief general physical examination should be performed. Special note

**Table 4.5　Evaluation of Patients With Suspected
Increased Intracranial Pressure**

I. Brief history
II. Brief general physical examination
III. Neurological examination
   A. Level of consciousness
   B. Respiratory pattern
   C. Pupillary reaction
   D. Other brainstem reflexes
   E. Extremity tone, posturing and reflexes
IV. If evaluation suggests:
   A. Chronic, stable intracranial hypertension—
      obtain head CT scan
   B. Acute intracranial hypertension—
      stabilize with appropriate therapy
      (see Table 4.6)
      obtain head CT scan

must be made of the vital signs. Papilledema should be carefully looked for on funduscopic examination, and any evidence of nuchal rigidity must be carefully sought.

Next, the neurological examination should be undertaken with particular emphasis given to the patient's level of consciousness, respiratory pattern, pupillary reaction, other brainstem reflexes, extremity tone and posturing, and deep tendon reflexes. Abnormalities of these selected neurologic parameters should be interpreted in light of the discussion in the preceding section.

If the history and examination indicate a state of chronic intracranial hypertension without any evidence of acute decompensation, then the patient can safely be evaluated with routine laboratory studies and a head CT scan. However, if the evaluation indicates an intracranial catastrophe with acutely evolving intracranial hypertension, the patient must be stabilized with appropriate therapeutic measures (see next section) and taken immediately for a head CT scan.

In any patient suspected of having acutely or severely increased intracranial pressure, a lumbar puncture should not be performed initially. As discussed in Chapter 3, lumbar puncture in the face of intracranial hypertension may precipitate sudden decompensation. Head CT scan should always be procured as the initial diagnostic study. Thereafter, lumbar puncture may be done, if indicated, so long as the CT scan shows no large mass or other cause of severely increased intracranial pressure.

When intracranial hypertension is suspected on clinical grounds (especially when a focal mass lesion may be present), careful observation of the patient and institution of therapy at the earliest signs of herniation are imperative. These patients may deteriorate suddenly and unexpectedly and should not be left unattended. A common mistake is to send the patient alone to CT scan. This should be avoided; a physician must accompany such patients when they are sent for any type of study or procedure.

TREATMENT OF INCREASED INTRACRANIAL PRESSURE

Neurological or neurosurgical consultation should be obtained in all cases of suspected intracranial hypertension. However, because some delay will occur before the consulting physician arrives, the emergency room or general physician must be adept at the recognition and acute management of increased intracranial pressure.

The principles of treatment are outlined in Table 4.6. As with other neurological emergencies, the primary concern is that pulse, blood pressure and respirations be adequately maintained. The treatment of acute intracranial hypertension is three-pronged including the administration of hyperosmolar agents and corticosteroids, and intubation with controlled hyperventilation.

In emergent situations where acute intracranial hypertension is clearly

**Table 4.6 Acute Management of Increased
Intracranial Pressure**

  I. Maintain cardiac and respiratory functions
 II. Intubate and hyperventilate—maintain Pa CO_2
     between 20 and 25 mmHg.
III. Administer hyperosmolar agent and/or diuretic
     A. Mannitol (25% solution) 1.0 to 1.5 gm/kg IV
        every 4 to 6 hours
     And may administer
     B. Furosemide 20 to 40 mg IV every 4 to 6 hours
 IV. Administer corticosteroids—dexamethasone 10
     mg IV initially followed by 4 mg IV every 6 hours

---

present with impending or ongoing herniation, hyperventilation is the most
rapid means of reducing intracranial pressure. The decrease in $PaCO_2$ associated
with hyperventilation causes cerebral vasoconstriction with a marked
decrease in cerebral blood volume and intracranial pressure. For effective
control of intracranial pressure, the $PaCO_2$ should be maintained between
20 to 25 mmHg.

Hyperosmolar agents also act quickly to reduce intracranial pressure by
decreasing the water content of brain. They should, therefore, be administered
concurrently with intubation and hyperventilation. Although several
hyperosmolar agents are available, mannitol is the agent most commonly
administered. Mannitol is given in a 25 percent solution at a dose of 1.0
to 1.5 gm/kg by intravenous bolus injection; this dose may be repeated
every 4 to 6 hours as needed. The diuretic, furosemide (Lasix), is employed
by some neurologists and neurosurgeons in addition to Mannitol to reduce
intracranial pressure. Furosemide appears to inhibit CSF production in addition
to causing a significant diuresis. The dose employed is 20 to 40 mg
by intravenous bolus injection every 4 to 6 hours as needed.

In acute situations, corticosteroids are generally administered in addition
to a hyperosmolar agent and hyperventilation. Although corticosteroids are
administered acutely, they do not begin to work to reduce cerebral edema
until several hours later. Dexamethasone is the usual corticosteroid employed
and is given in an initial dose of 10 mg intravenously followed by
4 mg intravenously every 6 hours thereafter. Note that corticosteroids reduce
cerebral edema and associated intracranial hypertension only under
certain circumstances. Corticosteroids are particularly effective in reducing
vasogenic edema associated with brain tumor, abscesses, epidural and subdural
hematomas; however, they are less effective in reducing the edema
that occurs with cerebral contusion, cerebral infarction and intraparenchymal
hemorrhage. Nevertheless, it is common practice to administer dexamethasone
under the latter circumstances when intracranial hypertension
is present. The evidence that corticosteroids are helpful in anoxic/hypoxic
brain injury where the edema is of the cytotoxic variety is controversial

at best. Accordingly, these agents are not generally given to patients with increased intracranial pressure secondary to anoxia.

The above approach to the treatment of intracranial hypertension refers to the management of patients who require acute therapy. Such therapy must often be given to stabilize the patient even before a head CT scan can be obtained to discover the underlying etiology. There are certainly instances where patients present with signs of increased intracranial pressure but without evidence of acute decompensation. Such patients may be evaluated without acute therapy. Once the CT scan has been performed and the underlying process is identified specific therapy may be instituted. For example, if the CT scan reveals metastatic tumor, corticosteroid therapy is usually the only treatment required to control cerebral edema and associated intracranial hypertension until radiation therapy can be instituted.

REFERENCES

1. Cooper, P.R., Moody, S., Clark, W.K., et al: Dexamethasone and severe head injury; a prospective double-blind study. J. Neurosurg., 51:307, 1979.
2. Fishman, R.A.: Brain edema. N. Engl. J. Med., 273:706, 1975.
3. Fishman, R.A.: Cerebrospinal Fluid in Diseases of the Nervous System. W.B. Saunders Co., Philadelphia, 1980.
4. Hooshmand, H., Dove, J., Houff, S., et al: Effects of diuretics and steroids on CSF pressure. Arch Neurol., 21:499, 1969.
5. James, H.E., Langfitt, T.W., Kumar, V.S., et al: Treatment of intracranial hypertension. Acta Neurochir., 36:189, 1977.
6. Mulley, G., Wilcox, R.G., and Mitchell, J.R.A.: Dexamethasone in acute stroke. Br. Med. J., 2:994, 1978.
7. Plum, F. and Posner, J.B.: The Diagnosis of Stupor and Coma. 3rd Ed. F.A. Davis Co., Philadelphia, 1980.
8. Zervas, M.T. and Hedley-Whyte, J.: Successful treatment of cerebral herniation in five patients. N. Engl. J. Med., 286:1075, 1972.

5

Coma in the Emergency Room

Allan H. Ropper, M.D.

INTRODUCTION

The comatose patient is among the most common confronting the emergency physician and certainly presents the most challenging neurological encounter in the emergency room (ER). It is estimated that 3 to 5 percent of ER admissions in large hospitals are due to diseases that alter consciousness. Moreover, coma is predominantly an ER problem since the onset of coma in an already hospitalized patient is a rare occurrence. Because coma is a syndrome (unfortunately a loosely defined one in many texts) it provides only a gateway to diagnosis. By careful attention to (1) the circumstances of history, (2) a specially contrived "coma examination" and (3) specific signposts of the diseases that commonly cause coma, a diagnosis can be derived within minutes in the majority of patients. In the remainder, a tentative clinical impression or limited list of possibilities is evident after the physical and laboratory examination. In recent years an overdependence on the CT scan has regularly produced diagnostic errors. Very few diagnoses in coma are apparent with the CT that are not uncovered by a careful examination. Moreover, abdicating the neurological examination for a CT scan loses the 30–60 minutes required to transport a patient from the ER to the scanning suite, perform the scan, view it and transport the patient back. This time is frequently better spent on a more careful examination. It has been observed that two-thirds or more of CT scans are normal in coma, and that the most important general therapeutic maneuver in coma is close observation. It therefore behooves the physician to master the examination of the comatose patient and the limited list of diseases that may cause coma. This chapter outlines a practical approach to coma and highlights the major causes with their associated signs. The principles apply equally to the evaluation of any comatose patient but are oriented towards the ER. General treatment of coma in the ER is outlined in the final section.

DEFINITION OF COMA

Coma is epitomized by the absence of arousal and thereby any meaningful purposeful reaction to environmental change. An exact narrative description of the patient and his reactions to testing are the best method of depicting coma and deciding where in the spectrum of "level of consciousness" between drowsy and comatose the patient lies. Terms such as stupor, semi-coma, obtundation are ambiguous, differ in meaning between observers, and have little place in clinical work. The pathologic implications of drowsiness are at times different from coma, but generally they may be considered relative degrees of the same phenomenon.

In distinction to arousal, or the level of consciousness, a host of terms are used to describe the "content of consciousness." The most common is confusion which denotes disorientation and inability to carry on intellectual activities normally. While many drowsy or less responsive patients are confused, confusion can exist without alteration in the level of consciousness. Nevertheless, from a practical standpoint diagnostic considerations should focus on the level of consciousness rather than confusion.

PATHOANATOMY AND PATHOPHYSIOLOGY OF COMA

Awakeness depends on the normal functioning of two neuronal systems, the reticular activating system (RAS) and the cerebral hemispheres. Damage or metabolic dysfunction in either system produces unresponsiveness. This is the fundamental principle of coma diagnosis and the initial neurological examination is oriented solely towards finding which one of the two systems is at fault. Coma, therefore, can result from damage to any component of the RAS, its projections to both cerebral hemispheres, or the hemispheres themselves. The RAS is a loosely organized system of neurons within the reticular formation of the brainstem tegmentum (the dorsal grey matter portion). The reticular formation extends from the thalamic region down through the medulla but only neurons from the midpons to the caudal thalamus are involved in maintaining arousal. Current evidence suggests that RAS neurons maintain arousal indirectly by inhibiting "non-specific" thalamic relay nuclei which in turn are inhibitory and project diffusely to the cerebral cortex. These relationships and the approximate location of the RAS are depicted in Figure 5.1. Electrical stimulation of the pontine and midbrain RAS desynchronizes the electroencephalogram (EEG), a pattern typically associated with arousal. The anatomic basis of behavioral arousal by environmental stimuli is the substantial number of connections between each of the sensory systems (visual, auditory, tactile) and the RAS. Lesions such as pontine or cerebellar hemorrhage and basilar occlusion with pontine stroke are the most common anatomical causes of coma in the posterior fossa.

While the specialized functions of the cortex such as language, vision,

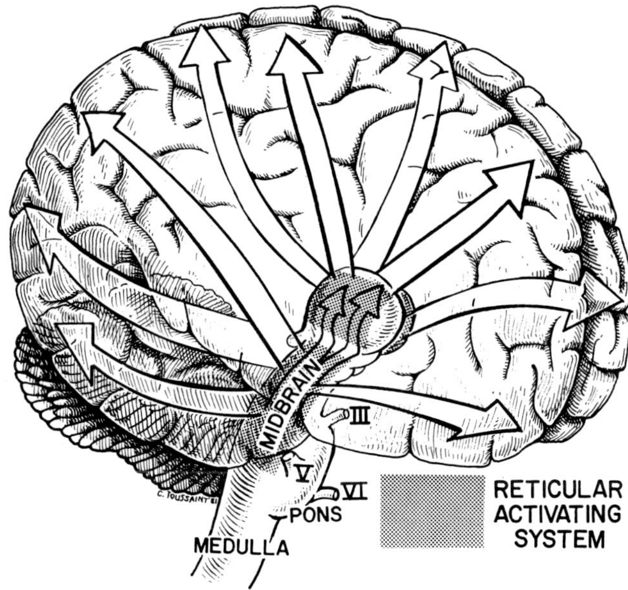

Fig. 5.1 Schematic representation of the brainstem RAS and its projections to the hemispheres. Only those portions of the RAS from the mid-pons rostrally are important for arousal.

sensation, etc., are localized, cortical functioning in alertness is not. Arousal is related only in a semi-quantitative way to the total mass of functioning cerebral hemisphere tissue. Lesions in the cerebral hemispheres may cause coma in one of three ways:

1. Bilateral, generalized lesions or metabolic derangements debilitate both hemispheres diffusely and prevent the expression of arousal even when the RAS is functioning. Examples would include hypotension-ischemia, generalized epilepsy, drug ingestion, hypoglycemia, subarachnoid hemorrhage, and encephalitis.

2. Large masses in one hemisphere may compress the contralateral hemisphere effectively creating bilateral lesions. This is probably an extremely infrequent mechanism of coma despite how frequently it is invoked.

3. Large lesions of one or both hemispheres may secondarily compress the brainstem-RAS and cause coma indirectly at the level of the RAS. It should be noted that large acute lesions of one hemisphere such as stroke or hemorrhage may cause substantial drowsiness, though not usually deep coma, even without contralateral hemispheres or brainstem compression.

Ultimately coma is caused by anatomical destruction of crucial areas of the RAS (or secondary impairment such as a cerebellar mass pressing on the brainstem), or lesions in both the hemispheres (anatomical coma), or widespread disruption of brain metabolic process (metabolic coma). The mechanisms of coma in metabolic encephalopathies and anesthesia are incompletely understood but a multifactorial effect on energy supply, membrane activities and neurotransmitters is likely. Some drugs and endogenous toxins suppress the activity of both the RAS and hemispheres while certain anesthetics probably act disproportionately on the RAS. These patterns are reflected in subtleties of the clinical coma examination.

EMERGENCY ROOM ASSESSMENT OF THE COMATOSE PATIENT

There is a rapid systematic way to evaluate the comatose patient.[6,7] Because resuscitation, respiratory and cardiovascular problems must be attended to prior to commencing the coma exam (see below for details), vital signs are obtained first. The neurological examination stands at the center of the evaluation and is performed next before obtaining a detailed history or performing a thorough general medical examination. Other elements of the general examination, except perhaps nuchal rigidity are best deferred until the severity and nature of coma have been assessed. The material below is presented as a practical guide for the evaluation of coma but not necessarily in the usual sequence of performance for emergency cases.

HISTORY

The important features of the coma history are (1) the exact circumstances and suddeness of onset, (2) details of any preceding neurological symptoms (headaches, seizures, weakness, brainstem symptoms such as dizziness, diplopia, dysarthria, vomiting), (3) drug or alcohol use and (4) history of liver, kidney, pulmonary, cardiac or psychiatric disease. (Table 5.1).

Unfortunately, the history in coma is usually either obvious and given by family members (e.g., trauma, previously known medical or neurological conditions) or is simply not available, the patient having been found unresponsive and brought by ambulance attendants. Sometimes a phone call to the location where the patient was found provides invaluable information (e.g., the patient complained of a headache to the bartender, or the patient spoke of suicide, etc.). From ambulance attendants two specific questions should be asked—was there vomitus at the scene and were the pupils enlarged initially. The former indicates one of the neurological catastrophes, particularly intracranial hemorrhage and the latter suggests recovery from global brain ischemia. Seizures are generally not witnessed by ambulance

Table 5.1 Historical Features Suggesting Structural vs. Metabolic Coma

Suggests Structural	Suggests Metabolic
Sudden observed onset	History of major medical illness
Preceding "hard" neurologic symptoms	Liver
Diplopia	Renal
Vomiting	Pulmonary
Vertigo	Previous history of overdose or severe depression
Hemiparesis	
Bleeding diathesis	Known drug abuse
Chronic alcoholism	
Previous anatomical brain lesion	
Stroke	
Tumor	
Subdural	

attendants but if such activity was observed by others it is usually transmitted to them. A most common error is to report as seizures the jittery extensor posturing movements associated with hypotension.

A history of chronic alcoholism offers a clue to subdural hematoma, occult head trauma or drug overdose. Alcoholism should also be taken into account when examining the eye movements since extremely high ethanol levels can alter these and speciously suggest a brainstem lesion. It is best to assume first that unresponsiveness is not due to alcohol, or alcohol alone, since alcoholic patients have such a high incidence of other CNS lesions, many of which are remediable.

THE BASIC ER COMA EXAMINATION

Because all subsequent decisions in the ER depend on the coma examination, each feature must be elicited assiduously and no question of the validity of examination findings allowed. A knowledge of the common pitfalls in the coma examination is also necessary.[1] These are set apart from the text for emphasis. With experience certain recurrent patterns in the examination become evident, thus simplifying precise diagnosis. There are two points which the examination can immediately settle and to which all attention is directed, namely: (1) are there findings of a brainstem lesion, which would indicate coma is due to disruption of the RAS, or, alternatively, is there damage to the hemispheres; and (2) is the examination pattern one of a structural or metabolic disease (Table 5.2). The coma examination has four basic parts: (1) a general assessment of the depth of coma or degree of unresponsiveness, (2) symmetry and nature of movements, and Babinski signs, (3) pupillary size and reaction, and (4) assessment of spontaneous and

**Table 5.2 Neurological Signs Suggesting a Structural
Cause of Coma**

I. Hemispheres
   A. Hemiparesis
   B. Unilateral facial weakness
   C. Babinski sign or asymmetric toe signs
   D. Cheyne-Strokes breathing
   E. Ocular dipping
   F. Absence of eye movement abnormalities

II. Brainstem—RAS
   A. Quadriparesis with extensor posturing
      (may be asymmetric)
   B. Eye movement abnormalities on oculocephalic
      or oculovestibular testing
      (especially major asymmetries)
   C. Ocular bobbing
   D. Corneal reflex abnormalities
   E. Irregular respiratory patterns

N.B. Pupillary enlargement and light unreactivity are usually due to compression of the brainstem by a large hemispheral lesion. However, primary brainstem lesions (e.g., infarction) may cause the same signs.

reflex eye movements. The examiner should recount these four items with each unresponsive patient. The whole examination takes less than 5 minutes though the number of abnormalities which may be encountered is large.

As already noted an exact description of the patient's state of consciousness is preferable to summary terms such as stupor, coma, etc. First, the patient is observed on the stretcher without examiner intervention. Likeness to sleep and apparent restful postures such as arm under the head, or one cheek resting on the hand while the patient is lying on the side, crossed legs or flexed hips are all suggestive of light coma from which arousal will be easy.[7] Unnatural positions such as arms thrown across the body or hanging over the side of the stretcher, slack jaw, wrist hyperflexion, tonic extension or flexion of the limbs, all indicate a deeper coma from which arousal will be difficult or impossible. Persistent asymmetries in the resting posture of the limbs are significant and almost always indicate a hemiparesis due to a unilateral hemispheral lesion. Lack of restless movements on one side also indicates a hemiparesis. One of the most helpful signs in the supine patient is a slightly out-turned leg which indicates either a hemiparesis or a hip fracture. (Fig. 5.2).

Sign: Out-turned leg when viewed from head of bed.

Pitfall: Usually hemiparesis but may be a hip fracture, or patient asymmetrically positioned.

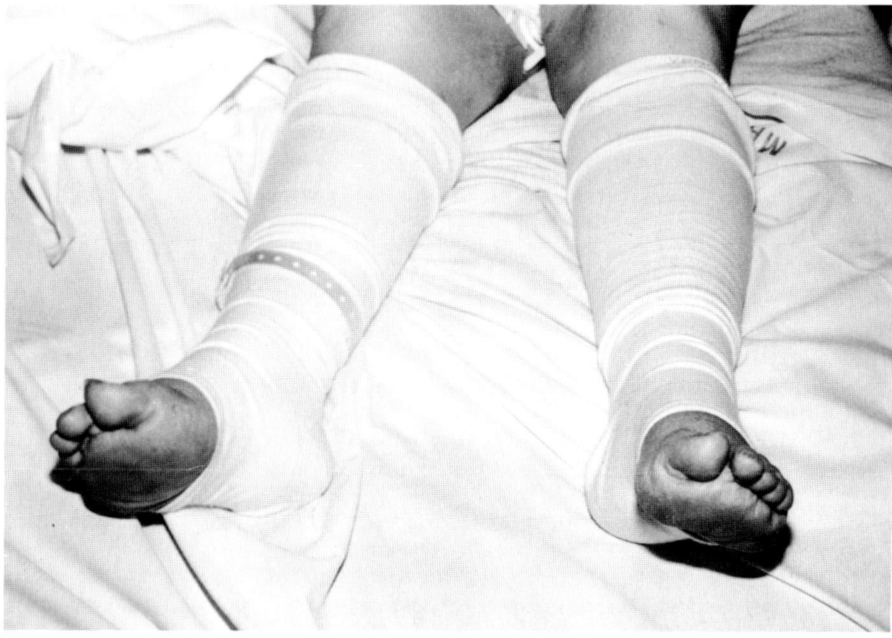

Fig. 5.2 Subtle out-turning of the right leg as a sign of hemiparesis in a comatose patient. Hip fracture produces a similar appearance.

A rapid technique for detecting hip fractures is to place a stethescope on the symphisis pubis and tap each patella listening for a difference in bone conduction of the sound.

Any unusual movements should be noted, especially if rhythmic, particularly small twitching movements of finger, toe or facial muscle. These may be the only indications of a seizure. It should be emphasized that small excursion clonic movements of extended limbs occur with hypotensive episodes such as Stokes-Adams attacks and should not be confused with epilepsy.

> **Sign:** Small, extensor shaking movements of limbs.
>
> **Pitfall:** Associated with hypotension, not epilepsy.

The terms decorticate and decerebrate posturing have been adopted from animal work to describe stereotyped tonic flexor and extensor forearm movements, respectively. The anatomical significance of various posturing is not as clear in humans as in animal preparations, and, as with level of arousal, an exact description of the patient's movements is more useful for describing the neurological condition than summary terms. It is said that flexion and supination of the arms (decortication) denotes a more rostral level of motor system damage than extension and pronation (decerebration), but acute lesions seen in the ER frequently cause decerebration regardless of location. The legs generally extend with both types of posturing, but a combination of knee and hip flexion combined with arm extension is sometimes caused by pontine lesions. Metabolic coma (especially ischemia and hepatic encephalopathy) may produce vigorous extensor posturing.

Sign: Posturing.

Pitfall: Poor localizing value and not always an anatomical lesion. May be caused by metabolic derangements.

Posturing often co-exists with more purposeful, well-integrated limb movements and simply indicates subtotal damage to the motor system.

After a few calm moments of observation the physician should attempt to arouse the patient by using increasingly harsher stimuli.[7] Conversational speech, then shouting, then mild pinching of the knuckles and finally strenuous pinching are attempted. All the while the patient's responses are observed in a manner similar to that outlined above. Specifically, stereotyped versus purposeful avoidance movements of the limbs and their symmetry are noted. The minimal stimulus necessary to elicit eye-opening or vocalization is gauged and clearly recorded as the best reflection of the depth of coma. Pinching of the skin is generally an unsatisfactory stimulus since it leaves unsightly ecchymoses and offers little advantage over pressure on the knuckles or other bony prominences except as noted below. The most useful noxious stimulus is a Hoffman clamp, commonly used to control IV drip rates, applied to the knuckle. By noting the number of turns required to elicit a response the depth of coma and any asymmetries can be gauged. One of the most difficult tasks is to determine if the movement of a limb is a stereotyped-obligatory (posturing) movement or one which demonstrates that the patient is purposefully fending off the stimulus. Most errors are made by calling primitive movements, particularly leg flexion, purposeful simply because the limb moves away from the stimulus. In comatose adults the only certain purposeful movement is abduction or withdrawal from a medially delivered stimulus (i.e., pinching the inside of arm or thigh). Any other movements are more than likely due to posturing.

Sign: Withdrawal of a limb from pain.

Pitfall: Only abduction is clearly a higher level purposeful movement (or the patient reaching with his hand to push away the painful stimulus).

A unilateral Babinski sign is a dependable marker of asymmetric damage to the brain, while bilateral signs may occur with metabolic disease.

Examination of the brainstem reflexes is the key to determining if the causative lesion is located in the midbrain-pontine area or in the hemispheres. However, many drugs and alcohol in large doses may obliterate these reflexes to varying degrees and speciously suggest anatomical brainstem lesions. In the extreme case, drug overdose can simulate brain death. Herein lies the major pitfall in coma diagnosis:

Sign: Abnormalities or absence of elicited brainstem reflexes.

Pitfall: Drugs may obliterate eye movements, pupillary reaction and breathing, but usually do so symmetrically.

The pupils are examined first. Round, symmetric and light reactive pupils of 2–5 mm diameter with few exceptions exonerate a midbrain RAS lesion as a cause of coma. A unilaterally enlarged (5 mm) unreactive or barely reactive pupil is a sign of midbrain–IIIrd nerve compression and is virtually always caused by asymmetric compression from a hemispheral mass above rather than an intrinsic brainstem lesion.

Sign: Unilateral dilated pupil.

Pitfall: Generally not primary brainstem lesion.

Solely because they are more common, enlarging hemispheral masses are the usual cause of dilated unreactive pupils. An upper brainstem infarction will rarely present as coma and dilated pupils.

Bilaterally dilated and unreactive pupils indicate severe midbrain–IIIrd nerve compression. However:

Sign: Dilated pupils.

Pitfall: Drugs with atropinic activity either ingested or instilled by a previous examiner can cause this as well as compression of the midbrain from above.

A test dose of intravenous physostigmine 1–2 mg will not cause the normally expected pupillary constriction if such drugs are present. This diagnostic test is not routinely recommended, but if physostigmine is used to control arrhythmias then the concomittant observation of pupillary size is very useful. Instillation of 2 drops of 1 percent pilocarpine will not affect the pupil if mydriatics were previously used. Third nerve damage is associated with full constriction to pilocarpine within 5–10 minutes. Before calling pupils unreactive they should be examined with a bright diffuse light and magnifying glass.

> **Sign:** Bilaterally unreactive pupils.
>
> *Pitfalls:* Weak light stimulus or light not diffuse enough (do not use ophthalmoscope beam).

Reactive symmetrical, small pupils (1–2.5 mm) are usually related to metabolic coma, but also occur with acute hydrocephalus or deep central hemispheral lesions. Large doses of barbiturates typically produce such small pupils and may, in extreme cases, make them truly unreactive to light (by that time spontaneous breathing has been totally suppressed). Tiny (1 mm) pupils are caused commonly by narcotics, even in subhypnotic doses but are also the hallmark of catastrophic pontine lesions (hemorrhage, infarction).

> **Sign:** Pinpoint pupils.
>
> *Pitfall:* Pontine lesions look the same as narcotics but the former can be distinguished by abnormal eye movements and pupillary light reactivity.

A unilaterally small pupil occurs on the side of large, deep hemispheral lesions such as hypertensive hemorrhage and is occasionally a part of a Horner's syndrome on the side of a carotid artery dissection. Hippus or (spontaneous fluctuation in pupillary size) is common in metabolic encephalopathy but if striking and/or unilateral should suggest subclinical seizures.

Eye movements are the most useful portion of the coma exam (Fig. 5.3), and both spontaneous and elicited movements provide important information. Horizontal eye movements are subserved by the pons and midbrain (IIIrd nerve) and are the key to determining if a brainstem lesion is the cause of coma. First, the lids are lifted and the resting position of the eyes are noted. Drowsiness produces slight horizontal divergence which should not be mistaken for a brainstem lesion. An excessively abducted eye at rest indicates a third nerve lesion, (particularly if associated with a dilated or poorly reactive pupil) while an adducted eye usually indicates a sixth nerve lesion. Vertical separation of the ocular axes, or skew, may be seen in mild form (2 mm) in many situations, but if greater usually indicates a cerebellar or pontine lesion. Spontaneous dysconjugate eye movements are always abnormal and are a dependable sign of pontine damage, strongly

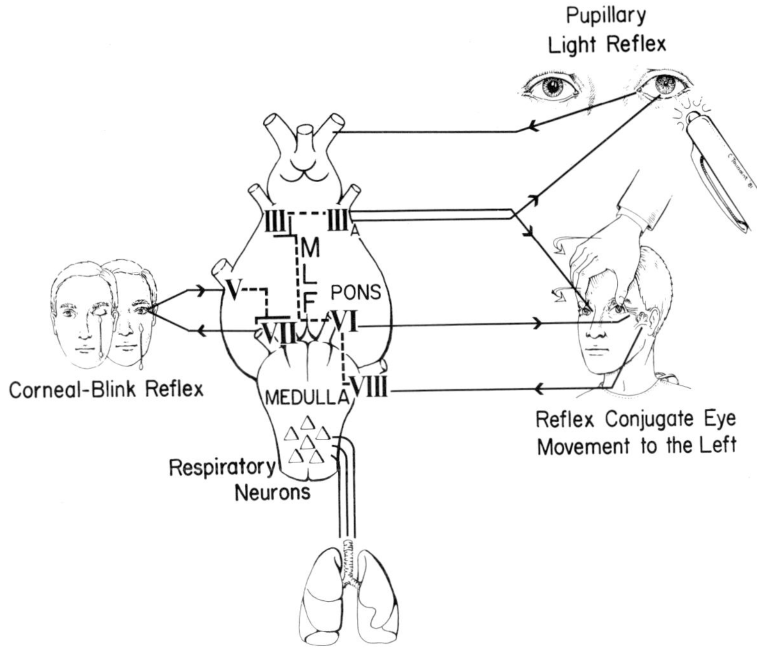

Fig. 5.3 Schematic representation of the major brainstem reflexes used in the coma examination. (from Ropper, A.H., Martin, J.B.: Coma. Ch. 20. In Harrison's Principles of Internal Medicine, 10th Ed., McGraw Hill, New York, 1983; reprinted with permission.)

suggesting that a lesion in that area is responsible for coma. On the other hand, spontaneous, full, conjugate horizontal roving eye movements indicate that the cerebral cortex is severely depressed or disconnected from the brainstem (i.e., the coma is caused by a bilateral hemispheral or diffuse process).

Two types of cyclic conjugate eye movements have fairly consistent localizing value. Ocular bobbing is a repetitive, arrhythmic brisk downward and slow upward movement usually resulting from pontine lesions. Horizontal eye movements, therefore, will be impaired when bobbing is present. Ocular dipping is the opposite slow downward, fast upward movement associated with global brain ischemia as after cardiac arrest. The eyes turn down and inward with lesions around the midbrain-thalamic junction. Traditionally this is associated with thalamic hemorrhages but it is also seen with basilar artery occlusion and ischemia of the top of the brainstem.

Sign: Eyes turned down and in.

Pitfall: Basilar occlusion, (occasionally embolus to top of basilar artery) as well as thalamic hemorrhage.

Eyes at rest which deviate tonically and laterally indicate either a large hemispheral lesion ipsilateral to the side of gaze or a small contralateral pontine lesion. In patients with coma the former is more likely the cause since small unilateral pontine lesions do not alter alertness.

While the direction of spontaneous gaze is usually a dependable marker of the side of a large hemispheral lesion (e.g., hemorrhage, stroke), on occasion it is misleading.

> **Sign:** Conjugate eye deviation towards the side of the lesion in hemispheral disease.
>
> *Pitfall:* Besides unilateral pontine disease (which is rarely a cause of coma), occasional thalamic hemorrhages or deep infarctions cause "wrong way eyes" (i.e., the eyes paradoxically gaze away from the deep lesion).

If the eyes rove freely and conjugately from side to side then the pontine and midbrain tegmentum are intact and this precludes coma of brainstem origin. However, most patients do not have such movements and the integrity of the eye movement pathways must be tested by head turning (oculocephalic response loosely called "Dolls-eyes") or caloric stimulation (oculovestibular response). It is not commonly recognized that two disparate pieces of information are derived from the reflex eye movements. The first, as mentioned above, is the extent to which the eye movement pathways in the pons-midbrain tegmentum are disrupted. Second, the ease with which the eyes move or seemingly glide towards the side opposite head turning are an indication of disinhibition of brainstem reflexes by damaged cerebral hemispheres above. In other words, freely moveable eyes are "decorticate" and confirm bilateral hemispheral disease as the cause of coma.

The oculocephalic maneuver consists of holding the head by the brow or crown, raising the lids and rolling the head from side to side, first slowly then more vigorously in an attempt to elicit horizontal eye movement (Fig. 5.3). It should not be performed if there is a question of cervical spine instability (the oculovestibular-caloric test should be used instead–see below). The same maneuver may be done by flexing and extending the neck to elicit vertical eye movements. On occasion the lids will open with neck flexion; hence the term "Dolls eyes." Drowsy patients may show a few contraversive eye movements, then arouse and follow the direction of head movements with the eyes demonstrating that they are awake. It should be noted that full adduction (medial motion) of an eye is by nature slightly more difficult to elicit than abduction.

Caloric stimulation of the labyrinths is a more vigorous stimulus than head turning and is saved for instances where no or incomplete responses are obtained with head turning or if there is cervical spine instability. Caloric stimulation is ideally performed with the head elevated 30 degrees from horizontal in order to maximally stimulate the horizontal semicircular canal which is closest to the tympanic membrane. Generally 30 ml of ice water is used and squirted into the external canal over about 20 seconds through a soft tube that may be obtained by cutting the needle off a 19 gauge butterfly intravenous device. Both ears are tested with at least a 3–5 minute hiatus between sides. The lids are lifted lightly to observe the eyeballs. Before commencing, there should be no evidence of tympanic membrane rupture and the external canals should be free of wax. Performing the test in the presence of basilar skull fractures, even with intact tympanic membranes, is controversial, because of the risk of inducing bacterial meningitis.

In the comatose patient the normal response to cold water caloric stimulation is conjugate deviation of both eyes towards the irrigated ear. This response vindicates much of the brainstem as the cause of coma. If the hemispheres are functioning, as in the alert patient, there will be a compensatory rapid nystagmus away from the side of tonic deviation and the stimulated ear. In catatonia and hysterical coma the nystagmus will be present. By observing the eyes carefully, ophthalmoplegias may be found (see below). If there are no calorically induced eye movements then extensive brainstem damage is suggested, but calorics may also be obliterated by CNS suppressant drugs or previous VIIIth nerve damage. This latter pitfall should not be overlooked considering how many people have labyrinthine or VIIIth nerve disease, have received high doses of ototoxic aminoglycosides or loop diuretics or have petrous bone fractures with VIIIth nerve damage.

Sign: Absent oculovestibular (caloric) response.

Pitfall: CNS suppressant drugs in large doses or afferent VIIIth nerve damage from trauma or ototoxic drugs.

On occasion the eyes will tonically deviate upward or downward in metabolic-drug coma after unilateral caloric stimulation.

Abnormalities of elicited horizontal eye movements are interpreted similarly to spontaneous ones; namely, faulty abduction of one eye is due to a VIth nerve lesion, faulty adduction due to a IIIrd nerve or internuclear (i.e., medial longitudinal fasciculus) lesion and conjugate gaze paresis, or the inability to get the eyes well over to one side, is due to a large hemispheral lesion contralateral to the paresis, or less likely a pontine lesion ispilaterally. Most pure third nerve lesions (adductor paresis) are accompanied by pupillary dilation and are due to compression by a mass above, not a primary brainstem lesion. With completely absent reflex eye movements drugs should be suspected, rather than presuming that eye movement mechanisms are destroyed by an anatomical lesion. Phenytoin, barbiturates, tricyclic antidepressants and occasionally alcohol and phenothiazines can cause varying degrees of ophthalmoparesis. The presence of normal to small diameter pupils distinguishes drug overdose from a large lesion in, or compressing, the midbrain.

The corneal reflexes are good indicators of pontine function since their afferents are the Vth nerve and efferents the VIIth nerve (Fig. 5.3), but they add little to the information derived from eye movements in the acute ER situation. They may also be obliterated or dulled by drugs.

Respiratory patterns are often touted as helpful in coma diagnosis, but practical experience suggests they are of inconsistent localizing value. As with eye movements, apnea or virtual apnea indicates either severe anatomical brainstem (medullary) damage (frequently brain death) or drug-metabolic suppression of respiratory neurons. Shallow, slow regular breathing most often is associated with metabolic coma. A rapid, deep (Kussmaul) pattern is an attempt to compensate for metabolic acidosis as in diabetic ketoacidosis or ethylene glycol intoxication but is also seen with large, bilateral pontine lesions or acute pulmonary diseases and in mild form with hepatic encephalopathy. Cheyne-Stokes respirations are due to bilateral, mild hemispheral disease and are not a cause for concern about a structural brainstem lesion.

The plantar response is (surprising to many physicians) only an ancillary part of the coma examination. A Babinski sign is most helpful if present only on one side where it signifies a contralateral lesion but does not aid localization. Bilateral Babinski signs may be due to metabolic disease, most frequently hepatic or ischemic encephalopathy, and severe drug overdose is rarely a cause.

Other useful tests include forced eyelid lifting which exposes psychogenic unresponsiveness (trance) by the appearance of Bell's phenomenon. This is an upward and slightly outward movement of the globes occuring when the patient is truly awake and resisting eyelid opening. In most unresponsive patients the eyelids feel flaccid when lifted upwards, frequently more so on the side of a facial paralysis.

In patients who are arousable an attempt should be made to elicit a hemianopia by threatening the visual fields with outstretched fingers.

The fundoscopic examination is helpful in detecting several specific causes of coma, among them subarachnoid hemorrhage (subhyaloid hemorrhages), hypertensive encephalopathy (exudates, vasospasm), methanol intoxication (disc swelling), as well as detecting papilledema if the intracranial lesion is a subacute or chronic one. At the end of the neurological examination the physician should have a firm idea of localization or suspect a more global process like intoxication. If the diagnosis is unclear or a metabolic-drug cause is suspected then certain points in the general examination are noteworthy.

THE GENERAL PHYSICAL EXAMINATION IN A COMATOSE PATIENT

Fever in a comatose patient suggests a systemic infection, frequently pneumonia and a low-grade fever is common in recent aspiration. Subarachnoid hemorrhage also causes a low-grade fever. When no source of fever is obvious the temptation to attribute it to a "neurogenic" cause should be avoided since this is rare and is usually associated with very high temperature levels (44–45°C) and other signs of excessive hypothalamic-diencephalic function. Very high temperatures, should also suggest heat stroke as a possible reason for unresponsiveness. Hypothermia is most frequently related to bodily exposure subsequent to the comatose state. This is exacerbated by, or may be primarily due to, myxedema, alcohol, phenothiazine or barbiturate overdose or shock. Hypothermia causes coma directly only at extremely low levels, probably below 31°C.

Hypertension, particularly in patients not previously known to be hypertensive, often is caused by large, acute intracranial masses with their attendant intracranial hypertension. The most common causes are intracerebral and subarachnoid hemorrhage. Hypertensive encephalopathy is a consideration when preceding hypertension, renal failure and/or seizures are present.

Hypotension is the hallmark of unresponsiveness due to low cardiac output as in myocardial failure, peripheral vasodilation as in septic shock, or internal hemorrhage. More obscure causes such as Addisonian crisis should be considered with compatible serum electrolyte abnormalities. In severe brain injuries concomittant with the onset of brain death, hypotension is common. Diabetes insipidus due to any large hemispheral lesion or aneurysmal rupture of the anterior communicating artery will exacerbate hypotension by producing intravascular volume depletion.

The skull and tympanic membranes should be inspected for subtle signs of trauma. It is very useful to percuss the skull to detect an acute subdural hematoma in the elderly. This sign was described by McKissock over 40 years ago and is underutilized in ERs.[5] The tongue should be inspected for lacerations due to seizures.

In cases where the cause of coma is still not evident a search should be made for petichiae (thrombocytopenia, fat embolism, SBE), ecchymosis (excessive anticoagulation and related intracranial hemorrhage), skin color changes (intense cyanosis-methemoglobinemia, mucosal rubor-carbon monoxide, yellow skin-myxedema), mucosal corrosive burns (heavy metal intoxication), general flushing (atropinic-drug overdoses, especially antidepressants) and needle marks. Absence of sweating suggests the hyperosmolar non-ketotic syndrome if there is no fever and heat stroke or atropinic-drug overdose if high fever is present.

An enlarged liver or signs of chronic liver disease raise the question of hepatic encephalopthy. (Remember that metabolic encephalopathies can cause Babinski signs and subtle focal findings.)

The patient's breath odor is most useful when alcohol is detected. This alerts the clinician to three potential situations: (1) coma is due to deep alcohol or other simultaneous drug anesthesia, (2) some of the neurological signs, particularly eye movements, may be obliterated or altered by alcohol or drugs thus confounding the exam, or (3) there is occult head trauma and possible subdural hematoma. On occasion the ketotic odor of diabetic ketosis is detected (also seen with alcoholism) or other similar characteristic odors such as fetor hepaticus. Even rarer are the characteristic ingestion odors such as cyanide or paraldehyde.

COMA SCALES AND PROGNOSTICATION

In recent years several numerical scales to gauge the depth of coma have been proposed. These are of little diagnostic value but do serve other useful functions. First, they have some prognostic value and may be useful in resource allocation. In this country, however, it has not been generally accepted that early prostication should guide medical decisions except in extreme cases. Second, they are a useful way for medical and nursing personnel to transmit succinct, reproduceable neurological examination information.

The ER physician should be familiar with the best studied and most popular of these scales, the Glascow Coma Scale, originated by Jennet, Teasdale and co-workers.[3] Their scheme is simple, has been well-tested for reproduceability between observers, and offers some empirical early prognostic information in head trauma, perhaps less so, in medical coma. There are three categories from which a total coma score is derived (Table 5.3). In head trauma the major early prognostic features are absent pupillary reaction or absent reflex eye movements 6 hours after onset suggesting a 95 percent death rate. Other combinations have less early predictive value.

Prognostication in non-traumatic coma is more difficult because of the heterogeneity of diseases but a large multicentered study found that coma due to vascular catastrophies (subarachnoid and other hemorrhage) had the worst outcome, cardiac arrest was intermediate and hepatic and other miscellaneous (metabolic) causes the best.[4] In the first hours, 97 percent of patients lacking any two of corneal, pupillary and oculovestibular responses died or remained unresponsive. If any two of these responses were present but there was no verbal or motor response, 80 percent died or remained unresponsive. Beyond these combinations, the ability to discriminate a poor outcome was limited, approaching 50/50 in most instances. In both head trauma and medical coma, signs at one day and beyond give more prognostic information but are of little direct use to the ER physician. The patients age also has a great influence on outcome. We feel that the

**Table 5.3 Glascow Coma Scale Scoring System Total Score =
E + M + V (Score of 3–15 possible)**

Observations		Points
Eye opening (E)	Spontaneous	4
	To speech	3
	To pain	2
	Nil	1
Motor response (M)	Obeys	6
	Localizes	5
	Withdraws (flexion)	4
	Flexion posturing	3
	Extension posturing	2
	Nil	1
Verbalization (V)	Oriented	5
	Confused conversation	4
	Inappropriate words	3
	Incomprehensible sounds	2
	Nil	1

coma scales and prognostic systems should be viewed with some skepticism
in the ER because of the uncertainty which is always involved in acute
situations (see Chapter 1, Principle 14). Similarly, it is inadvisable to make
a determination of brain death in the ER. It seems best to be aggressive
within reason until the facts and cause of an individual case of coma are
clarified. However, as prognostication becomes more sophisticated and resources more limited, the ER physician will likely be involved in major
early triage decisions and should therefore become acquainted with these
coma grading systems and their prognostic value.

LABORATORY EXAMINATION IN THE ER

Four laboratory tests are used in the ER diagnosis of coma: CT scan, CSF
analysis, toxicologic analysis and routine chemistry-hematology determinations. The EEG, which is frequently helpful, is not often obtained until
the patient reaches the ward, but in rare specific circumstances such as
subclinical epilepsy ("spike-wave stupor") it may be the central diagnostic
test.

In coma of unknown etiology the CT scan, if available, should be planned
for early in the evaluation, but not before a careful neurological examination.
It is now common practice to do a CT before a lumbar puncture. An apparently normal CT by no means excludes an anatomical lesion as the cause
of coma and, conversely, abnormalities on CT do not always explain coma.
The examination findings correlated with the CT are the most dependable
guide to diagnosis. A partial listing of anatomical lesions which may be
missed by CT includes early infarction; brainstem lesions of various types
but most notably pontine-midbrain infarction due to basilar thrombosis;

encephalitis including early Herpes simplex; subdural hematoma (especially bilateral) in an intermediate stage when it is isodense to adjacent brain; small contusions and axonal shearing lesions due to closed head trauma; cortical vein thrombosis; and the absence of cerebral perfusion associated with brain death. CT is an effective way to confirm the diagnosis in most acute subarachnoid hemorrhages and then precludes lumbar puncture. However, if subarachnoid hemorrhage is suspected, a lumbar puncture should be performed even with a negative CT.

When one thinks critically about the information gained from a CT scan, it becomes apparent that most radiologic abnormalities simply confirm the clinical diagnosis. This is certainly true for cerebral hemorrhage, subarachnoid hemorrhage, sub- or epidural hemorrhage, pontine hemorrhage, Herpes encephalitis, brain tumor, etc. The real value of CT is frequently in its normality (the caveats above should be noted). The majority of causes of coma in fact are associated with a normal CT (Table 5.4).

Skull X-rays are not useful as a routine part of the coma evaluation unless CT is unavailable. They may, however, give important information in head trauma, indicating the severity of impact and likelihood of an underlying hematoma or contusion.

Lumbar puncture is now used mostly for the diagnosis of suspected meningitis-encephalitis and in those cases of suspected subarachnoid or pontine hemorrhage if the CT fails to show blood. For the information gathered by lumbar puncture to be useful a careful examination for xanthochromia is necessary. The CSF should be centrifuged in a test tube, not a microhematocrit tube, and the color of the supernatant compared to a tube of water. Yellow coloration indicates the presence of pre-existing blood or very high protein in the CSF and fairly well excludes a traumatic puncture. Hyperbilirubinemia causes a similar coloration and very high CSF protein content may do likewise. If a questionable traumatic puncture is performed the first and last tubes of collected CSF should be sent for cell count. A significant decrement in the number of red blood cells suggests traumatic blood but red cell counts above 10,000 in the last tube are always suspect for subarachnoid hemorrhage. Lumbar puncture performed in the first 60 minutes or less after a subarachnoid hemorrhage will occasionally be bloodless. Focal neurological signs, particularly aphasia and seizures, with the finding of CSF lymphocytes should suggest Herpes virus encephalitis. On occasion, vigorous seizures alone, without an infectious process can cause several CSF lymphocytes. A few red cells (20–500/mm3), if not traumatic, are consistent with Herpes encephalitis, a hemorrhagic infarction, as from cortical vein thrombosis, very early subarachnoid hemorrhage, or an intracerebral hematoma. Oxalate crystals may be seen in ethylene glycol intoxication and are associated with an aseptic meningeal reaction. It is strongly recommended that the physician performing the lumbar puncture do his own CSF examination as soon as possible after the procedure.

Toxicologic analysis is required in any case of coma of unclear origin.

Table 5.4 The Value of the CT Scan in the Diagnosis of Coma

I. Normal brainstem reflexes/No lateralizing signs
  A. Diagnosis facilitated by CT scan
    1. Bilateral subdural hematomas
    2. Subarachnoid hemorrhage
    3. Bilateral traumatic contusions or brain swelling
    4. Hydrocephalus
  B. CT normal or unhelpful
    1. Drug ingestion
    2. Endogenous metabolic encephalopathy
    3. Shock
    4. Hypertensive encephalopathy
    5. Meningitis
    6. Non-herpetic encephalitis
    7. Generalized epilepsy
    8. Reyes' syndrome
    9. Psychiatric states

II. Normal brainstem reflexes/lateralizing motor signs
  A. Diagnosis facilitated by CT scan
    1. Cerebral hemorrhage
    2. Large infarction with edema
    3. Herpes virus encephalitis
    4. Sub- or epidural hematoma
    5. Brain tumor with edema
    6. Brain abscess with edema
    7. Traumatic contusion
    8. Pituitary apoplexy
    9. Metabolic encephalopathy superimposed or
       pre-existing stroke
  B. CT normal or unhelpful
    1. Metabolic encephalopathy with focal signs
       (especially hyper-hypoglycemia)
    2. Isodense subdural hematoma
    3. Thrombotic thrombocytopenic purpura

III. Brainstem reflex abnormalities
  A. Diagnosis facilitated by CT scan
    1. Pontine, midbrain hemorrhage
    2. Cerebellar hemorrhage
    3. Cerebellar infarction with brainstem compression
    4. Hemispheral mass causing advanced brainstem compression
  B. CT normal or unhelpful
    1. Basilar artery occlusion—brainstem infarction
    2. Severe drug overdose
    3. Brainstem contusion—hemorrhage
    4. Brain death

(from Ropper, A.H., Martin, J.B.: Coma and other disorders of consciousness. Ch. 20. In Principles of Internal Medicine, 10th Ed., McGraw-Hill, 1982; reprinted with permission).

Quantitative assays are preferable to qualitative ones since the presence of drugs in the stomach or blood does not prove intoxication as the cause of coma. The extent of commercial assays vary but most screen for ethanol, barbiturates, benzodiazepines, and narcotics. Fresh blood is the best specimen but basic drugs such as amphetamines and phenothiazines are frequently easier to detect in urine.

Qualitative drug screening is useful in the ER because of simplicity and the rapidity of results. The heated ferric chloride test for salicylate detection in urine gives falsely positive results with phenacetin and ketonuria (from starvation or diabetic ketoacidosis). Boiling the urine eliminates acetoacetic acid and with it the latter source of error. Falsely negative results occur with acidic urine containing large amounts of phosphates but this may be eliminated by using an excess of ferric chloride reagent. Phenastix testing for phenothiazine intoxication is relatively dependable but the reagent stripes become rapidly outdated.

STATES TO BE DISTINGUISHED FROM COMA

Other states simulate coma and the first diagnostic step after a thorough physical examination is to determine if one of these is present. Pseudocoma or the "locked in syndrome" is perhaps the most important because it has specific patho-anatomic significance. This is a state in which an awake person has lost most of the efferent (output) from the nervous system and therefore appears unresponsive because of an inability to react. It occurs in 2 varieties. First, and more commonly in the ER, basilar artery occlusion with infarction of the base of the pons causes transection of all descending motor fibers while leaving the midbrain tegmentum intact. This leaves unharmed the reticular activating system which is crucial to alertness. Locked in patients appear unresponsive because they cannot move their limbs, mouth or face but are fully awake and are capable of responding appropriately with blinking and vertical eye movements. The reason for selective preservation of vertical eye movements and alertness is the preservation of midbrain and pontine tegmental areas while the descending motor fibers in the pons are heavily damaged. The distribution of infarction also serves to emphasize one of the basic principles of coma, discussed further above; only that portion of the reticular formation above the mid pons is necessary for arousal. Failure to recognize this state and thus carry on discussions in the patient's presence may create an agonizing situation. The second rarer type of the de-efferentation occurs in profound neuromuscular paralysis due to Guillain-Barré syndrome, myasthenia gravis or with neuro-muscular blocking drugs. Here, vertical eye movements are not selectively spared.

Catatonia is the summary term for peculiar motor activities associated with the major psychoses. In its hypomobile form it simulates coma but most patients appear awake with the eyes open, blinking spontaneously and appearing comfortable. There may be an associated "waxy flexibility" in which the limbs maintain their posture and position after being moved by the examiner. After recovering, these patients have recall of the period of unresponsiveness. Hysterical unresponsiveness (trance) is not uncommon in the ER. These patients demonstrate signs of voluntary attempts to appear comatose, primarily the Bell's phenomenon (bilateral elevation and abduction of the globes when the eyelids are forcibly opened). Caloric stimulation of the external auditory canal causes the expected response for an awake patient, namely slight conjugate eye deviation and brisk nystagmus in the opposite direction. These physical signs are discussed in detail above and it is necessary for the moment only to recognize that psychogenic unresponsiveness should enter into the differential diagnosis of coma.

Akinetic mutism and vegetative state have unfortunately been variously described by different authors but are still useful when used in their original sense. Akinetic mutism is an awake state in which the patient is immobile and silent though the limbs will withdraw appropriately to pain. It appears to be the severest form of the loss of spontaneity and impulse due to frontal lobe lesion or hydrocephalus and may appear acutely. Abulia is a milder form of akinetic mutism in which there is only a delay in all responses, though they are correct, or nearly so, when they come. The vegetative state is a chronic syndrome which occurs weeks after ischemia or other global brain injury and is therefore not likely to be seen in ER. It consists of an awake appearing patient with eyes open and roving about, stereotyped posturing and frequently spells of excessive sympathetic nervous system activity.

DIFFERENTIAL DIAGNOSIS OF COMA IN THE ER

In many instances the cause of coma is due to an obvious problem such as trauma, hypoxia, liver or kidney failure or known drugs ingestion. In these cases the examination in the ER serves to delimit the extent of damage and establish a neurological baseline. The details of most of the diseases which cause coma are covered elsewhere but certain general guidelines are helpful (see Table 1.2). Sudden coma is due to one of the neurologic catastrophes: hemorrhage, ischemic-hypoxia, or trauma. Subacute onset coma is related to preceding medical illness, encephalitis, or secondary brain swelling surrounding a major pre-existing neurological lesion (tumor, stroke). In these instances the primary lesion or underlying illness has been present for some time and the ER diagnosis is not difficult.

It is therefore with the catastrophic lesions that most diagnostic problems arise and a familiarity if not memorization of the archetypal coma syndromes is necessary for the ER physician. The major features of the catastrophic lesions are summarized as follows:

1. Subarachnoid hemorrhage—instantaneous onset with severe headache, neck stiffness, vomiting, transient loss of consciousness in 25 percent, extensor posturing, notable lack of focal signs;

2. Basal ganglionic or thalamic hemorrhage—acute but not instantaneous onset, vomiting, complete hemiplegia and hemisensory deficit, characteristic eye signs;

3. Pontine hemorrhage—sudden onset, loss of reflex eye movements, ocular bobbing in some, extensor posturing, hyperventilation, diaphoresis, pin-point pupils;

4. Cerebellar hemorrhage—occipital ache, vomiting, severe ataxia or inability to stand, gaze paresis, signs of hydrocephalus;

5. Basilar artery thrombosis—neurological warning TIAs (some), reflex eye movement abnormalities, abnormal corneal responses, asymmetric limb paresis.

The commonest stroke, infarction in the carotid-middle cerebral artery territory does not cause enough brain swelling acutely to cause coma. Occlusive anterior circulation stroke is therefore not a primary consideration in the ER diagnosis of coma (while basilar occlusion obviously is). A rote listing of the other diseases which cause coma serves little purpose. The physician should arrive at a generic diagnosis first (e.g., brainstem, hemispheral, metabolic) and the differential diagnosis then becomes greatly limited. This also points the way to the most expedient laboratory testing.

Table 5.4 is partial listing of the causes of coma which may be seen in the ER, cross referenced by neurological signs and CT scan abnormalities.

TREATMENT OF COMA IN THE ER

The immediate goal in the ER is to prevent further brain damage. This requires that resuscitation take precedence over diagnosis but to a large degree both of these take place simultaneously. In approximate order of urgency hypoxia, hypotension, hypercarbia, hypoglycemia, hyperglycemia and severe hyperthermia should be anticipated and rapidly corrected.

An intravenous access is established and naloxone and dextrose given, each in a bolus if the cause of coma is not otherwise obvious. The routine use of thiamine is suggested because the use of dextrose might precipitate acute thiamine deficiency and Wernicke's disease in an alcoholic patient. The veins of intravenous drug abusers are frequently sclerosed and difficult to cannulate. If the pupils are small and narcotic overdose is suspected, narcotic antagonists can be administered sublingually through a small gauge needle.

Maintenance of a patent airway is the next priority.[8] Drowsy patients typically have pharyngeal and glossal hypotonia that is sometimes evident by gutteral breathing sounds or snoring. Partial pharyngeal obstruction is overcome by a flexible oro-pharyngeal airway. It is wise to routinely place one in patients who cannot be aroused. These patients are incapable of protecting the trachea from aspiration of gastric-oral contents and if vomiting is occurring, firm backward pressure on the larynx will occlude the upper esophagus thus transiently preventing gastric contents from reaching the airway (the Sellick maneuver).

Tracheal intubation is performed in those patients with (1) obvious apnea, (2) labored respiration or (3) if aspiration is highly likely (e.g., spinal cord injury with gastric atony, or cerebral hemorrhage with likely vomiting, or bulbar paresis from brainstem infarction). Mechanical ventilation is dictated by hypoventilation, cyanosis or the need for therapeutic hyperventilation in cases of increased intracranial pressure. The use of intravenous fluids for resuscitation takes on a special dimension in coma because most intracranial catastrophes predispose to brain swelling which is exacerbated by the administration of water. In most patients normal saline should be used as the intravenous solution because it is least hypotonic after glucose in other solutions has been metabolized and is also preferred as the vehicle for phenytoin administration. Fluids are generally kept to a minimum though the need for volume to treat hypotension obviously takes precedence over fluid restriction. If readily available, albumin solutions are preferred first for hypotension.

Treatments for specific intracranial catastrophies must often be started on an anticipatory basis so that potentially valuable time is not wasted. One of the most common such situations is suspected brainstem ischemia from basilar thrombosis in which heparin is administered. Here the diagnosis should be quite firm since cerebellar and pontine hemorrhages resemble brainstem ischemia and preclude anticoagulation. A history of basilar TIAs is most reassuring in excluding cerebellar or brainstem hemorrhage.

Physostigmine has isolated uses in the ER. It may be used to awaken patients with atropine-related drug overdoses such as tricyclic antidepressants. However, the risks of 1–2 mg intravenously is probably justified only when there are concomitant serious cardiac arrhythmias. The putative beneficial effects of physostigmine on other drug overdoses, particularly benzodiazepines, is still argued. The purely diagnostic use of intravenous physostigmine is discouraged (the pupils should constrict unless there are high levels of intoxicants with atropinic activity).

The generic problem of precipitously raised intracranial pressure (ICP) is dealt with in a uniform manner regardless of cause[8] (see Chapter 4 for more extensive discussion). Raised ICP is signaled by unilateral (occasionally bilateral asymmetric) pupillary enlargement and light unreactivity. (The one pitfall here is in coma due to subarachnoid hemorrhage where a posterior communicating artery or similar aneurysm causes third nerve damage without raised ICP.) Immediate medical reduction of ICP is required while awaiting more definitive therapy (e.g., removal of a subdural hematoma). The rate of intravenous fluids is first slowed. Next hyperventilation, preferably by hand ambu bag is used to reduce PCO_2 to 32 torr or lower. This is then sustained by a mechanical ventilator. An osmotic agent is administered simultaneously. In the ER situation an initial dose of mannitol 1gm/kg is recommended though smaller subsequent doses (0.25–0.5 gm/kg) every 2–3 hours will maintain the effect.

If all of these fail to reduce ICP, a single bolus of short or intermediate acting barbiturate (methohexital 25–50 mg or pentobarbital 1.5–3 mg/kg respectively) may be administered. Obviously, secure mechanical ventilation is required prior to the use of barbiturates. Barbiturate boluses frequently produce a profound and rapid ICP reduction when other therapies have failed but are limited by the side effect of hypotension. Their beneficial effects on ICP may not be sustained but may nonetheless be helpful in the emergent situation. Because of the novelty of high dose barbiturate therapy it is best instituted with the aid of an experienced anesthesiologist, intensive care specialist or neurosurgeon. Finally, ventricular puncture for removal of intracranial CSF may be attempted by a neurosurgeon in selected patients with hydrocephalas as a stop-gap maneuver. By these means virtually all comatose patients who reach the ER may be supported until definitive therapy is possible or at least until the cause of coma can be determined.

REFERENCES

1. Finklestein, S., Ropper, A.H.: The diagnosis of coma: its pitfalls and limitations. Heart Lung, 8:1059, 1979.
2. Fisher, C.M.: The neurological examination of the comatose patient. Acta Neurol. Scand., 45 (suppl 6): 1, 1969.
3. Jennet, B., Teasdale, G., Braakman, R., et al: Predicting outcome in individual patients after head injury. Lancet, 1:1081, 1976.
4. Levy, D., et al: Prognosis in nontraumatic coma. Ann. Int. Med., 94:229, 1981.
5. McKissock, W., Richardson, A., Bloom, W.: Subdural hematoma: a review of 389 cases. Lancet, 1:1365, 1960.
6. Plum, F., Posner, J.: The Diagnosis of Stupor and Coma. 3rd Ed., F.A. Davis, Philadelphia, 1980.
7. Ropper, A.H., Martin, J.B.: Coma and other disorders of consciousness. Ch. 20. In Principles of Internal Medicine, 10th Ed., McGraw-Hill, 1982.
8. Ropper, A.H., Kennedy, S.K., Zervas, N.T.: Neurological and Neurosurgical Intensive Care. University Park Press, Baltimore, 1982.

6

Emergency Management of Seizure Disorders

Paul A. Hwang, M.D., C.M., F.R.C.P.(C.)

CLINICAL PRESENTATIONS

The patient with a seizure disorder may present in many ways. He may have a brief lapse of consciousness with or without any accompanying movements (a "blackout"). There may have been a fall, perhaps accompanied by some head trauma. Sometimes, there has been a warning (an "aura") consisting of an unusual sensation, feeling or movement prior to the loss of consciousness. The patient may also present in a dazed, confused state after having had a seizure, which may or may not have been witnessed. Often, there is a past history of similar episodes suggesting recurrent seizures, perhaps related to alcohol consumption or withdrawal. Occasionally, the patient presents in a rather dramatic fashion to the Emergency Room in a continuing epileptic status ("status epilepticus") requiring immediate medical treatment. Rarely, a condition of intermittent unresponsiveness (a "twilight state") lasting for minutes to hours may represent non-convulsive status epilepticus. Other typical presentations (particularly in children) include absences (brief episodes of blank staring) and automatisms (semi-automatic motor manifestations accompanied by impaired consciousness). Atypical representations include enuresis, nocturnal seizures, apneic episodes, acute psychotic and aphasic episodes and, possibly, aggressive behavior.[1]

Case 1

W.T. was a 28-year-old right-handed man who had always been in good health. The evening prior to admission, he was returning home from a party where he had a few drinks. Suddenly he collapsed and lost consciousness. He was noted to turn pale in the face, and, as his head hit the ground, his limbs made a few clonic movements. He did not bite his tongue, nor was he incontinent of urine. The episode lasted about 2–3 minutes, following which he was confused for about a minute, felt rather weak generally, but was responsive. He had no aura, and no past or family history of seizures. Physical exam in the emergency room 2 hours after the ictus was completely normal, including a detailed neurological examination.

Is It A Fit, A Faint Or A Fall?

Often, when the patient has had an episode of loss of consciousness, it is unclear if he had an epileptic seizure (a paroxysmal discharge of neurons resulting in altered consciousness, memory, sensation or movement) or a syncopal episode (due to impaired cardiac function, or poor cerebral circulation) or perhaps a simple fall with concussion (i.e., a transient loss of consciousness). The patient himself is usually not helpful, and accurate assessment depends on the observation of the event by witnesses, and on the clinical examination (see Clinical Exam below). The differential diagnosis of a blackout is difficult and relies primarily on an accurate history, including the circumstances of the episode, the prodrome (if any), the aura (the first warning signs or symptoms), the ictus or event itself and the post-ictal events following the acute episode (Table 6.1).

Other conditions to be considered in the differential diagnosis of blackouts include:

1. Migraine, particularly the basilar artery variety, resulting in symptoms of vertebro-basilar ischemia with loss of consciousness;

2. Narcolepsy, a disorder of sleep characterized by daytime sleepiness, sleep paralysis, hypnagogic hallucinations and cataplexy;

3. Transient Ischemic Attacks (see Chapter 8); and,

4. Breath holding spells in children of preschool age who have episodes of pallor or cyanosis, usually provoked by pain or stress; (see Chapter 16).

Some Definitions

An epileptic seizure is a paroxysmal discharge of a group of neurons resulting in a transient impairment of sensation, movement, consciousness or memory.

Epilepsy is a chronic disorder characterized by recurrent seizures of cerebral origin.

The term seizure disorder refers to a condition characterized by a single seizure or recurrent seizures, epileptic in nature. It is often used to refer to epilepsy without some of the social stigma attached to the latter term.

Recurrent seizures due to an underlying known process or lesion are called symptomatic seizures, (e.g., hypoglycemia, brain tumor) and are not usually classified as epilepsy, which refers to idiopathic recurrent seizures with unknown etiology and minimal or no pathology.

Table 6.1 Differential Diagnosis of a "Blackout"

	Seizure	Syncope	TIA	Concussion	Hysteria
Setting	May have had previous seizures Family history	Fatigue Stress Hunger	Cardiovascular disease Hypertension	Head trauma	Attention-getting Secondary gain Dramatic, with anxiety
Prodome	Sleep-deprivation Hyperventilation Photic stimulation Stress	Light-headed Dizziness Palpitations	None	None	Hyperventilation Paresthesias Indifferent expression
Aura	None (absences, "grand mal") Fear, déjà vu Hallucinations Forced thinking (complex partial)	Tinnitus Dimming of vision Dizziness Pallor	Localized or lateralized paresthesiae, weakness, language deficit Brainstem signs	None recalled (retrograde amnesia)	Perioral and limb paresthesias
Ictus	Blank stare Unresponsiveness Automatisms Tonic movements Clonic movements Tonic/clonic convulsions Incontinence Tongue-biting	Collapse Sweating Bradycardia or other arrhythmia Motionless (usually) Pulse weak	Hemiparesis Hemianesthesia Language deficit Brainstem or cranial nerve signs	Head trauma with fall and loss of consciousness	Tetany Hyperventilation, "Seizure" or loss of consciousness only Dramatic and bizarre
Duration	Seconds (absences), 1–2 minutes (complex partial)	Usually < 1 min.	Prolonged, min. to hours (usually < 24 hours)	Seconds to hours	Seconds to hours
Post-Ictal	Immediate recovery (absence) Confusion Paresis, dysphasia, amnesia (partial or generalized tonic/clonic seizures) Somnolence	Clear sensorium, General weakness, Pallor	None or minimal neurological deficit	Retrograde and antegrade amnesia, Signs of head injury	None

International Classification Of Epileptic Seizures (Table 6.2)

Notice that this is a classification of epileptic seizures and not of the epilepsies, as there is inadequate knowledge of the etiology and pathophysiologic mechanisms to provide a logical classification of the epilepsies at present. Epileptic seizures are classified according to clinical and electrographic (EEG) criteria, as recently defined by the Commission on Classification and Terminology of the International League Against Epilepsy.[6] Clinicians accustomed to the previous International Classification may find some of the changes noteworthy (Table 6.2).[2]

In general, seizures are still classified into two broad categories: partial and generalized. Those that show clinical and/or electrographic evidence of focal onset are partial seizures, whereas those that show synchronous involvement of all cerebral regions in both hemispheres are generalized seizures. Partial seizures occurring without impairment of consciousness are simple partial seizures and they may be sensory, motor, autonomic, or psychic, depending on their symptomatology. It should be pointed out that simple partial seizures with psychic symptoms are very unusual. Almost always, there is an accompanying change in consciousness, which puts them in the complex partial category. By definition, complex partial seizures (also known as psychomotor or temporal lobe seizures) have clinical or EEG evidence of focal onset (usually involving the temporal lobe, but occasionally the frontal lobe), but, in the new classification, are always accompanied by impairment of consciousness. They are usually accompanied by psychic symptoms (e.g., hallucinations, déjà vu, amnesia), automatisms (motor mani-

Table 6.2 International Classification of Epileptic Seizures

I. Partial seizures
   A. Simple partial (consciousness retained)
      1. Motor
      2. Sensory
      3. Autonomic
      4. Psychic
   B. Complex partial (consciousness impaired)
      1. Simple partial, followed by impaired consciousness
      2. Consciousness impaired at onset
   C. Partial seizures with secondary generalization
II. Generalized seizures
   A. Absences
      1. Typical
      2. Atypical
   B. Generalized tonic-clonic
   C. Tonic
   D. Clonic
   E. Myoclonic
   F. Atonic
III. Unclassified Seizures

(from ILAE: Proposal for revised clinical and electroencephalographic classification of epileptic seizures. Epilepsia, 22:489, 1981 Raven Press, New York; reprinted with permission.)

festations in a semi-automatic manner), or abnormal sensory or autonomic symptoms (e.g., epigastric aura). Partial seizures, simple or complex, may progress to generalized tonic-clonic seizures by the epileptic discharges spreading from the primary focus to other brain regions via cortico-cortical pathways, including the commissures connecting the two hemispheres. Simple partial seizures may become complex partial prior to secondary generalization into tonic-clonic seizures.

Generalized seizures, by definition, do not have a focal onset, but involve both hemispheres synchronously, by clinical and EEG criteria. The typical absence (previously called "petit mal") is well known, consisting of a brief episode (usually less than 30 seconds) of blank staring, accompanied by rhythmic blinking or fluttering of the eyes. But they are often accompanied by minor motor manifestations including slight head nodding, chewing or lip-smacking, myoclonic jerking of extremities or other minor automations. There is no preceding aura, and recovery of consciousness is abrupt and complete, without post-ictal symptoms, unlike complex partial seizures. General physical and neurological examination is usually normal, but there is often a family history of similar seizures. The EEG shows the characteristic 3 cycles per second (Hz) spike-wave discharges either at rest or provoked by hyperventilation or photic stimulation. The background activity is normal giving the EEG picture of a primary corticoreticular epilepsy, implying an absence of gross cerebral pathology.[4]

The atypical absence is characterized by similar episodes of brief staring and minor automatisms but the patient has other types of seizures as well: myoclonic, atonic (also known as akinetic seizures or "drop attacks"), tonic and generalized tonic-clonic seizures. These are often refractory to medical therapy and almost always there is an associated developmental delay or mental retardation. The EEG shows a pattern of irregular or slow spike-wave complexes at 2–2½ Hz in the presence of an abnormal background activity. This has been called a secondary corticoreticular epilepsy, implying diffuse cortical pathology.[4]

Generalized tonic-clonic seizures (previously called "grand mal" or "major motor seizures") are easily recognized, beginning with bilateral tonic extension of the extremities at the onset perhaps accompanied by a cry, followed by rhythmic jerking movements in a bilaterally synchronous manner. There may be associated foaming at the mouth, tongue-biting and urinary or fecal incontinence. Not all tonic-clonic seizures are generalized at onset, as partial seizures (simple or complex) may become secondarily generalized. A patient observed to have generalized clonic movements late in a seizure should not be presumed to have generalized tonic-clonic seizures unless a reliable report of the onset of the seizure indicates lack of focal onset. Tonic or clonic seizures show only one phase, either generalized tonic or clonic movements rather than the more common initial tonic posturing and then clonic movements of a tonic-clonic event. Some seizures are characterized as tonic-clonic-tonic because of the clinical sequence of movements recorded.

The EEG during a seizure may show only movement or muscle artifact which obscures the underlying electrographic changes or an epileptic recruiting rhythm consisting of an initially generalized attenuation of background activity, followed by an incremental-decremental pattern of gradually increasing amplitude rhythmic sharp discharges and gradually decreasing amplitude and frequency slower rhythmic discharges. The ictus is followed by a generalized depression of cerebral electrical activity.

Myoclonic seizures are clinically characterized by a synchronous and asymmetric brief jerking movements of a muscle or muscle group in one or more extremities. They may involve the trunk, causing flexion or, less commonly, extension movements characteristic of "infantile spasms" of early childhood (West's syndrome). Myoclonic seizures are also seen in generalized metabolic encephalopathies (e.g., uremia, hepatic failure), degenerative disorders (progressive myoclonic epilepsy, Lafora's disease, and cerebral lipidosis) and infectious disease (e.g., subacute sclerosing panencephalitis, SSPE, due to measles virus). The EEG may show only evidence of generalized encephalopathy with or without EEG discharges synchronous with the myoclonic jerking movements, or may have periodic complexes or high amplitude discharges occurring at regular intervals (e.g., SSPE).

Atonic seizures are attacks of sudden loss of postural tone, resulting in a fall to the ground (previously "akinetic seizures" or "drop attacks"). There is usually loss of consciousness, but the attack may be so brief that the patient is unaware of any "blackout."

Unclassified seizures are epileptic seizures that cannot be classified by clinical or EEG criteria into any of the above categories. Often, data is inadequate for accurate classification and careful observation is necessary, perhaps on an in-patient basis. Occasionally, intensive monitoring with continuous EEG and concomittant videotape monitoring is necessary to classify some of these seizures accurately.

Only when the epileptic nature of a seizure and its proper category is accurately established can therapy be rationally based.

Status Epilepticus

By definition, status epilepticus is a state of recurrent seizures without recovery of baseline neurological status in between the seizures. The International Classification of Epileptic Seizures proposes that this includes any type of seizure that "persists for a sufficient length of time or is repeated frequently enough that recovery between attacks does not occur".[6] In general this includes clinical or EEG seizure activity that lasts 30 minutes or more. The Classification of Status Epilepticus (Table 6.3) follows closely the International Classification of Epileptic Seizures as recently modified and is divided into convulsive status epilepticus and non-convulsive status epilepticus (Table 6.3).

The most common and most serious type is generalized tonic-clonic status epilepticus. This carries a mortality of about 10 percent even with the best

Table 6.3 Classification of Status Epilepticus

I. Convulsive Status
  A. Generalized tonic-clonic status
  B. Partial motor status ("epilepsia partialis continua")
II. Non-Convulsive Status
  A. Absence status (petit mal status)
  B. Complex partial status (psychomotor status)
  C. Partial sensory status

(Modified from ILAE: Proposal for revised clinical and electroencephalographic classification of epileptic seizures. Epilepsia, 22:489, 1981 Raven Press, New York; with permission).

current management. Neurological morbidity is also considerable. Once clinically diagnosed by observation of a generalized tonic-clonic seizure prior to recovery of full consciousness from the preceding seizure, aggressive medical therapy should be instituted in an attempt to terminate the status within the first 30 minutes. This is considered a critical time period, following which time oxygen tension in the brain falls, together with exhaustion of metabolic substrates, which may lead to irreversible brain damage. The treatment is discussed below under Management of Seizure Disorders.

Interpretation of cerebrospinal fluid (CSF) findings requires some caution as status epilepticus is known to give rise to fever (usually of a mild to moderate degree, unless pathologic hyperthermia is present), as well as CSF pleocytosis (usually mononuclear cells in small numbers) and increased CSF protein. Before therapy is initiated for meningitis, a careful microscopic examination of a Gram stain preparation of the CSF and comparison of CSF glucose with blood glucose (normal ratio is greater than 0.6) is warranted. If in doubt, antimicrobial therapy with penicillin and chloramphenicol is warranted, until bacterial culture results are available. (see Chapter 19).

Non-convulsive status epilepticus may present with a "twilight state" of decreased responsiveness, either continuously or intermittently (as in complex partial or psychomotor status). The diagnosis is often confirmed by EEG recordings which can also provide confirmation of a therapeutic response (although temporary) to IV diazepam 5–10 mg IV over 2–5 minutes.

Case 2

Mrs. M.T. was a 56-year-old right-handed woman with a past history of absences (called "petit mal") in her childhood, but without any recurrence since her adolescence. At breakfast one morning her husband suddenly noticed that she was only intermittently responsive, answering his questions with a "yes" or a "no." Occasionally she fumbled with her clothes and appeared dazed. In the office, her physician noted intermittent confusion, with delays in answering questions lasting up to several seconds. She was disoriented and had marked impairment of recall and memory. Occasionally, eyelid flutter was noted as well as automatisms including a few chewing movements and a fine jerking of the outstretched hands. An EEG showed slightly irregular generalized spike-wave complexes at 3 Hz, which responded promptly to diazepam 5 mg IV with normalization of the EEG. Her "twilight state" also cleared dramatically within a few seconds, although she was completely amnesic for the episode.

It should be noted that absence status (exemplified by Case 2) may also occur *de novo* in an adult, without a prior history of seizures.

Atypical Presentations

The patient with a seizure disorder (previously known or unknown) may present in a twilight state of fluctuating impaired consciousness. The differential diagnosis includes non-convulsive status epilepticus (absence status or complex partial status), metabolic-toxic encephalopathy, transient global amnesia and conversion reaction. An EEG is very helpful and is often diagnostic, particularly in cases of non-convulsive status epilepticus.

Other unusual presentations of seizure disorders include:

1. poor school performance

2. frequent automobile accidents

3. "day-dreaming" episodes

4. myoclonic jerking

5. hypersomnolence on arousal in the morning

6. enuresis

7. "nightmares" or "night terrors"

8. "hypoglycemic" attacks

9. aphasic or dysphasic episodes

10. acute "psychotic" episodes

Alcohol-Related Seizures ("Rum Fits")

These are usually generalized tonic-clonic seizures occurring in adults who abuse alcohol. They may occur during bouts of heavy drinking, or within a few hours to days of cessation of drinking. Most alcoholics with "rum fits" do not have epileptic seizures. A minority may have epileptic seizures precipitated by alcohol consumption or withdrawal, or may have complications of alcoholism resulting in cerebral injury (e.g., head injury from falls) and subsequent epileptic seizures. But in most cases, the EEG is non-epileptiform, although an exaggerated response to photic stimulation (photomyoclonic response) may occur.

These are not usually treated with anti-epileptic drugs (AEDs). The commonly used drugs have not proved efficacious. However, status epilepticus precipitated by alcohol withdrawal should be treated as a medical emergency. The drugs of choice include paraldehyde, valproic acid, vitamin B replacement (Thiamine) and fluids. Exclusion of a more life-threatening underlying cause (e.g., subdural hematoma) is necessary and requires admission, particularly if this is a first episode.

Post-Traumatic Seizures

Seizures that occur within the first week of non-penetrating head trauma, including the immediate post-traumatic period, are not considered epileptic and do not necessarily predispose to recurrent seizures. They may require short-term AED therapy for control of seizure activity. Although useful, the EEG is not necessarily diagnostic of an epileptic tendency.

After the first week, however, the occurrence of post-traumatic seizures is associated with a significant tendency towards chronicity and recurrence, particularly in the presence of significant neurologic deficit, an epileptiform EEG pattern or a positive family history of epilepsy. Such patients should be treated with the usual AED used for control of partial seizures: carbamazepine, phenytoin, primidone or phenobarbital.

Penetrating head injuries are associated with a high incidence of post-traumatic seizures (most studies suggesting about 50 percent incidence). Anti-epileptic therapy is usually indicated, as well as the management of the local cerebral injury (debridement, evacuation of clot, closure of meninges and skull defect, etc.).

Seizures In The Elderly

These often indicate the presence of an underlying neurological disorder affecting this age group, most commonly cerebrovascular in origin (cerebral infarction). Other causes include degenerative diseases (e.g., Alzheimer's or Parkinson's disease), post-traumatic scars, tumors or systemic disorders. For instance, epilepsia partialis continua may be the first manifestation of non-ketotic hyperosmolar coma in diabetics.

Symptomatic Seizures[13]

> **Case 3**
> Mr. G.D. was a 45-year-old right-handed construction worker who was well until his first seizure. This was preceded by an aura of a "horrible smell," followed by a "foul taste in my mouth," lasting a

few seconds. Then he lost consciousness. He was noted to make rhythmic chewing and swallowing movements, while staring blankly for about 1½ minutes. He returned slowly to responsiveness, but complained of a throbbing right-sided headache. His examination revealed mild left facial weakness most notable during involuntary facial movements. There was also a left superior visual field defect on confrontation. EEG showed a moderate number of spikes recorded from the right temporal region with nasopharyngeal electrodes. CT scan revealed a hypodense lesion in the right temporal lobe, near the region of the uncus. This proved to be a low-grade glioma at operation.

PRINCIPLE 1: It should be remembered that seizures are a symptom of cerebral disease and not a disease entity in themselves.

THE CLINICAL EXAM[14]

The important questions to try and answer during the history taking and physical examination are:

1. Is it an epileptic seizure?

2. What type of seizure is it?

3. Is there an underlying cause (symptomatic seizure) or is it idiopathic epilepsy?

4. Are there any complications of the seizure (e.g., scalp laceration from a fall, aspiration, etc.)?

History

Because there is often loss or impairment of consciousness during the seizure, the patient may not be able to give a full account of the ictus itself. However, his recollection of pre-ictal events is extremely important to elicit. An aura of abnormal sensation, emotion, thought or movement almost always signifies that the seizure has been focal or partial in onset, despite a subsequent "generalized tonic-clonic" seizure (due to secondary spread of the paroxysmal discharge from the focus). The presence of amnesia for the events preceding the seizure may point to temporal lobe pathology involving the hippocampus, or may reflect a retrograde amnesia of cerebral concussion if this occurred when the patient fell.

The ictal events are best described by a reliable witness who should be questioned closely for details. Where did the movements first begin? Did the eyes or head move in any particular direction at the onset of the seizure? Was the patient responsive or were there automatisms? Automatisms, including lip-smacking, swallowing, chewing and biting movements, strongly suggest the presence of a complex partial seizure involving limbic structures. On the other hand, pure motor or sensory symptoms, with or without spread (Jacksonian march) may be well described by the patient as consciousness is retained. Generalized tonic-clonic movements are not recalled by the patient, unless they are hysterical or due to malingering.

Post-ictal changes are also important. Was the patient able to move both sides of his face equally well? Was his head or were his eyes deviated toward one side? Did he move his arms and legs equally well on both sides? When the post-ictal confusion had cleared was there persistent impairment of speech or language expression or comprehension? Was he able to recall any aura (e.g., déjà vu, hallucinations, fear, epigastric sensation)? The duration of the seizure and of post-ictal changes is ascertained. Witnesses tend to exaggerate the duration of anxiety-provoking events such as seizures. If seizures are recurrent, a reliable family member or friend can be taught to observe and time these episodes objectively.

Physical Exam

The general physical examination provides important clues about the possible cause of the seizure disorder. Characteristic skin changes may suggest a neurocutaneous syndrome (e.g., Sturge-Weber with a facial hemangioma and underlying cerebral angiomatosis). An asymmetry of facial features or of the extremities (best assessed by comparing thumbnails, hands and feet) with a hemiatrophy points to an early-life contralateral hemispheric damage. A cranial bruit in a young patient with partial seizures suggests an underlying arteriovenous malformation. Evidence of underlying cardiac, hepatic, renal or pulmonary disease suggests the possible symtomatic nature of the seizure disorder (Table 6.4).

The neurological exam should be thorough and directed towards the presence of any possible asymmetry of functions (Table 6.4). Facial asymmetry during voluntary or involuntary movements (e.g., flattened naso-labial fold)

Table 6.4 Clues Suggesting Possible Structural Etiology of Seizure Disorder

---

I. History:
  A. The first seizure in adult life, whether of the partial or secondarily generalized type.
  B. Presence of an aura at seizure onset suggests focal pathology.
  C. Uncinate fits (complex partial seizures with olfactory or gustatory aura) may be associated with a high incidence of glioma in the temporal lobe.
  D. Post-ictal focal symptoms (e.g., hemiparesis, dysphasia, unilateral hypethesia).
  E. Associated neurological symptoms of recent onset: headaches, nausea or vomiting, dysphasia, weakness or numbness.

II. Examination:
  A. Signs of raised intracranial pressure (e.g., papilledema, lethargy, irritability).
  B. Signs of meningeal irritation (e.g., stiff neck, Kernig's or Brudzinski's signs).
  C. Focal neurological deficits (e.g., hemiparesis, hemianesthesia, dysphasia or dyspraxia, visual field defect, hyperreflexia, Babinski's signs).
  D. Unilateral post-ictal (Todd's) paralysis.

---

suggests cortical involvement contralateral to the side of diminished movements. A mild hemiparesis may be seen only as a decreased arm swing while walking or as impaired rapid alternating digital movements. Any asymmetry of the muscle stretch reflexes should be carefully noted. Sensory findings may be present only on double simultaneous stimulation. A superior visual field defect may point to a structural lesion in the contralateral anterior temporal lobe, involving Meyer's loop of the optic radiations. Language disturbances (dysphasias) direct one's attention to the dominant hemisphere. Specific impairment in verbal memory reflects involvement of the dominant medial temporal region (including the hippocampus), whereas a similar deficit of non-verbal materials suggests non-dominant (almost always right-sided) temporal involvement. An initial post-ictal examination may be misleading and repeat assessment is often indicated. Signs of anti-convulsant toxicity (nystagmus, ataxia) are also important to note.

INDICATIONS FOR ADMISSION

The First Seizure

As a general rule, the adult patient who presents with a first seizure should be admitted for detailed investigation in the hospital. This applies not only to generalized tonic-clonic seizures (previously referred to as "grand mal" or "major motor seizures") but particularly to partial seizures because of the increased risk of a structural brain lesion being present. In cases of generalized tonic-clonic seizures related unequivocally to alcohol consumption, a reasonable alternative is to observe the patient closely overnight in the emergency room, reassess thoroughly when the patient is alert and able to cooperate with a full neurological examination, and discharge only when there is no question of an intracranial lesion, such as a subdural hematoma, precipitating the seizure. When there is any doubt, the wisest choice is to admit, observe carefully in hospital and conduct a thorough investigation including a CT scan and EEG and appropriate biochemical and CSF studies. Alcohol-withdrawal seizures should be managed in a similar manner if there is the slightest doubt regarding their nature or any suspicion of the presence of possible intracranial pathology.

On the other hand, the occasional adult who presents with unquestionable simple absence seizures, reproducible by hyperventilation for 2–3 minutes and has a normal neurological examination and a positive family history of the same condition, may be safely followed in the office or outpatient clinic with an EEG and a prescription for ethosuximide (Zarontin).

Loss Of Consciousness Of Undetermined Origin

These patients are also best investigated as in-patients, particularly if the question of cardiac syncope ("Stokes-Adams" attacks) vs. seizures arises. Often they need detailed cardiovascular *and* neurologic investigations to resolve the issue, including EKG, EEG, CT scan, echocardiography and biochemical tests to rule out conditions such as hypoglycemia, hyponatremia, hypocalcemia. At times, intensive monitoring with continuous recording of EEG and EKG for 24–72 hours may be necessary for a firm diagnosis, using a portable cassette recorder (e.g., Oxford Medilog), similar to the Holter monitor for EKG monitoring.

Symptomatic Seizures

These are associated with evidence of an underlying cause of the seizure, whether partial (e.g., due to a cerebral tumor or other space-occupying lesion in the brain) or generalized (e.g., due to a systemic disorder such as hypoglycemia). Almost always these require further investigations that are best performed on an in-patient basis, followed by the most appropriate therapy.

Intractable Seizures

These constitute another indication for admission. Sometimes, an underlying systemic problem (e.g., infection) may have exacerbated the seizure tendency. Recently the technique of *intensive monitoring* has been used to study these problems better.[10] This consists of continuous EEG and video-tape recording up to 24 hours at a time, recording interictal and ictal EEG and behavioral changes, as well as frequent assessment of plasma AED levels. Often, the information obtained is of great aid in defining the seizure type(s) and establishing the best possible drugs and doses needed to control the seizures.

The well-known chronic epileptic, however, who has a long history of poor compliance with medical treatment need not be admitted for every seizure. Careful physical assessment when the immediate post-ictal state is resolved, a blood sample for AED levels, and an estimated partial loading dose of the missed AED(s) may be all that is required. The partial loading dose is calculated from the formula: *Additional dose* $= V_D \times$ weight (in kg) $\times$ change in plasma level desired. V_D is the volume of distribution of the drug. For phenytoin V_D is 0.6 and this times the body weight equals 42 liters for a 70 kg man. Hence, the partial loading dose of phenytoin(Dilantin) or PHT needed to increase plasma level from 5 to 15 μg/L is given by 42 L $\times$ 10 μg/L $= 420$ mg. Table 6.5 shows the V_D for several other drugs. However, it should be remembered that even chronic epileptics may develop complications from falls (e.g., subdural hematoma), infections (perhaps from bone marrow supression caused by AEDs) or metabolic disorders (e.g., hyponatremia). Hence, a careful and thorough assessment is necessary, before discharging such a patient from the emergency room.

Status Epilepticus

Status epilepticus should always be managed as a neurologic emergency, followed by hospitalization to determine precipitating causes (e.g., AED withdrawal, central nervous system (CNS) infection, neoplasm, cerebrovas-

Table 6.5 Volume of Distribution (V_D) of Common Anti-Epileptic Drugs*

Drug	V_D (liters/kg)
Carbamazepine	0.8
Clonazepam	1.9
Diazepam	1.0
Ethosuximide	0.7
Phenobarbital	0.8
Phenytoin	0.6
Primidone	0.6
Valproate	0.18 (adults); 0.36 (children)

* Values are approximations of best studies available.

cular disease), and possible complications of the status (e.g., vertebral compression fractures, hypoxia, metabolic acidosis), and of the therapy (e.g., respiratory depression due to barbituates, heart block due to phenytoin). Even non-convulsive status epilepticus should be assessed by EEG (and CT scan for complex partial or psychomotor status) and clinical follow-up to ensure full recovery without relapse.

Psychosocial Admissions

Commonly, the patient with chronic epilepsy encounters numerous psychological and social stresses that may necessitate admission. Some develop pseudo-seizures or hysterical seizures, which are "intractable" to medical therapy and may be surprisingly difficult to distinguish from epileptic or "real" seizures.[7,8] These may require an experienced neurologist and a psychiatrist to diagnose, followed by supportive psychotherapy.

An intolerable family situation may result from an inability to cope with a member having frequent seizures requiring hospitalization of that member until the rest of the family has the time and opportunity to adjust to the new situation, perhaps through family therapeutic sessions.

Although aggressive behavior is rarely ictal, poorly directed violent behavior may accompany complex partial seizures, especially in the post-ictal period.[1] This may necessitate admission and appropriate management until such violent "acting-out" has subsided or adequately controlled by tranquilizers (e.g., haloperidol, Haldol).

LABORATORY INVESTIGATIONS[14]

These should be designed to discover the underlying cause of the seizures. The most common causes are naturally age-related. In childhood, seizures are commonly related to perinatal trauma or asphyxia, congenital malformations, metabolic, toxic or traumatic conditions but may be idiopathic. In adolescence, trauma, intoxications and infectious disorders are likely. In young adults, trauma and neoplasms are common, whereas in older adults, cerebrovascular disease (stroke), tumors and degenerative diseases are seen. Due to such a variety of causes, neither the traditional "4-pack" (EEG, brain scan, skull x-ray and lumbar puncture) or the newer "3-pack" (including CT scan, plain and with contrast enhancement replacing the skull X-ray and isotope brain scan) is adequate in all cases, although the latter may serve as a starting point in most cases presenting with their first seizures.

Biochemical Tests

Additional investigations to consider include biochemical tests for hepatic and renal functions, blood glucose, calcium, magnesium, electrolytes, hematological (complete hemogram including platelet count and sedimentation rate) and serological or immunological tests (e.g., VDRL, ANA). Occasionally, assessment of metabolites such as amino acids, organic acids and sialooligosaccharides in the urine may be necessary, particularly in children. A careful lumbar puncture with analysis of the CSF for cells, protein, glucose (with corresponding blood glucose), cultures and serology for syphilis is often indicated as well, particularly in cases of first seizures.

Radiological

Skull X-rays

Skull X-rays are usually not of much help in the diagnosis or management of patients with seizure disorders. In the acute setting they may be useful in ruling out a fracture or a shifted pineal, suggesting the presence of a mass lesion intracranially. In the epileptic with recurrent seizures, skull films may show pathological calcifications (in slow-growing tumors or congenital vascular malformation, such as Sturge-Weber). In patients with temporal lobe epilepsy an asymmetry of the cranium with thickening of the hemicranium on one side, elevation of the petrous pyramid and a smaller middle cranial fossa suggest an atrophic process affecting the ipsilateral cerebral hemisphere (e.g., perinatal injury). However, with the availability of the CT scan, skull X-rays are no longer a useful diagnostic test in most cases.

CT scan

The patient with a first seizure, generalized or partial, should have a CT scan as part of the initial assessment for underlying pathology. An exception is the patient with simple absence seizures ("petit mal") who has a normal neurological examination, and the characteristic 3 Hertz (Hz) spike and wave complexes on the EEG. Otherwise, both the plain CT and the contrast-enhanced CT scan should be obtained to increase the detection rate for cerebral lesions, and determine their vascularity and possible etiology.[3] Even patients with known epilepsy, who present with a change in the pattern of their seizures (frequency or type of seizures), or have new neurological symptoms (e.g., unexplained headaches) or signs should have CT scans. Epileptics are by no means immune from the cerebral afflictions of non-epileptics, and tumors may appear 5 or even 10 years after the onset of seizures. Moreover, many epileptics who have had a "complete work-up" in the pre-CT days may only have had a "4-pack" investigation, which is now considered inadequate without a CT scan.

Electroencephalography (EEG) [2,9]

The EEG is one of the few tests which is sensitive to cerebral function as opposed to structure (e.g., radiological investigations). Since epilepsy is primarily a disorder of function, it is to be expected that the EEG would be the diagnostic test of choice. However, certain points should be remembered:

1. Almost all EEGs are inter-ictal recordings, made when the patient is *not* having a seizure. Ictal EEGs in the routine 30–40 minute recording are rare but may be very informative. The usual interictal EEG may be disappointingly "non-diagnostic" or "non-epileptiform" in almost half the cases of clinical epileptic seizures. When clinically indicated, repeat EEGs can increase the probability of detecting epileptic activity.

2. Activation procedures performed in most EEG laboratories include intermittent photic stimulation and hyperventilation which tend to provoke generalized epilepsies of the absence type. These procedures are simple and with low risk, and should be part of most routine EEG tests.

3. In children and adolescents sleep deprivation for 24 hours followed by a spontaneous sleep EEG study may activate both generalized and partial epileptic seizures, including temporal lobe foci. In adults, sleep deprivation is less useful than pharmcologically induced sleep, using a short-acting barbituate (e.g., pentobarbital) and/or a phenothiazine (e.g., chlorpromazine), particularly for suspected temporal lobe epilepsy.

4. The use of special electrodes, such as nasopharyngeal or sphenoidal, permits the recording of electrical activity from infero-medial regions of the temporal lobes which are inaccessible to the usual scalp electrodes. These are indicated in cases of complex partial seizures when the routine EEG is non-diagnostic or non-epileptiform.

5. The diagnostic yield from several EEGs using the above activation procedures and electrodes is about 75 to 80 percent in patients with

epileptic seizures. The remainder may be diagnosed in special epilepsy centers by intensive monitoring,[10] withdrawal of AEDs or using depth electrodes implanted in the brain.

6. The possibility of pseudoseizures or hysterical seizures has to be considered when the EEG is normal during a generalized convulsion.[7,8]

MANAGEMENT OF SEIZURE DISORDERS[5,12]

General Principles

The principles to be kept in mind in the treatment of seizure disorder are summarized in Figure 6.1 and Table 6.6 (modified after Sherwin [12] and Goldberg [5]). Remember that seizures are a symptom of brain dysfunction, and an underlying cause has to be looked for in all new cases before a diagnosis of "idiopathic epilepsy" can be accepted. In cases with a demonstrable cause:

> **PRINCIPLE 2:** The proper treatment of symptomatic epilepsy is the treatment of the underlying cause.

The choice anti-epileptic drugs depends heavily on the seizure type. For partial seizures, whether simple or complex partial, with or without secondary generalization, the drugs of choice include carbamazepine, phenytoin, primidone and phenobarbital, although some studies have suggested that valproate, clonazepam and chlorazepate and methsuximide may be useful in some refractory cases of complex partial seizures. For generalized seizures of the tonic-clonic type, the primary drugs are the same as for the partial seizures.

However, for the other types of generalized seizures, the order of preference changes. For simple absences (typical "petit mal") ethosuximide is the drug of choice, with phenobarbital a second drug. Valproate should be reserved for refractory cases, because of possible fatal hepatoxicity. For atypical absences, atonic seizures and myoclonic seizures, valproate or clonazepam is recommended. Myoclonic seizures including infantile spasms, may respond to ACTH and/or a ketogenic diet. The combination of valproate and clonazepam should be used only with great caution because of possible precipitation of absence status epilepticus. Acetazolamide (Diamox) may be tried in children with generalized seizures which are intractable to the usual AEDs, or in women whose seizures are exacerbated in the perimenstrual period (catamenial epilepsy). The usual dose is 500–1000 mg/day in two to four divided doses. Electrolyte and fluid balance should be monitored regularly.

The value of monitoring plasma levels of anti-epileptic drugs has been established. It serves to detect poor compliance, drug preparations with

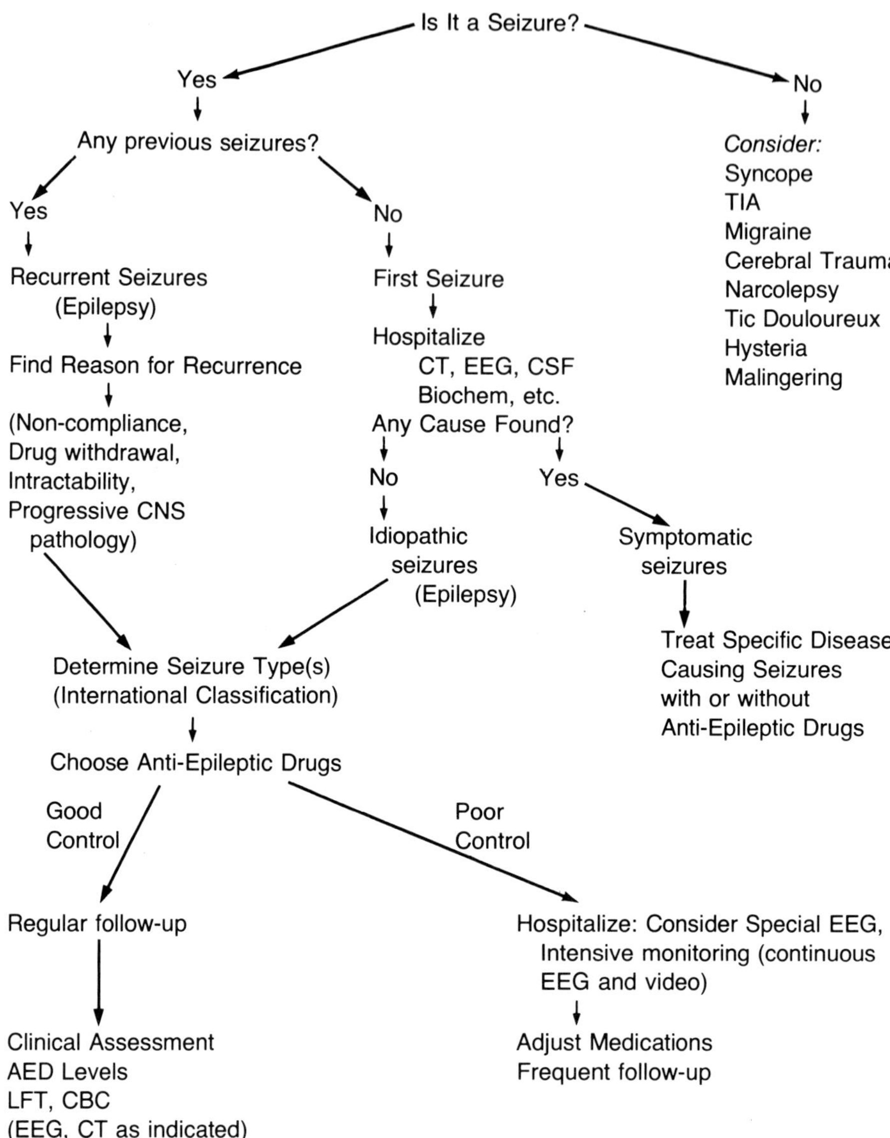

Fig. 6.1 Management flow chart for a suspected seizure.

decreased bioavailability, malabsorption, rapid or slow drug metabolizers, and interactions with other agents (AEDs as well as other drugs) and provide laboratory confirmation of suspected drug toxicity. This is particularly important in chronic epileptics who have "escaped" control or have proven "refractory" to medical therapy. Occasionally, such patients have to be admitted, and their plasma levels of AEDs carefully monitored, together with EEG

Table 6.6 Principles of Treatment of Seizures

   I. Establish the diagnosis and rule out underlying cerebral pathology.

  II. Classify seizure type, using clinical and EEG criteria.

 III. Select AED of first choice for seizure type.

 IV. Increase dose slowly till end-point is reached:
    A. Complete seizure control,
    B. Optimum plasma drug level, or
    C. Toxic side effects appear

  V. If poor seizure control, gradually withdraw first drug while replacing with second drug of choice for seizure type; monotherapy is preferable to polypharmacy.

 VI. If improvement is only partial, other drugs may be necessary.

VII. Adjust dose gradually according to plasma levels, keeping in mind:
    A. Pharmacokinetics of each drug
    B. Potential drug interactions

VIII. If best medical therapy is unsuccessful, refer to specialized epilepsy center for intensive monitoring and possible surgical therapy.

(Modified after Sherwin, A. L.: Pharmacological principles in the management of patient with epilepsy. p. 211. In Meinardi, H., Rowan, A.J., eds.: Advances in Epileptology, 1977, Swets and Zeitlinger, B.V., Amsterdam, 1978; with permission).

and behavioral changes by "intensive monitoring." [10] Some characteristics of commonly employed AEDs are provided in Table 6.7. Notice that most AEDs may be taken once or twice daily and still provide adequate plasma levels because of their long half-lives. Exceptions are valproate and primidone (the parent compound). Factors causing low serum levels include: poor bioavailability of a particular drug preparation and malabsorption by the gastrointestinal tract of the patient or competition with other agents being ingested at the same time. Abnormal degrees of protein binding may affect total plasma level of AED measured (e.g., renal or hepatic failure). Rapid metabolism due to genetic influences ("fast metabolizers") or drug interaction (e.g., phenobarbital induces phenytoin metabolism by the liver) may occur. Total body water or the volume of distribution of the drug can change in edematous states and in pregnancy. Finally, perhaps most commonly, non-compliance on the part of the patient is a serious problem requiring much effort in education.

Management Of Status Epilepticus

> **PRINCIPLE 3:** Generalized status epilepticus is a neurologic emergency and should be treated immediately.

The principles of management are outlined in Table 6.8. A vigorous attempt should be made to control the seizure activity within 30 minutes, before falling tissue O_2 concentration results in irreversible brain damage, particularly to hippocampus, cerebral cortex and cerebellum. Once the ABC's of resuscitation (*A*irway, *B*reathing, *C*irculation) are assured and appropriate

Table 6.7 Characteristics of Common Anti-Epileptic Drugs (AED)

Drug	Trade Name	Usual Adult Dosage mg/day (mg/kg/day)	Therapeutic Plasma Level (µg/ml)	Approximate Half-Life (hrs)	Remarks
Carbamazepine (CBZ)	Tegretol	600–1200 (10–20)	4–12	8–24	Risk of blood dyscrasia Requires CBC, platelets, LFTs
Phenytoin (PHT)	Dilantin	300–500 (4–7)	10–20	16–24	Gingival hyperplasia, hirsutism drug interactions Saturable enzyme kinetics Requires LFTs, CBC
Primidone (PRM)	Mysoline	750–1500 (10–20)	6–12	6	Metabolized to PB
Phenobarbital (PB)	—	90–250 (2–4)	15–30	96	Learning disability, hyperactivity, sedation, lethargy
Valproate (VPA)	Depakene	1000–2500 (15–30)	50–100	6	Hepatotoxicity, interacts with PHT and PB, tremor, alopecia, GI up-set
Clonazepam	Clonopin Rivitrol	1.5–20 (0.02–0.3)	0.015–0.075	30	Sedation, ataxia, personality change;
Ethosuximide (ESM)	Zarontin	500–1000 (7–15)	40–100	50	GI upset, drowsiness, ataxia, rarely hematological suppression. May increase generalized tonic-clonic seizures.

Table 6.8 Treatment of Generalized Tonic-Clonic Status Epilepticus in Adults

I. Ascertain diagnosis of status epilepticus, and determine cause if possible.

II. Baseline blood tests: antiepileptic drug plasma levels, biochemistry, hemogram, arterial blood gases.

III. IV infusion: 50 ml 50% glucose solution (with Thiamine 100 mg if vitamin deficiency is suspected, e.g. alcoholics).

IV. Diazepam 10 mg IV at 2 mg/min infusion. Monitor respirations, blood pressure, heart rate. Repeat in 10–20 minutes if seizures recur. Maximum 20 mg.

V. Phenytoin (Dilantin) 18 mg/kg IV at a rate of not more than 50 mg/min, with EKG monitoring and frequent vital signs as above. Usually a dose of 1200 mg is used (for 70 kg man). If seizures continue 20 minutes after initial loading dose, a further 7 mg/kg may be given (usually about 500 mg additionally) to give a total of 25 mg/kg.

VI. Phenobarbital at a rate of no more than 100 mg/min may be infused until the seizures stop, or a maximum of 20 mg/kg (average 1400 mg for 70 kg adult) is given. Intubation and respiratory assistance is required at this point.

VII. General anesthesia should be administered if status continues 30 minutes after the phenobarbital infusion. The choice of agents include:
 A. Short-acting barbituate with antiepileptic action that can be measured in the plasma (e.g., sodium amytal);
 B. Inhalation anesthetics (e.g., halothane);
 C. Neuromuscular blocks may be necessary to control motor manifestations and allow adequate ventilation. The response to AEDs can then be determined by EEG monitoring.

VIII. Other agents to consider in intractable status epilepticus:
 A. Valproic acid (rectal administration of suspension)
 B. Lorazepam (Ativan)
 C. Paraldehyde solution (15 ml with equal volume of mineral oil) rectally administered, particularly for status epilepticus precipitated by alcohol withdrawal, and for children;
 D. Hypothermia, using external cooling (e.g., blanket with circulatory coolant) to lower body temperature to about 32° C.
 E. Steroids to control cerebral edema resulting from status epilepticus (e.g., Dexamethasone 10 mg IV initially, then 4 mg every 6 hours).

blood studies initiated, diazepam is infused intravenously. Both diazepam and phenytoin should be injected separately and directly in the tubing close to the IV site, but each drug may also be dissolved in a small volume of isotonic saline and infused slowly at the rates indicated. Cardio-respiratory depression should be watched for closely, as well as possible heart block with phenytoin. The combination of diazepam and phenobarbital is particularly liable to cause respiratory depression, and intubation with respiratory assistance is often necessary. Paraldehyde may be administered rectally while waiting for the anesthesiologist to provide general anesthesia, when the above measures have not been successful in terminating the status within about 30 minutes. The search for an underlying cause or precipitating factor must not be forgotten, as localized lesions such as brain tumors or subdural hematomas may present with convulsive status epilepticus.

Non-convulsive status epilepticus almost always requires the use of an EEG for definitive diagnosis. Diazepam 5–10 mg IV administered during the EEG produces the characteristic abolition of epileptic activity which is diagnostic. The appropriate long-term AED is then begun: ethosuximide or valproate for absence status, phenytoin or carbamazepine for complex partial status. The above regimen may be modified in cases of drug withdrawal status epilepticus, when the anticonvulsant withdrawn should be used first.

It should be remembered that an underlying acute CNS insult often is a precipitating cause. The ominous causes include acute cerebrovascular injury, anoxia, trauma, infections and neoplasms. As soon as the acute emergency is under control, an attempt to uncover the underlying pathology should be made. This may require the use of EEG, CT scan (plain and with contrast enhancement), CSF studies (including cells, cultures, protein, glucose and appropriate immunological studies), biochemical and microbiological studies (see "Intractable Seizures" above).

CONCLUSION

Inasmuch as most epileptics have a number of problems of everyday living, in addition to the seizures, the medical treatment of their seizures is not adequate in itself. Often, the patients have problems understanding and adjusting to their illness with the accompanying social stigma. They need assistance in obtaining education, employment, automobile licenses, and in establishing social relationships. Adequate follow-up includes attention to all these areas, and often the help of a social worker or psychologist or the resources of the local epilepsy association (which may be a branch of the Epilepsy Foundation of America) may be necessary. But supervision by an understanding and knowledgeable physician in the overall care of a patient with a seizure disorder is indispensable, for both acute emergencies and subsequent long-term management.

ACKNOWLEDGMENTS

Supported in part by an NIH grant for Biomedical Research Support (BRSG-0537) to University of Colorado Health Sciences Center, and by the Pearce Bailey Foundation for Neurological Research.

REFERENCES

1. Delgado-Escueta, A.V.: The nature of aggression during epileptic seizures. N. Eng. J. Med., 305:711, 1981.
2. Gastaut, H.: Epilepsies. p. 1. In Rémond, A., ed.: Handbook of EEG and Clinical Neurophysiology, Vol. 13, Part A, 1975.
3. Gastaut, H., Gastaut, J.L.: Computerized axial tomography in epilepsy. p. 5. In Penry, J.K., ed.: The Eighth Epilepsy International Symposium, Raven Press, New York, 1977.

4. Gloor, P.: The 1977 William G. Lennox Lecture. Epilepsia, 20:571, 1979.
5. Goldberg, M.A.: Pharmacological strategies in the treatment of epilepsy. Semin. Neurol., 1:81, 1981.
6. ILAE: Proposal for revised clinical and electroencephalographic classification of epileptic seizures. Epilepsia, 22:489, 1981.
7. King, D.W., et al.: Pseudoseizures: Diagnostic evaluation. Neurology, 32:18, 1982.
8. Massay, E.W., Riley, T.L.: Pseudoseizures: recognition and treatment. Psychosomatics, 21:987, 1980.
9. McIntyre, H.B., Goldberg, A.S.: The knowledgeable use of the EEG in seizure disorders. Semin. Neurol., 1:77, 1981.
10. Penry, J.K.: Intensive monitoring of epileptic patients. p. 29. In Wada, J., Penry, J.K. eds: Advances in Epileptology: The Tenth Epilepsy International Symposium, Raven Press, New York, 1980.
11. Rasmussen, T.: Cortical resection for medically intractable refractory focal epilepsy: results, lessons and questions, p. 253. In Rasmussen, T., Marino, R. eds.: Functional Neurosurgery, Raven Press, New York, 1979.
12. Sherwin, A.L.: Pharmacological principles in the management of patient with epilepsy. p. 211. In Meinardi, H., Rowan, A.J., eds.: Advances in Epileptology, 1977, Swets and Zeitlinger, B.V., Amsterdam, 1978.
13. Treiman, D.M.: Seizure types and causes of epilepsy. Semin. Neurol., 1:65, 1981.
14. Walter, R.D.: Evaluation of the patient with a suspected seizure disorder. Semin. Neurol., 1:61, 1981.
15. Walter, R.D., Ed.: Epilepsy. Semin. Neurol., 1:1, June, 1981.

7

Emergency Diagnosis and Management of Brain Infarctions and Hemorrhages

Michael P. Earnest, M.D.

"When I woke up I had a bit of a headache and thought I must have been sleeping with my right arm under me because it felt all pins-and-needly and numb and I couldn't make it do what I wanted. I got out of bed but I couldn't stand; as a matter of fact I actually fell on the floor because my right leg was too weak to take my weight. I called out to my wife in the next room and no sound came—I couldn't speak. . . . I was astonished, horrified. I couldn't believe that this was happening to me and I began to feel bewildered and frightened and then I suddenly realized that I must have had a stroke."*

INTRODUCTION

Cerebrovascular disease is the third-leading cause of morbidity and mortality in the United States. Each year in the United States over 500,000 persons suffer a stroke ("cerebrovascular accident"). Only one-third return to normal function or regain enough function to be self-sustaining in activities of daily living. These statistics emphasize that stroke is a common disease, and one the general physician must often treat.

Unfortunately, patients with strokes have been too often considered by the physician to have an untreatable disease. So the management plan has consisted of bed rest, some routine admission laboratory tests, a few days' observation and nursing care, some physical therapy, and then discharge to home or to a nursing home. That management schema may be appropriate in a few cases, but is grossly inappropriate in the vast majority. The

---

* (Gardner, H.: *The Shattered Mind - The Person After Brain Damage*, p. 402. Alfred A. Knopf, New York, 1975.)

physician has an urgent responsibility whenever he faces a stroke patient to understand the process as completely as possible and to reverse it or, failing to reverse it, preserve as much functioning brain tissue as possible. Physicians treat cardiovascular emergencies immediately and vigorously; even more so should they treat a cerebrovascular emergency, a stroke.

The reasons for vigorously treating an acute stroke are:

1. Brain damage from cerebrovascular disease is not immediately lethal to the nervous tissue. It often progresses over the first few hours. It also may be reversed by aggressive treatment, in some instances.

2. Dysfunctional brain tissue surrounding the dead area can be preserved until normal healing processes (e.g., development of collateral circulation) can restore its function.

3. The brain sometimes responds to cerebrovascular lesions in self-destructive ways (e.g., edema and arterial vasospasm). Those harmful reactions can sometimes be prevented or treated.

Unfortunately, there are no means currently available to totally reverse the damage done by a brain infarction or hemorrhage. However, every gram of brain tissue preserved by aggressive treatment increases the patient's chances for survival and recovery of a meaningful life. Every neurologic function retained improves the patient's chances for successful rehabilitation.

THE ANATOMY AND PATHOPHYSIOLOGY OF BRAIN DAMAGE FROM CEREBROVASCULAR DISEASE

The brain is supplied by two major vascular systems, the carotid system, or anterior circulation, and the vertebrobasilar, or posterior circulation (Figs. 7.1 and 7.2). Each system originates from the aortic arch as a pair of vessels, the right and left common carotid arteries and right and left vertebral arteries. The common carotid arteries ascend in the anterior neck and bifurcate at about the angle of the mandible into the external carotid and internal carotid arteries. The external vessels supply the face, pharynx, mouth and scalp. The internal carotid arteries enter the skull and are the major suppliers of blood to the respective cerebral hemispheres. Just after entering the skull, each internal carotid artery gives off a branch to the orbit, the ophthalmic artery (shown, but not labelled, in Fig. 7.1), which supplies the optic nerve and retina. This vessel is an important one for clinical diagnosis of cerebrovascular lesions (see below).

Each vertebral artery ascends in the posterolateral neck and enters the vertebral canal, running through the transverse processes of the first six cervical vertebrae. It then enters the intracranial cavity through the foramen

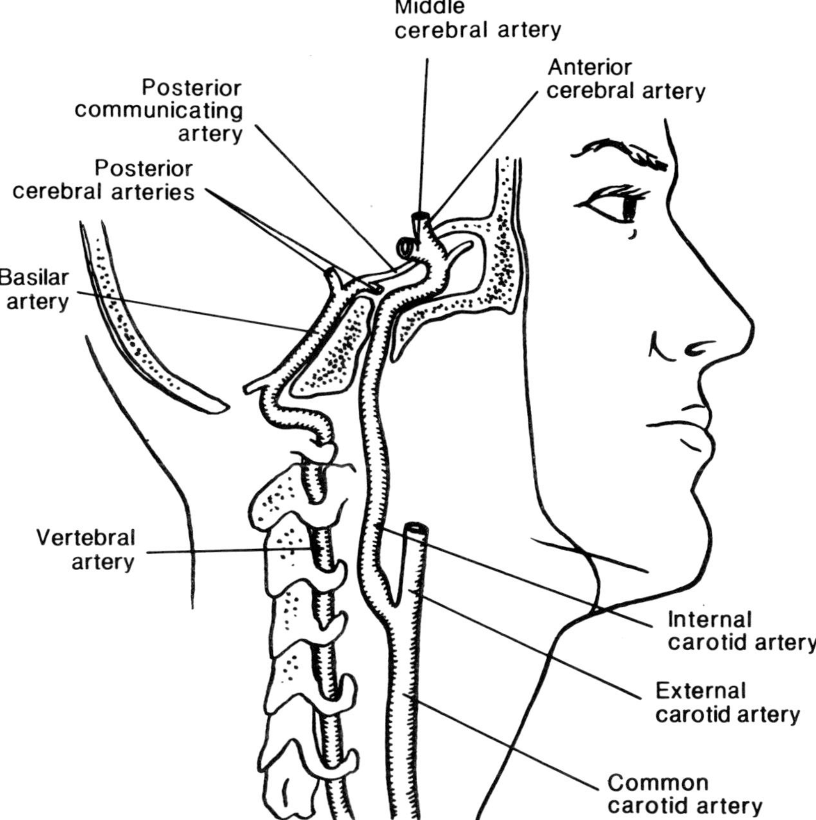

Fig. 7.1 The major vessels to the brain. The internal carotid, anterior and middle cerebral arteries comprise the anterior circulation. The vertebral, basilar and posterior cerebral arteries and branches comprise the posterior circulation. (Adapted from an original painting, by Frank H. Netter, M.D. from The CIBA Collection of Medical Illustrations, copyright by CIBA Pharmaceutical Company, Division of CIBA-GEIGY Corporation; reprinted with permission).

magnum. The two arteries join to form the basilar artery at the junction of the medulla with the pons. The basilar artery then divides into the two posterior cerebral arteries (Fig. 7.2).

The anterior and posterior circulations communicate with each other, and the right and left carotid system communicate as well, by the Circle of Willis (Fig. 7.2). This network of vascular connections at the base of the brain is usually an anatomically complete channel that allows blood to flow from the anterior circulation into the posterior territory, or vice versa, or from the right or left carotid to the opposite hemisphere whenever the primary vessel is occluded or severely stenosed. However, there are frequent normal variations of this collateral system so one or more communicating

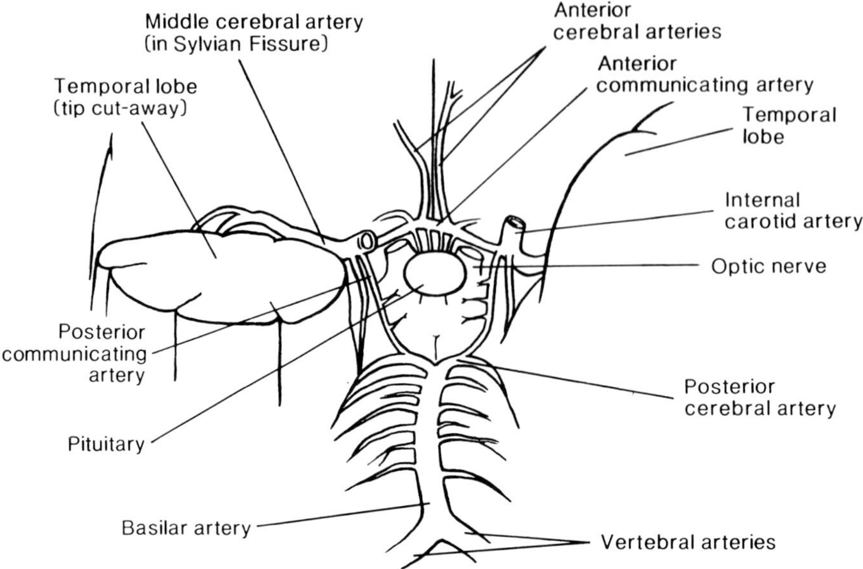

Fig. 7.2 The Circle of Willis seen from below the brain. (Adapted from Truex and Carpenter, Human Neuroanatomy. 6th Ed. Williams & Wilkins Co., Baltimore, 1969; reprinted with permission).

channels are atrophic or even absent. Such variations explain some of the clinical differences between patients with the same vascular lesion. A carotid occlusion in a person with a fully patent Circle of Willis can be totally asymptomatic, but in the person with an incomplete Circle is more likely to produce a massive cerebral infarction.

There are two major vascular processes causing the clinical syndrome physicians call "a stroke" (Table 7.1). These are vascular obstruction, causing ischemic brain infarction, and vascular rupture, causing intracranial hemorrhage. Within each of these two broad categories there are two distinct subgroups of mechanisms. Vascular obstruction and ischemic brain infarction can be caused either by a vessel developing an *in situ* thrombus, or an embolus may travel from a source more proximal in the blood stream and then lodge in a vessel of the cerebrovascular system, thus blocking blood flow to a part of the brain. Intracranial hemorrhage also has two distinctly different causes. One type of hemorrhage, the subarachnoid hemorrhage, occurs in the subarachnoid space, on the surface of the brain, and is caused by rupture of an aneurysm. Such aneurysms usually result from congenital weakness of a vessel wall at a branching junction, but may result from localized infection or trauma. The second type of intracranial hemorrhage, the intracerebral hemorrhage, occurs because of the rupture of a small vessel within the substance of the brain.[21] Such hemorrhages usually occur deep within the cerebral hemisphere but may occur elsewhere. The

Table 7.1 Pathologic Mechanisms Causing a Stroke

Ischemic Infarction	Intracranial Hemorrhage
Thrombosis of an artery *in situ*	Subarachnoid hemorrhage
Embolism from a distant site	Intracerebral hemorrhage
Spasm (rare)	

most common cause of such hemorrhages is chronic systemic hypertension, which has damaged the small penetrating arterioles of the brain.

Initial Management Of The Stroke Patient

Transient stroke-like symptoms may occur and then resolve within a few hours. (Those syndromes are discussed in Chapter 8.) However, when the physician faces the patient with a stroke syndrome in the emergency room, he cannot predict the future and must assume that the patient's symptoms will persist and he must worry that the symptoms will get worse. When faced by such a patient the clinician should have a method for managing the patient that is comprehensive and detailed. He should have a clear differential diagnosis, know how to make a specific diagnosis and then should be able to effectively manage the specific problem diagnosed.

Table 7.2 outlines a rational process that is a helpful framework for managing a stroke patient. The steps outlined give a comprehensive management plan and the appropriate sequence in which they should be taken.

The first step in managing the stroke patient is to prove that, indeed, the patient does have a stroke. A definition of stroke must be clear in the physician's mind: a focal neurological dysfunction of acute onset caused by cerebrovascular disease. The dysfunction usually lasts more than 24 hours.

A stroke, then, is initially defined by: (1) a sudden onset (usually the course

Table 7.2 Management of the Stroke Patient—Requirements for Comprehensive Care

I. Emergency management
  A. Prove it's a stroke
  B. Define the mechanism of damage
  C. Localize the lesion
  D. Preserve brain tissue
  E. Consider an angiogram
II. Management in the next few days
  A. Prevent progression
  B. Look for associated conditions
  C. Prevent complications
  D. Rehabilitate early
  E. Plan discharge
  F. Prevent future strokes

from the onset of symptoms to development of clinically obvious signs requires a few hours or less); and (2) focal neurological signs, (a hemiparesis, hemianopsia, aphasia, hemisensory deficit, cranial nerve, cerebellar signs, etc.). As mentioned above, the physician cannot predict if the patient's symptoms will persist or will be transient, but he must prove that the patient's problem is being caused by cerebrovascular disease. Other diseases that can present with stroke-like syndromes, but which must be distinguished from stroke, are brain tumor, brain abscess, encephalitis and subdural hematoma. These must be diagnosed early in the patient's course because failure to diagnose them will result in inappropriate treatment (i.e., treatment as a stroke) and may lead to permanent brain injury or death from the nonstroke lesion.

The first tool to use in making an early, presumptive diagnosis of stroke, and ruling out the other lesions, is the history. The age of the patient is usually helpful. Strokes usually occur in older people, so a young patient with a stroke-like presentation must be carefully screened for a non-cerebrovascular lesion. The nature of the onset of symptoms is also helpful. Cerebrovascular disease usually presents with an acute onset. From the first mild symptoms to maximum symptoms, or until the patient is brought to the physician, is usually only a few hours. A good rule of thumb is: *Any stroke-like syndrome with a duration of onset (i.e., the time from first symptoms to the maximum symptoms) of longer than 24 hours is unlikely to be due to cerebrovascular disease.* Other etiologies must be ruled out.

Another helpful type of onset is the very acute onset. If the patient's symptoms progressed from no symptoms to severe ones within minutes, or less than 1 hour, the most likely diagnoses are embolic ischemic brain infarction or intracranial hemorrhage. The nonvascular processes of tumor, abscess, subdural hematoma, encephalitis rarely progress that rapidly.

The general physical examination may also be helpful in distinguishing cerebrovascular lesions from non-vascular ones. Fever suggests possible brain abscess, meningitis or encephalitis. A stiff neck also suggests nervous system infection. The examination of the cardiovascular system may also help, but is seldom definitive. For example, the presence of atrial fibrillation or a carotid bruit or an absent carotid pulse suggests a stroke but does not rule out a brain tumor or any other non-vascular etiology for the neurologic syndrome.

The neurologic examination is mainly helpful in distinguishing vascular from non-vascular etiologies by focusing on the patient's level of consciousness. Ischemic cerebrovascular disease usually does *not* cause depression of consciousness. If the patient has prominent focal signs and yet is alert, the most probable cause is a brain infarction from ischemic cerebrovascular disease. However, if the patient has a depressed level of consciousness, the non-vascular lesions, as well as intracranial hemorrhage, must be considered and ruled out.

Next, the physician should consider the possible mechanisms of the patient's stroke.

What Is The Mechanism Of The Stroke?

When an older patient presents with an acute-onset hemiparesis and the patient is alert, the doctor can reasonably diagnose a stroke. However, the physician should also try to discover the mechanism of the cerebrovascular event. Does the patient have a brain infarction, and if so, was it caused by an embolus or an *in situ* thrombus? Or does he have an intracranial hemorrhage, and is it primarily a subarachnoid hemorrhage or an intracerebral one?

Table 7.3 outlines some historical clues and findings on examination that help distinguish ischemic infarctions from intracranial hemorrhages. However, the clinical distinction, without use of laboratory tests, between embolic or thrombotic infarctions and between subarachnoid and intracerebral hemorrhages, is often very difficult. Also, no one of the clues and signs suggesting brain infarction or intracranial hemorrhage is diagnostic; they merely help guide the physician's thinking.

The history of a typical intracerebral hemorrhage illustrates the distinctions. The patient usually has onset of a severe headache that within minutes progresses in severity and is accompanied by nausea and vomiting, depression of alertness and focal signs, often a hemiparesis. The onset commonly is while the patient is up and active. The physician finds the patient has severe hypertension, and often has a history of chronic hypertension. In contrast, the patient with an ischemic infarct usually has the onset at rest or while asleep and has a stepwise or remitting, waxing and waning symptom course for the first few hours. The patient is alert and usually has no headache. The presence, on examination, of cardiac valvular disease or atrial fibrillation suggests the probability of an embolus to the brain.

However, as when trying to rule out a non-vascular etiology, the physician, to be sure of the nature of the vascular process, should employ a radiologic test.

Table 7.3 Historical Clues and Signs on Physical Examination that Help Distinguish Brain Infarction from Intracranial Hemorrhage*

Brain Infarction	Intracranial Hemorrhage
History	
Stepwise onset and progression of symptoms	Sudden onset of severe symptoms
Onset at rest or while asleep	Onset while active
Prior similar, but transient, focal symptoms	Prominent headache, nausea or vomiting
General Examination	
Obvious cardiac valvular disease	Severe hypertension
Cardiac arrhythmia	
Neurologic Examination	
Patient is alert	Patient obtunded
	Large hemorrhages in the retina

* These features are common but not invariable

Radiologic Tests In The Early Management Of The Stroke Patient

The three radiologic tests most helpful in the early management of a stroke patient are the computerized tomograms of the head (the CT scan), the radioisotope brain scan and the arteriogram. The quickest and most definitive test is the CT scan. It can, in most instances, clearly distinguish between cerebrovascular lesions and nonvascular ones, and can often define the actual mechanism of a cerebrovascular event.[11,27] Table 7.4 describes the features shown on CT scan by the various lesions. Figures 7.3, 7.6 and 7.7 illustrate common vascular lesions.

A specific clinical problem illustrates the use of the CT scan. A 55-year-old alcoholic patient presents with a right hemiparesis and aphasia. He is drowsy, so the physician must be concerned about an intracranial mass as well as cerebral infarction. If the CT scan is normal, a mass, including intracerebral hemorrhage, brain tumor or abscess, and subdural hematoma, is

Table 7.4 CT Scan Findings in Different Brain Lesions Which Present as Stroke-Like Syndromes

Lesion	CT Scan
Cerebral infarction	No CT abnormalities for several hours (up to 48 hours). Then shows low density lesion that often has contrast enhancement. Cannot distinguish thrombus from embolus. (Figs. 7.3, 2.1, 2.3)
Subarachnoid hemorrhage	Extensive increased density (blood) in the cerebral sulci and subarachnoid cisterns at the base of the brain. Sometimes the enhanced CT scan shows an aneurysm. (Figs. 7.6, 2.4)
Intracerebral hemorrhage	Circumscribed high density lesion within the substance of the brain. No change with contrast enhancement. (Fig. 7.7)
Brain abscess	Diffuse low density mass (edema) within brain substance around a center that has marked contrast enhancement, often in a ring shape (Figs. 2.8, 19.1).
Brain tumor	
Primary	Low or high density irregular mass with variable contrast enhancement. Distribution doesn't fit known vascular supply territories.
Metastatic	One or more low density areas with nodular, contrast enhancing centers.
Subdural hematoma (Subacute or chronic)	Low density, lunar- or lens-shaped space between brain and skull over cerebral hemisphere (Fig. 2.10).
Encephalitis	Usually poorly demonstrated low density area with variable enhancement. Often primarily in one or both temporal lobes.

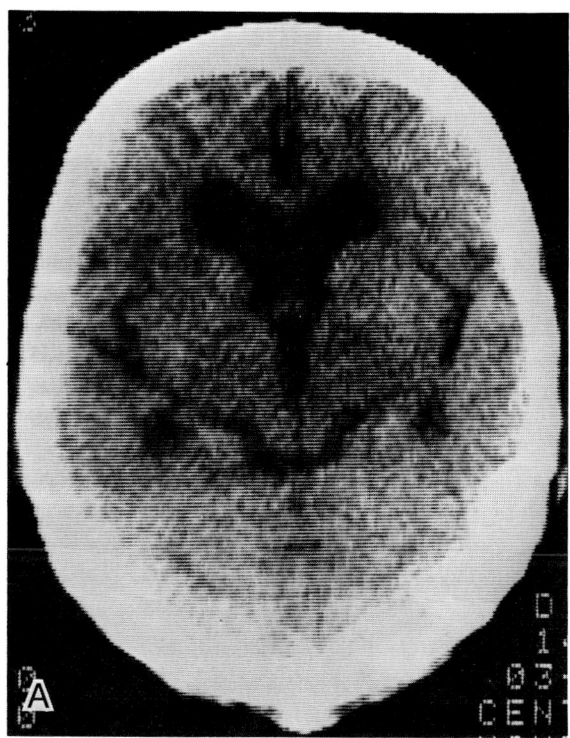
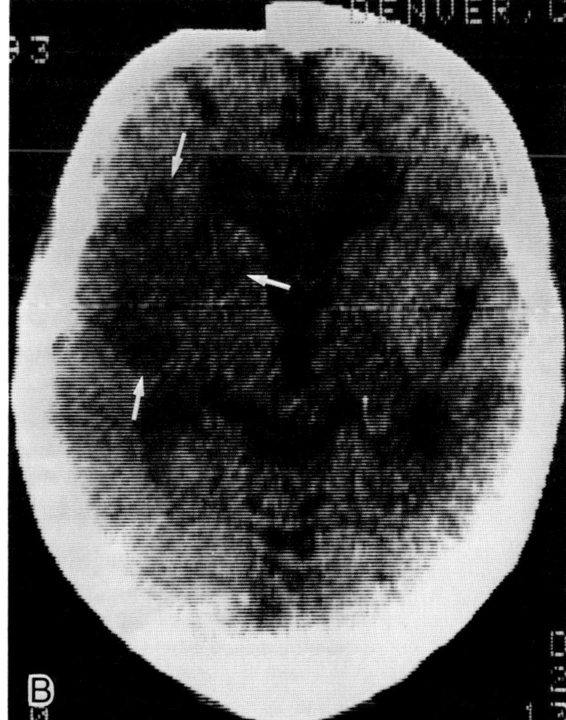

Fig. 7.3
CT scans of a left frontal lobe cerebral infarction on day 1(A) and day 10(B) showing appearance of low density lesion (dark) in the left hemisphere.

ruled out, and a cerebral infarction is likely. However, subarachnoid hemorrhage, encephalitis and meningitis are still possible, so a lumbar puncture must be done. If the CT scan is abnormal, it will show the intracerebral hemorrhage, tumor, abscess, etc., and so guide the physician's subsequent management.

The isotope brain scan can be used, if CT scanning is not possible. However, it has very limited value in the acute setting: it is helpful only if it is positive. If the brain scan is done within 24 hours of the onset of the patient's symptoms, and the static images show a lesion, the process is usually *not* a vascular one. If the scan is negative, the diagnoses of brain abscess, subdural hematoma and tumor are unlikely, but are not completely ruled out. The isotope brain scan is usually negative in intracranial hemorrhage.

Before the advent of CT scanning, angiography was often required to adequately distinguish cerebrovascular lesions from the non-vascular ones. There was no other way in the emergency setting to visualize brain structure. CT scanning has reduced the need, and has helped define more limited indications for angiography. Those will be discussed when the management of specific cerebrovascular lesions is presented.

EARLY MANAGEMENT OF BRAIN INFARCTION
Immediate Management To Preserve Brain Tissue

The immediate task of the physician in any emergency is to preserve the patient's life. In a neurologic emergency, the next step is to preserve the brain. When the physician first evaluates the patient with a cerebral infarction, the infarction has at it's center a portion of brain tissue that has been irreversibly damaged and so is already dead or is dying and cannot be salvaged. However, surrounding the infarcted area is a region of dysfunctional but viable, recoverable brain tissue. It is this portion of the brain that the physician must be most concerned with.

The dysfunctional, damaged tissue has three main requirements: glucose, oxygen and blood flow. The glucose and oxygen are the fuel and oxidant required to maintain the life of the cells. Blood flow is necessary to bring the glucose and oxygen, and to remove normal metabolic waste products. Blood flow is especially necessary in damaged tissue for removing other products, such as lactic acid, hemorrhage, edema fluid, arising from the damaged and infarcted tissue.

The physician should thus check a blood glucose and assure that the glucose is maintained in the normal range. If there is any clinical suspicion of inadequacy of the patient's ventilation the physician should draw a sample for arterial blood gases and then give the patient oxygen. If the blood gases show hypoxemia, the physician should continue administering oxygen.

The management of cerebral blood flow is a more complex task. Cerebral perfusion depends on the cardiac rate and rhythm, systemic blood pressure, intracranial pressure and cerebrovascular autoregulation. The latter cannot be controlled by the physician, and increased intracranial pressure is rare early in the course of a patient with brain infarction. So the physician must try to aid brain perfusion by managing the cardiac rate and rhythm and the systemic blood pressure. Any serious arrhythmia should be corrected by appropriate medication, so cardiac output and thus cerebral perfusion are increased. Atrial fibrillation is common in old persons with vascular disease, and, if present, any excessively fast or slow ventricular response should be corrected. Attempting electrical conversion of atrial fibrillation to normal sinus rhythm is not appropriate because of the excessive risk of inducing periods of bradycardia or other arrhythmias that would impair cardiac output and thus increase the damage in the infarcted region of the brain.

The treatment of serious abnormalities in systemic blood pressure is also important. If the patient is significantly hypotensive, that should be corrected. Often older stroke patients are dehydrated and correction of their volume deficit will restore an adequate blood pressure. If some other cause of hypotension is found, it must be corrected.

The treatment of hypertension in the early management of the patient with brain infarction is more controversial. Patients with modest hypertension, for example, systolic pressures up to 200 mm mercury or diastolic pressures up to 110 mm, probably should not be treated in the acute phase of the illness. If the patient is already on antihypertensive agents, those should be maintained, but an attempt to rapidly lower the blood pressure further risks increasing the ischemia in the damaged brain. However, if the patient's blood pressure is significantly higher, the high blood pressure may cause further damage to ischemic brain tissue by causing added edema, localized hemorrhages or vasospasm of cerebral vessels. Thus, the physician should probably institute treatment of the hypertension. However, he should not treat with any drug that has a risk of inducing hypotension, which could seriously further damage the already impaired brain. A reasonable goal is to reduce the diastolic blood pressure to approximately 105 mm mercury. Control of the systolic pressure is probably less critical. An effective medical regimen to use is to use a continuous infusion of nitroprusside (Nipride), beginning at an infusion rate of 0.5 µg/kg/min and increasing the rate in 0.5–1.0 µg/kg/min increments every 3–5 minutes until the blood pressure is adequately controlled.[2,18]

Cerebral vasodilating medications or inhaled carbon dioxide are probably not helpful in treating brain infarction. In fact, there is theoretical and experimental evidence that such methods may be harmful. The vasodilating agent probably affects only the healthy cerebral vessels but does not dilate the damaged vessels in the ischemic area. As a result, blood may actually be shunted away from the ischemic region. There are no other agents that beneficially affect the blood flow, function or recovery of ischemic brain tissue.

Anticoagulants and antiplatelet drugs are not helpful in reversing a completed infarction and should not be used until the physician has fully explored the indications and contraindications for their use. The use of anticoagulants to prevent progression of an infarction or to prevent subsequent embolic infarctions will be discussed later.

Localizing The Infarction

The physician's major concern should be with trying to infer the location of the lesion in only a gross anatomic fashion. The major distinction that should be made is whether the infarction lies in the distribution of the anterior, carotid circulation or in the posterior, vertebral-basilar circulation territory. If the lesion is in the anterior circulation, then is it on the right or the left? These distinctions tell the physician which major vessels may be occluded and so guide him and the radiologist in interpreting a CT scan or isotope brain scan. The location of the lesion also influences the decision about doing an angiogram. If the lesion is in the carotid circulation, an angiogram is safer and more likely to disclose a surgically treatable lesion than if the lesion were in the vertebral-basilar circulation.

The localization of the lesion can be decided, usually rather easily, from the clinical syndrome. Table 7.5 lists the important clinical features that localize an infarction to either the carotid or vertebral-basilar circulation. The most common brain infarction is one in the lateral cerebral hemisphere, the portion of the brain supplied by the middle cerebral artery, the main intracranial branch of the internal carotid artery. A lateral hemisphere infarction usually produces a contralateral hemiparesis and hemisensory loss.[14] If the infarction is in the left hemisphere, aphasia usually is produced. If there is also acute total loss of vision in the eye contralateral to a hemiparesis, carotid artery disease is most likely. The visual loss is due to occlusion of the ophthalmic artery, the first major intracranial branch of the internal carotid artery.

A hemiparesis with cranial nerve or cerebellar signs is the most common presentation of a brain stem stroke.[14] The "brain stem" encompasses the

Table 7.5 Clinical Signs that Localize the Infarction to a Specific Circulation

Carotid (Anterior) Circulation	Vertebral-Basilar, (Posterior) Circulation	Poorly Localizing
Hemiparesis and hemisensory loss together	Hemiparesis with cranial nerve signs	Hemiparesis with no other signs
Aphasia (usually a left hemispheric infarction)	Cerebellar signs	Hemianopsia with hemiparesis or hemisensory loss
Acute monocular loss of vision contralateral to a hemiparesis	Hemianopsia alone	

midbrain, pons and medulla. Cranial nerve signs refer to findings of ophthalmoplegia, pupillary abnormalities, isolated facial sensory loss or weakness (i.e., not associated with an ipsilateral hemiparesis or hemisensory loss), or unilateral abnormalities of the gag reflex, pharynx movement or tongue strength. This is strong evidence for vertebral-basilar circulation vascular disease, if the physician has already ruled out an intracranial mass causing a herniation syndrome. The classic syndrome is that of the "alternating hemiplegia," in which the hemiplegia is of the limbs contralateral to the cranial nerve signs. However, cranial nerve signs may be bilateral or, rarely, ipsilateral to the hemiparesis. Cerebellar signs, with or without a hemiparesis, mean vertebral-basilar disease. Hemianopsia alone is usually caused by infarction of the visual cortex or optic radiation of one occipital lobe. This portion of the hemisphere is supplied by the posterior cerebral artery, the main terminal branch of the basilar artery. A depressed level of consciousness often occurs with brain stem strokes because of damage to the reticular activating system. The combination of depressed consciousness with cranial nerve signs implies a brain stem lesion, if a cerebral mass lesion with herniation has been ruled out.

Hemiparesis with no associated sensory or cranial nerve signs can be a small infarction (a lacune) in the deep cerebral white matter or in the pons, and so doesn't indicate a specific circulation.[14] Hemianopsia with hemiparesis or hemisensory loss can also occur with infarctions due to anterior or posterior circulation vascular lesions.

The physician should try to decide the anatomic location of the lesion based on the neurologic examination. However, early in his management he need not be too concerned about localization. Other management decisions are more important.

What About Doing An Angiogram?

In ischemic cerebrovascular disease the indications for doing angiography in the acute setting are not widely agreed upon. In some institutions with special interest and expertise in the diagnosis and management of cerebrovascular disease, and that have experienced angiographers, angiograms are often done in acute ischemic events. However, in community hospitals with little specialized expertise in cerebrovascular disease or cerebral angiography, an angiogram may rarely be done. The institution in which the physician is working and the expertise of the radiology staff and technicians are important factors to recognize when considering angiography in the acute phase of an ischemic stroke.

However, there are clinical situations in which angiography should be done, or seriously considered. In some of these, the patient should be transferred to another institution if the hospital in which the physician is seeing the patient cannot provide adequate cerebral angiography. The most frequent indication for early angiography in a stroke patient is suspected intracranial hemorrhage. That will be discussed in a later section. For ischemic cerebrovascular disease the most pressing indications for early angiography, that is within the first hours of the work-up, are:

1. Rapidly progressing neurologic signs. In the patient who is having increasing neurologic signs, it is mandatory to know the mechanism for the stroke and to define the specific vascular lesion.[13] This is especially true when the symptoms and signs suggest a carotid, anterior circulation infarction. Carotid arteriography has a relatively low risk of morbidity and mortality and a reasonable probability of finding a significant vascular lesion.[3,23] Vertebrobasilar angiography is more hazardous than carotid and the vertebro-basilar circulation has a very low incidence of surgically accessible lesions.

The physician must first be sure the CT scan shows no mass and no intracranial hemorrhage. If the CT is negative, then the progressing neurologic signs could be due to worsening ischemia caused by a severe (greater than 90 percent) stenosis of the internal carotid artery, a dissecting aneurysm of the aorta or of the carotid artery alone, an intraluminal clot in the carotid artery attached to an atherosclerotic plaque, or some other unusual lesion that may require emergency surgery to repair (Figs. 7.4 and 8.1).

The younger the patient, the safer the angiogram and the more likely the radiologist will find an unusual or surgically treatable lesion. Very old (i.e., over 70) patients have a higher risk of morbidity or mortality from the procedure and a lower probability of finding a treatable lesion.

2. The patient with a suspected acute carotid occlusion. The clinical settings in which an acute carotid occlusion should be suspected are stroke following trauma to the anterior neck, as from a karate blow or trauma in an automobile accident, stroke following surgery on the carotid artery or in the region, a major stroke following angiography of the carotid, an acute stroke accompanied by anterior neck pain or tenderness, a hemispheric stroke plus acute blindness of the eye contralateral to the hemiparesis, or an acute stroke accompanied by the disappearance of a known bruit in the carotid artery ipsilateral to the infarction. When acute carotid thrombosis is suspected, an angiogram should be done immediately to prove the diagnosis. If carotid occlusion is confirmed, emergency thrombectomy within a few hours may be effective to reverse the process.[7,16] Again, the younger patient is the better candidate.

3. The young patient with a suspected embolic stroke, but the physician is not certain the mechanism was an embolus. This is a less powerful indication than the prior two. However, if one or more emboli are seen on an angiogram the physician then knows he must anti-coagulate the patient acutely and chronically and he must also launch an exhaustive search for a source of the embolus. Figure 7.5 shows the appearance of emboli on an angiogram. The angiogram is the only test to prove the

Fig. 7.4
Right carotid artery angiogram showing the internal carotid with severe stenosis and an intraluminal clot (lucent area above stenosis) in a 67-year-old woman with a mild stroke.

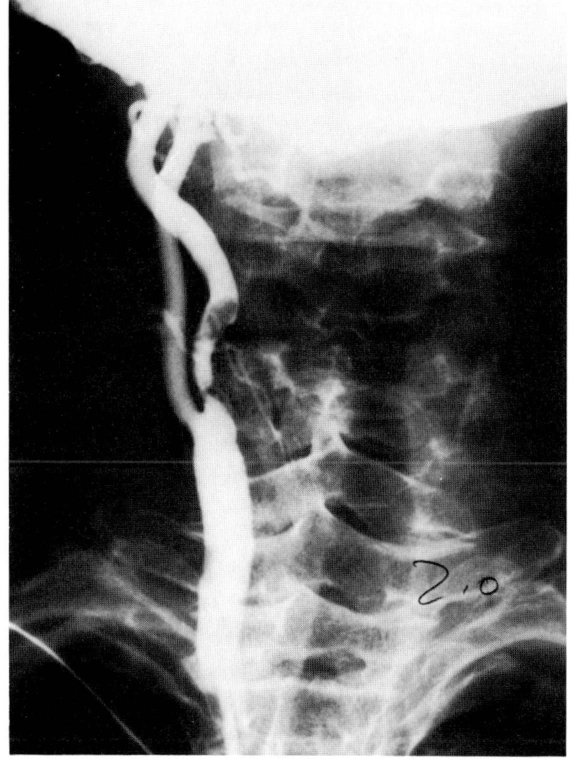

presence of emboli and it must be done promptly because emboli can break up and disappear within hours.

Preventing Or Halting Progression Of An Infarction

The section "Early Management of Brain Infarction" outlined the basic steps to preserve as much viable brain tissue as possible by assuring that the brain receives adequate glucose, oxygen and blood flow. However, sometimes, in spite of compulsive early management, the patient's symptoms and signs worsen. The physician must then aggressively seek the cause for the patient's deterioration.[13] Has the blood pressure, cardiac rate and rhythm, ventilation or blood glucose changed? Perhaps a hemorrhage has occurred in the infarcted area, so the CT scan should be repeated and a lumbar puncture done. Maybe the patient has a high fever or sepsis, thus further impairing brain function. However, if those factors are ruled out, the clinician's diagnosis must be "stroke in progression," and he must presume a worsening vascular lesion. As described above, angiography is, in most cases, the next step to define the cause of the patient's decline. However, if one is done and fails to uncover a surgically correctable lesion, the physician must institute anticoagulation.

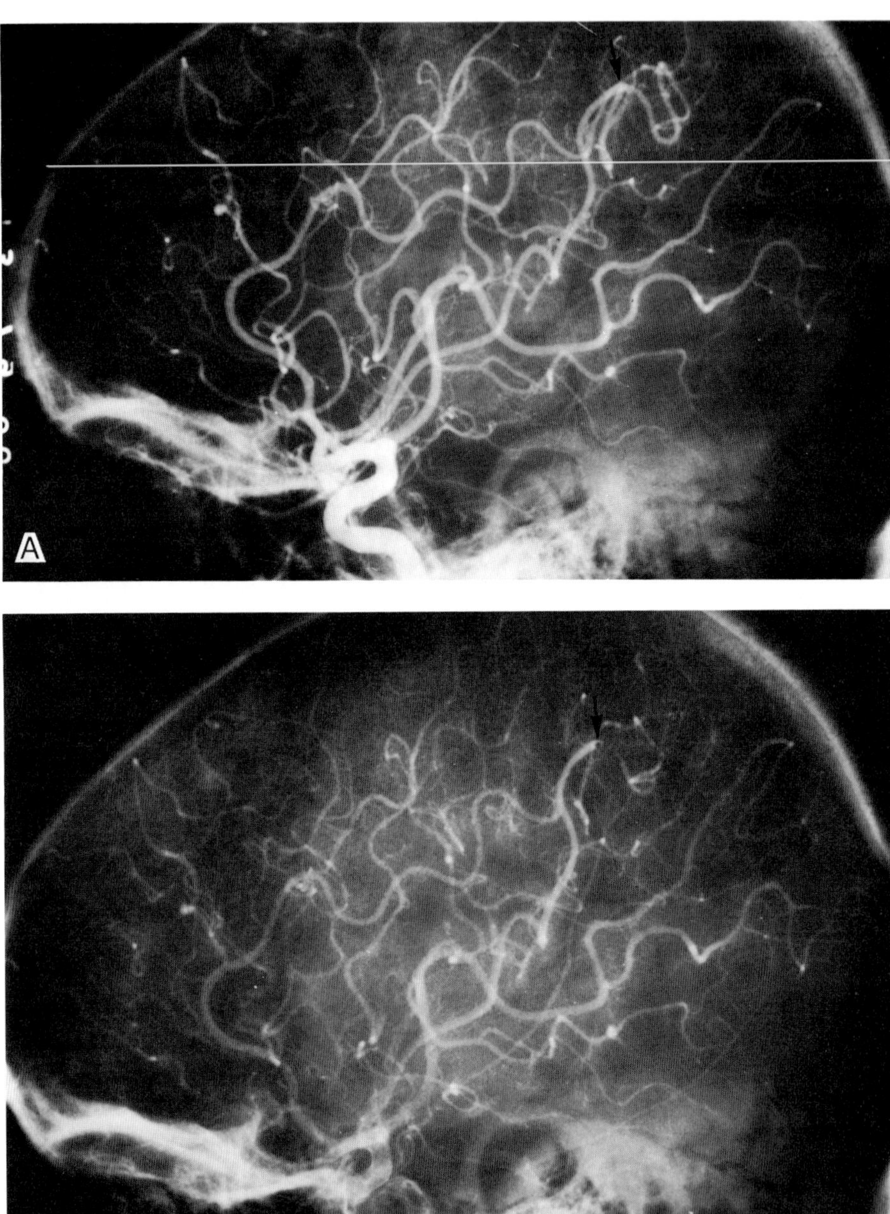

Fig. 7.5 Left middle and anterior cerebral arteries before (A) and after (B) occurrence of cerebral embolus. The proximal, rounded end of the embolus is indicated by an arrow. The embolus extends several millimeters distally.

Two rigid criteria *must* be met before anticoagulants can be safely given. First, a CT scan, done within the last few hours, must show no blood. *Also,* a lumbar puncture (LP), done within the last few hours, must have shown no blood in the cerebrospinal fluid (CSF). Both tests are necessary because the CT scan can fail to show low concentrations of blood in the CSF and the LP often does not show blood when there has been intracerebral hemorrhage.[15,26] Anticoagulation cannot be done safely until both tests are negative for blood.

Once the physician is sure there is no intracranial or spinal fluid blood, he should begin anticoagulation. A widely used, and most immediately effective method for anticoagulation is to give an intravenous bolus of heparin (2,500 to 7,500 units) followed by a continuous intravenous infusion of 5,000 units in a modest volume of diluent every 4 hours. The adequacy of anticoagulation may be judged by obtaining an activated partial thromboplastin time (aPTT). An aPTT of 1½ to 2½ times control is considered therapeutic.[5] Some authorities recommend checking venous blood clotting times to measure the anticoagulant effect.[25] This method may be used if the aPTT is not available.

The patient should be closely observed after anticoagulation. If his condition deteriorates further, a repeat CT scan and LP should be done to rule out hemorrhage precipitated by the anticoagulation. If hemorrhage is found, the anticoagulant must be stopped and the heparin effect reversed with protamine.[5]

If the patient stabilizes or improves, heparin anticoagulation is continued for several days and then is changed to oral anticoagulation with warfarin (Coumadin).

Progression of neurologic signs in the acute stroke patient is rarely due to brain edema during the first 24 hours. After the first day, significant brain edema does occur in and around large infarctions to cause clinical deterioration. Unfortunately, there are no good means to prevent or reverse infarction-induced brain edema. The general measures of keeping the patient slightly dehydrated, elevating his head and avoiding giving excessive salt are probably helpful, but won't reverse clinical deterioration. Dexamethasone (Decadron), so helpful in tumor-induced brain edema, has not been proved to be effective but is still often used. Osmotic diuretics, such as mannitol, will temporarily reverse brain herniation caused by infarction-induced brain edema, but mannitol does not seem to prevent or effectively treat the edema itself.

The Role Of Lumbar Puncture (LP) In Acute Management Of Brain Infarction

The two major reasons for performing an LP early in the course of an acute stroke patient are:

1. To prove that there is no infection (meningitis, encephalitis or neurosyphilis) present.

2. To rule out blood in the cerebrospinal fluid. Blood in the CSF would indicate intracranial hemorrhage and would change the physician's understanding of the mechanism of the stroke and so guide his subsequent management.

The author believes that an LP should be done early on for almost every patient with a suspected brain infarction. The knowledge of CSF blood or evidence of infection is important information to include in further management decisions. Patients in whom an LP may not be indicated are the very old stroke patient with an uncomplicated stroke syndrome and no signs of infection.

Management Over The Next Few Days

Once the emergency decisions have been made and immediate management has been instituted, the physician must begin the process toward helping the patient make as full a recovery as possible. The detailed subsequent management is beyond the scope of this article. However, management over the next several days should include:

1. A thorough search for any underlying conditions that may have precipitated the patient's stroke-cardiac disease: blood lipid disorders, diabetes mellitus, hypertension, blood clotting disorders, neurosyphilis, birth control pills, etc. (Table 7.6)

2. Careful daily observations and compulsive nursing care to prevent or detect early the common complications of stroke: aspiration pneumonia, decubitus ulcers, joint contractures, urinary tract infections, thrombophlebitis, depression, etc.

3. Begin ambulation and physical rehabilitation as soon as possible. Early involvement of physical, occupational and speech therapy is important.

4. Discharge planning should begin early in the patient's course, so his home can be adequately prepared or another disposition can be found. The hospital stay will thus be minimized.

5. The physician should consider every possible way to prevent a future stroke. Treatment of hypertension or other conditions predisposing the patient to having a stroke must be done. Continued anticoagulation may be necessary. The role of antiplatelet drugs such as aspirin, sulfinpyrazone (Anturane) or dipyridamole (Persantin) is uncertain. If an arteriogram was not done early in the course, perhaps one should be done later to look for surgically correctable extracranial vascular lesions. Non-invasive vascular studies, such as ultrasound arteriography, Doppler studies or oculoplethysmography might be done to look for significant stenoses of the carotid arteries.

Special Situations In Patients With Ischemic Cerebrovascular Disease

The Younger Stroke Patient

Patients under 60 years old with brain infarctions have different etiologies for their strokes than the older patients.[6,8] Cerebral emboli from cardiac disease, coagulation and blood lipid disorders, dissecting aneurysms of the carotid artery, neurosyphilis, and other treatable, underlying conditions are more common (Table 7.6). The physician should be especially diligent to search for predisposing factors in the young stroke patient. Lumbar puncture, arteriography, cardiac ultrasound, non-invasive vascular studies of the carotid arteries and all other relevant tests should be more seriously considered and more often done in the younger patient.

The Limited Role of Surgery In Acute Ischemic Cerebrovascular Disease

Carotid endarterectomy, thrombectomy and embolectomy have a limited role in acute ischemic cerebrovascular disease. Although controversial, emergency surgery is probably indicated when an acute carotid occlusion

Table 7.6 Medical Conditions to be Sought in a Young Patient with Cerebral Infarction

I. Cardiac Disease
   A. Valvular disease (rheumatic, congenital)
   B. Atrial fibrillation
   C. Atrial myxoma
   D. Myocardial infarction
   E. "Click murmur" syndrome (prolapsing mitral valve)

II. Coagulation Disorders
   A. Hypercoagulability
   B. Thrombocytosis

III. Infection
   A. Neurosyphilis
   B. Bacterial endocarditis

IV. Vasculitis
   A. Lupus erythematosus
   B. Polyarteritis nodosa
   C. Other large vessel arteritis

V. Carotid Artery Disease
   A. Carotid artery dissection
   B. Fibromuscular hyperplasia
   C. Premature atherosclerosis
   D. Carotid occlusion

VI. Other
   A. Hypertension
   B. Diabetes mellitus
   C. Birth control pills
   D. Sickle cell anemia
   E. Hyperproteinemia (e.g., cryoglobulinemia)
   F. Blood lipid disorders

is producing a stroke syndrome.[7,16] The surgery must be done within a few hours, probably less than 6 hours, of the occlusion. Surgery is contraindicated after 6 hours because of the risk of inducing hemorrhage in the infarcted hemisphere. Similarly, acute surgery to remove a severely stenotic lesion of the carotid artery or an intraluminal carotid blood clot or embolus in a patient with progressing neurologic deficit may reverse the process.[16,31] However, such patients comprise a small minority of all stroke patients.

The more common role for carotid surgery is several weeks later in the course, when the patient is recovering and an arteriogram has shown a stenotic or ulcerated lesion of the carotid artery. Surgical removal of the lesion may prevent future strokes.[23,28]

The newly developed technique of anastamosing an extracranial to an intracranial vessel, the extracranial-intracranial (EC-IC) bypass, may be useful to increase blood flow to an ischemic area of the brain. However, the value of EC-IC bypass to improve recovery from a previous stroke or prevent future strokes has yet to be demonstrated.[22,29]

The Small Intracerebral Hemorrhage

A small, deep intracerebral hemorrhage can produce a clinical syndrome identical to a cerebral infarction. The use of CT scanning in stroke patients has shown that about 25 percent of patients with apparent cerebral infarctions actually have had an intracerebral hemorrhage.[11] This finding makes it mandatory for the physician to do a CT scan on almost every patient with suspected cerebral infarction, especially if he is considering using anticoagulants.

The Large Cerebellar Infarction

Occasionally a cerebellar infarction will develop significant edema and will cause mass effect, obstructing CSF flow through the fourth ventricle, causing hydrocephalus, and also compressing the brain stem, causing respiratory and cardiovascular deterioration and even death. Any patient with a stroke and cerebellar signs, often also with cranial nerve signs, should be closely observed for deterioration of his levels of consciousness or change in his vital signs. If those occur, a repeat CT scan may be compared with the original one. If edema and mass effect are demonstrated in the cerebellum, vigorous management of the impending brain herniation should be begun. If the patient severely deteriorates, neurosurgical decompression of the posterior fossa and excision of a portion of the infarcted cerebellum may be required.[12]

The Asymptomatic Bruit

Although not truly a neurologic emergency, the discovery of a bruit in the neck creates anxiety for the physician and creates a sense of urgency about an impending stroke. Obviously, if the patient has neurologic symptoms or signs that are possibly related to a cerebrovascular lesion, that patient should be referred for further vascular tests. However, when the patient has had no related neurologic symptoms, what should be done? What is the risk of a stroke in the near future? Should angiography be done? If a significant vascular lesion is found, does surgery or medical management prevent stroke?

In an asymptomatic patient with a carotid bruit, there is an increased risk of future stroke. However, recent studies indicate that the future stroke often is in a vascular territory different from the vessel with the bruit or the stroke is a hemorrhage, unrelated to extracranial vascular disease.[9,30] These findings raise doubt about claims that surgery to correct a vascular lesion causing a bruit (a "bruitectomy," if you will) prevents future strokes.[4] The issue is still controversial, but medical neurologists generally favor conservative, long-term clinical follow-up of the patient with an asymptomatic bruit. If symptoms ever occur, the vascular work-up is done.

A low-risk alternative is to obtain non-invasive vascular studies, such as carotid Doppler and ultrasound imaging studies and oculoplethysmography. If those suggest a severe stenosis of the artery, then arteriography can be done. If a significant lesion is found, then endarterectomy can be performed. This management plan is a rational one, but has not been shown to reduce future strokes. It also exposes an asymptomatic patient to some risk of injury from the angiogram and surgery.

Hypoglycemia

Older patients with diabetes mellitus develop strokes. They also can become hypoglycemic. On rare occasions a patient with hypoglycemia alone will present with focal neurologic signs, looking like he has had a cerebral infarction or hemorrhage. More typically, an elderly diabetic patient with a prior cerebral infarction presents with obtundation and increased focal signs. However, he may not have had another stroke, but is merely hypoglycemic. The physician should consider hypoglycemia and should obtain a serum glucose sample in every patient with an acute stroke syndrome, and should treat the patient for hypoglycemia if clinical or laboratory evidence supports the diagnosis. However, the routine administration of large doses of glucose to every stroke patient is not indicated, and may be harmful.

MANAGEMENT OF PATIENTS WITH INTRACRANIAL HEMORRHAGE

The Nature Of Intracranial Hemorrhage

The patient with a typical intracranial hemorrhage has signs and symptoms different from those of brain infarction. Central nervous system hemorrhage is an intracranial catastrophe. When the aneurysm or other vascular structure ruptures, blood, under arterial pressure, is pumped into the suba-

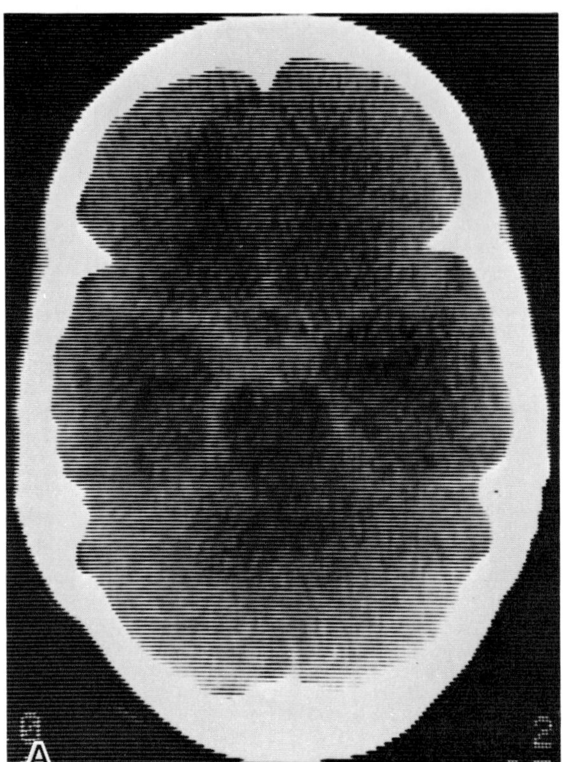

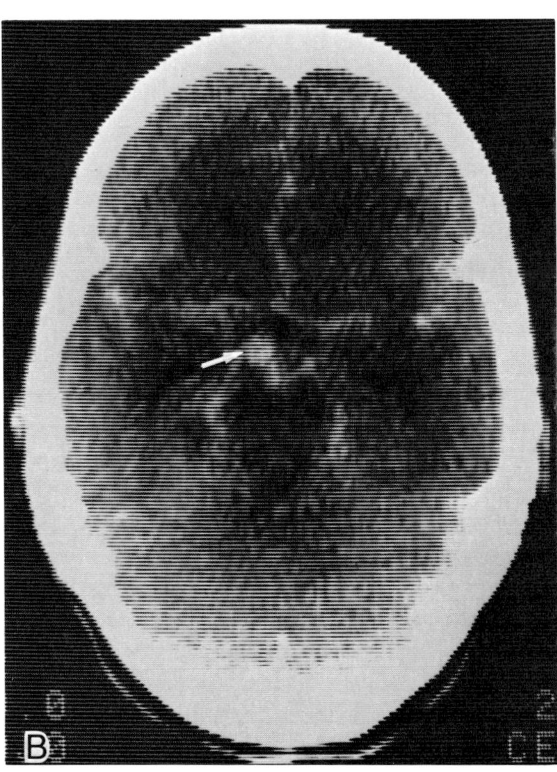

Fig. 7.6
Subarachnoid hemorrhage—CT scan before contrast injection (A), showing typical starfish-shaped distribution of blood at the base of the brain, and after contrast (B), showing the cerebral arteries and a large aneurysm (arrow) of the left posterior communicating artery.

rachnoid space or into the brain itself. Intracranial pressure increases, the patient has a sudden bad headache, nausea, vomiting, and soon has confusion and then develops a depressed level of consciousness. Because of the problems with intracranial pressure, toxic effects of the blood, vascular spasm and recurrent bleeding, intracranial hemorrhages have a worse prognosis for survival or for a good, functional recovery than do the brain infarctions.

As previously discussed, intracranial hemorrhages occur in two common types, subarachnoid hemorrhage and intracerebral hemorrhage. A subarachnoid hemorrhage is caused by rupture of an aneurysm into the CSF-containing subarachnoid space (Fig. 7.6). Because of the absence of focal brain destruction subarachoid hemorrhages often have no focal signs, that is, no hemiparesis, hemisensory loss, hemianopsia, etc. Intracerebral hemorrhages, on the other hand, are caused by rupture of a blood vessel within the brain substance, so focal tissue destruction occurs (Fig. 7.7). Thus, intracerebral hemorrhages usually have prominent focal signs. As with any clinical rule, the distinction of the two hemorrhages is not always clear. A ruptured aneurysm can produce a stream of arterial blood that dissects into the brain causing a secondary intracerebral hematoma. Also, occasionally an intracerebral hemorrhage occurs near the cerebral ventricles and so ruptures into the ventricular system, causing coma without prominent focal signs. However, the general distinction applies and is usually helpful: a pa-

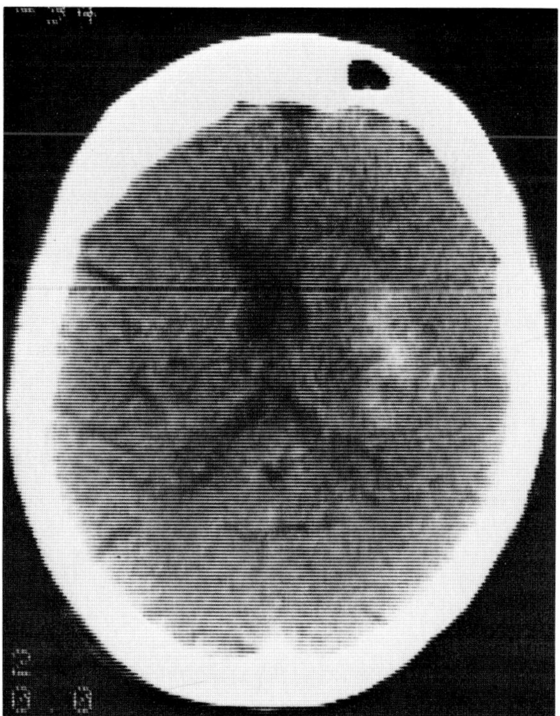

Fig. 7.7
CT scan of intracerebral hemorrhage into the basal ganglia of the right cerebral hemisphere (white area). Note the compression and shift of the ventricles to the left.

tient with suspected intracranial hemorrhage and prominent focal signs probably has had an intracerebral hemorrhage. The absence of prominent focal signs suggests a primary subarachnoid hemorrhage.

Early Management Decisions

A patient presenting with an intracranial hemorrhage often is critically ill. He has depressed consciousness and altered respirations, pulse and blood pressure. He may progress rapidly into coma, respiratory arrest and then cardiac arrest.

The physician's first step should be to place an intravenous line and order it as "keep open." An IV provides an easily accessible route for administering drugs. If the patient is comatose, he should be intubated. If ventilation is inadequate, it should be mechanically supported. An EKG should be done and any life-threatening arrhythmias treated (Table 7.7).

The administration of dexamethasone (Decadron), 10 mg intravenously, is probably helpful. The anti-edema effects of the drug may help reduce intracranial pressure. The drug may not begin its action for a few hours, but it should be given early in the course so its effect will begin as soon as possible. Osmotic diuretics, such as mannitol (0.5–1.0 g/kg, as an IV bolus) should be given if signs of brain herniation are present. Other rapid-acting diuretics, such as furosemide (Lasix), 20–40 mg, IV, may also help dehydrate the patient and so reduce intracranial pressure.

A decision must also be made about treating systemic hypertension. The blood pressure is often severely increased in a patient with an intracranial hemorrhage. If the systolic pressure is over 200 mm of mercury or the diastolic is above 110 mm, the pressure probably should be treated. However, the physician should avoid making the patient hypotensive because blood perfusion of the brain may drop, especially if there is a severe increase of intracranial pressure, and the patient's condition will be made worse. A reasonable approach is to use nitroprusside (Nipride) in a continuous IV infusion, beginning at a rate of 0.5 μg/kg/min and increasing the rate by 0.5–1.0 μg/kg/min increments until the blood pressure is adequately controlled.[2,18] A reasonable goal for control of blood pressure is a diastolic pressure of approximately 100 mm mercury.

As with brain infarctions, adequate blood oxygenation and blood glucose should also be confirmed. If either is below normal, it should be corrected.

The Role Of CT Scanning

After initially stabilizing the patient, the physician must obtain a CT scan. The CT scan will not only confirm the presence of blood and rule out other unexpected etiologies, such as a tumor, it will also help define the type of intracranial hemorrhage that has occurred. An intracerebral hemorrhage appears as a dense clot within the brain parenchyma, causing mass

Table 7.7 Management Scheme for Intracranial Hemorrhage

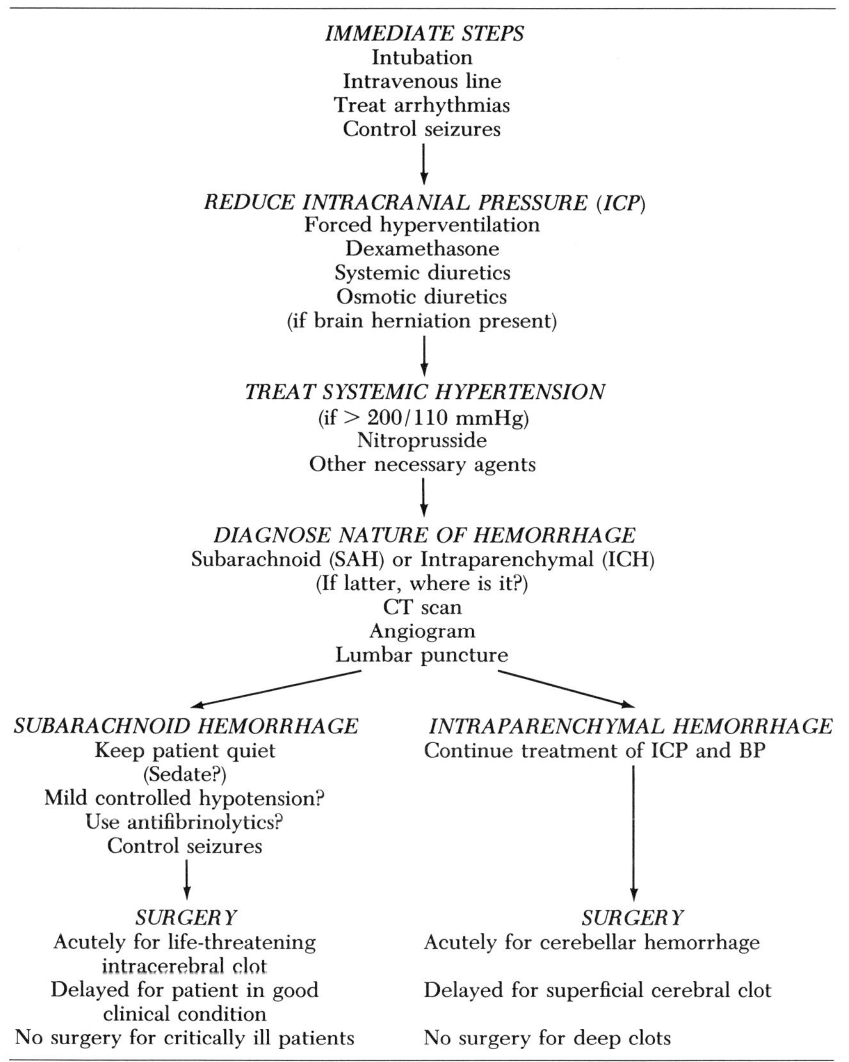

effect and shift of nearby brain structures (Fig. 7.7). Any subarachnoid blood is usually localized to the vicinity of the intracerebral clot. A subarachnoid hemorrhage usually appears on CT scan as large amounts of blood mixed with CSF diffusely present through the subarachnoid cisterns at the base of the brain (Fig. 7.6A). There is usually no associated clot in the brain substance. The contrast-enhanced scan may even show an aneurysm as a discreet, round enhancing lesion attached to a blood vessel at the base of the brain (Fig. 7.6B).

The CT scan is vital to confirm the diagnosis and to rule out other possibilities. It also is important because it shows the exact location of any intracerebral hemorrhage. Such clots in certain locations must be surgically removed as soon as possible to save the patient's life. (Those special situations are discussed below.)

What If CT Scanning Is Not Available?

The CT scan is, by far, the best early radiologic test, however, it will not always be available. In that situation, the decision by the physician must be made to either: (1) do a lumbar puncture, to prove the presence of subarachnoid blood; (2) order a cerebral angiogram to prove the presence of an intracerebral hemorrhage or an aneurysm; or (3) stabilize and then transfer the patient elsewhere for a CT scan and further management. The latter choice is probably best because the CT scan is such a valuable part of the early evaluation. However, if safe transfer is not possible, the physician should decide within a few hours whether to do the LP or an angiogram. A prompt decision is important so the physician can obtain the data to guide his further management. General guidelines that help in the choice of a test are:

1. If the patient has a severely depressed level of consciousness or other signs of severely increased intracranial pressure, an LP should not be done. The angiogram should be done.

2. If the patient has prominent focal signs, an LP should not be done. The angiogram is the safest test.

3. If the patient is only drowsy and has no prominent focal signs, the LP is safe and can be done.

A non-traumatic LP that shows blood in the CSF proves the patient has had an intracranial hemorrhage. However, an LP that produces a clear, colorless CSF with no blood does *not* rule out intracranial hemorrhage. It may be negative because the blood from a subarachnoid hemorrhage has not yet spread to the lumbar CSF. That diffusion of the blood may require up to 2 hours. The LP may be negative for blood in an intracerebral hemorrhage because the clot is totally within the brain parenchyma, and has not dissected out into the subarachnoid space. When a LP shows no blood, but the physician's strongest diagnosis is intracranial hemorrhage, a CT scan or angiogram or a repeat LP several hours later must be done.

Medical Management Of A Subarachnoid Hemorrhage

Once a patient with a subarachnoid hemorrhage has been initially stabilized the physician must consider two different questions: (1) How can a second hemorrhage be prevented?; and (2) Should an angiogram be done, and when? (Table 7.7)

The major risk for further morbidity and mortality of the patient with a subarachnoid hemorrhage is the risk of a second hemorrhage. The first hemorrhage occurred because the aneurysm wall weakened and then burst. That initial hemorrhage was halted, probably by two mechanisms: vascular spasm in the region of the aneurysm, reducing the blood pressure and flow through the aneurysm, and then the normal formation of blood clot in the aneurysm, sealing the hole. However, the thin-walled, friable aneurysm remains and normal fibrinolysis begins to slowly erode the clot, so a second hemorrhage is a serious threat.

Measures to prevent a second hemorrhage must be begun. The patient should be kept quiet, to avoid stress or agitation causing sudden systemic hypertension, thus rupturing the aneurysm. Sedation may be necessary for an agitated patient. Phenobarbital is a particularly good sedative because of its effects to cause sedation, lower systemic blood pressure to prevent convulsions, an occasional accompaniment of an SAH. If the patient's blood pressure is elevated, it should be carefully controlled. Some reports indicate that maintaining a slight systemic hypotension may reduce morbidity and mortality.[20]

The role of agents to slow intravascular fibrinolysis, and so retard lysis of the clot sealing the aneurysm, has not been unequivocally proven. Some studies indicate that such agents in high doses, specifically epsilon aminocaproic acid (Amicar, 48 gm/day) may be beneficial.[19] The possible benefits of such agents must be weighed against the increased risks of thrombophlebitis, pulmonary emboli and arterial thromboses.

Angiography should be considered in every patient with a SAH. The primary guidelines for the decision are:

1. A patient with a suspected ruptured aneurysm, or one documented by CT scan, who has an associated life-threatening intracerebral clot should have angiography. In that clinical setting emergency neurosurgery is indicated to try to save the patient's life. The surgeon must evacuate the clot, but may also have to occlude the aneurysm to stop intraoperative bleeding. An angiogram is necessary to define the location, anatomy and number of aneurysms to guide the surgeon's work.

2. A patient who has a SAH and no associated cerebral clot on CT scan, but who is comatose or has prominent focal signs, should not have angiography. That patient has a prohibitive risk of morbidity and mortality from surgery to correct the aneurysm, so an angiogram is not necessary for the surgeon. The angiogram may be done in subsequent days if the patient improves and becomes a good candidate for surgery.

3. The patient with a SAH who is alert or has only a modest depression of consciousness and no prominent focal signs, should have an angiogram within the first 24 to 48 hours. That patient is a good operative candidate. Defining the anatomic details of the aneurysm(s) will enable the surgeon to more intelligently decide when and how to operate.

Patients who don't fall clearly in one of those categories require individualized decisions based on the patient's clinical condition, the expertise of the radiologist and the carefully thought out medical judgements of the physician and his consultants.

The Role And Timing Of Surgery

Surgery to obliterate the aneurysm is the best treatment for most cerebrovascular aneurysms. However, the decision to do surgery must consider the risks to the patient. A prohibitive risk, contraindicating surgery, is a patient in bad clinical condition, especially one in coma or with prominent focal signs. Medical complications, such as pneumonia or cardiac disease, are serious risk factors, as is advanced age. The young, otherwise healthy patient with no, or modest, depression of consciousness and no major focal signs is the best candidate for surgery. However, the best time to operate has not been well established.[10,24]

Ideally, surgery should be done when the patient has made a full recovery from the effects of the first SAH. However, the risk of a second SAH forces the clinician to consider surgery as soon as possible. A commonly stated clinical axiom is that second hemorrhages most often occur from 7 to 14 days after the initial SAH. Therefore the aneurysm should be occluded before that time, if at all possible.

The one situation where immediate surgery is indicated for a patient with a SAH is the patient whose aneurysm has bled both into the subarachnoid space and into the brain parenchyma, causing a life-threatening intracerebral hematoma. That clot must be removed acutely, attempting to save the patient's life.

The anatomy of the aneurysm also influences the timing of surgery somewhat. A large aneurysm, over 8 mm, or one with multiple lobes, may have an increased risk of early second rupture. Finding such an aneurysm on the angiogram encourages the physician to recommend surgery relatively early in the course.

Medical Management Of Intracerebral Hemorrhages

The term "intracerebral" hemorrhages is not fully accurate. Hemorrhages into the parenchyma of the brain can occur in any part of the brain, including the brain stem and the cerebellum. However, about 75 percent of all parenchymal hemorrhages in the brain occur in the cerebral hemispheres, most commonly in the gray matter nuclei deep in the hemisphere.

The basic pathologic lesion underlying intracerebral hemorrhages is a chronic degeneration of the walls of small trunks. This degeneration is a normal part of aging, but is greatly accelerated by systemic hypertension.[21] The degeneration of the vessel wall leads to formation of microscopic aneurysms, and these may rupture, causing hemorrhage into the brain. Once the small hemorrhage begins, it stretches and ruptures other small vessels nearby and so produces a self-sustaining process that leads to a large clot. The process is probably arrested by the resistance of the brain tissue to continued expansion of the clot and also probably by increased intracranial pressure causing a tamponading effect on the ruptured vessels. In contrast to a ruptured aneurysm causing an SAH, the active hemorrhaging is probably arrested soon after it begins and second intracerebral hemorrhages rarely occur.

The medical management of primary intracerebral hemorrhages thus differs somewhat from that of a SAH (Table 7.7). There is no need for quiet, sedation, induced hypotension or antifibrinolytic drugs to prevent a second hemorrhage. However, there is a greater need to control intracranial pressure and the effects of the local mass. The patient's blood pressure is also often severely elevated, and so may require vigorous treatment. The specific methods of treatment were outlined in the previous section, "Early Management Decisions." Repeated doses of dexamethasone and diuretics, every 4 to 8 hours, may be necessary to control brain herniation.

The Role Of Angiography And Surgery

Angiography is not necessary for the diagnosis; the CT scan can definitively prove an intracerebral hemorrhage. An angiogram is necessary only if the physician suspects either a ruptured aneurysm in the subarachnoid space (and a secondary intracerebral hematoma) or a congenital arteriovenous malformation. The indications and timing then are the same as those for angiography for the subarachnoid hemorrhage patient.

Unfortunately surgery, for the majority of patients with intracerebral hemorrhage, is not helpful. The initial hemorrhage has done the damage and the hematoma must be slowly lysed and resorbed. However, there are two indications for acute surgery:

1. A patient with an intracerebral hemorrhage that is located in a superficial location (e.g., the frontal, temporal or occipital lobe). If the patient's clinical condition suggests his life is in danger, removing the hematoma may be life-saving. If the patient is clinically stable and not apparently in danger of dying, even a superficial hematoma is probably best left undisturbed in the acute phase of the illness.

2. A hemorrhage into the cerebellum. Cerebellar hematomas are an extreme emergency and require surgery. This distinct problem is discussed below.

Hemorrhages deep in the hemisphere and hemorrhages in the brain stem cannot be removed without causing excessive damage to overlying brain. Attempts to remove the deep hematomas in the acute illness are almost universally fatal. However, in some patients with deep hemisphere hematomas, poor clinical recovery, and a continuing depressed level of consciousness, surgery later in the course, after 2 weeks, may produce some clinical improvement. Those patients often on CT scan show continuing mass effect and poor resorption of the hematoma.

Cerebellar Hematoma—An Extreme Emergency

About 10 percent of all intraparenchymal brain hemorrhages occur in the cerebellum (Fig. 7.8). A hemorrhage in that location can be rapidly fatal because it can compress the nearby respiratory and cardiovascular centers in the medulla and cause a respiratory or cardiac arrest. However, early diagnosis and prompt surgery to remove the hematoma can prevent medullary compression, and the patient often makes a complete recovery. Every physician should be aware of the uncommon but very distinctive clinical syndrome caused by a cerebellar hemorrhage. The patient usually has a history of hypertension. He has the sudden onset of a severe occipital head-

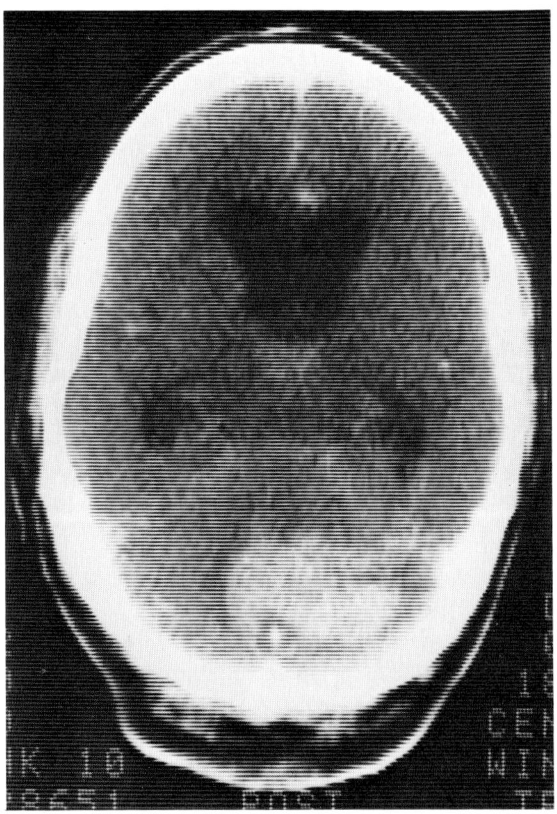

Fig. 7.8
CT scan showing large hemorrhage into the right cerebellum extending to the left of the midline, obstructing the 4th ventricle and causing hydrocephalus.

ache, often accompanied by nausea, vomiting and vertigo. He cannot walk because of severe ataxia. He may then become drowsy. On examination there is often severe hypertension, a reflex response to the hematoma causing pressure on the medulla, but there are few cranial nerve signs and no limb weakness. The patient's gait, if tested, will demonstrate severe ataxia.

Some cases with classic symptoms and signs and a rapidly deteriorating course should be taken directly to the operating room for a posterior fossa craniotomy to remove the suspected hematoma.[1] However, in most suspected cases, a CT scan should be quickly obtained, and the diagnosis verified before surgery is done. The physician should accompany the patient to any radiologic test and should be prepared to treat cardiac or respiratory arrest. The physician should also clearly direct the radiologist's attention to the cerebellum. The region of the cerebellum and brain stem are especially hard to visualize on a CT scan, and often have serious artefact. The radiologist often must use special views to adequately demonstrate or rule out a cerebellar lesion.

If a cerebellar hemorrhage is demonstrated the patient should be taken to the operating room and the clot removed. Surgery should probably be done even if the patient is in good clinical condition. A fully alert patient may suddenly have a respiratory arrest and die.

The Problems Of Hypertensive Encephalopathy And Eclampsia

Hypertensive encephalopathy is often diagnosed in a patient with severe hypertension, confusion, depressed level of consciousness, and focal neurologic signs and convulsions. Hypertensive encephalopathy is a medical emergency, and the dangerously increased blood pressure must be rapidly lowered to a safe level.

Unfortunately, intracranial hemorrhages, especially intracerebral hemorrhages, often produce an identical syndrome. When the cause of the signs and symptoms is a hemorrhage, treatment should focus on management of that lesion. Treatment of the blood pressure is a secondary consideration, although severe hypertension should be treated.

Whenever the general physician sees a patient with severe hypertension and neurologic signs he should consider hypertensive encephalopathy, but he must also rule out an intracranial hemorrhage. A CT scan should be done and, if that is negative, an LP should follow. If those two tests show no signs of intracranial hemorrhage, then the diagnosis of hypertensive encephalopathy is acceptable.

Similarly, a woman late in pregnancy who develops severe hypertension, confusion, depression of consciousness, seizures or other neurologic signs may well have eclampsia. However, intracranial hemorrhage must be ruled out by performing a CT scan and LP.

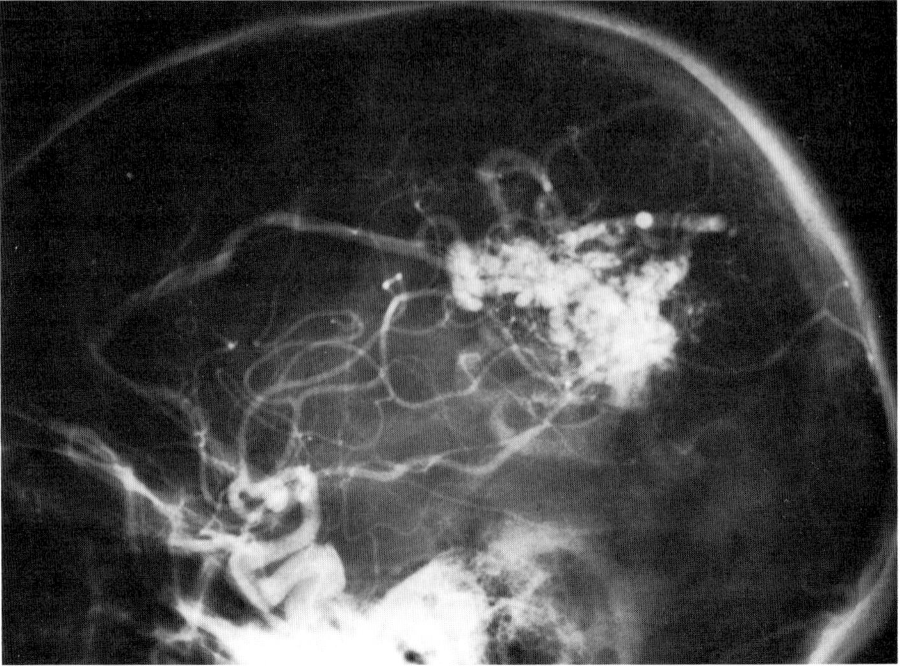

Fig. 7.9 Cerebral arteriogram showing large tangle of abnormal vessels, an arteriovenous malformation (AVM) deep in the brain. This 37-year-old woman had a hemorrhage into the right thalamus.

Arteriovenous Malformations

An arteriovenous malformation (AVM) is a congenital malformation of the cerebrovascular system in which there is an anomalous connection of the arterial system with the venous one. The connecting vessels are usually themselves abnormal and have thin, nonelastic and fragile walls. These weak vessels contain blood flowing under arterial pressure and so may rupture and cause an intracranial hemorrhage (Fig. 7.9). The hemorrhage may occur into the subarachnoid space or may occur within the brain tissue itself. Hemorrhages from AVMs generally have a lower morbidity and mortality than those caused by aneurysms or hypertensive vascular disease. Management of the hemorrhage should be guided by the location of the hemorrhage, either subarachnoid or intraparenchymal. The principles discussed above for management of hemorrhages caused by aneurysms or hypertensive vascular disease apply also to management of a hemorrhage from an AVM.

CONCLUSION

Cerebrovascular disease is a common cause of acute neurologic disease. The general physician must have the knowledge to rule out other etiologies and prove the diagnosis of cerebrovascular disease. He must be able to define the exact nature and location of the vascular lesion and then he must manage it effectively. The brain tissue destroyed by infarction or hemorrhage cannot be restored. However, the physician must do everything possible to preserve every gram of viable tissue and so improve the patient's chances for survival and a meaningful recovery.

REFERENCES

1. Brennan, R.W., Bergland, R.M.: Acute cerebellar hemorrhage-analysis of clinical findings and outcome in 12 cases. Neurology 27:527, 1977.
2. Cohn, J.N., Burke, L.P.: Nitroprusside. Ann. Int. Med. 91:752, 1979.
3. Faught, E., Trader, S.D., Hanna, G.R.: Cerebral complications of angiography for transient ischemia and stroke: prediction of risk. Neurology 29:4, 1979.
4. Fields, W.S.: The asymptomatic carotid bruit—operate or not? Stroke 9:269, 1978.
5. Genton, E.: Guidelines for heparin therapy. Ann. Int. Med. 80:77, 1974.
6. Golden, G.S.: Strokes in children and adolescents. Stroke 9:169, 1978.
7. Goldstone, J., Moore, W.S.: Emergency carotid artery surgery in neurologically unstable patients. Arch. Surg. 111:1284, 1976.
8. Grindal, A.B., Cohen, R.J., Saul, R.F., Taylor, J.R.: Cerebral infarction in young adults. Stroke 9:39, 1978.
9. Heyman, A., Wilkinson, W.F., Heyden, S., et al.: Risk of stroke in asymptomatic persons with cervical arterial bruits. N. Engl. J. Med. 302:838, 1980.
10. Hunt, W.E., Hess, R.M.: Surgical risk as related to time of intervention in the repair of intracranial aneurysms. J. Neurosurg. 28:14, 1968.
11. Kinkel, W.R., Jacobs, L.: Computerized axial transverse tomography in cerebrovascular disease. Neurology 26:924, 1976.
12. Lehrich, J.R., Winkler, G.F., Ojemann, R.G.: Cerebellar infarction with brain stem compression—diagnosis and surgical treatment. Arch. Neur. 22:490, 1970.
13. Millikan, C.H., McDowell, F.H.: Treatment of progressing stroke. Stroke 12:397, 1981.
14. Mohr, J.P., Fisher, C.M., Adams, R.D.: Cerebrovascular Diseases. p. 365. In Isselbacher, K.J., Adams, R.D., Braunwald, E., et al., eds.: Harrison's Principles of Internal Medicine. 9th Ed., McGraw-Hill, New York, 1980.
15. Mutlu, N., Berry, R.G., Alpers, B.J.: Massive cerebral hemorrhage—clinical and pathological correlations. Arch. Neurol. 8:74, 1963.
16. Najafi, H., Javid, H., Dye, W.S., et al.: Emergency carotid thromboendarterectomy: surgical indications and results. Arch. Surg. 103:610, 1971.
17. New, P.F.J., Aronow, S.: Attenuation measurements of whole blood and blood fractions in computerized tomography. Radiology 121:635, 1976.

18. Physician's Desk Reference. p. 1519. 35th Ed., Medical Economics, Oradell, New Jersey, 1981.
19. Ramirez-Lassipas, M.: Antifibrinolytic therapy in subarachnoid hemorrhage caused by ruptured intracranial aneurysm. Neurology 31:316, 1981.
20. Ransohoff, J., Goodgold, A., Benjamin, M.V.: Pre-operative management of patients with ruptured intracranial aneurysms. J. Neurosurg. 36:525, 1972.
21. Ross-Russell, R.W.: How does blood pressure cause stroke? Lancet 2:1283, 1975.
22. Samson, D.S., Boone, S.: Extracranial-intracranial (EC-IC) arterial bypass: past performance and current concepts. Neurosurgery, 3:79, 1978.
23. Sundt, T.M., Sandok, B.A., Whisnant, J.P.: Carotid endarterectomy-complications and preoperative assessment of risk. Mayo Clin. Proc., 50:301, 1975.
24. Sundt, T.M., Whisnant, J.P.: Subarachnoid hemorrhage from intracranial aneurysms—surgical management and natural history of disease. N. Engl. J. Med., 299:116, 1978.
25. Toole, J.F., Cole, M.: Ischemic cerebrovascular disease. In Baker, A.B., Baker, L.H., eds.: Clinical Neurology. Vol. 1, Ch. 10. Harper & Row, Hagerstown, MD, 1975.
26. VanGijn, J., VanDongen, K.J.: Computerized tomography in subarachnoid hemorrhage: differences between patients with and without an aneurysm on angiography. Neurology, 30:538, 1980.
27. Weisberg, L.A., Nice, C.N.: Intracranial tumors simulating the presentation of cerebrovascular syndromes—early detection with cerebral computed tomography. Am. J. Med., 63:517, 1977.
28. West, H., Burton, R., Roon, A.J., et al.: Comparative risk of operation and expectant management for carotid artery disease. Stroke, 10:117, 1979.
29. Whisnant, J.P.: Extracranial-intracranial arterial bypass. Neurology, 28:209, 1978.
30. Wolf, P.A., Kannel, W.B., Sorlie, P., McNamara, P.: Asymptomatic carotid bruit and risk of stroke—the Framingham study. JAMA, 245:1442, 1981.
31. Yarnell, P., Earnest, M., Kelly, G., Sanders, B.: Disappearing carotid deficits. Stroke, 9:258, 1978.

8

Transient Neurologic Symptoms, Including Blackouts, Dizziness and Transient Ischemic Attacks

Michael P. Earnest, M.D.

INTRODUCTION

Transient neurologic symptoms are a common experience. We often experience transient lightheadedness, unsteadiness, unusual muscle twitches or cramps, fleeting numbness and tingling sensations, headaches and other pains, and briefly blurred vision. Patients often come to a physician with a history of these or other transient neurologic symptoms and ask the physician "What's happening?", "Am I having a stroke (brain tumor, multiple sclerosis, etc.)?" The physician must then try to answer these questions for the patient, and must also reassure himself that the symptoms are innocuous.

The causes of transient neurologic symptoms range from the benign, such as mild orthostatic hypotension, to life-threatening, such as vertebral-basilar system transient ischemia that is the first sign of an impending basilar artery occlusion. Usually the physical examination is normal by the time the physician sees the patient, and there are no laboratory tests that help.

TRANSIENT NEUROLOGIC SYMPTOMS IN GENERAL

The Many Causes Of Transient Neurologic Symptoms

Table 8.1 lists the many common causes of brief neurologic symptoms. Primary neurologic processes include transient ischemic attacks, migraine phenomena, partial seizures, multiple sclerosis and pressure-induced neuropathy. Non-nervous system causes are anxiety, hyperventilation, orthostatic hypertension, cardiac arrhythmias and labrynthine (inner ear) disease. These

161

Table 8.1 Causes of Transient Neurologic Symptoms

Neurologic Disorders	Other Processes
Transient ischemic attack	Anxiety
Partial seizure	Hyperventilation
Multiple sclerosis	Labrynthine disease
Pressure neuropathy	Orthostatic hypotension
Migraine phenomena	Cardiac arrhythmia
Small cerebral infarction or hemorrhage	Hypoglycemia

processes sometimes present with a characteristic syndrome well-known to the general physician. Others may not be familiar. A brief description of the typical clinical presentations may be helpful:

1. Transient ischemic attacks (TIA)—An elderly patient presents with a history of several hours of weakness or numbness of the body and limbs on one side. If the right body was affected, trouble speaking (aphasia) may have been present. The clinical presentations of different types of TIAs will be discussed later.

2. Partial seizures—When the cerebral cortex has a lesion, such as an old traumatic scar, that area can initiate partial seizures with symptoms appropriate to the normal function of that area of cortex. A lesion in the motor area may induce seizures with twitching of one hand or one side of the face. A lesion in the sensory cortex may produce seizures characterized by transient paresthesias of one part of the body. Aphasia, vertigo, and bizzare psychologic experiences can also be produced by lesions in or near the temporal lobe.

3. Multiple sclerosis (MS)—Demyelination of white matter in the central nervous system caused by MS usually causes neurologic symptoms and signs that last for days or months. These then only partially recover. However, many patients with MS describe transient sensory, motor and visual symptoms that last only a brief time and then resolve completely.[14] Some MS patients also initially present with recurrent unusual transient neurologic symptoms.[14] However, only later, when more classic symptoms and signs develop, is the diagnosis made. The mechanism of these fleeting symptoms is unknown.

4. Pressure neuropathy—Mechanical pressure or a sharp blow on a peripheral nerve can produce transient sensory symptoms or weakness in the distribution of the nerve. The classic example is one's foot "going to sleep" after prolonged pressure on the sciatic nerve. Similar dysfunction can be produced in the arm or hand by pressure on the ulnar or radial nerves or nerve trunks in the axilla. Patients complaining of a numb, weak hand on awakening have usually been sleeping in a position

that caused unusual pressure or stretching in the axilla of nerves to the hand.

5. Migraine phenomena—Migraine headaches are frequently accompanied or preceded by numbness of one hand, facial paresthesias, visual symptoms, aphasia or clumsiness and weakness of one hand or leg. In migraine sufferers, such symptoms can also occur without a headache developing.[8] Occasionally the neurologic symptoms will be the first and only symptoms of a migraine disorder, or will occur months or years after the full headache syndrome has abated. The mechanism of the neurologic symptoms is unknown, but may be related to focal vascular spasm in the nervous system.

6. Small cerebral infarction or hemorrhage—Usually these lesions produce symptoms and signs that last several days, or are permanent. However, CT scanning of patients with cerebrovascular symptoms has shown that some patients with classical TIA syndromes have actually had small hemorrhages or infarctions. Those patients must be managed as stroke patients (see Chapter 7).

7. Anxiety and hyperventilation—The general physician, better than the neurologist, recognizes the perioral numbness, tingling hands and feet, shortness of breath, band around the head, and palpitations of the classic anxiety-hyperventilation syndrome. However, severe anxiety can also cause blackouts, blurred or double vision, transient unilateral numbness of a limb, amnesia, trouble speaking and ataxia. Again, the mechanisms are not known.

8. Labrynthine disease—Middle ear or inner ear disorders often present with vertigo, nausea, vomiting and ataxia.

9. Orthostatic hypotension—This usually presents as lightheadedness or dizziness upon standing, relieved by sitting or lying down. Orthostatic hypotension very rarely causes focal neurologic symptoms.

10. Cardiac arrhythmia—Arrhythmias also usually produce faintness or blackouts, but very rarely focal, unilateral symptoms.

11. Hypoglycemia—Again, the general physician is familiar with the classic symptoms. However, hypoglycemia can on occasion present as a transient hemiparesis or some other focal neurologic syndrome. In those instances, the symptoms don't resolve unless the patient is given glucose.

Each process usually presents with the classic symptoms. But unfortunately, a clinical syndrome may have several possible causes. For example, numbness of one hand lasting several hours can be caused by a transient ischemic attack, or multiple sclerosis. Yet the physician must try to make a single clinical diagnosis and then, if that diagnosis has serious implications for the patient's health, prove it and treat the cause. The most helpful tool the physician has is a detailed, thorough clinical history.

The Clinical History—The Key To Diagnosis

Usually when the physician sees the patient the symptoms have disappeared and the patient has no obvious neurologic deficits. The physician should spend most of his time and energy gathering a detailed and thoughtful history.

The clinician begins by knowing the patient's age. Older patients are more likely to have cerebrovascular and cardiovascular disease, causing transient ischemic attacks or cardiac arrhythmias. Younger patients more often have anxiety symptoms and hyperventilation but also migraine phenomena and multiple sclerosis.

The detailed history of the transient event is very important. If there were several events, the physician should elicit details of the latest one or the worst one. The physician should try to reconstruct as completely as possible the entire event: When was it? What were you doing at the onset? Did anything bring it on? What was the first symptom? The next symptom(s)? Were there other associated symptoms? How long did it last (Table 8.2)? What did you do to get relief? How did you feel afterwards? Was this spell the same as your usual ones? How was it different?

If the patient reports only one event, the physician must carefully search for prior symptoms that may be related, but have been neglected by the patient. Important questions are: Have you ever had this problem before? Ever had symptoms even faintly resembling your recent ones? As a child or young adult did you have any neurologic symptoms? (An affirmative response may suggest multiple sclerosis, seizures or migraine.) The physician specifically should ask about any symptoms that might suggest a specific diagnosis. He should look for symptoms of multiple sclerosis by asking about its common presentations: Have you ever had blindness in one eye for several days? One arm, one leg or both legs, numb or paralyzed for a few days? Severe double vision or severe dizziness and ataxia for several days?

Table 8.2 Typical Duration of Transient Symptoms Caused by Several Neurologic Processes

Etiology	Duration
Partial seizures	Seconds to 10 minutes
TIA causing only monocular blindness	Seconds to 10 minutes
Pressure neuropathy	Seconds to hours
Transient ischemic attack with hemiparesis, aphasia, etc.	30 minutes to a few hours (rarely over 8 hours)
Migraine phenomena	30 minutes to a few hours (rarely over 8 hours)
Multiple sclerosis	8 hours to several months

Prior transient ischemic attacks can be suspected if the patient reports prior transient hemiparesis, hemianopsia or hemisensory loss or aphasia for a few hours. Cerebrovascular disease is also suggested by prior episodes of total blindness in one eye lasting a few minutes. The duration of the recent or prior symptoms may suggest a specific etiology, as listed in Table 8.2.

A careful past medical history may disclose previous cardiac disease, hypoglycemia, diabetes, mental illness or other disorder that will suggest to the clinician a current diagnosis. Concerning previous neurologic illness the physician should specifically ask about seizures, including seizures as a child, migraine headaches, strokes, head injuries, unexplained blackouts, meningitis, encephalitis or "Any other disease of the brain or spine?" Other history should be obtained relevant to the specific clinical problem; for example, a history of ear infections or surgery in the patient with vertigo.

The Value Of Following The Patient

Often the nature or cause of recurrent transient neurologic symptoms is not clarified initially by the history, physical examination or laboratory tests. In those cases, careful follow-up may be extremely helpful. The physician should instruct the patient to call immediately if the event occurs again. If the event does recur, a repeat detailed history may provide clearer understanding of the nature and cause of the problem.

COMMON TRANSIENT NEUROLOGIC SYNDROMES

The Clinical Analysis Of Blackouts

When a patient says "I blacked out," the first task for the physician is to define the exact nature of the event. A "blackout" usually indicates a sudden, brief loss of consciousness. However, some patients use the term, or similar ones, to describe a feeling of faintness, blurring or "blanking out" of vision, a sense of loss of touch with the environment (a psychologic dissociation reaction, usually caused by anxiety) or a brief period of amnesia (also usually due to anxiety). Careful probing by the physician will usually reveal if consciousness was lost: Did you totally pass out? Did you fall to the ground? While you were 'out' were you still vaguely aware of the people and things around you? How long were you totally 'out'? Can you remember anything, any voices, any events from when you were 'out'?

Once it is assured the patient was unconscious the physician must try to understand the mechanism of loss of consciousness. Two common mechanisms account for the large majority of non-traumatic blackouts: (1) cessation or severe reduction of blood flow to the whole brain, and (2) a seizure. Less common causes are hypoglycemia, severe anemia and vertebral-basilar transient ischemic attacks. Rare, but known causes, are severe headache and severe anxiety, possibly by causing a cardiac arrhythmia.

Inadequate blood flow to the brain can be caused by systemic hypotension, usually postural, or a cardiac arrhythmia. Seizures cause loss of consciousness by interrupting the physiologic functions of both cerebral hemispheres or of the brainstem reticular activating system. Distinguishing between these two mechanisms of loss of consciousness, or between these and other mechanisms can be difficult. However, certain clinical features are helpful:

1. Cessation of blood flow to the brain—The patient usually describes an initial feeling of faintness, vision dims, he hears "roaring in my ears," knows he is about to pass out and often feels himself falling. The next thing he recalls is awakening on the floor, after only a minute or two elapsed time. The event may have been precipitated by standing up (orthostatic hypotension), urination (micturition syncope) pain or an emotionally stressful event (vasovagal syncope) or coughing (tussive syncope). If the patient has himself experienced prominent tachy- or bradycardia or palpitations, or has known heart disease, a cardiac arrhythmia may be the cause.

2. Epileptic seizure—A convulsion is suggested by the absence of presyncopal symptoms, or the presence of loss of consciousness or loss of memory longer than 5 minutes, urinary or fecal incontinence, a lacerated (bitten) tongue, or prominent headache, sore muscles, confusion or sleepiness after awakening from the blackout.

3. Hypoglycemia—Hypoglycemia leading to a blackout usually occurs in the setting of known diabetes mellitus treated with insulin or other hypoglycemic agents. The premonitory symptoms of anxiety, tremulousness, hunger, cold sweating and confusion usually precede the blackout by several minutes or longer.

4. Severe anemia—A patient with severe anemia usually has had prior orthostatic faintness and gives a detailed account of the blackout similar to the patient with cessation of blood flow to the brain.

5. Vertebral-basilar TIA—This is an uncommon cause of a simple blackout. A blackout caused by such a TIA usually has prominent associated brain stem symptoms, such as vertigo, diplopia, dysarthria or ataxia, before or after the blackout.

Clinical And Laboratory Tests For Blackouts

Every patient presenting with blackouts should be examined for orthostatic blood pressure changes and should have performed a hematocrit, blood sugar and electrocardiogram. If a cardiac arrhythmia is suspected, prolonged cardiac monitoring should be done. If a seizure is suspected, an electroencephalogram must be ordered. Occasionally, a patient with recurrent blackouts must be admitted to the hospital for cardiac monitoring or for careful observation of the details of each blackout event. Patients who pass out, fall and are injured frequently should be admitted for an intensive work-up. Such patients, especially older ones, can sustain serious injuries from blackouts.

The Problem Of Dizziness

"Dizziness" is a much-used, poorly-defined term. The physician must be sure what the patient is referring to. Is he referring to a lightheadedness, faintness, "swimming" sensation in the head, or to true vertigo, a sensation of spinning, being himself physically moved or the environment moving. Sometimes even the most intelligent, verbal patient cannot define which it is, but the physician should always try to understand the exact nature of the symptom.

Three mechanisms can explain most syndromes of recurrent dizziness: (1) otologic, inner ear disease, (2) anxiety, and (3) postural hypotension (Table 8.3). Uncommon causes are multiple sclerosis, vertebral-basilar TIAs and partial seizures.[5] Tumors of the acoustic nerve are a rare cause of dizziness.

1. Inner ear disease—Labrynthine disease usually causes true vertigo with nausea and vomiting. During the episode the patient often remains immobile, finding that movement will cause worse symptoms. Walking is prevented by severe ataxia and fear of falling. In between attacks these patients often have tinnitus and hearing loss, which can be confirmed by the physical examination. During the attack they often have prominent nystagmus. One unusual type of labrynthine dizziness is benign positional vertigo, in which the patient has recurrent vertigo, often precipitated by lying down.

2. Anxiety—Dizziness of this type is the lightheaded, faintness variety. It is often accompanied by the symptoms of hyperventilation as well as

Table 8.3 Common Etiologies of Dizziness in 104 Patients

Etiology	Percent*
Peripheral vestibular disorders	38
Hyperventilation and other psychiatric	32
Multiple sensory deficits	13
Cerebro- and cardiovascular events	9
Specific neurological disorders (e.g., MS)	6
Unknown and miscellaneous	13

* The total is more than 100% because 12 patients had 2 diagnoses

(from Drachman, D.A., Hart, C.W.: An approach to the dizzy patient. Neurology, 22:323, 1971; reprinted with permission)

blurred vision and a psychologic sense of distance, dissociation from the environment.

3. Postural hypotension—Dizziness produced by postural hypotension is of the lightheaded faintness variety, and is brought on by the patient standing up. Orthostatic blood pressure changes can be demonstrated by taking lying and standing blood pressures.

4. Multiple sclerosis usually causes true vertigo, but the attacks usually last for days and are accompanied by other neurologic symptoms and signs. If the MS plaque is affecting the vestibular system, the neurologic examination usually shows dysarthria, disordered eye movements (in addition to nystagmus), facial numbness or weakness, or asymmetric reflexes or clumsy movements of the arm or leg.

5. Vertebral-basilar TIAs—Cerebrovascular disease can cause either true vertigo or a nondescript dizziness. However, to make a diagnosis of a vertebral-basilar TIA causing dizziness the physician should require a history of true vertigo accompanied by dysarthria, diplopia, weakness or numbness of the face or the limbs, or associated with a blackout.

6. Partial seizures—A lesion of the temporal lobe irritating the cerebral cortex can induce partial seizures that include vertigo. Such events are difficult to diagnose as seizures, but a seizure causing vertigo should be considered in a patient with known seizure disorder or a cerebral lesion and in patients with vertigo accompanied by an episodic behavioral disorder or psychologic experiences suggesting complex partial (temporal lobe, psychomotor) seizures.

Clinical And Laboratory Tests For Dizziness

The most important tests to perform on the physical examination are blood pressure, both lying and standing if the history suggests orthostatic hypotension, and a careful search for cranial nerve findings, such as nystagmus, disordered eye movements, a depressed corneal reflex, facial numbness or weakness, impaired hearing, a depressed gag reflex or unilateral tongue weakness. The patient's walking, balance, fine finger movements, strength and reflexes should also be tested if the patient has had true vertigo. If the main symptom was nondescript dizziness, a screening examination of the cranial nerves only will usually suffice.

Beyond the physician's initial physical examination there are few easily available tests to help diagnose the cause of dizziness. The most cost-effective next step probably is to refer the patient to an otolaryngologist, if the clinician specifically suspects inner ear disease, or to a neurologist.

The patient with several hours of severe, disabling vertigo, prominent nausea and vomiting, ataxia and falling, should probably be admitted to the hospital for observation and more intensive work-up. Those patients often require parenteral anti-emetic drugs, intravenous fluids, and bed rest until the symptoms resolve. Such patients may also fall and be injured if sent home.

Lancinating, "Ice Pick" Pains

Patients with migraine headaches often, apart from their usual headaches, have intense sharp, stabbing pains.[11] These often occur in or near the eye, but can occur elsewhere in the head. There are no precipitants, and the pains last only a few seconds or are instantaneous. Similar pains occur in patients without migraine headaches.[11] The mechanism for these pains is unknown. When a patient complains of such pains the history is characteristic. No treatment is necessary but the patient can be assured that the symptoms are benign.

TRANSIENT ISCHEMIC ATTACKS

The Pathophysiology Of TIAs

"Transient ischemic attack" is defined as a focal neurologic symptom, of sudden onset, lasting less than 24 hours, caused by cerebrovascular disease. The onset of symptoms, from no symptoms to the peak of severity, usually requires only a few minutes. The symptoms rarely last beyond 8 hours, but the traditional clinical definition allows up to 24 hours.

Many transient ischemic events, and maybe the majority, are probably caused by emboli to the brain vasculature.[6,10] Common sources are cardiac valvular disease, left atrial blood clots associated with atrial fibrillation, and atherosclerotic plaques at the origin of the internal carotid artery. However, some TIAs are probably due to focal brain ischemia caused by temporarily reduced blood flow through a severely stenotic artery.[6,10] Classic TIA syndromes can also be caused by tiny deep cerebral infarctions or hemorrhages.

Clinical Anatomy And Symptoms Of TIAs

Blood is carried to the brain by two pairs of arteries, the right and left carotid arteries and the right and left vertebral (Fig. 7.1). The two carotid arteries provide the major blood supply to the cerebral hemispheres. These arteries and their distal branches comprise the so-called anterior circulation. The vertebral arteries join to form the basilar artery. They comprise the posterior circulation, and supply the midbrain, pons, medulla and cerebellum, as well as the mesial occipital lobe (the visual cortex) of each hemisphere (Figs. 7.1 and 7.2).

TIA symptoms can be separated into two sets of syndromes: those comprising TIAs of the anterior circulation and those of the posterior circulation (Table 8.4). Anterior circulation TIA symptoms are characterized by hemi-

**Table 8.4 Neurologic Symptoms Produced by Ischemia in the Carotid
and Vertebral-Basilar Cerebrovascular Systems**

Carotid System	Vertebral-Basilar System
Hemiparesis	Diplopia
Hemi-sensory loss	Binocular visual loss
Aphasia	Vertigo
Transient monocular blindness	Tinnitus
	Ataxia
	Dysarthria
	Bilateral limb motor or sensory symptoms
	Loss of consciousness
	Drop attacks

paresis, monoparesis (weakness of one arm or leg), sensory loss in one or
both limbs on the same side of the body, aphasia, or transient total blindness
in one eye. Transient total loss of vision in one eye is usually caused by
an embolus passing up the internal carotid artery, then into the ophthalmic
artery and on to the central retinal artery of the eye. This symptom alone
is just as important a marker of carotid artery disease as is hemiparesis or
aphasia. These symptoms can occur singly or in combination.

Posterior circulation TIAs have less distinct, and more confusing (to the
physician) symptoms: double vision, dysarthria, ataxia, vertigo, tinnitus,
clumsiness of the limbs and blackouts. Two or more of these usually occur
together, and any may be accompanied by weakness or numbness of the
arms and legs. An unusual, but distinctive, TIA of the posterior circulation
is a "drop attack" in which the person falls down because of sudden bilateral
leg and arm weakness, but he doesn't lose consciousness. This syndrome
is caused by ischemia of the medulla or upper spinal cord.

The clinical importance of separating the two types of TIAs is based on
their different suitability for angiography and surgical treatment. Anterior
circulation TIAs often have associated atherosclerotic disease in the internal
carotid artery that can be angiographically demonstrated and surgically
excised (Fig. 8.1). However, surgery on the basilar or vertebral arteries
has a prohibitive morbidity and mortality.

The Natural History Of A TIA

A TIA alone rarely harms the patient. The symptoms can be temporarily
disabling and are often very emotionally distressing to the patient. However,
the symptoms pass within a few hours and the patient is well again. The
physician's concern about a TIA arises from his knowledge that a TIA may
be the first symptom of a crippling stroke.

The literature on the natural history of TIAs is varied, but generally indi-

Fig. 8.1
Right carotid angiogram showing a large intraluminal blood
clot. An underlying small atherosclerotic plaque was demonstrated at surgery. This 35-year-
old man had four TIAs over two
months and then a major stroke.

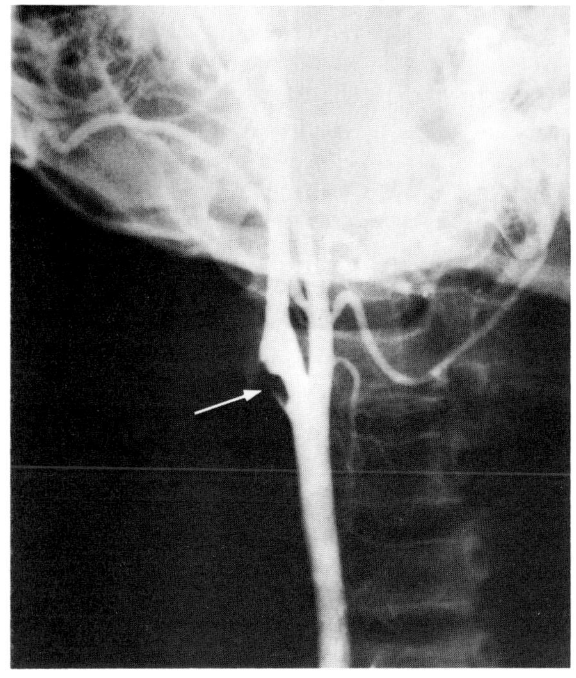

cates that, following a first TIA, the patient has a 20 to 30 percent risk of
having a stroke within 2 to 3 years.[2] It is this risk that demands every
patient with a TIA be thoroughly evaluated for conditions that may be
treated, and so a stroke prevented. But the physician's management must
also include the knowledge that 70 to 80 percent of TIA patients will not
have a stroke in the next few years.

Clinical Management Of The Patient With A Suspected TIA

Table 8.5 outlines a management plan appropriate for most patients with
a first TIA or recent onset of TIAs (i.e., onset within a few months). Some
patients must be managed differently, because of advanced age or severe
medical disabilities, but the questions outlined should be asked by the physician for every patient with a suspected TIA.

Many different processes can masquerade as a TIA (Table 8.1 and Ref.
6) so the physician must consider all the possible diagnoses and conduct a
detailed history to make a specific diagnosis, as previously described. A
CT scan should be done on almost every patient with a suspected TIA
because so many other important brain lesions can cause similar symptoms
(Fig. 8.2).[15]

After convincing himself of the diagnosis, the physician should try to
infer from the patient's symptoms which circulation, the anterior or poste-

Table 8.5 Questions to Consider in the Management of a Patient with Recent Onset of TIA Symptoms

Is it cerebrovascular disease?
Which circulation is involved?
Was it an embolus?
Admit the patient?
What are the predisposing conditions?
Do an arteriogram?
Is surgery appropriate?
What is the best medical management?
How long should treatment continue?

rior, was involved. If this decision cannot be easily made, the physician should manage the patient as if it were an anterior circulation event. Those TIAs are more often associated with surgically correctable lesions, and so the patient should more often be admitted to the hospital for angiography.

Several types of TIA patients should be promptly admitted to the hospital. The patient with his first anterior circulation TIA, and who is in good general health, should be admitted to have tests to diagnose any surgically treatable

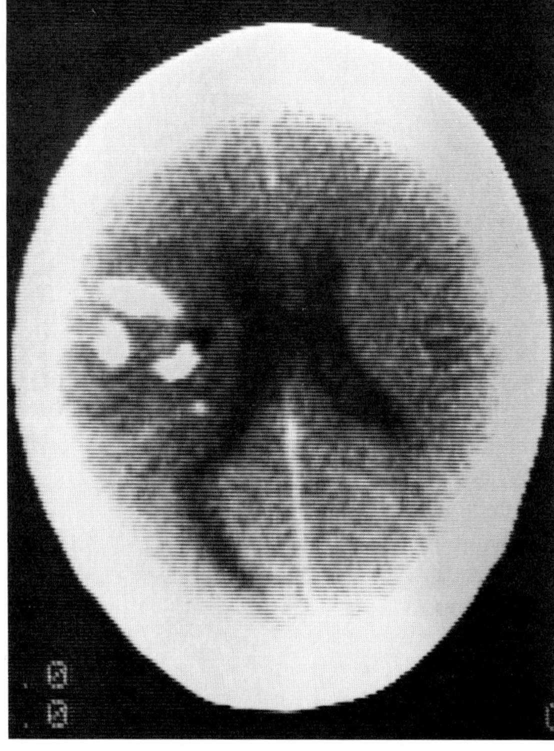

Fig. 8.2
CT Scan of a 39-year-old woman with recurrent aphasia and right body numbness. The large tumor has three densely calcified areas.

carotid artery lesion. The patient with a history of TIAs, regardless of which circulation is involved, who is now having more frequent TIAs has a high risk of a full-blown stroke in the near future. He should be admitted for aggressive work-up and treatment. A patient with prior TIAs who now presents with one whose symptoms and signs have not cleared as rapidly or as fully as before may have had a completed stroke, or may have one soon. He should be admitted for observation and further work-up.

Every patient, whether admitted or managed as an out-patient, should be thoroughly evaluated for conditions that may predispose him to having premature or progressive cerebrovascular disease. The causes to be sought are hypertension, diabetes mellitus, blood lipid disorders, coagulation or platelet disorders, syphilis, vasculitis, use of birth control pills, and abuse of amphetamines. A thorough history and appropriate laboratory tests should be done.

Many TIAs are probably caused by small thrombi or platelet clumps forming in the heart or on atherosclerotic plaques in the carotid or vertebral artery and then breaking loose and travelling to the intracranial circulation (see Fig. 8.1). The danger for the patient of an embolic TIA is the danger of a second embolus causing a major stroke. A patient with a TIA suspected to be caused by an embolus should be admitted to the hospital. If the source of the embolus was obvious, and is not surgically treatable, for instance rheumatic heart disease with atrial fibrillation, no angiogram is required, but the patient should be treated with anticoagulants. If the source of the embolus is not clear, or the physician wants to prove the diagnosis of an embolic TIA, an angiogram should be done to visualize the intracranial circulation, looking for intravascular filling defects caused by embolic material (see Fig. 7.5). The angiogram should also examine the origin of the internal carotid artery and the proximal common carotid artery, looking for a large or ulcerated atherosclerotic plaque that may have been the source of an embolus. If such a lesion is found, surgery can be done to remove it. If such a lesion is not found, the physician knows the embolus probably came from the heart.

Arteriography is also indicated in the patient who is having frequent TIAs. Arteriography is urgent if the patient has had several TIAs within the last few days. Frequently recurring TIAs can be a sign of a severe stenosis of the carotid artery, and a warning of impending carotid occlusion. They also may indicate a large ulcerated atherosclerotic plaque or an intraluminal blood clot in the carotid artery. Such lesions must be treated immediately. If surgery cannot be done, anti-coagulation must be begun.

The role of surgery in treating TIAs is controversial. The intent of surgery is to remove the vascular lesion causing the TIA and so prevent future TIAs and strokes. Surgery may prevent those future events, but it also entails significant morbidity and mortality, especially in the older or medically ill patient. Carotid artery surgery in community hospitals also has a higher morbidity and mortality than in large referral centers.[7] Surgery is indicated for the patients with severe vascular lesions and those with multiple TIAs. Surgery is not routinely indicated for patients with small carotid artery plaques who have one or rare TIAs. The role of surgery for patients with a history of several TIAs and a modest carotid artery stenosis or small ulcerated plaque is unclear. Unfortunately there have been no controlled studies comparing the present and future morbidity of surgical versus medical management.

A newly developed technique may eventually expand the role of surgery in the treatment of TIAs. With the advent of cerebrovascular surgery using the operating microscope, it is now possible to anastomose a superficial cranial vessel, most often the superficial temporal artery, with an intracranial one, usually a cortical branch of the middle cerebral artery.[1,16] This extracranial-to-intracranial (EC-IC) bypass then supplies added blood flow to the hemisphere. Use of this technique has given some highly selected patients good results by reducing subsequent TIAs.[13] It is unknown if future strokes will be prevented. A large cooperative study is currently evaluating the efficacy of this technique.[1]

Most patients with TIAs do not have surgery and are managed medically. General medical management should include control of hypertension and cardiac arrhythmias. Dehydration or congestive heart failure should be corrected to improve cerebral blood flow and anemia, hypoglycemia and other metabolic abnormalities should be reversed.

When a patient has had frequent, severe TIAs, anticoagulation should be begun immediately if angiography or surgery are not done and a CT scan and lumbar puncture show no evidence of an intracranial hemorrhage. Anticoagulants should also be used if there is a demonstrated source for emboli causing the TIAs. The role of anticoagulants in treating the patient with a first TIA or infrequent TIAs is less certain. Probably the patient with a first TIA, or recent onset TIAs, should receive anticoagulants for 3 to 6 months, the period in which he has the highest risk of having a stroke.[4] The physician must, however, also consider the risks of anticoagulation.[9] Elderly patients, patients with hypertension, and uncooperative or alcoholic patients, all have increased risks of systemic or intracranial hemorrhages induced by anticoagulation.[2]

After completion of the period of anticoagulation the physician should closely follow the patient for several months. If TIAs recur he must reconsider admitting the patient, doing an angiogram, or reinstituting anticoagulants.

Whenever anticoagulants are begun in the emergency setting, the first drug should be heparin. An initial intravenous bolus of 2,500 to 7,500 units will produce rapid anticoagulation.[9] Next, a carefully controlled intravenous drip of heparin at a rate of 5,000 units every 4 hours will probably maintain adequate anticoagulation.[9] This can be judged by obtaining an activated partial thromboplastin time (aPTT) test. A reasonable level of anticoagulation is shown by an aPTT of 1½ to 2 times the control value. The rate of infusion can be adjusted to ensure adequate but safe levels.

If heparin was begun initially, a second anticoagulant, warfarin (Coumadin) should be begun after a few days of heparin therapy. The best level of anticoagulation with warfarin for cerebrovascular disease is not well established, but the author and others use a prothrombin time (PT) of about 1½ times the control sample time. Prior clinical practice of maintaining the PT at twice the control value, about 25 seconds, seemed to have an excessive complication rate, possibly because the population of patients with TIAs is an elderly one.

The use of "antiplatelet" drugs has been recently touted as effective to reduce future stroke and death in TIA patients.[3] The purported protective effect is related to the drugs reducing the platelets' ability to aggregate and induce intravascular coagulation. The evidence for a beneficial effect is suggestive, but there is controversy. Which drug or drug combination and, what doses are best and how long to treat have not been unequivocally established. Aspirin, in doses of 1,300 mg per day, has been shown effective in one major study.[3] The combination of aspirin and sulfinpyrazone (Anturane, 800 mg per day) was not clearly superior but may have been slightly better than aspirin alone. Sex of the patient was important: only men had a beneficial effect. Women had no significant improvement in future morbidity and mortality. No final recommendation is currently possible, but a reasonable course is to treat a TIA patient, if not anticoagulated or after anticoagulants have been discontinued, with both aspirin and sulfinpyrazone. The author treats both men and women. Treatment should probably be continued 6 months to a year.[12] These recommendations will probably change as results of further studies are published.

CONCLUSION

Transient neurologic symptoms can be puzzling and threatening to the patient and to the physician. The physician must know the multiple possible causes of the symptoms and should be able, by taking a careful history, to choose the most likely cause. He can then reassure the patient of the benign nature of his symptoms, or he can launch an extensive work-up and treatment plan for a more life-threatening process.

REFERENCES

1. Barnett, H.J.M., Peerless, S.J.: The collaborative EC/IC bypass study. The rationale and a progress report. p. 271. In Moossy, J., Reinmuth, O.M., eds.: Cerebrovascular Diseases—Twelfth Research (Princeton) Conference. Raven Press, New York, 1981.
2. Brust, J.C.M.: Transient ischemic attacks: natural history and anticoagulation. Neurology, 27:701, 1977.
3. The Canadian Cooperative Study Group: a randomized trial of aspirin and sulfinpyrazone in threatened stroke. N. Engl. J. Med., 299:53, 1978.

4. Cartlidge, N.E.F., Whisnant, J.P., Elveback, L.R.: Carotid and vertebral-basilar transient cerebral ischemic attacks: a community study, Rochester, Minnesota. Mayo Clin. Proc., 52:117, 1977.
5. Drachman, D.A., Hart, C.W.: An approach to the dizzy patient. Neurology, 22:323, 1972.
6. Duncan, G.W., Pessin, M.S., Mohr, J.P., et al.: Transient cerebral ischemic attacks. Adv. Intern. Med., 21:1, 1976.
7. Easton, J.D., Sherman, D.G.: Stroke and mortality rate in carotid endarterectomy: 228 consecutive operations. Stroke, 8:565, 1977.
8. Friedman, A.P.: Headache. Ch. 13. In Baker, A.B., Baker, L.H., eds.: Clinical Neurology. Vol. 2. Harper & Row, Hagerstown, Md., 1974.
9. Genton, E.: Guidelines for heparin therapy. Ann. Int. Med., 80:77, 1974.
10. Pessin, M.S., Duncan, G.W., Mohr, J.P., et al.: Clinical and angiographic features of carotid transient ischemic attacks. N. Engl. J. Med., 296:358, 1977.
11. Raskin, N.H., Schwartz, R.K.: Icepick-like pain. Neurology, 30:203, 1980.
12. Sandok, B.A., Furlan, A.J., Whisnant, J.P., Sundt, T.M.: Guidelines for the management of transient ischemic attacks. Mayo Clin. Proc., 53:665, 1978.
13. Sundt, T.M., Siekert, R.G., Piepgras, D.G., et al.: Bypass surgery for vascular disease of the carotid system. Mayo Clin. Proc., 51:677, 1976.
14. Twomey, J.A., Espir, M.L.E.: Paroxysmal symptoms as the first manifestation of multiple sclerosis. J. Neurol. Neurosurg. & Psychiat., 43:296, 1980.
15. Weisberg, L.A., Nice, C.N.: Intracranial tumors simulating the presentation of cerebrovascular syndromes. Am. J. Med., 63:517, 1977.
16. Whisnant, J.P.: Extracranial-intracranial arterial bypass. Neurology, 28:209, 1978.

9

Trauma of the Head, Spine and Peripheral Nerves

Harold B. Vogel, M.D.

HEAD INJURIES

Initial Evaluation And Treatment

This subject was introduced in Chapter 1 with a reminder of the ABC's of emergency medicine: control of the airway, bleeding, and circulation. Another short but excellent elaboration of these points may be found in the American College of Surgeons' Manual, *Early Care of the Injured Patient.*[1]

It cannot be stressed often enough that control of the airway is paramount. The skull in the adult is a closed box and the injured brain must be accommodated within it. Anything which promotes further swelling, particularly hypercarbia from hypoventilation, may quickly cripple or kill a patient who might otherwise be saved. Perhaps the most important factors which have led to the recent improvement in mortality and morbidity in unconscious head injured patients have been rapid endotracheal intubation by ambulance personnel and the immediate institution of hyperventilation, enough to drop the arterial PCO_2 to the range of 25–30 mmHg.

Scalp lacerations may be deceptive. Torn galeal vessels may be in spasm in the ER and the wound may not bleed much there, yet one has no idea how much blood has been lost at the accident scene or in transit. In such cases an elastic bandage over some 4 × 4 gauze sponges usually will give temporary control until more formal debridement and closure may be carried out. Consider in all cases the possibility that blood loss may have been extensive and remember that it is possible for a patient to exsanguinate from a scalp laceration.

The source of hemorrhage, however, may not be so apparent and in the unconscious patient there are no complaints of pain to guide the examiner. Hypotension and tachycardia should suggest occult hemorrhage, and the abdomen is the most obvious site. Clinical signs of peritoneal irritation may be missing, particularly in children and the elderly. One should not hesitate to do an abdominal tap in suspicious cases.

An IV for infusion of fluids and withdrawal of blood for various studies (see below) should be placed as soon as the patient enters the ER, if it has not been done already in the field. Then a rapid physical exam is carried out to exclude life-threatening conditions, such as a sucking chest wound or cardiac tamponade.

The neurological exam should be thorough but need not be exhaustive. Three things need to be observed and *recorded* as baseline observations: (1) the level of consciousness, (2) the equality of the pupils and their reactivity to light, and (3) motion of the extremities.

> ***PRINCIPLE 1:*** The level of consciousness is the most important parameter in the evaluation of the head-injured patient.

The level of consciousness is obvious to the examiner at the patient's side, but conveying this information to others may be difficult. Fortunately the Glasgow Coma Scale (Table 9.1) has become a kind of international currency which facilitates communication, for instance, between ambulance personnel in the field and medical personnel at the hospital.[6,12]

Disparate pupillary size in an unconscious patient most often means one of two things: orbital trauma or intracranial hemorrhage on the side of the larger pupil. The former is usually, but not invariably, obvious. The latter reflects paralysis of the oculomotor nerve from downward herniation of the medial portion of the temporal lobe, impacting the oculomotor nerve and brain stem; if not relieved quickly, secondary brain stem hemorrhages may occur (see Chapter 4). As the affected pupil enlarges, its reactivity to

Table 9.1 The Glasgow Coma Scale

M	Best Motor Response	Obeys	6
		Localizes	5
		Withdraws	4
		Abnormal flexion	3
		Extensor response	2
		Nil	1
V	Verbal Response	Oriented	5
		Confused conversation	4
		Inappropriate words	3
		Incomprehensible sounds	2
		Nil	1
E	Eye Opening	Spontaneous	4
		To speech	3
		To pain	2
		Nil	1

light usually is lost also.

Check motion of the extremities to determine the presence or absence of hemiparesis or quadriparesis. Hemiparesis may follow from brain stem compression and may be ipsilateral or contralateral to the side of the dilated pupil. Quadriparesis suggests an associated cervical spine fracture. In the unconscious patient what would otherwise be a fairly painful stimulus may be required to evaluate the ability to move the extremities.

Bloodwork sent to the lab depends on the accident circumstances, but in general one wants to know right away what the hemoglobin and hematocrit are and to assure that blood is being set up for type and cross match. Other studies complete the workup: the rest of the CBC (white count and qualitative platelet estimate), arterial blood gases, serum electrolytes, blood sugar, a toxicology screen, and the blood alcohol level.

The unconscious patient needs a nasogastric tube, to empty the stomach and prevent aspiration, and a Foley catheter for accurate measurement of output. IV fluids should be run slowly, at 75 cc/hr initially but adjusted later according to the output. Some salt should be in the solutions given, since cerebral edema is promoted by 5 percent dextrose in water alone. Other lines include a central venous pressure or a Swan-Ganz catheter and frequently an arterial line as well.

Skull films in the ER usually are not much help, but a cross-table lateral cervical spine film is mandatory before the patient has been moved around much. If there is a suspicion of intracranial hemorrhage, further plain films are deferred until an emergency CT scan is obtained. Following this, the patient may go back to the ER for additional X-rays, to the floor, or to the OR. In some cases, particularly where acute traumatic arterial occlusion is suspected, the next step may be angiography.

Not many drugs are necessary or desirable in the initial management of the head injured patient. Dexamethasone (Decadron), 10 mg IV, is usually given, although its efficacy in the treatment of cerebral swelling is less clear in trauma than in other situations (e.g., where there is cerebral edema around a metastatic tumor). Other adjunctive measures for the control of raised intracranial pressure will be discussed below.

Since the level of consciousness and control of respiration are so important, one does not want to give drugs which will depress these functions. In the agitated, semicomatose patient, codeine is usually sufficient to control pain from associated injuries, such as fractures. Codeine is also the morphine derivative least likely to interfere with pupillary reactions, respiration, and level of consciousness. Sedation may be achieved with pentobarbital (Nembutal) or diazepam (Valium), but these must be used judiciously.

PRINCIPLE 2: Do not give morphine to patients with head injuries and use sedative drugs sparingly.

Specific Problems

Cerebral Concussion

These patients are usually wide awake and neurologically intact when seen in the ER. They give a history of head injury with a brief period of unconsciousness and, perhaps, amnesia for the event. Hospitalization is unnecessary in most cases, unless some other finding, such as a skull fracture, indicates that the injury has been more than trivial.

Linear Fractures

Linear fractures over the cranial vault generally are not important, except when they lie in specific locations, as will be described below. Most overlying scalp lacerations can be closed in the ER, but debridement must be thorough and some cases must be taken to the operating room, with curettage of the fracture line to remove impacted dirt and hair. The assumption is that the underlying dura is intact, but the possibility for later development of meningitis always exists.

Basilar Skull Fractures

Basilar skull fractures are difficult to visualize by X-ray studies. They may produce rhinorrhea by involvement of the frontal, ethmoid, or sphenoid sinuses, although the most common fracture site for this is through the ethmoids (Fig. 9.1A). Fractures extending through the petrous portion of the temporal bone may produce otorrhea or simply a hemotympanum (Fig. 9.1B). Otorrhea almost always stops spontaneously. Rhinorrhea stops sponta-

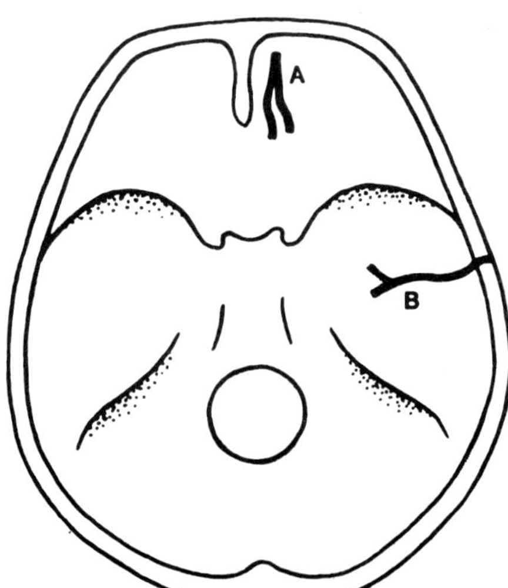

Fig. 9.1 Base of the skull. Fractures at A are the most common and may extend into the ethmoid sinuses, producing rhinorrhea. Fractures at B may produce otorrhea.

neously in 85 to 90 percent of cases; when it does not, repeated lumbar punctures or even surgical repair may be necessary. Because of the hazard of meningitis, patients with basilar skull fractures usually are put on a broad spectrum antibiotic, such as ampicillin.

Depressed Skull Fractures (Fig. 9.2)

These fractures almost always require surgery, but the timing for this depends on whether or not the overlying scalp has been lacerated; open skull fractures should be treated within 6–8 hours of injury. The surgical technique involves making a burr hole adjacent to the depression and then removing bone around it; extract the depressed fragments last. The reason for this is that the underlying dura and brain may be lacerated and the fragments may be tamponading torn cortical vessels. The principle is the same for any kind of surgery: hemostasis requires proper exposure.

Supratentorial Intracranial Hemorrhage

Acute Epidural Hematomas

These most often are apparent within 6 hours of injury and usually result from a torn middle meningeal artery. In the history one looks for the "lucid interval": a transient period of unconsciousness (concussion) at the outset; a period when function is regained; then a lapse into unconsciousness again as a result of the rapidly expanding clot. A linear skull fracture traversing the course of the middle meningal artery may be a clue (Fig. 9.3A). On CT scan the lens-shaped appearance is characteristic (Fig. 9.3B), caused by the attachment of the dura to the skull at the margins of the clot.

Traumatic intracranial hemorrhage in the subdural space and the frontotemporal brain is often caused by the greater sphenoid wing, the "dashboard" on which the brain impacts in head injuries (Fig. 9.4). The cerebrospinal fluid provides some protection for the brain, but its cushioning effect is easily dissipated.

Acute Subdural Hematomas

Acute subdural hematomas are frontotemporal in location and result from tearing of vessels in the region of the Sylvian fissure, that portion of the brain immediately subjacent to the greater sphenoid wing. The configuration of the clot conforms to that of the brain, because there is no constraint to its dissection in the subdural space (Fig. 9.5A), and, like any hemorrhage, after clotting the acute subdural hematoma is solid rather than liquid, so it cannot be drained adequately through burr holes (Fig. 9.5B). Its lethality stems as much or more from the swelling of associated cerebral contusion as from the clot itself.The sites most at risk for cerebral contusion are the anterior and inferior surfaces of the frontal and temporal lobes (Figs. 9.6A and B), since they border the greater sphenoid wing.

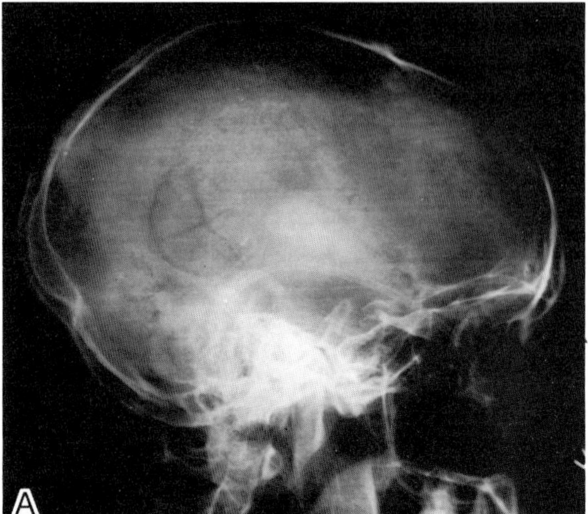

Fig. 9.2
(A) Lateral skull film. The patient had been struck with a hammer. (B) OR Photo. Same patient as in (A). Depression of the fracture fragments is obvious.

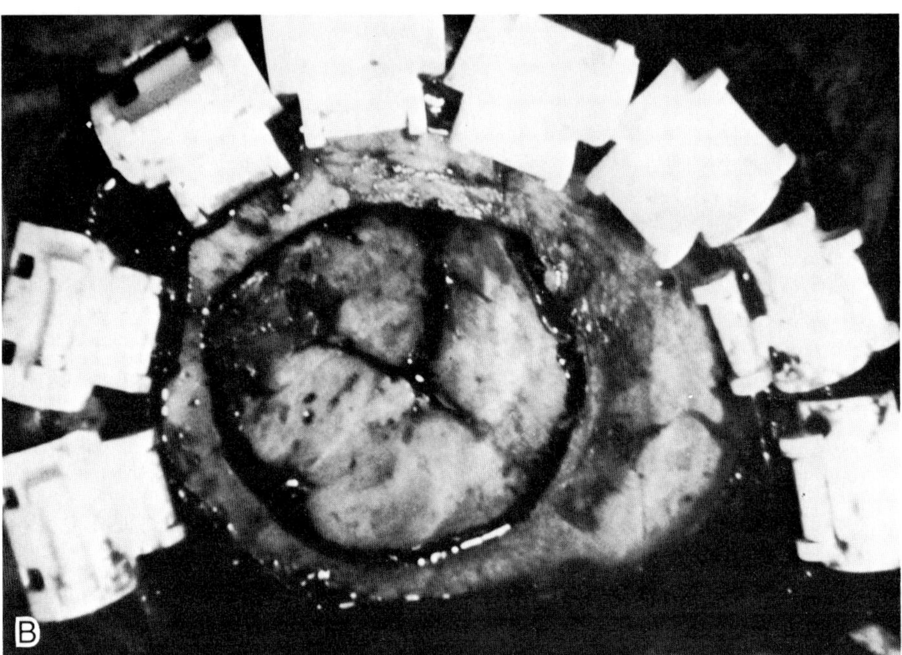

Intracerebral Hemorrhage

The bruising of the brain implies petechial hemorrhages at least; if they coalesce, areas of frank intracerebral hemorrhage occur, again most commonly in the frontal and temporal lobes (Fig. 9.7).

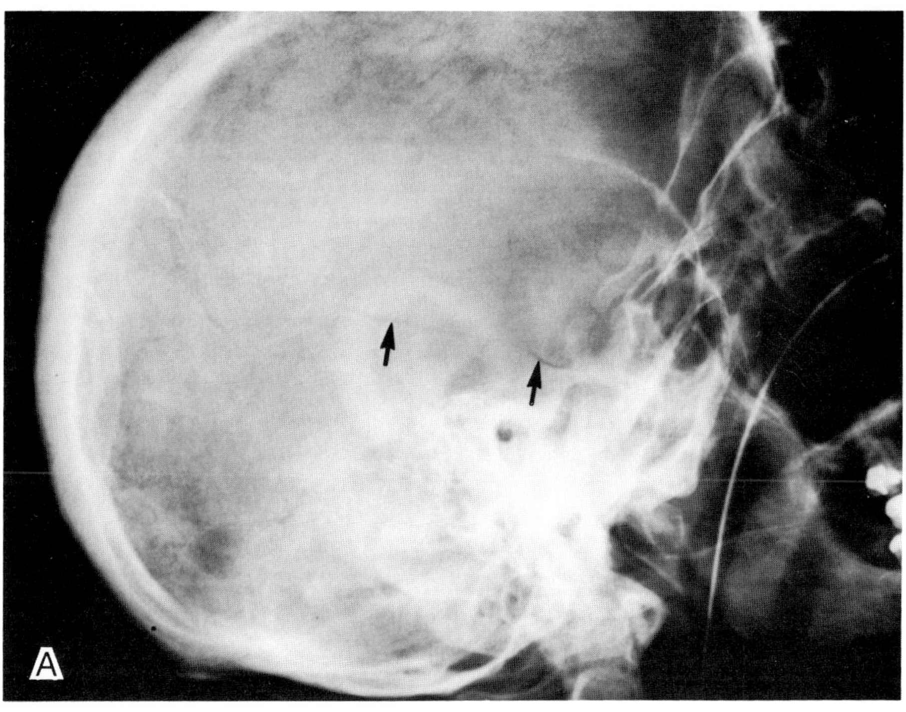

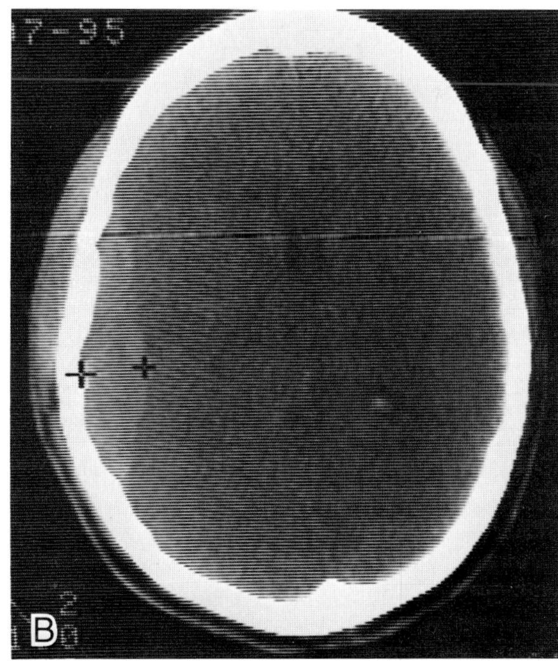

Fig. 9.3
(A) Lateral Skull Film. The arrows point to a fracture line which crosses the territory of the middle meningeal artery. (B) CT Scan. Same patient as in (A). The opaque clot has the lentiform shape characteristic of an epidural hematoma.

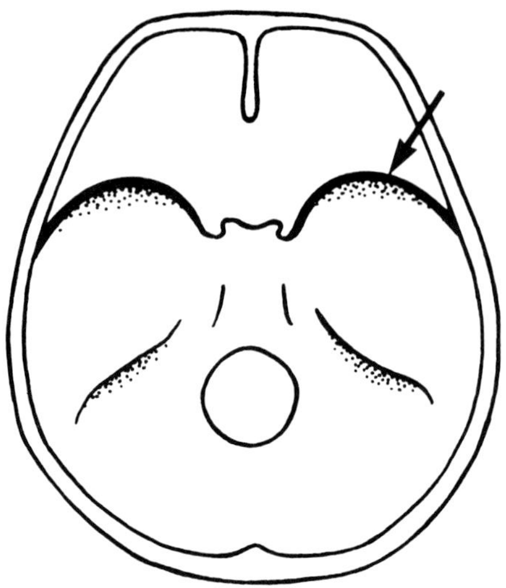

Fig. 9.4 Base of the skull. The arrow points to the greater sphenoid wing, the "dashboard" on which the brain is impaled.

Infratentorial Intracranial Hemorrhage

This condition is infrequent because of the relatively protected position of the posterior fossa, but diagnosis and treatment must be carried out quickly: this space is small and only a slight increase in pressure may result in respiratory arrest from medullary compression. A warning sign is the finding of a fracture line extending into the posterior fossa, particularly if it crosses one of the transverse sinuses (Fig. 9.8).

Gunshot Wounds of the Head

Gunshot wounds of the head in civilian practice very often are lethal. Sixty percent of them are self-inflicted and the common bitemporal trajectory is low enough that vital portions of the basal ganglia and hypothalamus are destroyed.[2] There is more of a chance for survival if the trajectory is anteroposterior and higher (Fig. 9.9). At surgery hemorrhage along the tract and bone fragments are suctioned away. If convenient, metallic fragments are removed; otherwise they are left alone, because the frictional heat resulting from the velocity of the bullet usually is sufficient to render them sterile.

Cranial Nerve Injuries

These injuries frequently occur in patients with head injuries. The most commonly injured is the olfactory nerve, but this may be overlooked if the patient is unconscious at admission and one may forget to check for it later. The clue to the injury comes with a comment by the patient that his food tastes "flat," because much of what we interpret as taste is actually

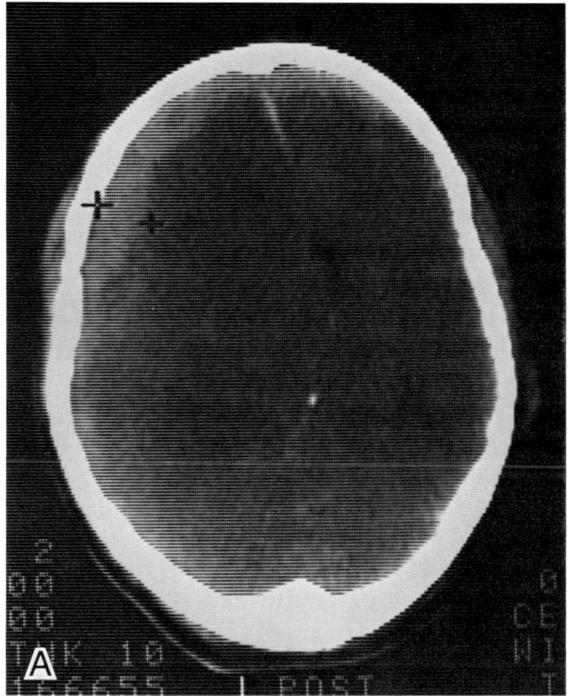

Fig. 9.5
(A) CT Scan. The brain has been shifted from left to right, not only because of the acute subdural hematoma, but also because of contusion of the subjacent brain. (B) OR Photo. The dura has been reflected and the underlying acute subdural hematoma has been exposed.

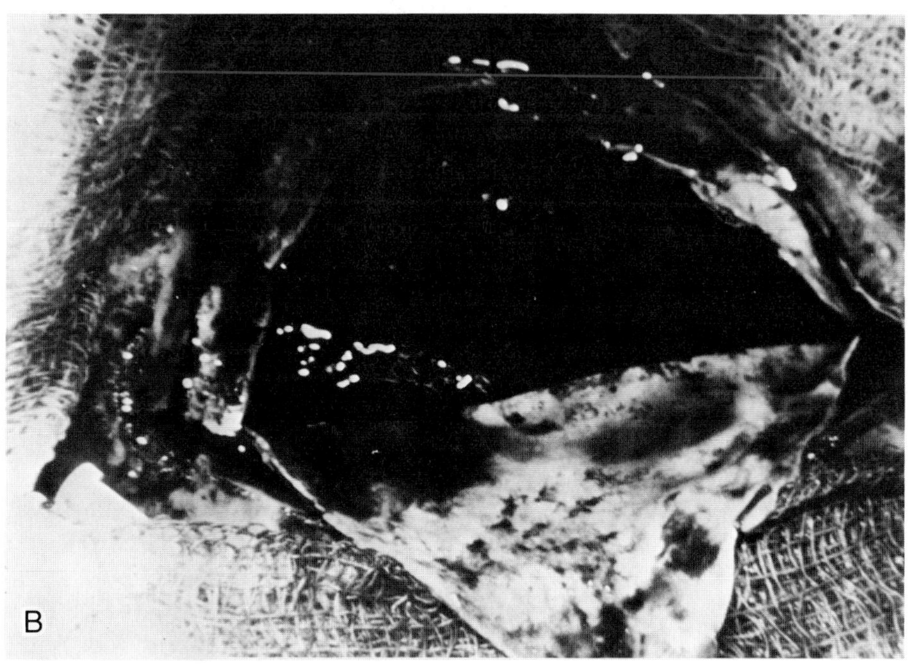

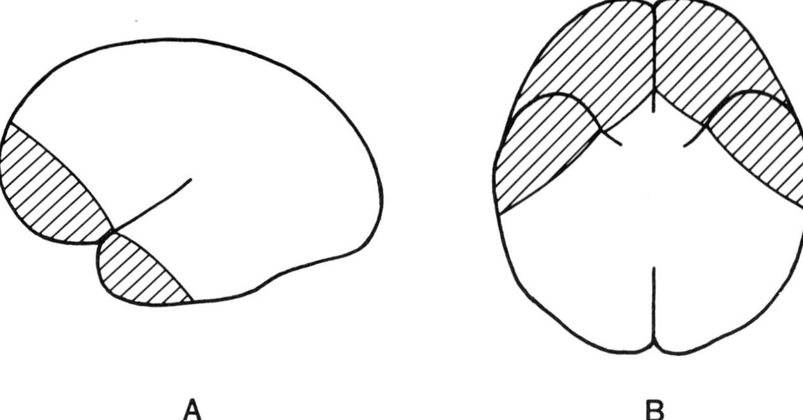

A   B

Fig. 9.6 (A) Lateral view and (B) Basal view of the brain. Areas most at risk for cerebral contusion are the anterior and inferior poles of the frontal and temporal lobes.

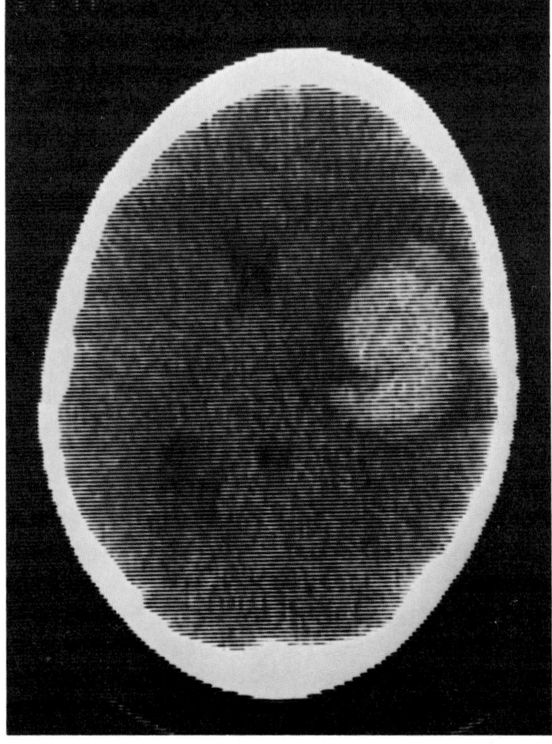

Fig. 9.7
CT Scan. The temporal lobe is a characteristic location for a traumatic intracerebral hemorrhage.

Fig. 9.8
Towne view of the skull. Fracture lines which pass into the posterior fossa of the skull are worrisome because they raise the possibility of infratentorial hemorrhage.

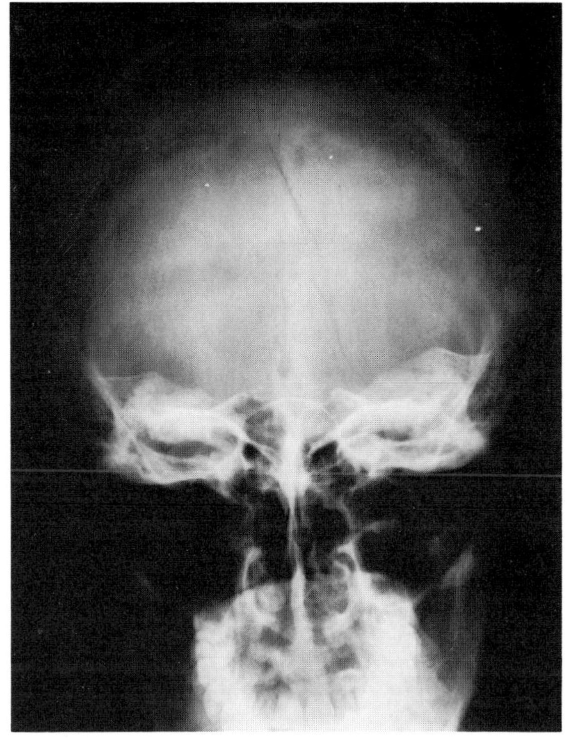

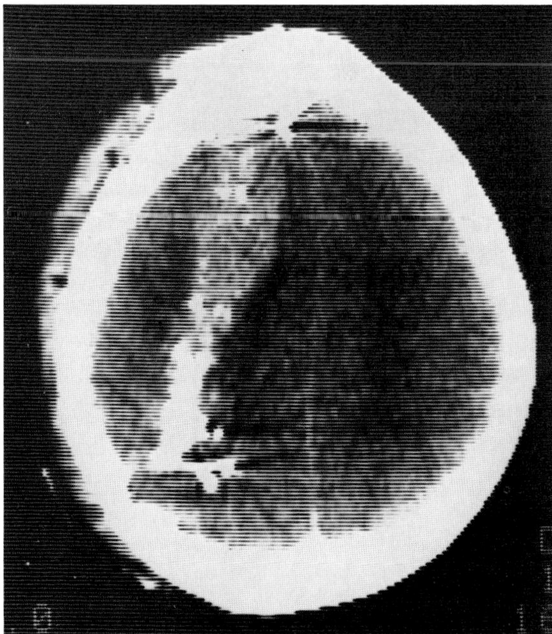

Fig. 9.9
CT Scan. The point of entry of this gunshot wound of the head was midfrontal. The patient survived, following ligation of the sagittal sinus anteriorally and debridement of the bullet tract.

the sense of smell. The second most commonly injured cranial nerve is the facial, or so it seems, because injury to the facial nerve is so apparent. Raised intracranial pressure may lead to secondary pressure on the oculomotor nerve, with resulting pupillary dilitation and loss of response to light, as mentioned earlier. Increased intracranial pressure may also cause diplopia due to abducens nerve palsy, since this nerve has the longest intracranial course of any of the cranial nerves.

Vascular Injuries

Injuries of this sort may lead to severe brain damage: hemiplegia, coma, and death can result from traumatic occlusion of the carotid artery in the neck. Another particularly striking condition results from tearing of the carotid artery as it passes through the cavernous sinus. The resulting carotid-cavernous fistula, with arterial blood reversing the flow in veins draining from the orbits (Fig. 9.10), can cause orbital edema and pain, extraocular muscle palsies, and a swishing noise which may be audible to the patient. The surgical remedy frequently requires carotid ligation, both intracranially and in the neck, to "trap" the fistula and reduce its arterial inflow.

Surgical Management

The importance of thorough debridement in the treatment of scalp lacerations, particularly when they overlie fractures, has already been mentioned. Whenever possible, scalp closure should be in two layers, with one row of sutures in the galea, which is the holding layer, and the other on the surface. The galea retracts a bit when cut, so eversion of the scalp may be necessary to visualize it when suturing.

In managing unconscious patients, measurement of intracranial pressure is very helpful. Inferences about intracranial pressure from the CT scan may be misleading, while precise data from the monitor permits better treatment and, it is hoped, a better prognosis.[8] Equivalent measurements can be obtained from the epidural, subdural, or intraventricular spaces.

Epidural pressure monitoring can be instituted quickly and presents no subsequent problems to the nursing staff. A burr hole is made in the skull and the fiberoptic sensor is slid between the dura and the skull. The distal cable is then brought out through the incision and is connected to the monitor, which provides a digital readout.

Subarachnoid pressure monitoring is the type most commonly in use today. Often the skull opening is done in the ER or on the ward with a hand-held twist drill. Then the dura is punctured and a hollow bolt is inserted which connects in turn to a transducer and then to the monitor. Cerebrospinal fluid pressure thus is directly measured. The problems with a fluid-filled system center around the potential for infection and the need for skilled nurses to keep the system accurate and functional.

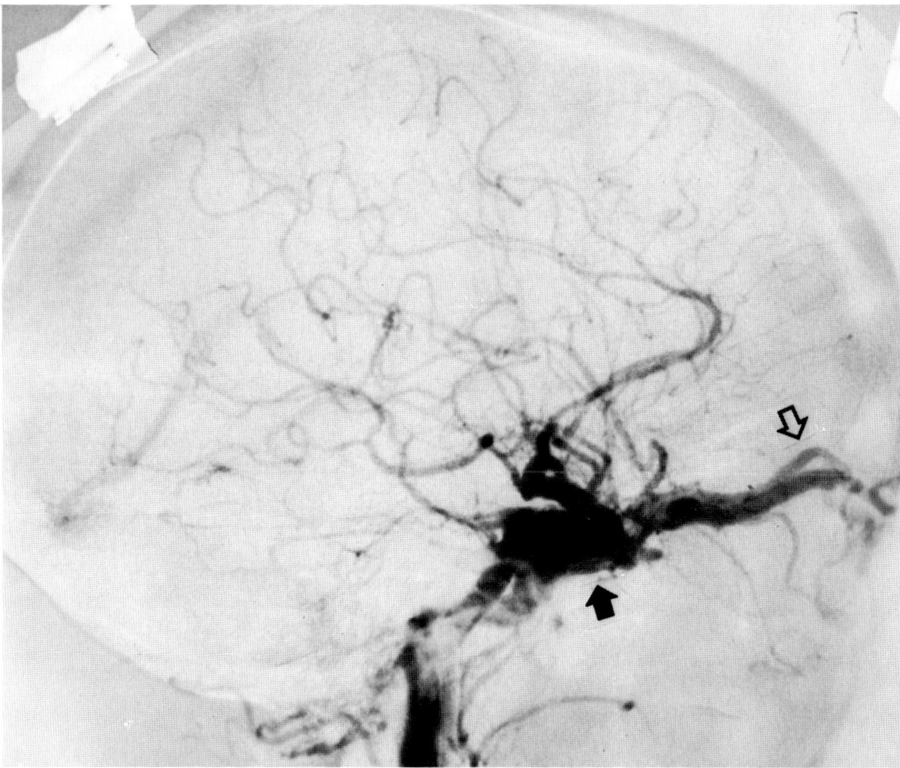

Fig. 9.10 Lateral carotid angiogram. This is the characteristic appearance of a carotid-cavernous fistula (dark arrow). The carotid artery is outlined as it enters the head and fills the intracranial vessels, but at the same time the dye is seen flowing forward from the cavernous sinus into the ophthalmic veins (open arrow) which normally return blood from the orbits. (See Fig. 7.5A.)

Ventricular pressure monitoring is much the same as subarachnoid pressure monitoring, except that fluid comes from the ventricular system through a catheter, rather than from the subarachnoid space. An additional problem with this method is that often in severely injured patients, where pressure monitoring is most critical, the ventricular system is compressed or shifted and so is hard to cannulate.

Burr holes (Fig. 9.11) in the treatment of acute head injuries are less necessary now than in the past, because the speed and accuracy of the CT scanner has lessened the need for exploratory procedures. They are placed over the association areas of the brain where iatrogenic cortical or subcortical damage would produce minimal permanent sequelae. *Burr holes are inadequate for the drainage of freshly clotted blood in epidural, subdural, or intracerebral locations,* because this blood is solid and cannot be

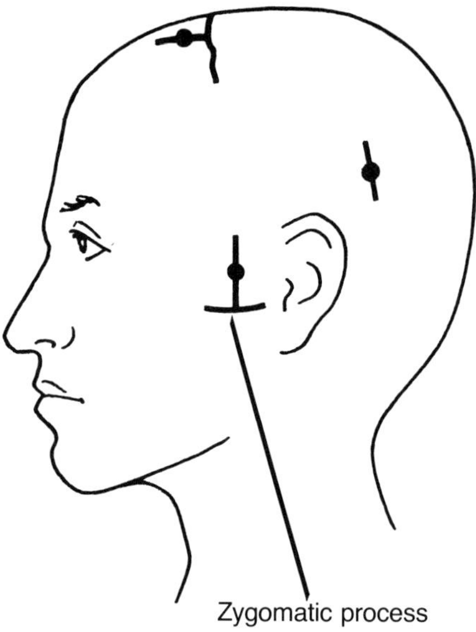

Fig. 9.11 Drawing of the standard locations for burr holes. These are placed over "silent" areas of the brain (i.e., away from the major motor, sensory, and speech areas). The frontal burr hole is made an inch from the midline, just in front of the coronal suture, where the head is somewhat flattened. The temporal burr hole is placed just above the zygomatic process. To get to the skull in this area, the superficial temporal artery usually must be ligated and the temporalis muscle must be incised. The parietal burr hole is made about an inch above and behind the tip of the ear. Note that, if necessary, all three incisions can be connected, a scalp flap turned, and a formal craniotomy performed (straight lines represent scalp incisions).

broken up sufficiently for extraction even using irrigation with a suction-catheter.

Harvey Cushing's subtemporal decompression does not decompress much brain, but this temporal craniectomy approach (Fig. 9.12) is good enough to enable the non-neurosurgeon to evacuate a considerable portion of the

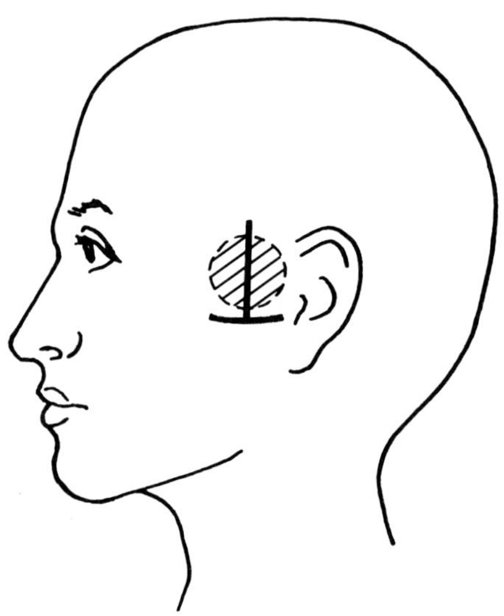

Fig. 9.12 Drawing of the location of a temporal craniectomy. The incision is a little longer, but the approach is the same as for a temporal burr hole. The skull opening is widened to the size of a silver dollar. When the patient is rapidly deteriorating, traumatic intracranial hemorrhage is suspected, and there is no time for definitive X-ray studies, this is the approach used. It will expose the usual acute epidural or subdural hemorrhage and most intracerebral hemorrhages as well.

Fig. 9.13 Drawing of a fronto-temporo-parietal craniotomy. This is the exposure most neurosurgeons use when the pre-operative CT scan has demonstrated intracranial hemorrhage in its usual relationship to the greater sphenoid wing. A question-mark incision is made (reverse question-mark on the right side), the scalp flap is turned, and a 4-hole free bone plate is removed. Further bone is rongeured away temporally and the dura is then opened.

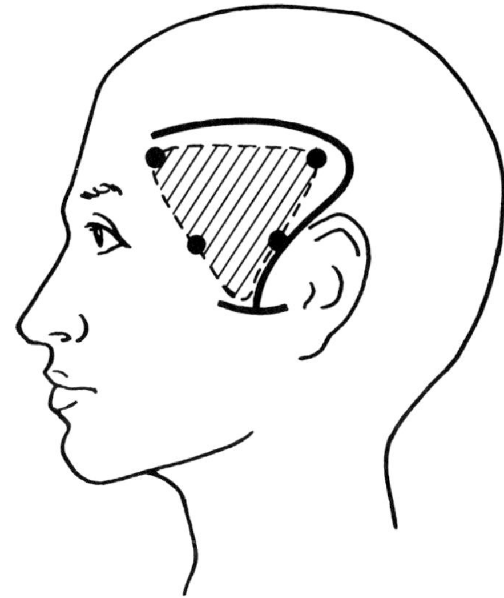

usual traumatic intracranial hemorrhage. A neurosurgeon probably would prefer the larger opening of a formal craniotomy (Fig. 9.13). If a head injured patient in the ER of a hospital without a CT scanner suddenly becomes comatose, with signs of brain stem compression from a rapidly expanding intracranial clot (a widely dilated pupil, hemiparesis), then whatever surgeon is at hand must decide whether mannitol will be given, to buy time for patient transport, or whether immediate temporal craniectomy on the side of the dilated pupil will be performed. People are alive today because of the courage shown by an orthopedist or general surgeon in carrying out this latter course of action.

Adjunctive Measures For The Control Of Elevated Intracranial Pressure

Almost as soon as the patient with a severe head injury is seen, measures should be instituted to reduce intracranial pressure, the most important being airway control by endotracheal intubation and hyperventilation to bring the arterial PCO_2 into the range of 25–30 mmHg. Many components of cerebral autoregulation of blood flow are lost following trauma to the brain, but responsiveness of cerebral blood vessels to PCO_2 is maintained almost until the time of brain death.

Dexamethasone is usually given at the time of admission, the initial dose being 10 mg IV and the maintenance dose 4 mg IV q 6 h. Because of the possibility of gastric or duodenal ulceration complicating this therapy over a period of time, patients are started on an antacid and/or cimetidine, 300 mg IV q 6 h.

Again, do not fluid-overload the head injured patient. Infusions should not run at more than 75 cc/hr initially and should contain some salt. One should try to estimate how much fluid has been given by ER personnel, and, if there is any question of overloading, the patient should be given furosemide, 20 mg IV, to diurese the excess fluid.

Mannitol is an excellent drug for reducing intracranial pressure, a hyperosmotic agent which rapidly removes fluid from uninjured portions of the brain. The initial dose is 1 gm/kg IV, run in as rapidly as possible. A relative contraindication to its use is the possibility of intracranial hemorrhage, yet paradoxically it is in just such cases that it is used most often. The reason for the prohibition is that a comatose patient may be given mannitol, improve because the pressure is relieved, and then lapse into coma again after 6–8 hours as the intracranial clot expands to increase intracranial pressure once more. It is that interval of improvement, however, that is relied upon in the emergency situation to get a CT scan or to transport the patient to a facility which has one.

> ***PRINCIPLE 3:*** Never give a head injured patient mannitol unless a definitive procedure, such as CT scanning or surgery, will immediately follow.

Barbiturates are now in vogue for the treatment of raised intracranial pressure. Pentobarbital is most often used, the loading dose being 2–300 mg (3–5 mg/kg) IV and then approximately 100 mg IV every hour, to produce blood levels in the range of 2.5–3.5 mg percent. These doses are near lethal but seem to be well-tolerated, providing the patient is intubated, on a respirator, and well-oxygenated.[7] This form of treatment, however, precludes neurological evaluation of the patient. Moreover, the patient is dependent on machinery for his survival, and the doctor is "instrument flying." Obviously, barbiturate therapy requires well-trained ICU nursing personnel if its benefits are to exceed its risks.

Complications

Most patients whose head injuries are not too severe do surprisingly well if their ventilation is adequately maintained. Consciousness is regained after several hours or days, and resumed oral intake re-establishes adequate nutrition. Intact kidneys usually compensate for therapeutic zeal with i.v. fluids.

One unpredictable condition which may show up quickly after injury, however, is that of inappropriate antidiuretic hormone secretion, which manifests itself clinically by a decrease in the level of consciousness or failure of mental status to improve. Urinary output may be no guide to the fact that the serum sodium is falling to a dangerous level. The lab picture shows an increased urine sodium, despite the hyponatremia. The treatment is fluid restriction, although in some cases hypertonic saline may be necessary also.

The reverse condition, that of diabetes insipidus, is not often seen, except terminally. Its presence suggests severe hypothalamo-hypophyseal damage and a dying brain. Treatment is by replacement of fluid lost with normal saline and aqueous pitressin, 5 units i.m., q 3–4 h. prn for urinary outputs over 200 cc/hr. One must be sure that the excess urine is not simply a reflection of fluid over-loading. The differential diagnosis is made by observing urinary response to fluid restriction, which will not change if the problem truly is diabetes insipidus.

The serum hemoglobin and hematocrit must be watched carefully, remembering that unconscious or semi-conscious patients cannot provide proper pain cues to sites of occult blood loss and that the damaged brain has an urgent need for an adequate supply of oxygen, which can only be transported by the blood. Appropriate transfusion has the additional effect of providing colloid, which by its osmotic effect helps reduce intracranial pressure.

In the patient who fails to improve or who worsens after several days in the intensive care unit, the possibility of delayed or recurrent intracranial hemorrhage must be considered and the CT scan should be repeated. Delayed vascular problems, such as cerebral vasospasm, thromboses, emboli, or initimal tears of the carotid artery, may necessitate angiography.

Infections are the most common type of complication seen in the unconscious patient. Pneumonia may follow quickly on the heels of atlectasis in the respirator-dependent patient, and bronchoscopy with extraction of atelectatic plugs should not be delayed if endotracheal suction proves ineffective. Prolonged urinary drainage obviously sets the patient up for urinary tract infection. Meningitis does not occur often but must be considered when other sources of fever have been ruled out, particularly if there is a basilar skull fracture.

Seizures occur in the first week following head trauma in about 5 percent of cases; as might be expected, the incidence increases with the severity of the injury.[5] Control usually can be achieved with the standard anticonvulsants, phenytoin (Dilantin) and/or phenobarbital.

SPINE AND SPINAL CORD INJURIES

Initial Evaluation And Treatment

The maxim, primum non nocere, "first, do no harm," has no greater application than to first-responders at an accident scene. Few victims will be found lying peacefully supine; even if they are, some motion is necessary during transport to the hospital and it is at such times that care must be taken to prevent permanent spinal cord injury.

> ***PRINCIPLE 4:*** Think spinal injury at the scene of an accident if the victim is unconscious or is complaining of neck or back pain or dysesthesias, numbness, or weakness in the extremities.

Such patients should have some sort of bracing applied, particularly if the problem seems to be a cervical spine injury, *before* they are moved, say, from a wrecked vehicle. A soft collar (Fig. 9.14) does not give much support, but it is better than nothing and may be the only thing which can be applied prior to removal; when free, better immobilization can be achieved before transport to the hospital (Fig. 9.15).

As with head injuries, one must consider associated life-threatening conditions, such as tension premothorax or cardiac tamponade. If there is paraplegia or quadriplegia, intra-abdominal hemorrhage can be difficult to diagnose: peritoneal signs may be minimal, the patient may not complain of abdominal pain, and the only clue may be hypotension.

A rapid neurological exam should be carried out as early as possible. This should include three observations: motion of the limbs, sensation (both pin-prick response and position and vibratory sense, since these travel up different spinal cord pathways), and reflexes. In trying to determine if a cord injury is "complete" (loss of all physiologic function below the level of the injury), it is particularly important to examine the perineal region, because sacral sparing may be the only guide to an "incomplete" injury, in which

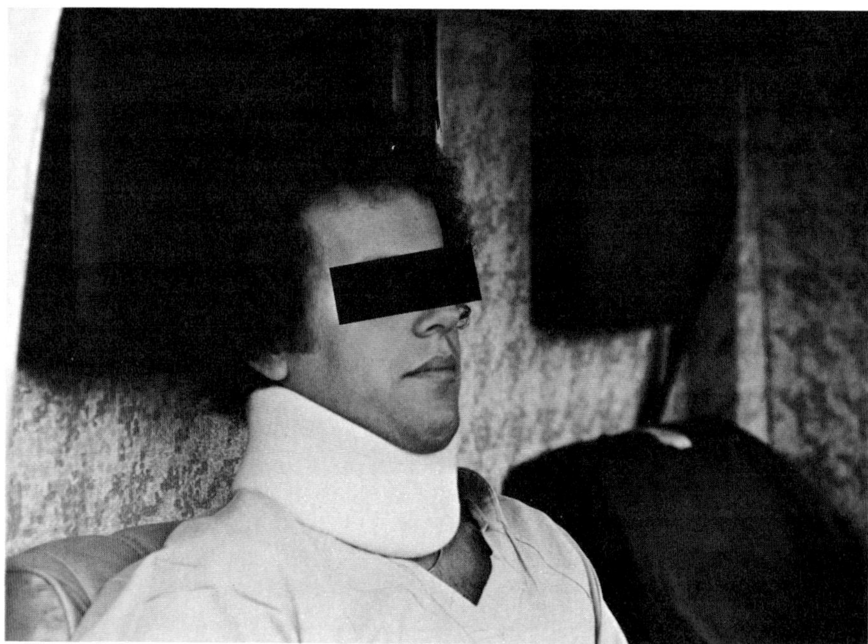

Fig. 9.14 A soft collar is applied prior to extraction of the accident victim with a neck injury from his wrecked vehicle. Care still must be taken, because this type of collar provides only partial support. If the circumstances permit, further stability can be achieved by slipping a board under the patient's upper back and head and taping him to it.

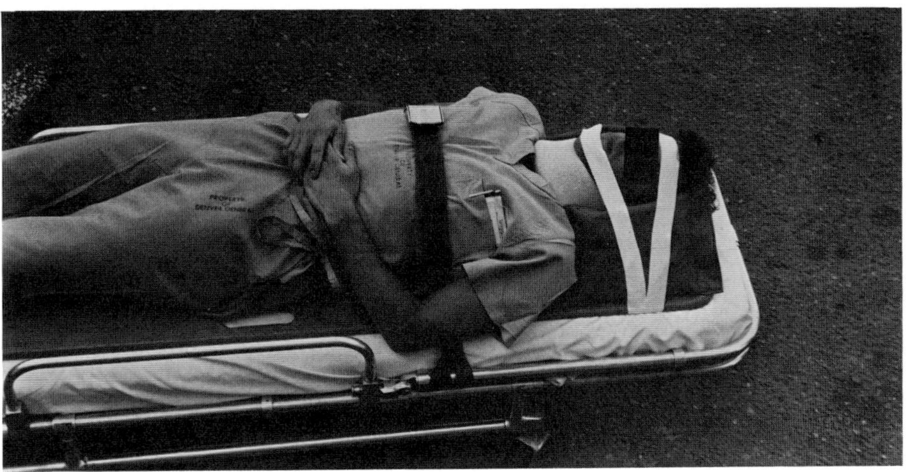

Fig. 9.15 Once free of the wreck, the patient with a neck injury is transported with the spine rigidly fixed, utilizing a back board (or scoop stretcher), sandbags, and tape.

the prognosis may be considerably better. One must discover if the patient can void, if there is any preserved perineal or perianal sensation, and the status of anal sphincter tone and the anal reflex.

> **PRINCIPLE 5:** Document in the patient's chart as early as possible and then at frequent intervals thereafter the results of the neurological exam. These findings not only help in establishing prognosis: evidence of a worsening neurological condition is one of the few indications for emergency surgery in cases of spinal cord injury.

Initial X-ray studies need not be complicated, but reasonable quality is important on AP, lateral, and oblique views. These films provide the basis for deciding whether or not to carry out more detailed studies, such as tomography and/or CT scanning. Flexion and extension films are almost never indicated on an emergency basis because of their obvious hazard.

The assumption generally is made that there is contusion and swelling of the spinal cord at the point of injury. Although its usefulness in treating this swelling remains to be critically evaluated, patients are usually given dexamethasone, 10 mg IV, as soon as possible after injury and then 4 mg IV q 6 h thereafter. Other measures that are effective in reducing intracranial swelling have not been shown to be helpful in treating spinal cord injuries.

Maintenance of blood pressure has been found to be important for the protection of the damaged spinal cord in the experimental setting. And since the patient with a cervical or high thoracic cord injury may be hypotensive because he has had the equivalent of a sympathectomy, his blood pressure probably should be brought back to a normal range, even though he may have no symptoms of hypotension. In this connection the protective effect of naloxone (Narcan) in the treatment of experimental spinal cord injury is being investigated, but its utility in the treatment of humans has yet to be demonstrated.

Spinal Cord Syndromes

"Concussion" implies transitory loss of function. It is common with head injuries but quite rare in spinal cord injuries. The picture with the latter is that of complete or nearly complete loss of function which rapidly clears in 24 hours. Because of such cases one should not attempt to give a prognosis until after the first few days of hospitalization.

The most common spinal cord injury, unfortunately, is that of complete transection. This is almost always physiologic rather than anatomic, but the result is the same:

> **PRINCIPLE 6:** With complete spinal cord transections, all function is immediately lost below the level of the lesion and does not return.

Frequently there is hematomyelia: bleeding within the central gray matter of the cord. Immobilization of the spine following injury is important even with complete transections to prevent this hemorrhage from increasing and to avoid its dissecting cephalad and adding to the neurological loss. This is particularly important in the cervical area, where ascent of even one segment can drastically alter the patient's potential for rehabilitation.

With a high cervical injury, consider also control of respiration: where there is complete transection, the intercostal muscles are not functioning, yet the patient can breathe because of the phrenic nerve supply to the diaphragm. But if hemorrhage within the cord ascends above the C4 level, the phrenics will be lost and the patient will suffocate, or at best will be transformed from a quadriplegic into a respirator quadriplegic, where the prognosis for extended survival is poor.

Fortunately, most complete cervical spinal cord injuries involve lower cervical segments. Table 9.2 provides a convenient guide to the level of injury.

One should not fall into the trap of moving up the trunk with a pin over anesthetic skin, discovering preserved sensation at about the level of the clavicles, and concluding that the level of injury is high thoracic: perusual of a dermatome chart will show that the lower cervical dermatomes are tightly clustered here and that accurate determination of the level requires pinprick testing in the arms and hands.

Following complete spinal cord transections, all descending nerve impulses are stopped at the level of the injury. The cord below this point is still viable, because of the segmental nature of the blood supply, but nevertheless at first this lower portion does not show any independent function.

Table 9.2 Guide to Cervical Spinal Cord Injuries

Fx/dislocation at	Lowest Preserved Roots	Motion Preserved	Sensation Preserved	Reflexes Preserved
C_4–C_5	C_5	Arm abduction Forearm flexion	Radial arm and forearm	Biceps jerk
C_5–C_6	C_6	Arm abduction Forearm flexion Supination	Radial arm and forearm Thumb and index finger	Biceps jerk
C_6–C_7	C_7	Arm abduction Forearm flexion Supination + pronation Wrist extension and flexion Finger extension	Radial arm and forearm Fingers 1–4	Biceps jerk Triceps jerk

In a case of paraplegia, for instance, the legs are flaccid, anesthetic, are flexic and the bladder is atonic. This is the syndrome of spinal shock. Then, after a variable period of 2–6 weeks, increased tone and reflex hyperactivity is seen, because of the loss of inhibitory impulses from above, but there still is no voluntary control of movement. There are also other signs of an "upper motor neuron" lesion: spasticity in the legs, ankle clonus, and Babinski signs. Mass reflex movements may occur (e.g., stroking the bottom of the foot may trigger a spinal cord reflex resulting in withdrawal of one or both legs). Gradually some moderation of these responses occurs.

Partial spinal cord injuries may show improvement with time. The general rule seems to be that the less the degree of impairment at the outset, the better will be the recovery. There are at least three recognizable partial cord injury syndromes:

1. The Brown-Séquard Syndrome (Figs. 9.16 and 13.1) is infrequently seen in the usual blunt trauma type of accident, because it represents a discrete hemisection of the spinal cord. Stab wounds are a more common cause. Incomplete variants of this syndrome are seen and the prognosis for improvement in such cases is fairly good.

2. The Central Cord Syndrome (Fig. 9.17) is seen with cervical spine injuries. Weakness in the hands can be quite marked at the outset, yet because so much of the rest of the cord is preserved, the prognosis for improvement with time is good also.

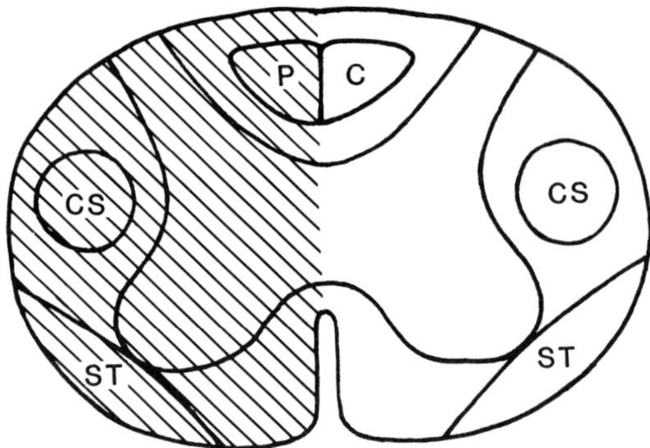

Fig. 9.16
Cross-section of the spinal cord to show the area involved in the Brown-Séquard Syndrome. There is hemiparesis and loss of position and vibratory sense on the side of the lesion, with contralateral loss of pain and temperature. PC: Posterior columns; CS: Corticospinal tract; ST: Anterolateral spinothalamic tract. (See Fig. 13.1)

3. The Anterior Cord Syndrome (Fig. 9.18) carries the worst outlook for recovery, because the damage to the corticospinal tracts is complete. Involvement of the spinothalamic tracts is complete also and all that remains is some functioning of the posterior columns.

Injuries of the conus medullaris occur most often with fractures at the thoracolumbar junction (T_{12}–L_1). They usually are devastating, because at this distal end of the spinal cord all of the lumbar and sacral segments are crowded into a very small area. To the extent that the terminating corticospinal tract fibers are involved, with preservation of the anterior horn cells, an "upper motor neuron" picture will be seen, with spasticity, hyperreflexia, and pathological reflexes. This is most often the case, but to the extent that anterior horn cells also are involved, there may be some degree of "lower motor neuron" involvement as well, with flaccidity and areflexia, and a patient may present with the confusing findings of weakness in the legs, hyperactive knee jerks, and yet absent ankle jerks.

Injuries of the cauda equina are infrequent, because the roots alone take up little space within the dural sac. Usually what is required for them to be affected is massive herniation into the spinal canal of a lumbar disc. A "lower motor neuron" type picture is produced and immediate surgical

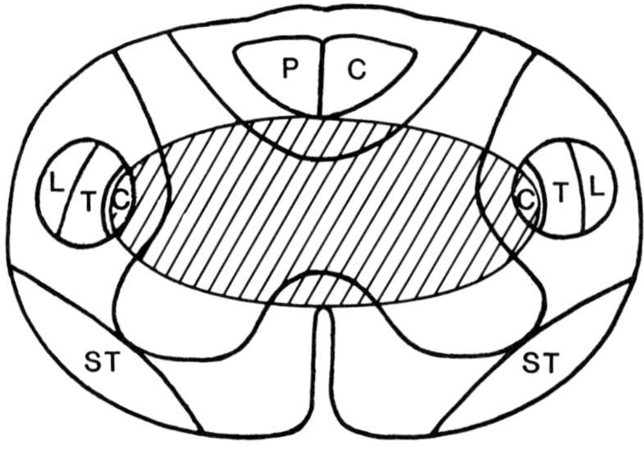

Fig. 9.17
Cross-section of the spinal cord to show the area involved in the central cord syndrome. Sensory loss typically is slight and weakness is greater in the arms and hands than in the legs, because of the distribution of nerve fibers in the corticospinal tracts. L: descending lumbar nerve fibers; T: thoracic nerve fibers; C: cervical nerve fibers.

Fig. 9.18
Cross-section of the spinal cord to show the area involved in the anterior cord syndrome. There is paraparesis and loss of pain and temperature to the level of the lesion (or just below it), but position and vibratory sense are relatively spared.

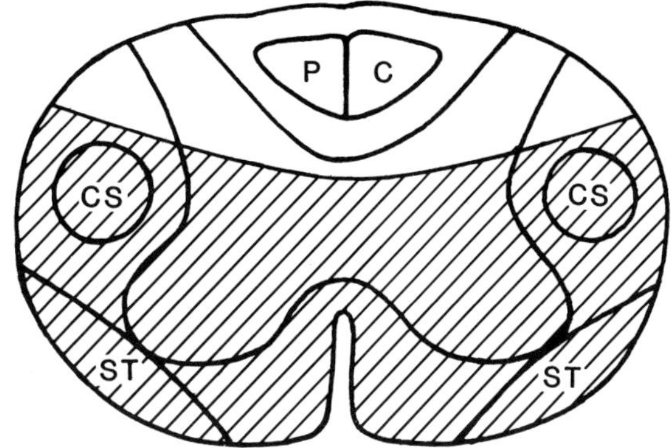

decompression is warranted, because the prognosis in such cases for return of function may be fairly good.

Gunshot wounds of the spinal cord (Fig. 9.19A and B) occur with distressing frequency. The velocities of the bullets involved in civilian wounds are sufficient to cause permanent cord damage if the spinal canal is entered, but there is not devitalization of a large amount of the surrounding tissue, and hence the need for debridement is not the same as in military wounds. Most civilian gunshot and stab wounds are not explored immediately, unless there are extenuating circumstances, such as a frank cerebrospinal leak.[11]

Spinal epidural and subdural hemorrhages usually are clinically unimportant, because they have relatively large spaces within which they can dissect up and down the spinal canal. Nevertheless, at times they may be significant and can represent one of the causes of a worsening neurological condition in the spinal cord injured patient. In such a circumstance emergency surgery may be necessary for their evacuation.

Finally, there are patients who for one reason or another following injury have hysterical paralysis. At times it is difficult to determine the realities of the situation, and often it is best to admit the patient to the hospital and watch him "recover," rather than provoking a scene in the ER where the patient (or the medical staff) will lose face. A clue to the hysterical nature of the condition is the preservation of reflexes in limbs where the patient complains of anesthesia and paralysis.

Vertebral Injuries

The typical "whiplash" injury is seen following a rear-end collision. The patient is neurologically intact but complains of neck pain which may last for months. The condition probably results from ligamentous tears, and the treatment is symptomatic. Great patience is needed on the part of both patient and doctor until time and nature resolve the problem.

Fractures involving the base of the skull and the first two cervical vertebrae generally do not produce a neurological deficit, because the ligaments

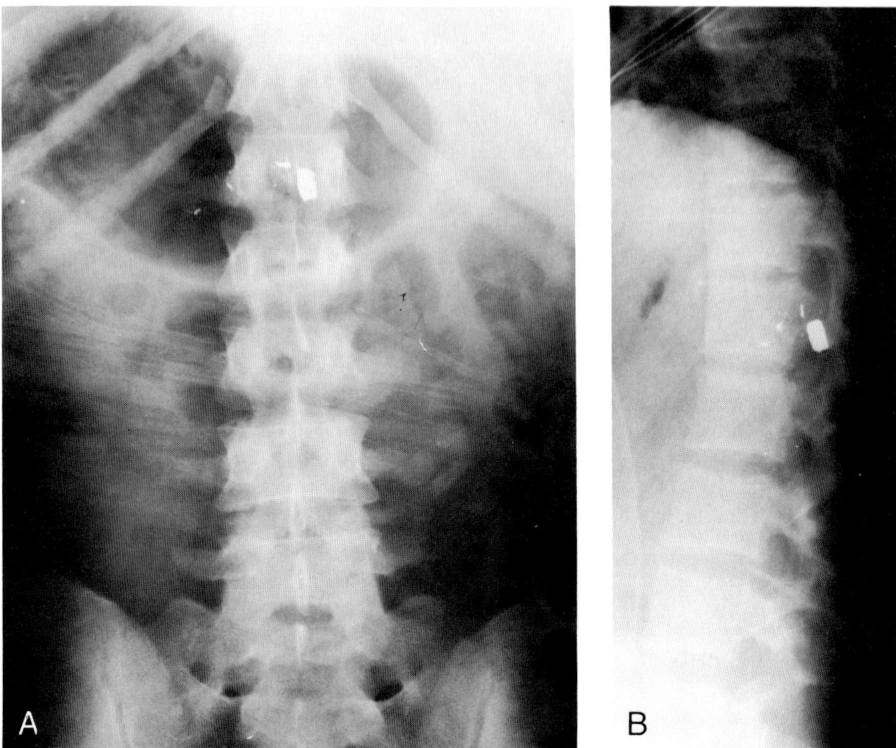

Fig. 9.19 (A) Anteroposterior and (B) lateral films of a patient with a gunshot wound of the spine. The point of entry was the chest anterolaterally and the bullet is seen in the spinal canal at L_1. Paraparesis was instantaneous and surgical removal of the bullet would not have changed this.

which bind these structures together are strong and the size of the spinal canal here is large in relation to the size of the spinal cord. This is fortunate because, as mentioned earlier, when the cord is injured at these levels the patient usually dies, since the lesion is above the nerve roots which provide the phrenic outflow.

Jefferson fractures involve C_1. They are axial-loading fractures and result from blows to the top of the head. The ring of this vertebra frequently is fractured in two places, but since there is no displacement, stabilization with a Philadelphia collar usually suffices until healing occurs (Fig. 9.27). An exception to this is seen when the transverse ligament holding the odontoid to the anterior arch of C_1 is also torn, resulting in instability between C_1 and C_2. In these cases more secure stabilization is required (see below).

The spine of C_2 is quite prominent. Fractures involving it and its associated laminae are called "Hangman's fractures," because this type of injury may be seen in judicial hangings. If fracture lines extend into the facets and pedicles of C_2, as is frequently the case, then stabilization with a halo brace is required (Fig. 9.25).

The embryological body of C_1 fuses with the body of C_2 in the adult to become the odontoid process, but the ligaments which bind the odontoid to C_1 are stronger than the bony union and so fractures across the base of the odontoid usually do not disturb its relationship to the anterior arch of C_1 (Fig. 9.20). Odontoid fractures do not heal well and posterior spinal wiring and fusion are often necessary.

Fractures involving the lower cervical spine which cause spinal cord injury usually are associated with subluxation of one vertebra on the other. Most of these occur from forced flexion of the head and there is bilateral facet damage (Fig. 9.21). Unilateral facet damage results from rotational injuries

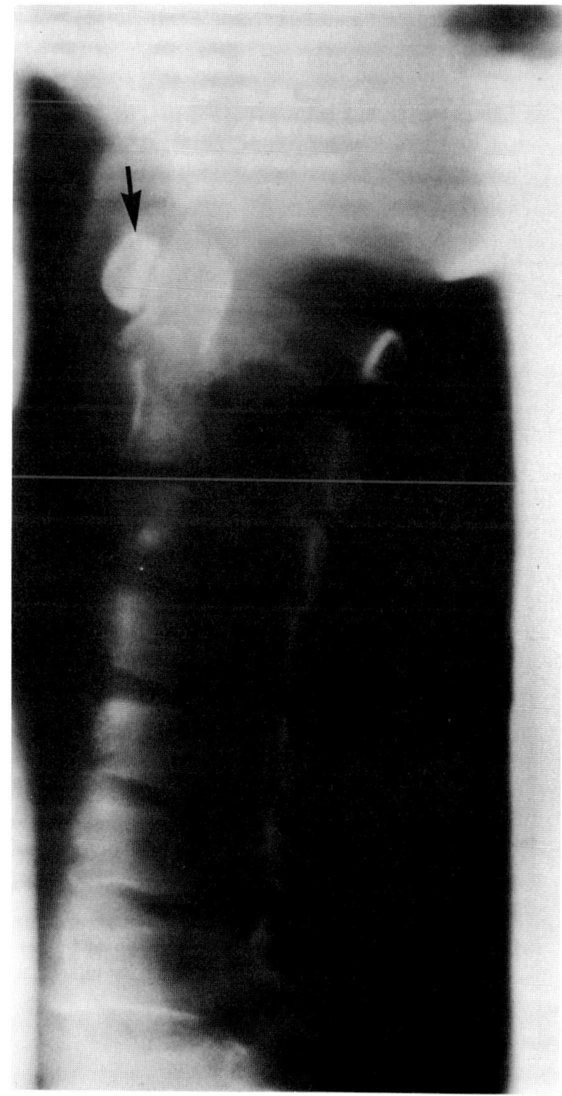

Fig. 9.20
Lateral cervical spine tomogram. Note that in spite of the fracture across its base, the odontoid has maintained its position with relation to the anterior arch of the atlas (arrow).

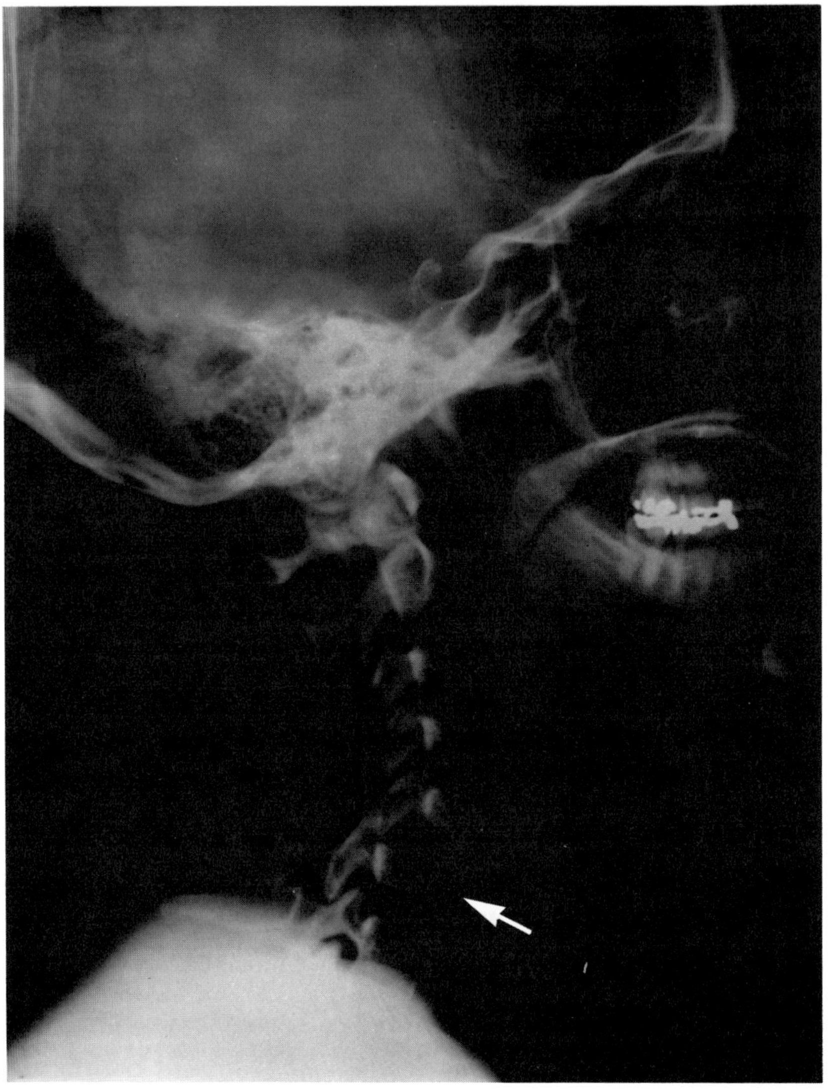

Fig. 9.21 Lateral cervical spine. Shown at C_5–C_6 is the typical flexion type cervical fracture-dislocation (arrow).

(Fig. 9.22 A and B). Extension injuries also are seen but with less frequency.

Thoracic spine fractures are uncommon, because of the buttressing effects of the rib cage, and when they do occur they are usually compression fractures only, with little subluxation. This is fortunate, because the spinal canal in this area is only slightly larger than the spinal cord.

A more common site for injury is the thoracolumbar junction, where the relatively fixed thoracic spine joins the relatively mobile lumbar spine.

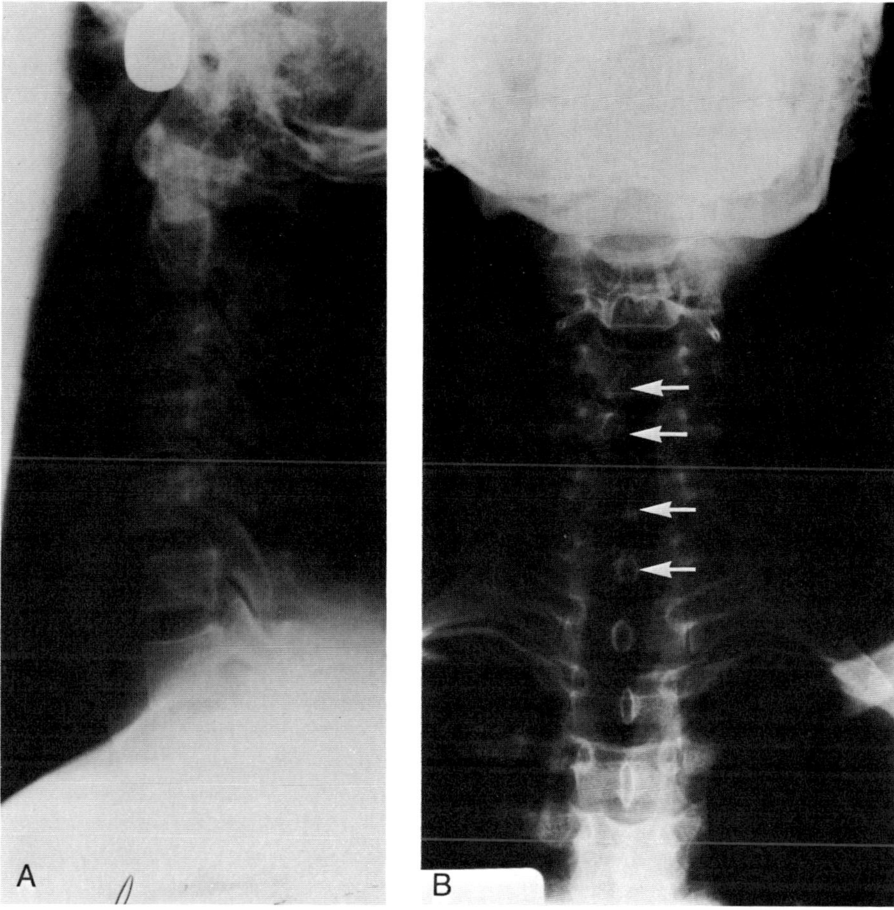

Fig. 9.22 (A) Lateral cervical spine. There is some subluxation of C_5 on C_6. The rotational component is less obvious but discernible. (B) AP cervical spine. Here the rotational component of the injury is brought out by the shift to the right of the spinous processes of C_4 and C_5 in relation to those of C_6 and C_7 (arrows).

But here too, because of the stabilizing effect of the surrounding tissues (the abdomen and its viscera, the thick lumbar muscles and their fascia), what occurs is a compression fracture with little or no subluxation and, consequently, no neurological involvement. Instability is suggested by inter-pedicular widening (Fig. 9.23) and treatment may be by Harrington rod or other fixation (Fig. 9.30).

Lower lumbar spine fractures may not sublux, but the force required to produce them may "burst" a piece of the centrum of the vertebral body back into the spinal canal, compressing the dural sac and cauda equina (see Fig. 2.11). Most commonly there is surprisingly little neurological loss, and decompression of the cauda equina usually is unnecessary.

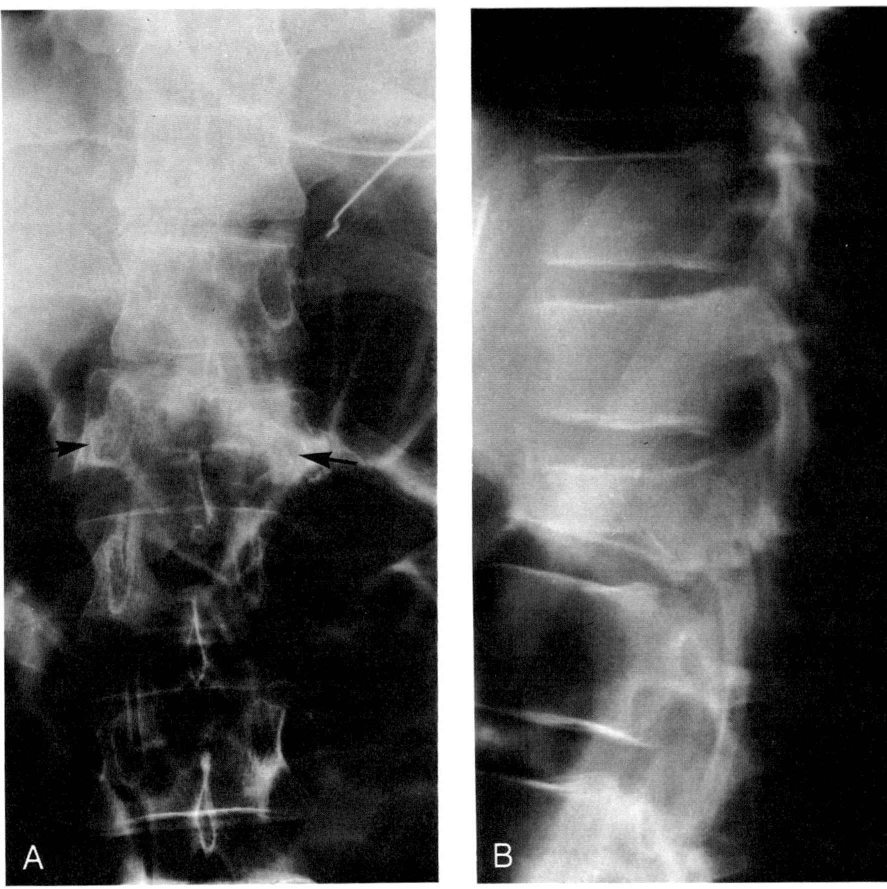

Fig. 9.23 (A) AP thoracolumbar junction. The vertebral body of T_{12} is crushed. Instability is indicated by widening of the pedicles when compared to those of T_{11} or L_1 (arrows). (B) Lateral thoracolumbar junction. The crushed vertebral body is wedged anteriorally, but there is little subluxation.

Management Of Spine And Spinal Cord Injuries

Treatment of spinal fractures requires reduction of dislocations and stabilization for about 3 months. Most dislocations occur in the cervical region and can be realigned by axial traction. Promptness in achieving reduction is important even with complete cord transections, because relief of pressure on otherwise compromised cervical nerve roots at the level of the dislocation may result in their regaining function and consequently improving the subsequent task of rehabilitation.

One of the first methods of achieving reduction by axial traction was the invention in 1933 of the Crutchfield tongs (Fig. 9.24). The patient lies

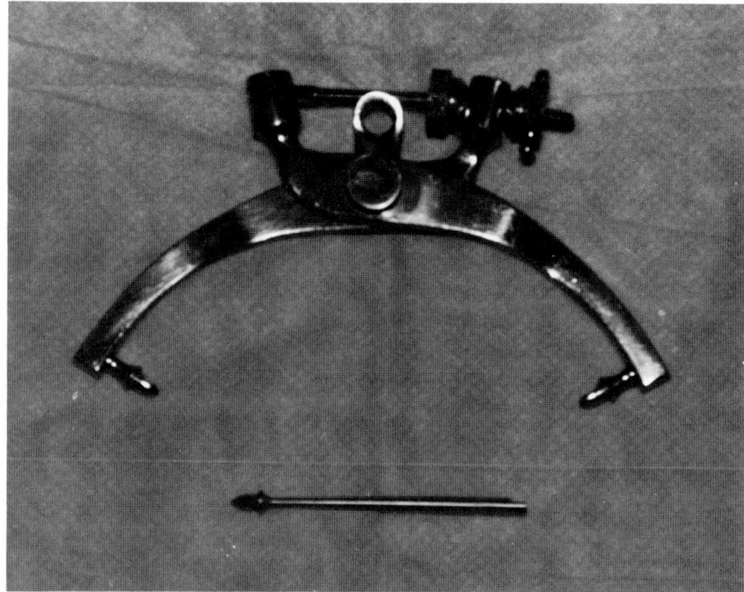

Fig. 9.24 Crutchfield tongs. Note the flange on the drill point, which permits only partial penetration of the skull.

supine on a frame which can be rotated on its long axis every 2 hours, thus relieving pressure on anesthetic skin. The tongs are placed biparietally in the skull, in line with the posterior margin of the helix of each ear, which puts them in line also with the cervical spine. A rope is attached to the tongs which goes over a pulley at the end of the frame and attaches in turn to a weight hanger. Starting with 15–20 pounds, weight can be increased until reduction is achieved. As much as 50 pounds may be needed to reduce locked facets, but with increasing weight vigilant attention is required, with repeat films (lateral cervical spine) and examination of the patient, because reduction may be followed by over distraction and the patient's condition may be worsened. This is particularly true if the fracture involves the upper cervical spine.

There are many variations of these tongs (Barton, Vinke, Gardner, etc.), but they all function basically in the same way. Following reduction, patients are usually kept on the frame with frequent turning for 6 weeks and then are placed in a hard collar for another 6 weeks. Tong traction is the safest way of handling cervical spine fractures, because with the patient supine the effects of gravity are obviated. The problem created is that rehabilitation is delayed, and early adequate rehabilitation is both physiologically and psychologically important.

For this reason, tong traction largely has been replaced by the halo brace (Fig. 9.25).[9] The ring around the patient's head is held in place by four

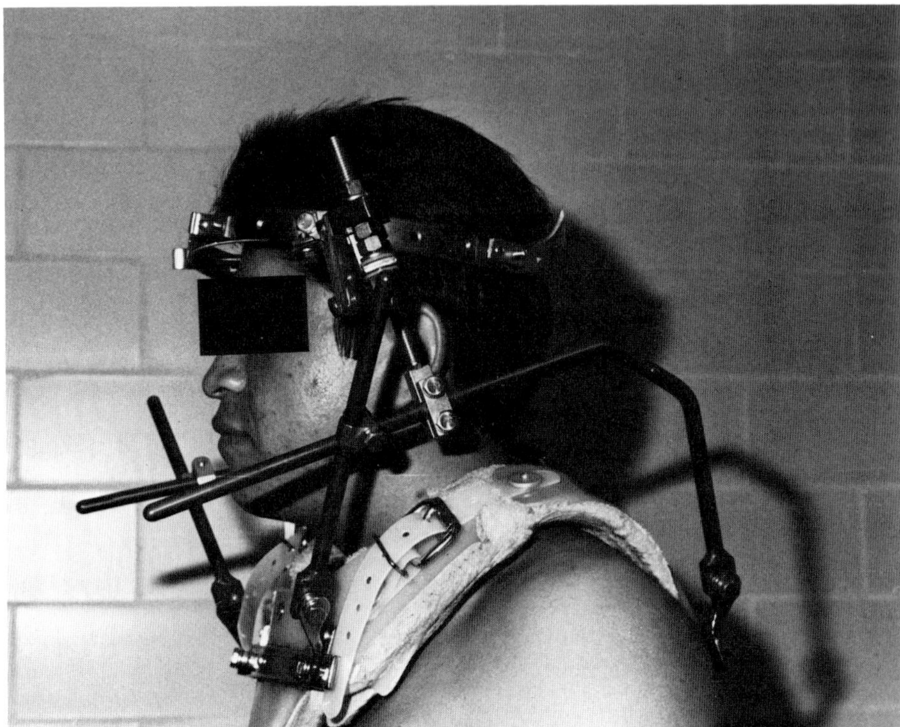

Fig. 9.25 Patient with a halo brace. Most cervical spine injuries can be handled conservatively by this means. The ring is held in place by four skull pins and the uprights are attached to a padded plastic vest.

skull pins and if axial traction for reduction of a fracture-dislocation is required, the patient can be put on a frame and weights can be applied, as with the Crutchfield tongs. Once reduction is achieved, the padded plastic vest is put on, its uprights are connected to the ring, and the patient is transferred to a regular bed, with early mobilization thereafter. The most important step here is the maintenance of some axial traction while the uprights are connected to the ring; if this is done properly, usually there is no re-subluxation when the patient is brought to a vertical position. Nevertheless, some cases do slip and for these there are only two recourses: one can keep the patient on a frame for 6 weeks or one can go to operative fixation, with posterior spinal fusion and wiring of the spinous processes across the fracture site. This latter procedure is generally preferred, because it permits faster rehabilitation of the patient.

Some degree of stability can be achieved with a 4-poster brace (Fig. 9.26) or a Philadelphia collar (Fig. 9.27). These are inadequate for treating unstable cervical spine fractures, but they are useful during emergency transport, when the patient is managed supine, and when subluxation is not a likelihood, as with Jefferson fractures. They are also useful when some degree

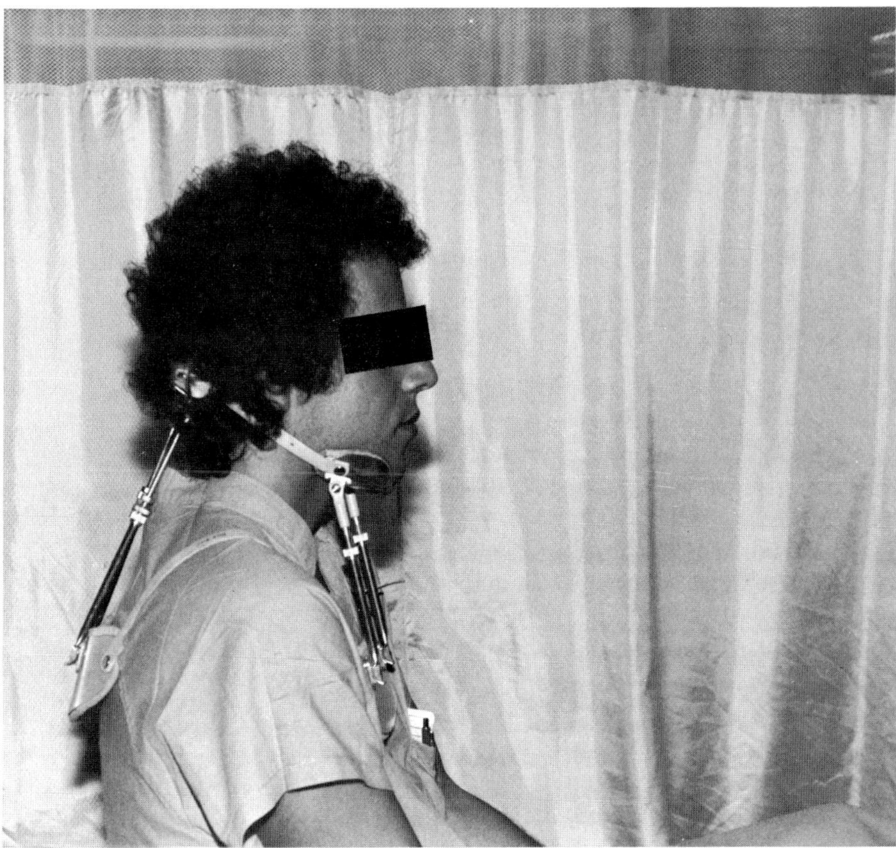

Fig. 9.26 Patient in a 4-poster brace. Stabilization is not as good as that obtained with a halo but it is better than that provided by a soft collar.

of stabilization already has been achieved (e.g., after anterior spine fusion or when a patient has been on a frame with Crutchfield tongs in place for 6 weeks).

Very little stabilization is achieved with a soft collar (Fig. 9.14). Extremes of motion are prevented, however, and this type of collar may provide useful symptomatic relief for the patient with a "whiplash" injury.

While early reduction of cervical fracture-dislocations is important, the indications for emergency surgery are few.

> *PRINCIPLE 6:* Operation will not help in cases where paralysis is immediate and complete and incomplete injuries may be made worse by early surgery.

There are some exceptions to this principle, although they occur rarely. Certainly neurological worsening is one. Massive disc herniation which catches the roots of the cauda equina is another. Open wounds represent

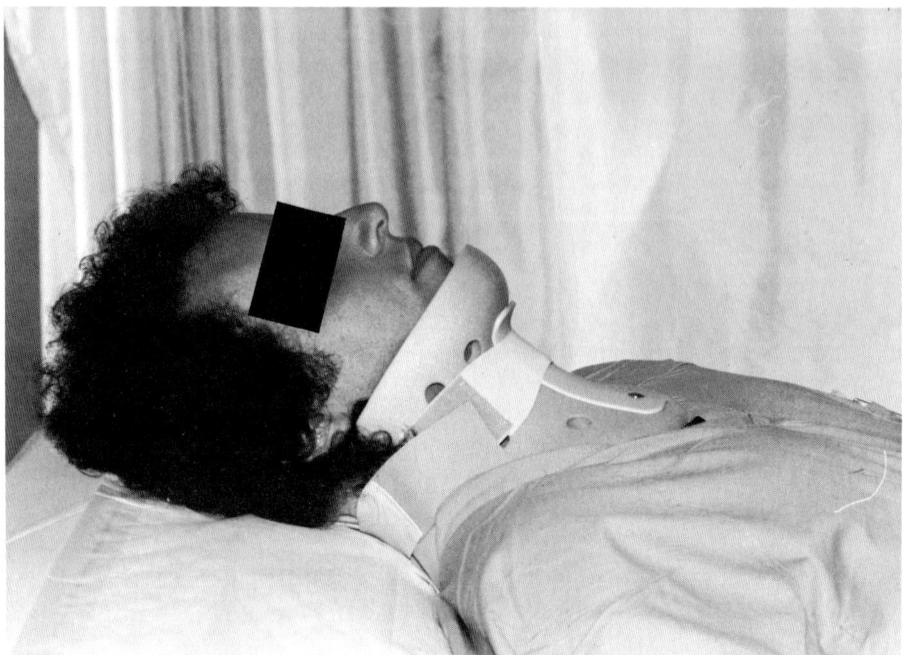

Fig. 9.27 Patient in Philadelphia collar. The degree of stability achieved is about the same as that of the 4-poster brace.

a third, although, as mentioned previously, most gunshot and stab wounds are now treated conservatively, unless the wound of exit or entrance is close to the midline and there is a cerebrospinal fluid leak.[11]

Surgically, the spine and spinal cord can be approached at any level either anteriorly or posteriorly. Anterior spine fusions (Fig. 9.28A and B) frequently are undertaken, but usually not in the acute phase of spinal injury and not in the specific instance of flexion injury of the neck with fracture-dislocation. This is because in such cases often the only remaining structure providing stability to the spine is the anterior longitudinal ligament and the anterior approach removes this.

The posterior approach, with interspinous wiring and fusion, is used particularly when the halo brace will not hold reduction of the fracture-dislocation. It may be combined with laminectomy (Fig. 9.29), if there is need for disc fragment removal or spinal cord decompression.

Harrington distraction rods are used in conjunction with fusion particularly in cases of unstable fractures at the thoracolumbar junction (Fig. 9.30). Their purpose is to reduce and stabilize the fracture and so permit early rehabilitation of the patient.

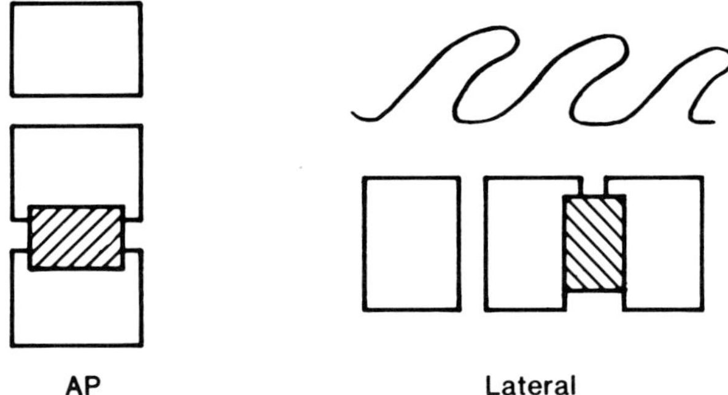

Fig. 9.28 AP and lateral diagrams of the cervical spine. Placement of the bone dowel in anterior spine fusion is shown.

Complications

Many of the complications of spinal cord injury seen in the past have been obviated through use of the halo brace and early mobilization. Patients with paraplegia or quadriplegia are always at risk for development of pulmonary emboli, but frequent turning and the early, vigorous physical therapy which the halo brace permits lessen the chance of this. It is unclear whether the use of "low dose" heparin (5,000 u. q 8–12 h) is helpful in these cases.

Bringing patients back into their usual relationship with gravity and mobi-

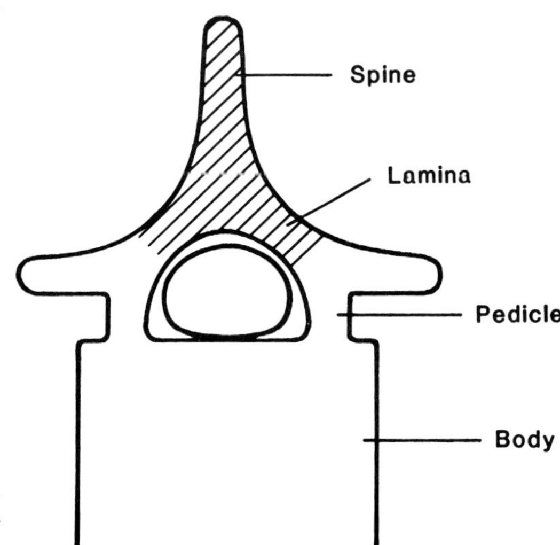

Fig. 9.29
Horizontal section through a vertebra. Demonstrated is the extent of bone removal in decompressive laminectomy.

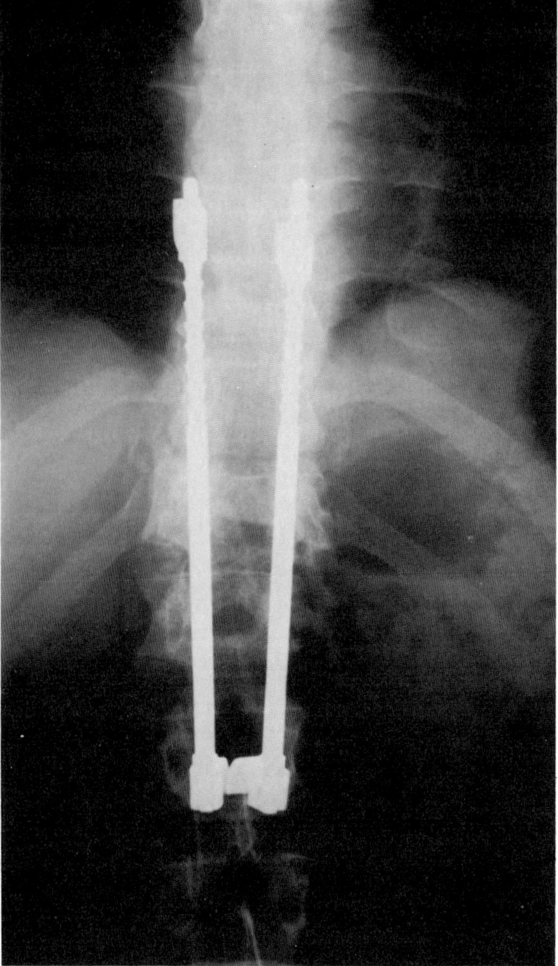

Fig. 9.30
AP film of the thoracolumbar junction. Same patient as in Figs. 9.23A and 9.23B. Harrington rods have been applied to stabilize the fracture at T_{12}.

lizing them also has cut down many of the nutritional and metabolic problems seen in the past, such as anemia, hypoproteinemia, and hypercalcuria with the attendant risk of formation of renal and bladder stones.

As mentioned earlier, quadriplegic patients and those with high thoracic cord injuries have had, in essence, a sympathectomy and the resulting loss of vasomotor control may present difficulties until some degree of automaticity in vasomotor tone is regained. Postural hypotension is one of these. Loss of temperature control is another. Especially in the early stages following injury it is important to remember that these patients are essentially poikilothermic, so they will assume the ambient temperature and so must be protected from overheating with too many blankets or chilling from not enough protection in the air-conditioned hospital.

If care is given to frequent turning, respiratory problems are infrequent, but it must be remembered that patients with complete high spinal cord injuries have lost the use of their intercostal muscles and so are breathing by means of the phrenic nerves alone. Hypoventilation may be insidious and blood gases must be checked. Atelectasis and pneumonia may develop rapidly.

The imbalance caused by loss of the sympathetic nerve supply and yet preservation of the parasympathetic through the phrenic nerves may cause temporary bradycardia. If necessary, this can be treated with atropine. Paradoxically, there may be loss of tone in the gastrointestinal tract, with resulting gastric distention and ileus. Such patients may need a nasogastric tube for a few days, until bowel sounds return and oral intake can be resumed.

Loss of bladder control in complete spinal cord injuries necessitates catheterization. A regimen of intermittent catherization usually results in a smaller incidence of infection than when continuous Foley cather drainage is used, but urinary tract infections still may occur and must be vigorously treated.

Pressure sores develop over bony prominences when patients are not turned frequently. The healing process when anesthetic skin breaks down is greatly retarded and multiple trips to the OR for debridement, skin grafting, and rotation of flaps then may be necessary. It is best not to let pressure sores develop in the first place. They should be rare if nursing care is vigilant.

Pain generally is not a problem in patients with spinal cord injuries. The notable exception to this occurs with gunshot wounds, where the partial damage caused by the blast effect of the bullet for some reason often is sufficient to provoke severe pain which is difficult to treat. Fortunately it usually subsides spontaneously over a period of days to weeks.

Spasticity developing after the period of spinal shock may be difficult to treat also. Of the many drugs available, diazepam perhaps is the best, but if the problem does not spontaneously abate orthopedic procedures, such as tenotomy, or neurosurgical procedures, such as rhizotomy, or even the use of intrathecal alcohol may be necessary.

Rehabilitation

The great improvement in the care of spinal cord injured patients which occurred during World War II was largely due to the creation of specialized spinal cord injury centers, first in Great Britain [3] and then in Australia, the United States, and elsewhere. A milieu is provided in such institutions for vital psychological support; medical specialists from various disciplines and therapists can focus on the problems these patients present; and vocational rehabilitation can be given appropriate emphasis. It is recommended that as soon as possible following initial resuscitation and treatment, which usually includes reduction and stabilization of spinal fractures, every effort be made to transfer these patients to a regional spinal cord injury center.

PERIPHERAL NERVE INJURIES[4,10]

Initial Evaluation And Treatment

The initial management of peripheral nerve injuries often is determined by other factors, such as the presence or absence of an open wound, arterial damage, lacerated tendons, or fractures. The reason for this is that, with the possible exception of sharply divided nerves, immediate exploration and repair is not necessary and even may be undesirable; nevertheless, if there is an open wound which must be debrided or an operation which must be carried out for some other reason, it may be quite feasible to explore the area of nerve damage at the same time. Advantage then may be taken of the fact that injured nerves do not lose their conductivity immediately, even if transected. This leads to:

> ***PRINCIPLE 7:*** When injured nerves are explored at early surgery, even if they cannot be sutured per primum, they should be identified, tested with a nerve stimulator, and tagged for future reference with fine guage stainless steel wire (which will show up on postoperative X-rays).

But whether surgery is immediate or delayed, early neurological exam is important, as it is with any other nervous system injury, and the pertinent findings of motor, sensory, and reflex impairment should be documented in the patient's chart, preferably with an accompanying diagram.

Types Of Nerve Injuries

Peripheral nerves may become functionless from a variety of causes and often in closed injuries one is left guessing what the precise nature and extent of the damage is.

Nerve Compression

Nerve compression implies a focal point of injury, which may be mild and reversible; moderate, with degeneration of axons distal to the injury but with preservation of axon sheaths so that regeneration is possible; or so severe that the whole nerve degenerates with no chance of recovery. Serial neurological exams, nerve conduction, and EMG studies often are required to demonstrate eventual return of function, or the lack of it.

Nerve Stretching

Nerve stretching occurs when the damaging force passes through the long axis of the nerves. Again, injuries may be mild but frequently they are severe because scarring may take place over wide segments, thus preventing axonal regrowth.

Nerve Lacerations

Nerve lacerations are the lesions surgeons prefer: the level of injury usually is clear, the problem is focal, and a surgical remedy may be possible. The rationale behind delayed nerve suture is that the extent to which the proximal nerve end will degenerate is not obvious initially; if suture is performed without trimming this end sufficiently, subsequent scarring may prevent growth of regenerating axons across the suture line. Nevertheless, experience with open civilian wounds has shown that many divided or partially divided nerves may in fact be reapproximated successfully per primum. A notable exception to this occurs with gunshot wounds, where segments of nerve may be missing and where the proximal extent of injury may be greater than expected because of the blast effect of the bullet.

Specific Problems

Root avulsions are seen most often in the cervical region. They occur in newborns as a birth injury from traction on the arm (Erb's paralysis) and in adults from violent downward pressure on the arm and shoulder (e.g., in motorcycle accidents). Such traction injuries also may stretch the brachial plexus and this frequently carries a poor prognosis.

The nerves to the extremities are fairly well-protected, which is fortunate, because they often run in conjunction with the major arteries and veins, forming neurovascular bundles. The brachial plexus comes close to the surface as it enters the arm. It actually lies lower in the neck than one might imagine and the precise level of a plexus injury may be difficult to determine. The clavicle is a useful landmark: injuries above it usually involve the roots and trunks of the plexus, while injuries below it more often involve the cords and peripheral nerves (Fig. 9.31).

The median and ulnar nerves are close to the inner surface of the upper arm. The radial nerve has by this time begun its circuitous course around the humerus, but this leaves it vulnerable to fractures. The ulnar nerve, of course, is exposed as it goes around the medial epicondyle of the humerus and the median nerve becomes exposed again at the wrist.

In the lower extremity, the femoral nerve is fairly superficial as it enters the anteromedial aspect of the thigh in the femoral canal. The lateral femoral cataneous nerve may be compressed as it passes medially to the anterior superior idiac spine, producing pain and numbness along the anterolateral aspect of the thigh, a condition known as meralgia paresthetica. The sciatic nerve is well protected by overlying muscles but may be injured by posterior dislocations of the hip. Finally, the superficial peroneal nerve is quite close to the surface as it comes around the head of the fibula.

Injuries to the peripheral sympathetic nervous system should not be forgotten. Horner's syndrome may be seen with traction injuries, and its presence adds to the poor prognosis in stretch injuries of the brachial plexus.

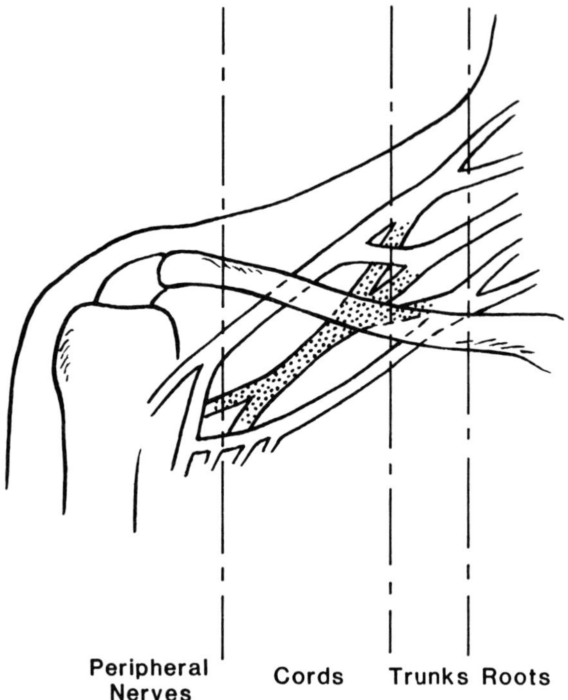

Fig. 9.31
Drawing to show relationships of the brachial plexus to the clavicle: Injuries above the clavicle are likely to involve roots or trunks, while injuries below usually affect cords or peripheral nerves.

The syndrome consists of ptosis of the eyelid and seeming enophthalmos, a small pupil (miosis), and ipsilateral loss of sweating over the face and neck.

Causalgia occurs from partial peripheral nerve injury. Apparently sympathetic nerve impulses are short-circuited at the point of injury and are routed centrally via sensory fibers and so cause pain. Sympathectomy may be curative. The syndrome is characteristic: constant, excruciating, burning pain; hyperesthesia; and sympathetic nervous system malfunction in the injured extremity.

Surgical Management

If exploration is carried out shortly after injury and clinically non-functional nerves are found to be contused but in continuity, they are handled as described earlier, by identifying them, stimulating distal to the point of injury for additional information, and tagging them with fine guage wire sutures in the epineurium. The reason for this is that if function does not return, it may be because of neuroma formation at the point of injury. "Neuroma" in this context means overgrowth of regenerating axons and scar tissue which at times is sufficient to block axonal regeneration distal to the point of injury. Neurolysis, or resection of this scar tissue, may be necessary in such cases.

If the nerves are found to be cut, a decision must be made whether or not to reapproximate the ends per primum or simply to tag them for suture at a later date. If the ends are ragged or if obvious contusion extends up the nerve for any distance, it is best to delay, because neuroma formation can be anticipated. The ideal situation for primary suture is the case where nerves have been cleanly divided, as in lacerations with sharp pieces of metal or glass.

Primary reapproximation is easy if it can be accomplished without tension. Guide sutures (later removed) are placed proximally and distally, the nerve ends are lined up, and reapproximation is carried out with fine suture material, 7–0 or finer and of silk or some permanent synthetic. Care must be taken to achieve the most accurate suturing possible and the best way to do this is for the surgeon to use magnifying loupes or the operating microscope. Tension is to be avoided at all costs, because otherwise one is creating the same condition which leads to stretch injuries. Avoidance of tension can be achieved by freeing up the proximal and distal nerve ends; by transposition (an obvious example would be the re-routing of the ulnar nerve in front of the elbow); or by flexing joints the nerves traverse. With this latter technique, the extremity post operatively can be put in a cast or splint and then gradually extended over a period of weeks. In general, the more distal the nerve injury, the greater the return of neurological function.

Delayed nerve suture (Fig. 9.32) involves identifying the cut ends and placing epineurial guide sutures, as before. The proximal neuroma and distal scar tissue then are palpated and trimmed back with a razor blade—proximally until healthy nerve fascicles can be seen and distally until the nerve is soft and the jumble of scar tissue seems to give way to a more orderly

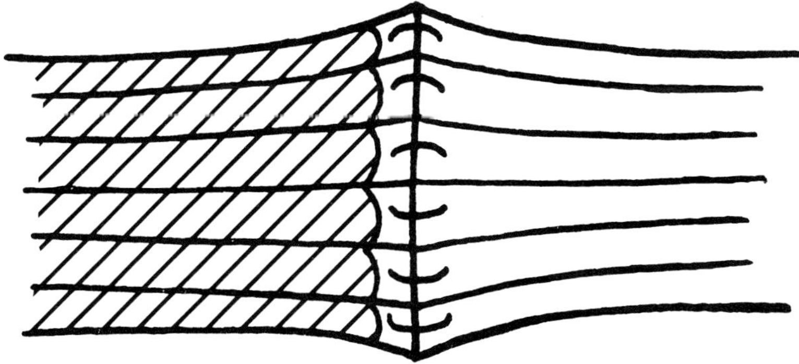

Fig. 9.32 Drawing which schematically indicates delayed nerve suture: the nerve ends are trimmed back with a razor blade until fasicles are seen proximally and a somewhat orderly arrangement of nerve tubules (as opposed to dense scar) appears distally. Temporary guide sutures (not shown) are placed to approximate the ends and fine sutures appropriate to the size of the nerve are used to suture the epineureum, under magnification.

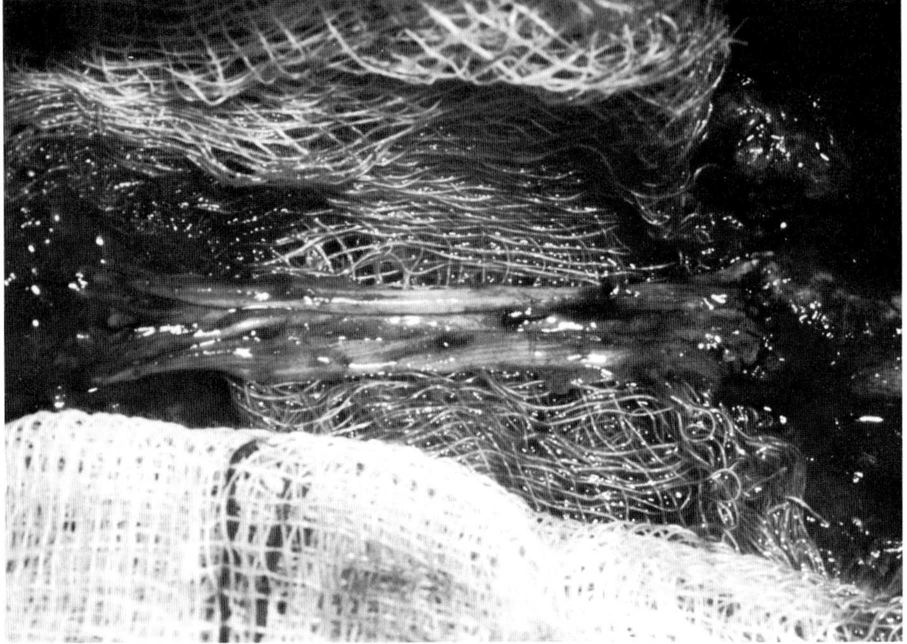

Fig. 9.33 OR Photo. The ends of the divided sciatic nerve could not be mobilized enough to permit direct reapproximation, so three sural nerve cable grafts were inserted to bridge the gap.

pattern of (empty) nerve tubules. Reapproximation then is with fine sutures and magnification.

If the gap between the nerve ends cannot be closed with the maneuvers mentioned above, consideration must be given to use of a nerve graft. Autografts are best, usually taken from a sensory nerve after its most important branches have been given off, so that the area of hypesthesia produced will be small. The sural nerve is ideal for this purpose. If the damaged nerve is small, one graft will be sufficient, but if it is large several strands ("cable grafts") may be necessary (Fig. 9.33).

Rehabilitation

Peripheral nerves regenerate from the point of injury at the rate of about 30 mm a month. It is clear, therefore, that the distal extremity must be protected, exercised regularly, and kept in a position of function until axonal regrowth occurs. Electrical signs of regeneration precede clinical detection, but a clinically useful test is Tinel's sign, the dysesthesia produced when a nerve is gently tapped. When encountered, the location of the sensitive area progressively extends down the arm or leg as the axons regenerate.

Splinting during this phase is very important. For the hand this means dynamic splinting with a cock-up splint that puts the hand in its position of function; for the foot this means a foot-drop brace.

Recent advances in the surgical treatment of peripheral nerve injuries have been made possible with the introduction of the operating microscope; nevertheless, our modern understanding of these problems, both in diagnosis and treatment, stem from the experiences of World War II, and the textbooks originating from that conflict have not been equaled.[4,10]

REFERENCES

1. American College of Surgeons: Early Care of the Injured Patient, 2nd Ed. Philadelphia, W. B. Saunders, 1976.
2. Freytag, E.: Autopsy findings in head injuries from firearms. Arch. Pathol., 76:215, 1963.
3. Guttmann, L.: Spinal Cord Injuries. 2nd Ed. Oxford, Blackwell Scientific Publications, 1976.
4. Haymaker, W., Woodhall, B.: Peripheral Nerve Injuries: Principles of Diagnosis. 2nd Ed. Philadelphia, W. B. Saunders Co., 1953.
5. Jennett, B.: Post-Traumatic Epilepsy, pp. 445–454. In Vinken, P.J., Bruyn, G.W., eds.: Handbook of Clinical Neurology. Vol. 24. New York, American Elsevier, 1976.
6. Langfitt, T.W.: Measuring the outcome from head injuries. J. Neurosurg., 48:673, 1978.
7. Marshall, L.F., Smith, R.N., Shapiro, H.M.: The outcome with aggressive treatment in severe head injury. Part II. Acute and chronic barbiturate administration in the management of head injury. J. Neurosurg., 50:26, 1979.
8. Miller, J.D., et. al.: Further experience in the management of severe head injury: J. Neurosurg., 54:289, 1981.
9. Prolo, D.J., Runnels, J.B., Jameson, R.H.: The injured cervical spine: immediate and long-term immobilization with the halo. JAMA, 224:591, 1973.
10. Seddon, H.: Surgical Disorders of the Peripheral Nerves. Baltimore, Williams and Wilkins, 1972.
11. Stauffer, E.S., Wood, R.W., Kelly, E.G.: Gunshot wounds of the spine: the effects of laminectomy. J. Bone and Joint Surg., 61A 389, 1979.
12. Teasdale, G.T., et al.: Assessment and prognosis of coma after head injury. Acta Neurochir., 34:45, 1976.

10

Neuromuscular Emergencies

David B. Simon, M.D.
Steven P. Ringel, M.D.
Joseph R. Lacy, M.D.

INTRODUCTION

Neuromuscular disorders often impair such vital functions as speaking, swallowing, and breathing, as well as all voluntary movement. In cases of acute onset weakness, immediate identification of the weakness and properly directed therapy may be lifesaving. It is also common for patients with a previously diagnosed neuromuscular disease to present with acute complications of their illness. These complications may be emergent, for example, in a patient with myasthenia gravis in acute respiratory failure. The physician's task then is to understand the nature of the complication and reverse it.

This chapter is organized with particular emphasis on neuromuscular complications that require prompt treatment. However, for the reader to comprehend the spectrum of neuromuscular disease, a more comprehensive overview is included. The first sections of the chapter outline the anatomy and physiology of the neuromuscular system and describe several laboratory techniques particularly useful in diagnosis. In the next section, individual neuromuscular disorders affecting either the lower motor neuron, peripheral nerve, neuromuscular junction or muscle are presented in sufficient detail to allow the reader an understanding of the major features of each disease. The final part of this chapter is designed to assist the clinician in systematically approaching a patient who seeks medical attention because of a particular neuromuscular symptom. That review of the common clinical presentations of neuromuscular disease should be particularly useful to the non-neurologist since it focuses on differential diagnosis and immediate therapeutic strategies that can be undertaken prior to obtaining neurological consultation.

ANATOMY AND PHYSIOLOGY OF THE NEUROMUSCULAR SYSTEM

The peripheral nervous system (PNS) includes all nerve tissue outside the brain and spinal cord as well as the lower motor neurons (LMN) which are located in the gray matter of the brainstem (cranial nerve motor neurons) and spinal cord (anterior horn cells). Fibers mediating volitional control of muscles descend from cortical and subcortical structures in the central nervous system (CNS) and synapse directly, or via interneurons, upon these LMNs. Afferent sensory fibers provide sensory input to the CNS, but also convey information from muscle spindles to the LMN about the length and tension of the muscle. This sensory input modifies the outflow activity from motor neurons and is important in regulating appropriate muscle tone. Elicitation of the myotatic stretch (deep tendon) reflex tests the integrity of this circuit.

The functional unit of the PNS is the motor unit, which includes the anterior horn cell, its axon, and all the muscle fibers innervated by that axon (Fig. 10.1). The number of fibers controlled by a motor neuron (the innervation ratio) varies widely; in general, the finer the control exerted over a movement, the smaller the innervation ratio.

Efferent axons of motor neurons combine with afferent sensory axons to form peripheral sensory-motor nerves, which contain fibers of varying diameters and conduction velocities. The fastest conducting fibers are surrounded by myelin, which serves as an insulator and permits a type of rapid "jumping" conduction (saltatory) from gap to gap (nodes of Ranvier) between the myelinated segments of the axon. The largest myelinated fibers, which conduct the fastest, consist of motor axons, and sensory fibers mediating position, touch, and muscle length and tension. Medium-sized myelinated fibers carry motor and sensory information to and from muscle spindles and also vibratory and pressure sensation. Small, lightly myelinated and unmyelinated fibers subserve pain and temperature and autonomic information. Involvement of specific fiber types or sizes may be seen in peripheral nerve disorders.

In addition to conducting electrical impulses, motor nerves have a nourishing (trophic) influence on muscle. If a muscle fiber is deprived of its nerve supply, it will atrophy despite the presence of an intact blood supply. If reinnervated by a nearby nerve twig, the muscle fiber may regain its normal size.

The synapse between nerve and muscle (neuromuscular junction; end plate) converts electrical transmission to chemical transmission so that conduction occurs in only one direction (Fig. 10.1). When a nerve action potential reaches a nerve terminal, the neurotransmitter, acetylcholine, (ACH) is released, diffuses across the synaptic cleft, and stimulates receptors in the post-synaptic membrane. Excess ACH is rapidly metabolized by acetylcholinesterase, a soluble enzyme present in post-synaptic folds. Permeability

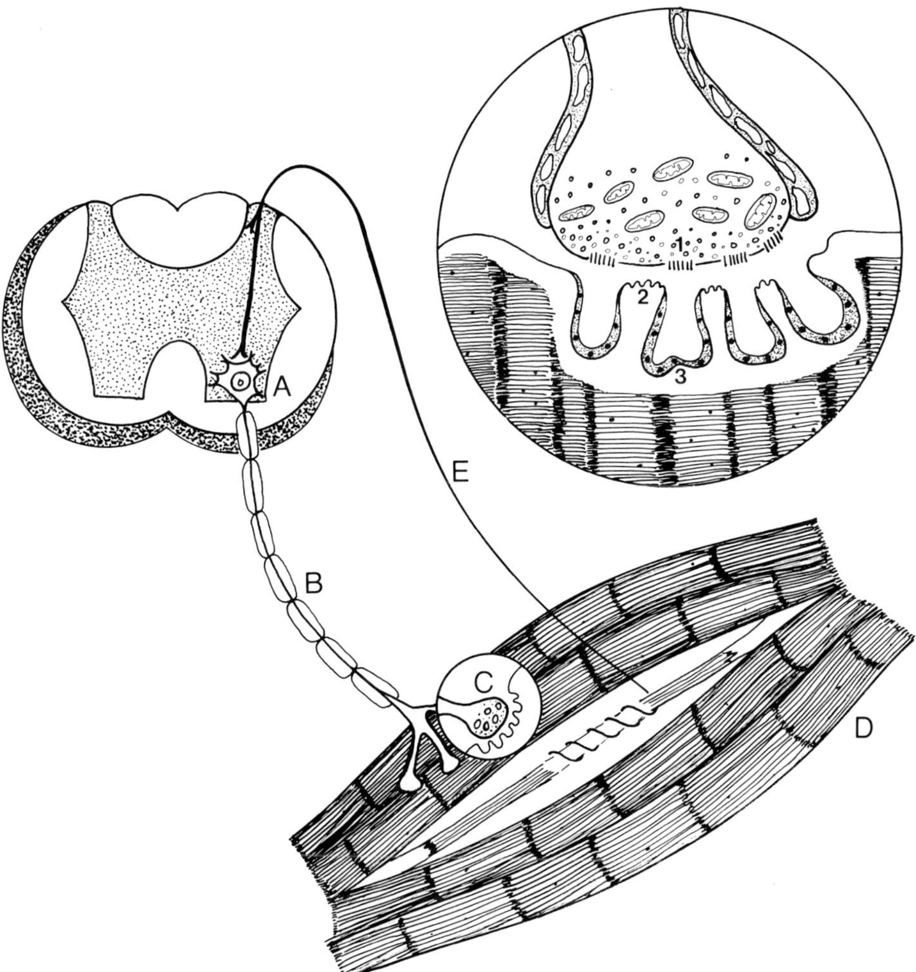

Fig. 10.1 Anatomy of the Neuromuscular System. Lower motor neuron diseases can effect any part of the motor unit which consists of an anterior horn cell (A), axon (B), neuromuscular junction (C), and numerous muscle fibers (D). Afferent fibers arising from the muscle spindle (E) provide a feed-back loop for monitoring muscle tension and length. The neuromuscular junction (inset) can malfunction if presynaptic release of acetylcholine is prevented (botulism) (1); if the acetylcholine binds to a damaged post-synaptic receptor (myasthenia gravis) (2); or if excess acetylcholine is not metabolized by acetylcholinesterase (organophosphate poisoning) (3).

changes to sodium and potassium in the end plate region of the muscle membrane lead to a wave or cascade of depolarization along the muscle membrane in a manner analogous to nerve depolarization.

The actual contractile force of muscle is produced by the contractile proteins actin and myosin. The complex process of muscular contraction, initiated by muscle membrane depolarization, begins with the release of calcium from the sarcoplasmic reticulum. Binding of this calcium to several regulatory proteins (tropomyosin, troponin) allows cross-bridges to form between the actin and myosin filaments. The process of muscle fiber shortening and lengthening (sliding filaments) requires large amounts of energy, which is produced from metabolism of glycogen and lipids and is stored in the muscle as high energy phosphate bonds (ATP, creatine phosphate).

Two major types of muscle fibers, slow twitch (red, aerobic, type I) and fast twitch (white, anaerobic, type II) are relatively evenly distributed in all human skeletal muscles. Type I fibers, rich in oxidative enzymes, maximize energy production and utilization via aerobic metabolism (Krebs cycle). Type II fibers are rich in glycogen and phosphorylase but poor in oxidative enzymes. These glycolytic fibers are larger and more powerful, but fatigue more quickly since anaerobic metabolism is less complete and lactic acid accumulates more readily. The muscle fiber type is determined by the motor neuron that innervates it so that all fibers belonging to a motor unit are of the same type. A fiber does not ordinarily convert from one fiber type to another unless it is separated from one type of motor neuron and reinnervated by another.

SPECIAL TECHNIQUES FOR DIAGNOSIS OF NEUROMUSCULAR DISORDERS

In addition to more routine laboratory investigations, electrodiagnostic studies and pathologic examination of muscle and nerve can help to establish a specific diagnosis and are often useful in following the course of certain neuromuscular diseases.

Electrodiagnostic Studies[5]

Routine electrodiagnostic studies include nerve conduction velocity (NCV), electromyography (EMG), and repetitive stimulation. NCVs are determined by electrically stimulating a sensory or motor nerve and recording the generated action potential distant from the stimulation site. Conduction along sensory fibers in the arms (i.e., median and ulnar nerves) is tested by stimulating the digital nerves in the fingers and recording at the wrist (orthodromic). Sensory conduction in the sural nerve is tested by stimulating the lateral calf and recording behind the lateral ankle (antidromic). Motor velocities are tested by stimulating a motor nerve and recording the action potential over the belly of the muscle that is activated. The time between the start of the stimulus and the onset of the response is called the latency. The conduction velocity along a nerve segment can be calculated by dividing the distance between the stimulus points by the difference in latencies (Fig. 10.2).

Conduction along a nerve may be slowed due to local compression or

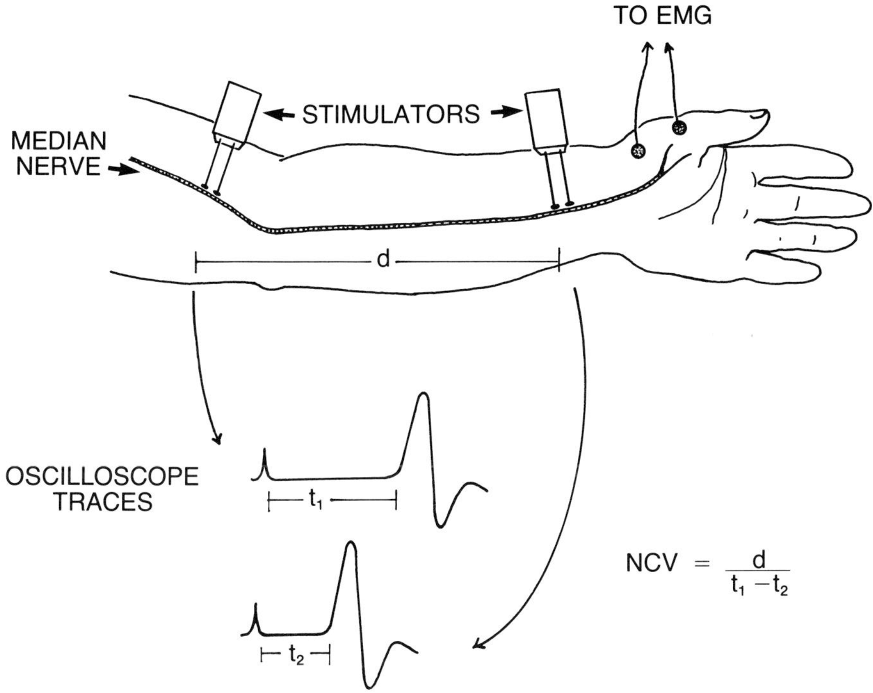

$$NCV = \frac{d}{t_1 - t_2}$$

Fig. 10.2 Nerve Conduction Velocity Determination. A peripheral nerve is stimulated proximally and distally and a muscle action potential is recorded. The distance between stimulation points divided by the difference in latencies provides the conduction velocity.

from diseases affecting either the nerve axon or its myelin covering. Axonal neuropathies demonstrate mild slowing of velocities with reduced response amplitudes. Disorders primarily affecting the myelin produce more marked slowing (<60 percent of normal velocity) with a reduced and dispersed response.

Electromyography involves insertion of a fine needle into a muscle and recording electrical impulses during several types of activity: upon insertion of the needle, with the muscle at rest, with minimal contraction and with full muscular effort. The electrical activity (motor unit potentials) is both viewed on an oscilloscope screen and heard audibly. Insertion of the needle normally causes a brief burst of electrical activity due to mechanical stimulation or injury of the muscle fibers. At rest, normal muscle is electrically silent. Abnormal spontaneous activity in the form of fibrillations or positive waves can be seen with denervation and in some primary muscle diseases. During minimal muscle contraction, individual motor unit potentials can be evaluated for their configuration, amplitude, and duration. Abnormally small, brief units with multiple phases (polyphasic potentials) occur most frequently with primary muscle disease, whereas, large, long polyphasic units are seen with chronic denervation (Fig. 10.3). With maximal contraction, the pattern of many motor unit potentials is observed (recruitment pattern) to see if there is a reduction or increase in the number of units necessary for a given effort. Diseases of the lower motor neuron and nerve usually show a reduced interference pattern while diseases of muscle may show early recruitment of a full interference pattern.

The neuromuscular junction is assessed by repetitive stimulation studies in which the action potential over a muscle is recorded while the nerve is repeatedly excited at rates of 2 to 50 per second. Normally, there is no

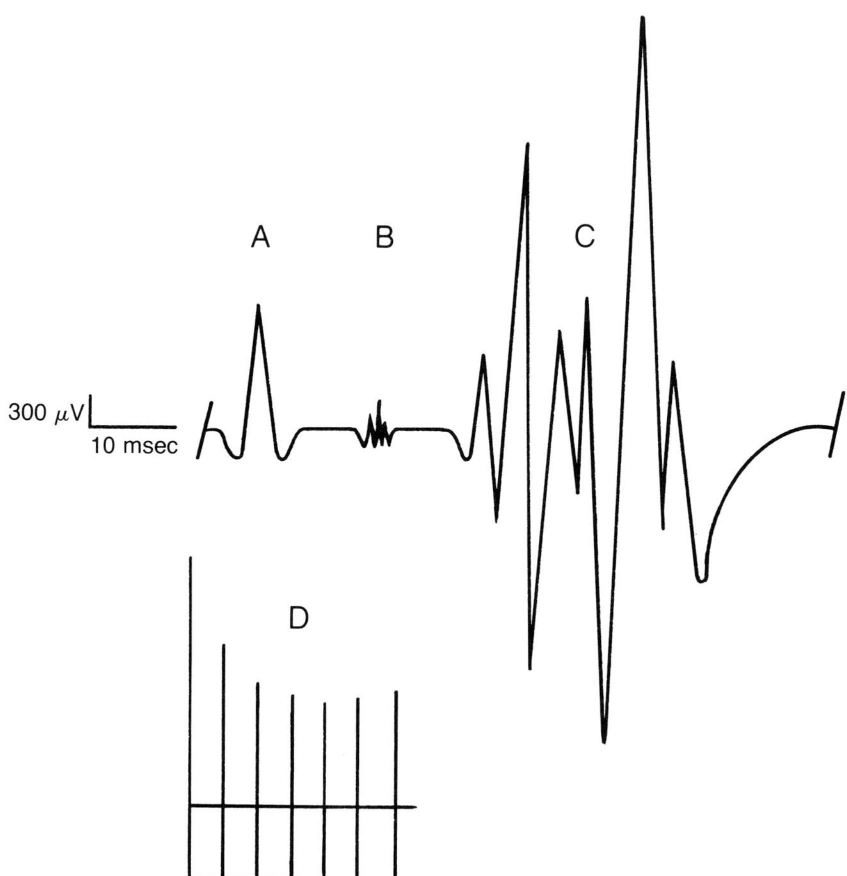

Fig. 10.3 EMG Motor Unit Action Potentials. Single motor unit potentials (MUP) in normal muscle (A), myopathy (B), and motor neuron disease (C). Note the striking difference between the small amplitude, brief duration polyphasic myopathic MUP (B) and the large amplitude, broad polyphasic neuropathic potential (C). A 2/second repetitive stimulation of a motor nerve in a patient with myasthenia gravis produces a normal amplitude first response, but a decremental response in subsequent motor unit action potentials (D).

significant decrease or increase in the amplitude of consecutive evoked muscle action potentials following repetitive stimulation. A decrease (decrement) of greater than 10 percent in amplitude is characteristic of myasthenia gravis. In botulism or in the facilitating syndrome of Eaton-Lambert (myasthenic syndrome), the initial action potential has low amplitude but it increases with repetitive stimulation.

Muscle And Nerve Biopsies[3]

Pathological interpretation of muscle biopsies has been greatly improved in the last two decades with the advent of histochemical techniques. A small piece of muscle (about the size of a pencil eraser) is surgically excised under local anesthesia, quick frozen, and processed with a variety of histological and histochemical stains. The latter reactions readily distinguish between type I and type II fibers and are useful in determining a host of enzyme deficiencies (Fig. 10.4). Detailed discussion of muscle biopsy findings is beyond the scope of this chapter, but suffice it to say that present techniques have provided biochemical as well as morphologic information that has led to the recognition of many new metabolic myopathies.

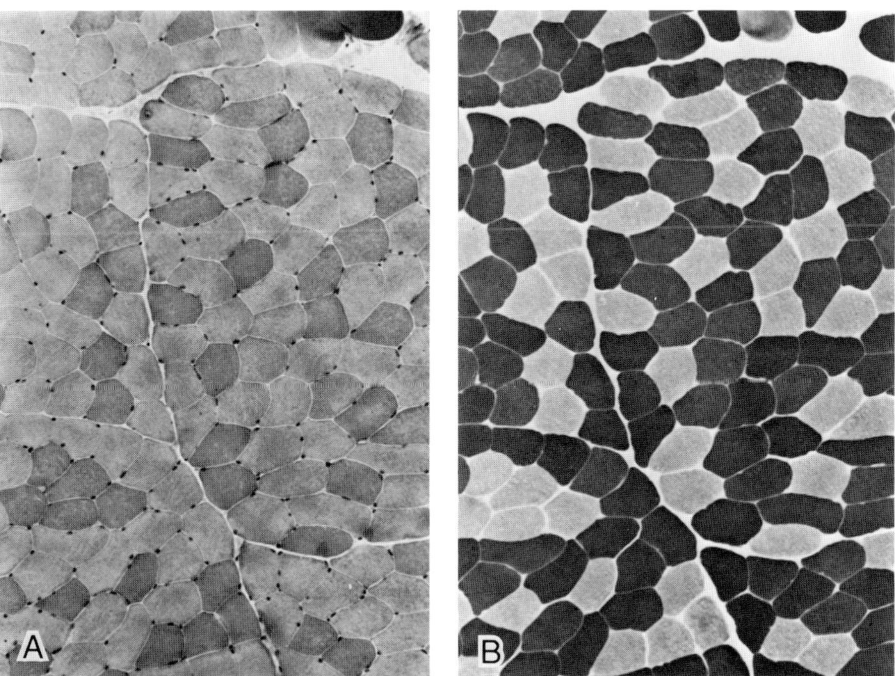

Fig. 10.4 Normal Muscle Biopsy. Serial 10 micron cryostat sections X 140. (A) Histologic stains (modified trichrome) demonstrate fibers of uniform size and shape with normal subsarcolemmal nuclei. (B) Histochemical stains (pH 9.4 myofibrillar ATPase) reveal a normal checkerboard distribution of Type I (light) and Type II (dark) fibers.

Although nerve biopsy is occasionally useful in distinguishing particular neuropathies (sarcoidosis, amyloidosis, vasculitis), it does not provide enough clinical information to be used routinely in the evaluation of patients with peripheral neuropathy. Ordinarily, a fascicle of the sural nerve is removed at the level of the lateral malleolus, leaving the patient with a small area of numbness over the lateral aspect of the foot.

DISEASES OF THE NEUROMUSCULAR SYSTEM[1,2,10]

Diseases Of The Lower Motor Neuron (Table 10.1)

Diseases affecting the lower motor neuron include the inherited spinal muscular atrophies (SMAs), amyotrophic lateral sclerosis (ALS), and poliomyelitis.

Spinal Muscular Atrophies (SMAs)

The spinal muscular atrophies are a clinically heterogeneous group of familial disorders characterized by weakness and muscle wasting. Pathologically one sees degeneration of anterior horn cells and cranial nerve motor nuclei without corticospinal or sensory tract involvement. The inheritance pattern is most frequently autosomal recessive, although X-linked recessive or dominant transmission occurs in 10 percent of cases.

The SMAs are classified according to the age of onset and severity of involvement. In the infantile form of SMA (Werdnig-Hoffmann disease) babies are either hypotonic and weak at birth or become weak within the first few months of life. These infants have a weak cry, a poor respiratory effort, and frequently aspirate when fed. Eye movements are unaffected and the infants commonly have very alert expressions. Fasciculations are usually not seen in the limbs, but are common in the tongue. Absent stretch reflexes are the rule. Treatment involves careful monitoring of nutrition to avoid aspiration and early recognition and treatment of pneumonia. Differential diagnosis includes hypotonic cerebral palsy, severe mental retardation, and a host of uncommon congenital myopathies or enzymatic deficien-

Table 10.1 Diseases of the Lower Motor Neuron

   I. Spinal muscular atrophies (SMAs)
      Infantile SMA (Werdnig-Hoffman)
      Intermediate SMA
      Juvenile SMA (Kugelberg-Welander)
  II. Amyotrophic lateral sclerosis (Motor Neuron
        Disease)
      Progressive bulbar atrophy
      Progressive muscular atrophy
      Primary lateral sclerosis
 III. Poliomyelitis

---

cies. Muscle biopsy is most helpful in diagnosis, since electrodiagnostic studies are difficult to interpret in infants. An intermediate form of SMA becomes apparent in children who fail to achieve normal motor milestones. These children are often able to sit unsupported, occasionally stand, but very rarely walk. Contractures and kyphoscoliosis are major complications. Proper wheelchair positioning, the use of body jackets, and in selected cases, spinal fusion will delay progressive spinal collapse.

Death in both the acute and intermediate forms of SMA is often due to respiratory insufficiency. Children with the acute form of SMA usually succumb within 1 to 2 years, whereas those with the intermediate form may survive into the second and occasionally third decade. How aggressive physicians should be in treating the inevitable respiratory decompensation is best discussed with the family prior to a panic-filled situation in the emergency room.

The juvenile form of SMA (Kugelberg-Welander) typically begins between the ages of 5 and 15 years. Walking becomes increasingly difficult with many patients requiring a wheelchair within 5–10 years of the onset of symptoms. As with all progressive neuromuscular diseases, stretching of extremity contractures will often prolong ambulation. Aggressive management of progressive kyphoscoliosis and respiratory infections, with careful attention to pulmonary toilet, is rewarding in these patients, who often live well beyond the third decade.

Amyotrophic Lateral Sclerosis (Motor Neuron Disease)[7]

Amyotrophic lateral sclerosis (ALS) is among the more devastating diseases to afflict mankind. Because of the degeneration of motor neurons and corticospinal tracts throughout the nervous system, patients develop progressive weakness, wasting, and spasticity of bulbar and extremity musculature. The majority of patients succumb within 2 to 3 years although up to 20 percent of patients have a milder illness and are alive at 5 years.

Bulbar motor neurons, anterior horn cells or corticospinal tracts may be primarily affected in ALS for which, respectively, the specific terms progressive bulbar palsy, progressive muscular atrophy, and primary lateral sclerosis have been applied. However, in most cases, as the disease progresses, some involvement of bulbar, lower and upper motor neurons is seen, justifying the inclusive term, ALS.

The disease, which is more common in men, may begin anytime during adulthood, but is most usual in later years. Although there is a familial form, 95 percent of cases are sporadic. Weakness and clumsiness of a limb are common early complaints, although speaking and swallowing problems may first bring the patient to a physician's attention. Intellect, ocular motility, sensation, and bowel and bladder function are spared. Loss of corticobulbar pathways produce pseudobulbar symptoms such as a hyperactive cough reflex, spastic dysphagia, and inappropriate outbursts of laughter or crying.

Examination of the patient with ALS will usually demonstrate a combination of upper and lower motor neuron dysfunction. Weakness, atrophy, and fasciculations of the tongue and limb muscles may be found along with a mixture of hypo- and hyperactive stretch reflexes. Laboratory data may show an elevated serum creatine phosphokinase (CPK), but most other blood chemistries are normal. Electrodiagnostic studies are usually very helpful in demonstrating fasciculations and other changes of denervation and reinnervation, in weak as well as clinically unaffected muscles.

Although ALS usually presents a distinctive picture, it is imperative to rule out treatable disorders that may mimic it. Wasting in the arms with leg spasticity may be caused by a cervical cord lesion and should be excluded by myelography, if indicated. Intoxication with mercury or lead and hyperparathyroidism have rarely been reported to produce an ALS-like picture. Although many predisposing factors have been linked to the later development of ALS, the etiology remains undefined.

Emergency complications of motor neuron disease are generally due to either swallowing or respiratory dysfunction. The combination of impaired tongue and pharyngeal function along with uncoordinated swallowing and a poor cough reflex, makes the patient with ALS susceptible to choking and aspiration (Fig. 10.5). Liquids and solid pieces of food become increasingly difficult to manage. Saliva may pool in the back of the throat when the patient is supine and cause choking. These symptoms are distressing and at times frightening to the ALS patient. Instruction to the family members on correct performance of the Heimlich maneuver may prove lifesaving (Fig. 10.6).

In addition to the risk of laryngeal obstruction and aspiration, problems with swallowing prevent a patient with ALS from maintaining adequate nutrition. Liquid nutritional supplements are often useful to prevent rapid weight loss. A variety of surgical procedures have been developed in an effort to obviate the complications of swallowing dysfunction. Surgical section of the nerves to the major salivary glands on one side (chorda tympani and Jacobsen's nerves) can reduce saliva production without causing sedation. Injection of a vocal cord with a Teflon substance can also reduce the risk of aspiration. In some cases, cricopharyngeal myotomy has been used to improve esophageal transport. Finally, placement of a pharyngostomy tube may be necessary to allow for adequate intake and lessen the risk of choking. The choice of procedures, all of which can be accomplished with local anesthesia, should be discussed at the appropriate time with the patient and an experienced otolaryngologist.

Respiratory complications due to aspiration pneumonia are generally reversible and are treated if the general quality of life is still acceptable. Terminal events in the ALS patient are usually due to respiratory insufficiency. Late in the disease, low flow oxygen may provide symptomatic relief for dyspnea.

Discussions as to the extent of measures to be taken in the late stages

Fig. 10.5 Aspiration. Anterior (A) and lateral (B) views of esophogram in a patient with recurrent aspiration pneumonia. The hypopharynx is dilated, barium pools in the epiglottal recesses, and contrast material outlines the vocal cords (arrows). (From Ringel, S. P., et al: Late-onset X-linked recessive spinal and bulbar muscular atrophy. Muscle and Nerve, 1:297, 1978; reprinted with permission).

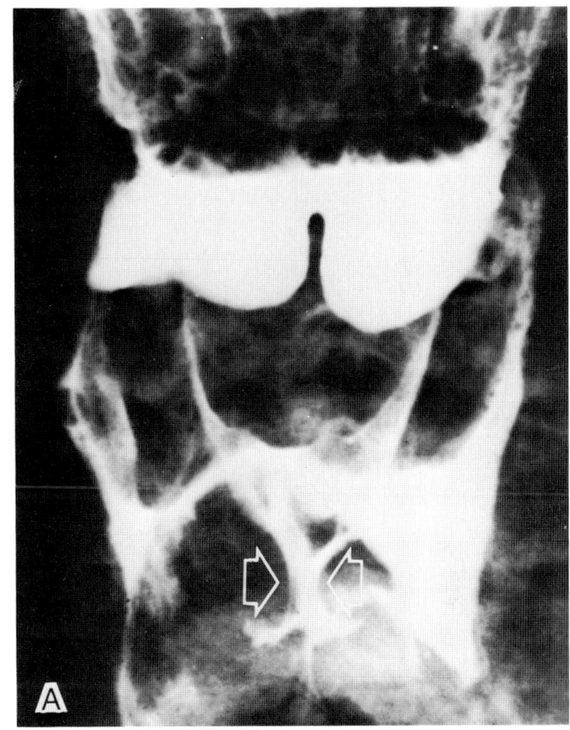

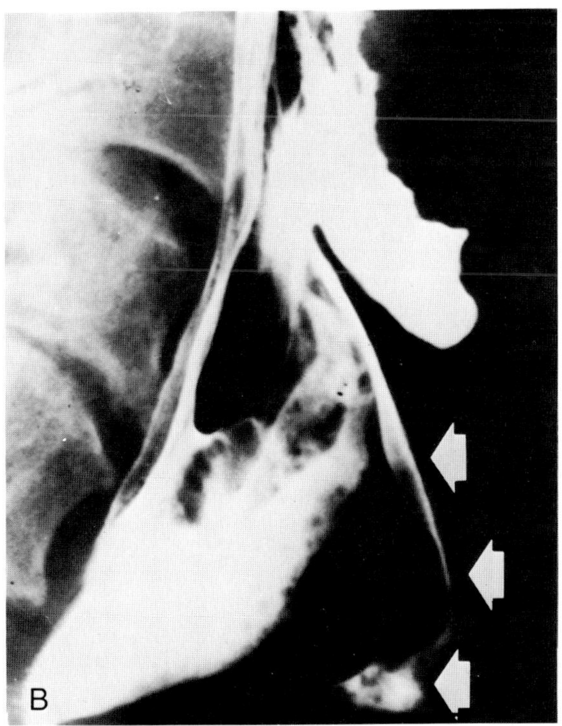

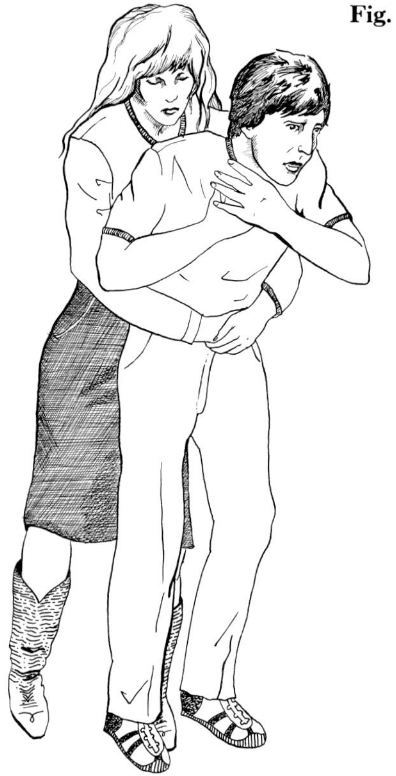

Fig. 10.6 Heimlich Maneuver. Forceful abdominal compression (standing or sitting) will dislodge an aspirated, obstructing particle of food and may be life-saving. The patient should be leaned forward during the thrust to prevent reaspiration of the dislodged particle.

of ALS should be undertaken before emergency decisions need to be made. Although, in our experience, the vast majority of patients do not desire heroic efforts to prolong life, there are individuals who demand intubation despite no prospect of being weaned from a ventilator. Discussions of these issues should emphasize that the patient's comfort is the foremost concern throughout the course of this terrifying disease.

Poliomyelitis

Fortunately, poliomyelitis has become a rare disease in the United States since the introduction of the Salk and Sabin vaccines. However, the reduced incidence of poliomyelitis has promoted a more casual attitude toward immunization and increases the likelihood of sporadic outbreaks. In any case of rapid bulbar or spinal paralysis, the diagnosis of polio should be considered. Clues to diagnosis include a viral prodrome, progressive asymmetrical weakness with retained sensation, and cerebrospinal fluid pleocytosis.

Diseases Of Peripheral Nerve (Table 10.2)

Peripheral nerve disorders may be classified into four categories: mononeuropathies, multiple mononeuropathies (mononeuritis multiplex), plexopathies, and polyneuropathies (peripheral neuropathies).

Table 10.2 Peripheral Neuropathies

I. Axonal neuropathies
  A. Diabetes
  B. Alcohol related
  C. Uremia
  D. Hypothyroidism
  E. Sarcoidosis
  F. Collagen vascular diseases
    1. Systemic lupus erythematosus
    2. Rheumatoid arthritis
    3. Wegener's granulomatosis
  G. Paraproteinemias
  H. Drugs
    1. Isoniazid
    2. Hydralazine
    3. Nitrofurantoin
    4. Vincristine
  I. Heavy metals
    1. Lead
    2. Arsenic
    3. Mercury
    4. Thallium
  J. Industrial toxins
    1. n-hexane
    2. n-butyltketone
    3. Acrylimide
    4. Organophosphate
  K. Amyloidosis
  L. Carcinoma (remote effect)
  M. Tick paralysis
II. Demyelinating neuropathies
  A. Guillain-Barré syndrome
  B. Diphtheria
  C. Porphyria

Mononeuropathy

The term mononeuropathy refers to damage of a single peripheral nerve. The most common causes of mononeuropathy are compression and traction. Any patient who is seen in an emergency room with trauma to an extremity should be carefully assessed for peripheral nerve damage. Common mononeuropathies include (Fig. 10.7):

1. Carpal tunnel syndrome, perhaps the most frequently occurring mononeuropathy, involves compression of the median nerve in the carpal tunnel at the wrist. A patient experiences numbness of the first three and one half digits of the hand, and pain in the hand, wrist, forearm and even upper arm. The pain typically awakens the patient from sleep. Weakness of median innervated muscles of the thenar eminence ensues if the compression is not relieved by splinting, hydrocortisone injection, or surgery.

2. Ulnar neuropathy results from acute or chronic injury of the nerve in the ulnar groove at the elbow.[4] Sensory loss over the last one and

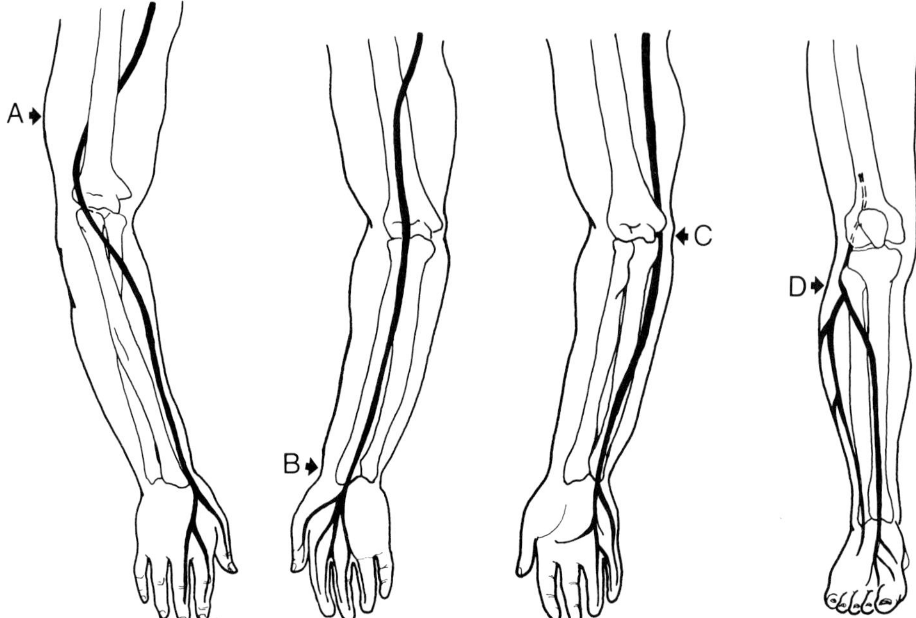

Fig. 10.7 Compression Neuropathies. Common sites of peripheral nerve compression include the radial nerve at midhumerus (A), median nerve at the wrist (B), ulnar nerve at the elbow (C), and peroneal nerve near the head of the fibula (D).

one half digits of the hand, together with weakness and atrophy of the intrinsic hand, hypothenar, and medial forearm flexor muscles is seen.

3. Radial nerve palsy is usually produced by compression of the nerve in the spinal groove of the humerus. Paralysis of extensors of the forearm and hand produce wrist and finger drop. Occasionally, sensory loss over the "snuff box" area of the thumb is present.

4. Peroneal palsy results from compression of the peroneal nerve as it crosses below the fibular head. This results in foot drop and diminished sensation over the dorsum of the foot.

Moneuritis Multiplex

Multiple mononeuropathy is a condition in which two or more isolated peripheral nerves are damaged. It is most commonly associated with diabetes and the collagen vascular diseases, particularly polyarteritis nodosa, and less frequently with ischemic vascular disease or sarcoidosis. Ischemic infarction is the usual mechanism of injury.

In diabetes, the femoral nerve is most commonly affected, producing a typical clinical picture referred to as diabetic amyotrophy (diabetic proximal neuropathy). A patient develops severe, persistent pain in the thigh followed within several weeks by weakness and atrophy of femoral innervated thigh muscles. As a result, the patient cannot flex the leg at the hip or extend the leg at the knee. Pain tends to slowly subside and strength generally returns over the course of a year or more. Days to months after the femoral nerve on one side is infarcted, the femoral nerve on the opposite side may become involved in a similar manner.

Plexopathy

The term plexopathy refers to injury of the brachial or lumbosacral plexuses. Although this may result from trauma, infection, or tumorous invasion of the plexus, several distinct syndromes are also recognized. Idiopathic brachial neuritis is a common cause of damage to the brachial plexus, usually involving the upper trunks and cords of the plexus. Initially, patients with brachial neuritis experience severe pain in the shoulder followed within several weeks by atrophy and weakness of the upper arm. Less commonly, the lower portion of the plexus is involved with resultant wasting and weakness of the muscles of the hand and forearm. A history of antecedent trauma, infection or immunization can often be obtained. The weakness and atrophy associated with brachial neuritis tend to recover completely over the course of 1 to 3 years as the damaged nerves slowly regenerate. Occasionally, with dislocation or injudicious relocation of the humerus, a partial brachial palsy occurs. In contrast to idiopathic brachial palsy, paralysis is immediate.

Lumbosacral plexopathy may occur in diabetes in cases where infarction involves the plexus rather than being limited to the femoral nerve. As in the more typical diabetic amyotrophy, the patient may experience severe pain in the upper leg for several days or weeks followed by weakness. When the entire lumbosacral plexus is involved, weakness and atrophy develop in muscles of the buttocks, and posterior and lower leg in addition to the femoral innervated muscles of the anterior thigh. The pain and weakness of this form of lumbosacral plexopathy usually resolve slowly.

Polyneuropathy

Peripheral or polyneuropathy is the condition in which progressive sensory loss and weakness develop in the legs and arms in a symmetrical fashion. Although the clinical picture is conveniently divided into axonal neuropathies and demyelinating neuropathies, some overlap of symptoms occur. With axonal neuropathies, the nerve fiber, (axon) is damaged, while in demyelinating neuropathies, the covering of myelin is stripped away. Common etiologies for the polyneuropathies are listed in Table 10.2. Axonal polyneuropathies, which are more frequently encountered, have a wide variety of toxic and metabolic causes, of which diabetes and alcohol abuse (probably including nutritional deficiency) are the most common. A careful history of chronic exposure to industrial toxins, household solvents, or medications should always be elicited, and in older patients, occult malignancy should also be considered.

Axonal polyneuropathies evolve in a distal symmetrical fashion and are predominantly sensorimotor in nature. The earliest symptom is sensory loss in the feet with later progression up the legs. Motor weakness usually follows sensory loss and similarly progresses from most distal to more proximal. Hands are usually affected later and to a lesser degree. Deep tendon reflexes are generally diminished with absence of ankle reflexes. Although axonal polyneuropathies tend to progress slowly, rapid progression may be seen with tick paralysis and rarely in the neuropathies associated with poorly controlled diabetes, alcoholism, uremia, and with high levels of exposure to heavy metals or industrial toxins.

Investigation of patients should include nerve conduction studies and appropriate serologic and urinary tests to determine the underlying etiology. The course of an axonal polyneuropathy is variable and depends upon the underlying cause. For example, the neuropathy associated with alcoholism or toxin exposure may be completely reversible if the offending agent is removed. However, in conditions such as diabetes, the neuropathy is irreversible and, at best, can be stabilized or slowed by better control of the diabetes.

In contrast to the axonal neuropathies, demyelinating polyneuropathies tend to be rapidly progressive and involve motor weakness more so than sensory loss. The most common variety, the Guillain-Barré syndrome (GBS), is an immunologically mediated disorder which in 50 percent of patients develops following infection, immunization, surgery, or trauma. The syndrome often begins with evanescent paresthesias of the extremities followed by rapidly ascending weakness and arreflexia, first in the legs and then in the arms. Weakness reaches its peak within 1 to 3 weeks at which point the patient may be totally paralyzed, requiring respiratory assistance in 20 to 30 percent of cases. Autonomic disturbances such as transient hyper- and hypotension, and brachy- and tachyarrhythmias may occur. Cranial nerves muscles are often affected, sometimes early on, resulting in facial weakness, difficulty swallowing, and rarely in impaired eye movements and pupillary reactivity.

Nerve conduction velocities are usually markedly slowed in GBS, confirming the presence of a demyelinating polyneuropathy. Cerebrospinal fluid protein is often increased above 100 mg percent. Despite the protein elevation, few or no cells are found (albuminocytologic dissociation).

The treatment of GBS is primarily supportive. The physician should be particularly alert for aspiration pneumonia from bulbar dysfunction and/ or respiratory failure. Intubation or tracheostomy is often necessary when vital capacity falls to less than 30 percent of predicted. While corticosteroids and plasmapheresis have been advocated by some for the treatment of GBS, these have generally not proved to be beneficial. Although the recovery phase is protracted in certain cases, most patients improve within a matter of months and 90 percent recover without significant residual disability.

Rarely, patients with diphtheria or porphyria may also develop a rapidly evolving motor neuropathy indistinguishable from GBS. In diphtheric neuropathy, the patient has a characteristic pharyngeal membrane and a mousey odor of his breath. Paralysis of bulbar muscles and loss of ocular accomodation occur early, but extremity weakness does not occur until 4–6 weeks after the acute illness. Porphyria should be suspected when a progressive neuropathy is accompanied by abdominal pains and mental changes. It is confirmed by the finding of excessive amounts of porphobilinogen and delta aminolevulinic acid in the urine.

Impaired nerve transmission is seen in tick paralysis. Progressive weakness typically occurs in children after an unrecognized tick (female Dermacentor andersoni) remains embedded, often near the hairline, for 4–5 days. Patients improve within hours of removal of the engorged tick.

Patients with inherited sensorimotor neuropathies do not develop rapidly evolving weakness requiring emergency attention. Both axonal (neuronal) and demyelinating (hypertrophic) varieties can occur and are usually categorized as Charcot-Marie-Tooth disease. The clinical expression is variable, but usually milder in dominantly inherited forms, and more severe with recessive inheritance.

DISEASES OF THE NEUROMUSCULAR JUNCTION (Table 10.3)

Disturbances of the neuromuscular junction may result from disorders which interfere with release of acetylcholine from the presynaptic membrane, which disrupt the postsynaptic membrane, or which interfere with inactivation of acetylcholine. (See Fig. 10.1 inset)

Myasthenia Gravis

The most common neuromuscular junction disorder is myasthenia gravis (MG), an autoimmune disorder in which acetylcholine receptor antibodies bind to the postsynaptic membrane, interfering with neuromuscular trans-

Table 10.3 Neuromuscular Junction Disorders

Myasthenia gravis
Botulism
Eaton-Lambert syndrome
Pseudocholinesterase deficiency
Organophosphate intoxication

mission. Although its role is not entirely clear, the thymus seems central to the genesis of this disease. A majority of patients have thymic hyperplasia and an additional 10 percent harbor thymic tumors. Approximately 15 percent of patients with MG have evidence of a concommitant autoimmune disease (rheumatoid arthritis, SLE, etc), particularly of the thyroid (Graves disease, Hashimoto's thyroiditis).

The peak incidence of MG is between 20 and 30 years of age with women affected two or three times as frequently as men. The ratio of females to males becomes more equal and thymomas are more common with onset after age 40. The disease occasionally begins in childhood and may occur as a transient disturbance in infants born to myasthenic mothers (neonatal myasthenia).

Symptoms of MG fluctuate throughout the day and are worse in frequently used muscles or after sustained activity. Typical symptoms affect cranial muscles and include ptosis, diplopia, nasal or slurred speech, and difficulty chewing and swallowing (dysphagia). The extremities are often weak, but to a lesser extent. Examination often reveals significant facial and neck muscle weakness as well.

Although the onset and progression of weakness associated with MG is usually insidious and occasionally limited to the eye muscles (ocular MG), patients with this disorder may experience sudden deterioration with life-threatening dysphagia and aspiration or severe respiratory compromise. This sudden decline is often precipitated by an infection, hypokalemia, emotional stress, unrecognized thyroid dysfunction, or with the administration of certain antibiotics (especially aminoglycosides and tetracyclines).

The diagnosis of MG can be confirmed by the use of the edrophonium (Tensilon) test, repetitive nerve stimulation, and by detection of acetylcholine receptor antibodies. Edrophonium hydrochloride is a short acting acetylcholinesterase inhibitor which temporarily improves the neuromuscular blockade of MG. Following the intravenous injection of 10 mg (1 cc) of edrophonium, a visible improvement in the patient's weakness becomes apparent within 30 to 60 seconds and remains for 4 to 5 minutes. Because an occasional patient will suddenly collapse after injection of the drug, a test dose of 2 mg should be given initially and atropine, an ambu bag, and an oral airway should be readily available. Repetitive nerve stimulation (see section on laboratory tests and Fig. 10.3) produces a decremental response in 70 percent of patients with generalized MG (40 percent of ocular MG) and acetylcholine receptor antibodies are detected in 90 percent of patients with generalized symptoms (50 percent of ocular MG).

In the past, the mainstay of treatment for MG was cholinesterase inhibitors such as pyridostigmine (Mestinon) or neostigmine (Prostigmine). These agents, by prolonging the activity of acetylcholine at the neuromuscular junction, provide temporary, incomplete symptomatic relief and often produce disturbing cholinergic side effects including excessive salivation, abdominal cramps, and diarrhea. In more recent years, concurrent with recognition of the autoimmune nature of MG, corticosteroids have been used as the first line of therapy. The effect of corticosteroids is often dramatic even when anticholinesterase agents have failed. Caution must be exercised during the first 5–10 days of steroid administration, since many patients become transiently weaker and may even require respiratory assistance. Thymectomy, which has always been undertaken in patients with a thymoma, is now routinely performed in adults under the age of 65 with generalized symptoms. In preparation for surgery, corticosteroids are administered for 6 to 8 weeks. Post-thymectomy, a majority of patients either experience complete or significant remission of symptoms. Recently, plasmapheresis has been employed in patients with MG who acutely deteriorate. This technique is expensive and the improvement is temporary (2–3 weeks), but it can be life-saving in a patient profoundly weak and on a respirator. Occasionally, other immunosuppressive medications (azathioprine, cyclophosphamide) and plasmapheresis are intermittently employed to improve function in patients who are unresponsive to more conventional therapy.

Botulism

Botulism, a rare but epidemiologically important disorder of neuromuscular transmission, often presents as an acute medical emergency requiring immediate attention. In adults, symptoms begin 6–24 hours after the ingestion of preformed botulinum toxin, the usual source of which is improperly canned foods. The toxin binds to presynaptic terminals where it blocks the release of acetylcholine, interfering with neuromuscular and cholinergic autonomic transmission. In infants, botulism may result from ingestion of the organism *Clostridium botulinum* rather than the toxin. Unlike the adult, the infant's intestinal environment allows the toxin to be formed in the gut and then absorbed.

Usually several hours after ingesting botulinum toxin, a patient develops severe nausea and vomiting. Over the next several hours to days the eyes and mouth become dry, the pupils may become dilated and fixed to light, and severe constipation develops. Descending neurologic dysfunction quickly ensues with paralysis of eye movements, difficulty swallowing and chewing, weakness of muscles of the neck, arms and legs, and finally, respiratory paralysis. The evolution of infantile botulism is slower, since toxin is not ingested, with neurologic and autonomic signs progressing over 8 to 10 days. In both forms, sensation remains intact, the spinal fluid is normal, and reflexes are preserved unless severe weakness develops.

The diagnosis of botulism may be confirmed by repetitive nerve stimulation. At rates much higher than those used to diagnose myasthenia gravis (50/second), a typical increase in the size of the motor response (incremental response) develops. The botulinum toxin can also be isolated from samples of serum, stool, or contaminated food. Since the latter test generally takes several days while other individuals may continue to be inadvertently exposed to the same source of toxin, repetitive stimulation should be attempted immediately in anyone suspected of botulism.

The treatment of botulism is primarily supportive. As with all acutely weak patients, this includes respiratory support, prevention of aspiration, fluid balance, and early treatment of infections. Antibiotics and enemas to rid the gut of toxin are frequently employed but are of uncertain value. In recent years, botulinum antitoxin has become available, although its usefulness is not yet established.

Other Neuromuscular Junction Disorders

The facilitating myasthenic syndrome (Eaton-Lambert syndrome) is similar to botulism in that there is a defect in the pre-synaptic release of acetylcholine. This disorder occurs in adults, most commonly in association with an underlying carcinoma, particularly oat cell carcinoma of the lung. Symptoms consist of mild weakness limited to the proximal muscles of the arms and legs with sparing of extraocular muscles. Deep tendon reflexes are diminished. The diagnosis is suggested by the finding of an incremental response similar to that seen with botulism following repetitive nerve stimulation. This condition may be improved by the administration of guanidine hydrochloride, an agent which facilitates release of acetylcholine from presynaptic terminals.

Organophosphates, which are commonly used in insecticides, have a marked anticholinesterase effect. Following exposure to such agents, patients experience immediate headache, vomiting, pupillary constriction, sweating, and weakness and twitching of muscles. These symptoms respond to the administration of atropine but if left untreated, weakness may result in respiratory failure and death.

In patients with plasma pseudocholinesterase deficiency, prolonged paralysis and apnea may follow administration of succinylcholine. Most patients will recover in 4–6 hours if artificial ventilation is maintained. If available to administer intravenously, a purified preparation of serum cholinesterase may terminate the paralysis.

DISEASES OF MUSCLE (Table 10.4)

A diverse array of disorders may affect the voluntary skeletal muscles. These include the dystrophies, inflammatory myopathies, metabolic, toxic, and endocrine myopathies, and several nonprogressive congenital myopathies. This section will focus on the more common disorders, highlighting distinguishing features and emphasizing when the patient is more likely to require emergency attention at some point in the natural history of the disease.

Table 10.4 Diseases of Muscles

I. Muscular dystrophies
   A. X-linked (Duchenne, Becker)
   B. Fascioscapulohumeral (FSH)
   C. Scapuloperoneal
   D. Limb girdle
   E. Progressive external ophthalmoplegias
   F. Myotonic

II. Inflammatory myopathies
   A. Infectious (viral, bacterial, parasitic)
   B. Immune mediated
      1. Polymyositis
      2. Dermatomyositis
      3. Myositis associated with other connective tissue disorders (Systemic lupus, polyarteritis nodosa, Sjogren's, rheumatoid arthritis, scleroderma)

III. Endocrine/metabolic myopathies
   A. Hyper-/hypothyroidism
   B. Hyper-/hypocalcemia
   C. Hyper-/hypoadrenalism

IV. Toxic myopathies
   A. Alcohol
   B. Amphotericin B
   C. Vincristine
   D. Chloroquine

V. Inherited metabolic myopathies
   A. Glycogen storage disorders
      (McArdle's, Phosphofructokinase and acid maltase deficiency)
   B. Lipid myopathies
      (carnitine and carnitine palmityl transferase deficiency)
   C. Periodic paralyses (Hypo-/hyper-/normokalemic)
   D. Malignant hyperthermia

The Dystrophies

A variety of muscular dystrophy syndromes have been characterized despite our generally inadequate understanding of etiology. Duchenne muscular dystrophy (DUD) is an X-linked recessive disorder characterized by progressive weakness, markedly elevated serum CPK, and the presence of necrotic, fibrotic muscle on biopsy. The onset of symptoms is insidious, but walking is usually noted to be clumsy by age 4–5. Pseudohypertrophy of the calf muscles and a tendency toward toe walking as heel cords shorten are characteristic. As the child loses strength in hip girdle muscles, he resorts to his arms to help arise from the floor or a chair, but even this maneuver (Gower's sign) soon becomes inadequate. Most boys require a wheelchair by age 10. The combination of respiratory muscle weakness plus scoliosis predisposes patients to pulmonary failure and infection, so that survival beyond 20 years is rare. If infection is the primary cause for respiratory decompensation, treatment, including temporary mechanical ventilation, may provide quality survival time. Eventually, however, ventilation becomes inadequate due to irreversible muscle weakness. Electrocardiographic abnormalities are present in 75 percent of patients. Cardiac enlargement, congestive heart failure, and cardiac dysrythmias (commonly tachyarythmias) may arise in the advanced stages.

Becker's dystrophy is another X-linked disorder that resembles DUD but is milder and progresses more slowly. Mean age of onset is 11 years with loss of ambulation usually by the late twenties. Survival is reduced due to respiratory complications or heart failure, although patients may live into their sixties with good medical care.

Other progressive muscular dystrophies are named according to the distribution of muscle involvement. Facioscapulohumeral and scapuloperoneal dystrophies cause progressive difficulties with daily life activities but generally do not shorten lifespan. Occasionally, patients have onset in infancy, are more severely affected, and may develop respiratory complications. Limb girdle dystrophy has become an all-inclusive term for a number of disorders resulting in progressive proximal weakness and wasting (limb girdle syndrome). The most common form of limb girdle dystrophy has its onset during the second or third decade with hip and shoulder weakness. Progressive involvement usually results in the need for a wheelchair 5 to 20 years after onset. Those patients with respiratory muscle involvement are susceptible to pneumonia and respiratory failure.

In ocular myopathies (Progressive External Ophthalmoplegia) weakness is often confined to the extraocular muscles and face. Some of these patients develop heart block so that electrocardiographic monitoring is important.

Myotonic muscular dystrophy (MYD) is a multisystemic disorder with an autosomal dominant inheritence. Skeletal muscle weakness, wasting, and myotonia are usually mild, so that patients remain ambulatory throughout life. Early cataracts, endocrine dysfunction, intellectual deficits, hypersomnolence, and gastrointestinal complaints are common. Potentially life-threatening problems include cardiac conduction defects and hypoventilation. First degree AV block may progress to complete heart block. Careful, regular monitoring of electrocardiograms will identify those patients that require pacemakers and protect against sudden death. Pulmonary insufficiency may be the result of muscle weakness, aspiration or respiratory center dysfunction. Reversible life-threatening events should be aggressively treated, as prolonged survival in MYD is anticipated if cardiopulmonary complications are controlled.

Inflammatory Myopathies

Muscle may be the site of infectious (viral, bacterial, parasitic) or immune-mediated inflammatory reactions. Myalgia and mild weakness are the most common symptoms in typical viral inflammatory myopathies and are usually self-limited, subsiding within 1–2 weeks. Rarely, fulminant rhabdomyolysis develops and can be fatal. In immunological disorders of muscle, the weakness usually progresses over weeks to months, although occasionally it may produce severe paralysis in a matter of days. Bulbar symptoms are uncommon except for dysphagia, which may necessitate nasogastric feedings. An aching, deep pain is described by many patients with myositis, and the muscles are often tender though rarely swollen. Muscle atrophy is unusual except when the disease is advanced. An elevated serum CPK is usually present and spontaneous activity (fibrillations, positive waves) and small, brief polyphasic potentials (myopathic units) are seen on EMG. A muscle biopsy is usually diagnostic, demonstrating inflammatory cell infiltrates with muscle fiber damage. Serological studies, including antinuclear antibody (ANA), rheumatoid factor, and sedimentation rate, may be elevated.

Myositis occurs in all ages and may be present in isolation (primary polymyositis), in association with a characteristic skin rash (dermatomyositis), or in association with other connective tissue disorders, such as lupus erythematosus, polyarteritis nodosa, Sjorgen's syndrome, rheumatoid arthritis, or scleroderma. Patients who are over the age of 50 years and who develop polymyositis or dermatomyositis are at a significant risk of having an occult malignancy (10 to 20 percent).

Potential emergent complications of the inflammatory myopathies include rapidly progressive weakness with swallowing dysfunction, respiratory insufficiency, and, rarely, cardiac muscle involvement with conduction defects. Pulmonary interstitial fibrosis with consequent diffusion problems is rarely seen. Prolonged vigorous support of the patient with an inflammatory myopathy is indicated, as the commonly used antiinflammatory and immunosuppressive agents (corticosteroids, azathioprine, methotrexate) may take several weeks to show a therapeutic effect.

Another presumed although unproven immunologic disorder that can mimic myositis is *polymyalgia rheumatica*. This disorder of adults produces pain, aching, and stiffness of extremities and trunk, aggravated by movement and constitutional symptoms including fever and weight loss. An elevated sedimentation rate and prompt response to corticosteroids supports the diagnosis. One-third of patients have associated temporal arteritis and can become blind so that temporal artery biopsy may be necessary if the patient develops visual impairment.

Endocrine/Toxic/Metabolic Myopathies

Muscle is sensitive to a number of systemic and local metabolic derangements. Hyper- and hypothyroidism may both lead to weakness. Reflexes are usually brisk in hyperthyroidism and muscle twitching may be present. Cramping, delayed relaxation, and tense, swollen extremities are seen with hypothyroidism along with a markedly elevated CPK. Abnormalities in calcium metabolism may also lead to muscle dysfunction with hypocalcemia causing tetany and hypercalcemia producing weakness and aching that may mimic motor neuron disease. Nonspecific muscle weakness may be seen in states of hyper- and hypoadrenalism. Changes in potassium levels due to adrenal imbalance, renal disease, or diuretic therapy may produce acute muscle weakness, but usually only at the extreme serum concentrations (<2.5 mEq/l, >7.0 mEq/l). Consideration of endocrine and electrolyte imbalances is critical in assessing a patient with acute or subacute neuromuscular symptoms because rapid correction may prove immediately therapeutic.

Muscle is also susceptible to a variety of exogenous drugs and toxins. Both acute and subacute weakness has been described with alcohol. A heavy bout of drinking may be followed by muscle swelling, tenderness, weakness, and myoglobinuria. Dehydration, electrolyte imbalances and nutritional deficiency may increase the sensitivity of muscle to the effects of alcohol. Therapy should be directed at maintaining adequate urine flow and fluid and electrolyte balance. Repeated low-grade insults lead to a subacute alcoholic myopathy.

Enzymatic defects in either glycogen or lipid metabolism may produce weakness and/or exercise intolerance. In McArdles disease (myophosphorylase deficiency) and phosphofructokinase deficiency (PFK), two disorders with impaired glycogen metabolism, severe muscle cramps, rhabdomyolysis, and myoglobinuria occur following brief, strenuous exercise. Repeated episodes may eventually lead to persistent weakness. Failure to produce lactate following ischemic exercise is diagnostic. The particular enzyme deficiency can be determined by muscle biopsy using histochemical reactions. Dietary supplementation with food products metabolized below the level of the enzymatic defect are surprisingly ineffective. Although most patients with these disorders spontaneously limit their activity to avoid cramping, overexertion can lead to significant rhabdomyolysis and myoglobinuric renal failure.

Acid maltase deficiency is a lysosomal glycogen storage disease that may present in adult life with respiratory failure due to selective, severe involvement of respiratory muscles. An underlying limb girdle distribution of weakness should tip-off the clinician to consider this diagnosis.

Deficiency of muscle carnitine, a substance essential for fatty acid transport, may cause weakness and rarely cardiac failure. Muscle biopsy demonstrates lipid containing vacuoles. Deficiency of the enzyme carnitine palmityltransferase (CPT) produces muscle cramps and myoglobinuria following a fast or exertion. Failure to produce ketone bodies after a prolonged fast and a normal lactate ischemic exercise test differentiates CPT deficiency from the glycogenoses.

Acute attacks of weakness associated with spontaneous fluctuations in serum potassium levels are designated the periodic paralyses. Hypokalemic periodic paralysis is an autosomal dominant disorder that usually presents in the second decade. Exercise, a carbohydrate load, alcohol or cold may precipitate an attack of weakness which often begins when first awakening, starts in the back and thighs and may progress within minutes to hours to completely immobilize a patient. Respiratory and bulbar muscles usually remain uneffected. Potassium levels as low as 1.5 mEq/1 may be seen, but patients may become weak at levels that a normal patient could easily tolerate (e.g., 3.0 mEq/1). Acute attacks are best treated with oral potassium in doses of 5 to 10 grams. Daily treatment with acetazolamide (Diamox) is helpful in some patients to diminish the frequency of attacks.

In hyperkalemic periodic paralysis, which may be dominantly or recessively inherited, attacks are usually provoked by rest after activity or cold, and may develop with remarkable rapidity. Serum potassium levels may be only mildly elevated. Intravenous calcium gluconate or sodium chloride may be used to treat a severe attack; milder attacks are usually self-limited. Acetazolamide has also been useful prophylactically in some patients.

A rare but life-threatening reaction to general anesthesia is the syndrome of malignant hyperthermia. The reaction is triggered by inhalation anesthetics (halothane, ether, cyclopropane) or succinylcholine. In susceptible persons, tachycardia, sweating, blood pressure fluctuations, and muscle rigidity precede a rapid rise in body temperature (up to 1° C. every 5 minutes). Acidosis, hyperkalemia, rhabdomyolysis and myoglobinuria may follow. Convulsions are common prior to death. Immediate therapy is critical; untreated patients usually die. All anesthetic agents should be discontinued and replaced with 100 percent oxygen. Dantrolene should be given intravenously 1 to 2 mg/kg every 5 to 10 minutes up to a total of 10 mg/kg. The patient should be cooled and sodium bicarbonate given to correct the acidosis. Careful attention to urine flow is important as myoglobinuric renal failure may result from the significant muscle breakdown. This disorder should not be confused with pseudocholinesterase deficiency, another condition which produces prolonged paralysis following the use of succinylcholine (see neuromuscular junction disorders).

There is a familial tendency to develop malignant hyperthermia. Individuals at risk often have an elevated serum CPK and mild, non-specific muscle weakness. Patients with certain known neuromuscular disorders (myotonic dystrophy, myotonia congenita, central core disease) may be at increased risk and should be carefully evaluated before receiving general anesthesia.

CLINICAL PRESENTATIONS IN NEUROMUSCULAR DISEASE

When a patient with an acute neuromuscular complication first seeks medical attention, the diagnosis is not often immediately apparent. Our main goal in this section is to organize the clinically emergent presentations of neuromuscular disease so as to assist the physician in prompt and accurate diagnosis and treatment of his patient. To avoid repetition, we have not elaborated on individual diseases. Rather, the reader should refer back to the more comprehensive discussion of each disease provided in earlier sections of this chapter. Although the most emergent problems are emphasized, some discussion of less serious presentations seems necessary, since undiagnosed, a more benign symptom can subsequently evolve into a serious, life-threatening complication.

Weakness (Table 10.5)

Because weakness is such a common symptom with neuromuscular disease, detailed consideration should be given to all aspects of this subject. A patient's disability depends not only on the particular muscles involved, but also on how this weakness affects his particular life style. Patients can be entirely unaware of rather profound weakness if they do not ordinarily use the muscle to full capacity or if the weakness has been developing insidiously. Acute paralysis, on the other hand, is justifiably alarming to both the patient and physician. While immediate measures are being taken to assure stable cardiorespiratory function, a rapid, sequential diagnostic evaluation must be vigorously pursued, since prompt and specific treatment will enhance the patient's recovery.

Patterns Of Weakness

Proximal weakness (shoulders, hips) is most characteristic of myopathies. Patients have difficulty elevating arms over the head, climbing stairs, or getting up from a chair or the floor (Fig. 10.8). They often walk with a waddling, lordotic gait, and with longstanding weakness, marked wasting can be a prominent feature. Associated deformities are common and include contractures, winging of the scapulae, scoliosis, hypertrophied calves, and a range of foot abnormalities (club foot, equinovarus and pes cavus). Proximal weakness without atrophy or deformity is more usual in myasthenia gravis, the inflammatory myopathies, and many metabolic and endocrine myopathies. The Guillain-Barre syndrome is the one neuropathy which may present with acute proximal weakness.

Distal weakness (hands, feet) is more characteristic of polyneuropathies (often with associated sensory disturbances) and motor neuron disease. Patients have difficulty with fine coordinated hand movements, such as buttoning a shirt, and with grip. With weakness in the lower extremities, patients walk with a characteristic "steppage" or slapping gait and frequently twist an ankle or trip over small objects.

Ptosis and/or ophthalmoparesis occurs in several dystrophies (FSH, myotonic, ocular myopathies) and is often a striking finding in neuromuscular junction disorders (botulism, MG, organophosphate poisoning). The pupils become fixed and dilated with botulism (and rarely GBS), are small and unreactive from organophosphate poisoning, but remain unaffected in the majority of neuromuscular diseases.

Facial weakness frequently goes unrecognized by patients when it pro-

Table 10.5 Differential Diagnosis of Acute Weakness

Disorder	Clinical Features	Laboratory
Lower motor neuron		
Poliomyelitis	Viral prodrome. Asymmetric paralysis Meningeal signs Bulbar signs	CSF pleocytosis
Peripheral nerve		
Guillain-Barré syndrome	Recent viral illness, immunization or trauma. Ascending paralysis and areflexia. Sensory symptoms but not signs.	CSF albuminocytologic dissociation. Markedly slow NCVs.
Tick paralysis	Typically in children. Weakness, areflexia, bulbar symptoms, numbness.	Find the tick and remove it.
Diphtheria	Recent membraneous pharyngitis. Palatal weakness. Eye accommodation weakness. (big pupils) Neuropathy late.	Culture C. diphtheriae organism.
Porphyria	History of psychiatric, abdominal or cutaneous symptoms. Guillain-Barré-like clinical picture.	Excretion of excessive porphyrins in urine.
Neuromuscular junction		
Myasthenia gravis	Fluctuating weakness. Ptosis, diplopia, dysphagia, dysarthria.	Positive Tensilon test. Decrement with repetitive stimulation EMG. Positive acetylcholine receptor antibody.
Botulism	History of recent home canned food ingestion. GI distress Rapid onset bulbar symptoms, paralysis, areflexia. Dilated pupils (rare)	Increment with repetitive stimulation EMG. Normal CSF. Toxin in food, blood or stool.
Organophosphate poisoning	History of insecticide exposure. GI distress, sweating, agitation, twitching, small pupils. Delayed neuropathy.	Identification of organophosphate containing substance.
Muscle		
Inflammatory myopathy (rapidly progressive)	Proximal weakness. Dysphagia, but not other bulbar dysfunction. Myalgia in 50%.	Elevated CPK. Myopathic EMG. Inflammation on biopsy.
Periodic paralyses	History of recurrent bouts of weakness. Family history. Speech, respiration spared.	High or low serum K.
Rhabdomyolysis	Recent strenuous overexertion. Trauma or toxin (ETOH) exposure. Swollen, tender extremities.	Elevated CPK. Myoglobinuria (positive benzidine test in urine without RBCs).

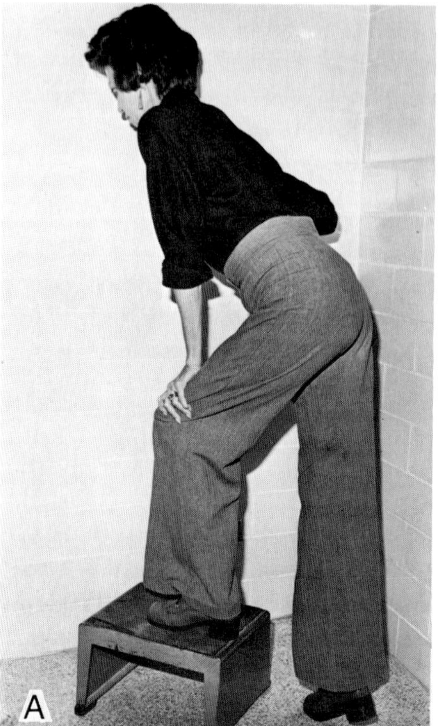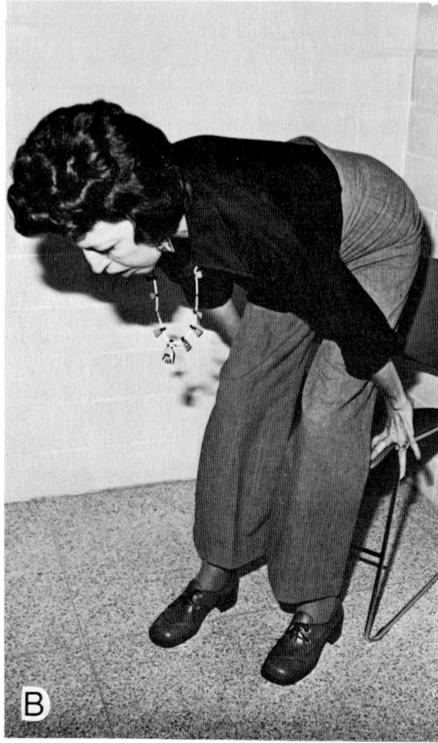

Fig. 10.8 Proximal Weakness. (A) In climbing stairs or stepping onto a stool, the patient with hip weakness supports the knee with one hand and uses the other for wall or hand-rail support. (B) In arising from a chair, both hands are used for support and the buttocks are elevated to allow knee extension before the upper torso is raised vertically. (From Ringel, S. P.: Clinical presentations in neuromuscular disease, p. 313. In Vinken, P. J., Bruyn, G. W., Eds.: Handbook of Clinical Neurology. Vol. 40, North-Holland Publishing, Amsterdam, 1979; reprinted with permission).

gresses slowly and symmetrically, although when questioned, the patient will often admit to longstanding inability to blow up a balloon, whistle, or drink through a straw. Facial weakness is usually a striking feature of neuromuscular junction disorders, can be pronounced in a few dystrophies (myotonic, FSH, congenital myopathies) and neuropathies (GBS, tick paralysis), but is mild or absent in most anterior horn cell diseases.

Any disturbance of palatal, pharyngeal, or lingual movement will result in dysphagia and dysarthria. Interruption of laryngeal muscle function produces hoarseness. Among the peripheral nervous system (PNS) disorders, myasthenia gravis (MG) most commonly produces this symptom complex. In MG, a patient's speech or swallowing becomes increasingly difficult with sustained effort. Acute speech and swallowing difficulties may occur also with GBS. Several of the slowly progressive dystrophies (myotonic, oculopharyngeal dystrophy), and anterior horn cell diseases (motor neuron disease, polio) are commonly associated with severe dysphagia and dysphonia. Over one-third of patients with an inflammatory myopathy complain of mild dysphagia, but they rarely aspirate and usually can speak clearly.

Onset And Development of Weakness

In evaluating a patient with acute weakness, the physician should determine the mode of onset, tempo of development, and distribution of weakness. In the periodic paralyses, botulism and MG, weakness can evolve in a matter of hours. In contrast, with polio, polyneuropathies, and most acute myopathies, weakness develops more slowly, usually not reaching a nadir for several days. Unlike poliomyelitis, where weakness is often asymmetrical (focal), a symmetrical ascending paralysis (feet-legs-arms) is more usual with a polyneuropathy, especially GBS. Descending (arms first) paralysis has also been described with porphyria and rarely GBS.

Several disorders are characterized by the acute onset of bulbar dysfunction, ptosis, ophthalmoparesis, and varying degrees of weakness of the extremities. These conditions include botulism, organophosphate poisoning, GBS, MG, tick paralysis, and diphtheria. An infectious prodrome typically occurs with polio, diphtheria, and viral myositis, and often with GBS. Infection also commonly initiates acute deterioration in patients with otherwise mild symptoms of MG.

Associated Problems And Findings

Isolated, severe gastrointestinal disturbance should suggest toxin exposure. Nausea and vomiting occur soon after exposure to arsenic, organophosphates, and botulism toxin. Organophosphates usually produce other acute cholinergic symptoms including miosis, profuse sweating, and muscle fasciculations. Reversal of muscarinic side effects is possible with large doses of atropine (2–4 mg prn). In botulism, mydriasis, drying of secretions, and constipation are more usual and occur along with weakness 6–24 hours after ingestion of the toxin. Antitoxin is usually ineffective.

Paralysis in association with acute rhabodomyolysis is seen in patients with enzymatic defects in glycogen (McArdle's, PFK) or lipid (CPT deficiency) metabolism. They often have a history of recurrent, severe, painful muscle cramps and dark urine (myoglobin) following exercise (glycogen defect) or fasting (lipid defect). Cranial muscles are spared and respiratory assistance is usually not required. Other neuromuscular disorders that produce weakness with rhabdomyolysis include acute polymyositis (often viral), alcoholic myopathy, and malignant hyperthermia states. The causes of rhabdomyolysis and myoglobinuria are considered in greater detail in a subsequent section.

Early absence of deep tendon reflexes and complaints of paresthesias or numbness in hands and feet with accompanying stocking/glove sensory loss points toward a neuropathy as the cause of acute weakness. The absence of these findings, however, does not exclude the diagnosis, since several neuropathies (GBS, tick paralysis) may result in extreme weakness without any apparent sensory loss. Likewise, with profound, longstanding weakness produced by primary muscle or anterior horn cell diseases, reflexes may become diminished and eventually absent.

Disturbances of bowel and bladder function are not typical of acute neuromuscular disorders, although in GBS and polio, transient urinary retention may occur several days after the onset of weakness. Rather, with acute urinary retention or incontinence in association with leg paralysis (arms spared), one should suspect spinal cord compression. Other support for this diagnosis includes a history of back pain, a dematomal level of sensory loss, hyperactive reflexes, and an extensor plantar response (Babinski) (see Chapter 13).

Laboratory Investigations

Electrodiagnostic studies are the single most useful test in differentiating causes of acute neuromuscular weakness and should be performed as soon as possible. Repetitive stimulation studies (see laboratory test section) produce a decremental response in MG and an incremental response in botulism. Demyelinating polyneuropathies (GBS, porphyria) often produce very marked conduction slowing which is patchy in distribution, whereas in axonal polyneuropathies (toxins), nerve conduction slowing is mild. In polio or other anterior horn cell diseases, conduction studies are normal, yet, as with neuropathies, denervation is apparent by electromyography (EMG). In acute muscle diseases, EMG reveals myopathic changes.

Other useful tests in differentiating causes of acute weakness include serum potassium (periodic paralysis), glucose (diabetic neuropathy), BUN (uremic neuropathy), acetylcholine receptor antibody (MG), viral titers to cytomegalovirus, mycoplasma and mononucleosis (GBS), CPK (myopathy), throat culture (diphtheria), urine for porphyrins, myoglobin, and heavy metals, and stool (or blood) for a botulinum toxicity assay. A lumbar puncture will help differentiate poliomyelitis (mildly elevated protein and pleocytosis) from GBS, in which the protein is often markedly elevated with few white blood cells (albuminocytologic dissociation).

Initial Management

Regardless of the cause of acute weakness, the physician must always be alert to unrecognized aspiration due to bulbar dysfunction and impending respiratory failure. Early intubation should be performed if either of these symptoms is developing. Similarly, during early recovery, aspiration and/

or pneumonia are constant threats. The physician should carefully observe the overzealous patient, so relieved to be free of a respirator that he hurries to resume eating to regain strength. Barium in a bronchus on cineesophagram or the presence of food coloring in the tracheal aspirate after a test meal will alert the physician that the patient is aspirating.

The prognosis of patients with acute weakness from neuromuscular disease is excellent, with frequent reversal of symptoms provided they do not succumb to pneumonia or another avoidable complication.

MUSCLE ACHES/CRAMPS (Table 10.6)

Patients commonly seek medical attention because of muscle aches and pains. In a large proportion of cases, no definite etiology can be determined and such non-specific terms as "fibrositis" or fibromyalgia have been applied.

Table 10.6 Muscle Pain and Cramps

I. Pain and tenderness
   A. Muscle
      1. Inflammatory myopathy
      2. Infectious—viral, parasitic
      3. Polymyalgia rheumatica
      4. "Fibromyalgia"
      5. Acute rhabdomyolysis
   B. Nerve
      1. Acute brachial neuritis
      2. Guillain-Barré syndrome
      3. Diabetic amyotrophy
      4. Other polyneuropathies
   C. Other
      1. Referred pain—arthritis, CNS
      2. Psychiatric—depression, hysteria
II. Cramps and stiffness
   A. Cramps
      1. Strenuous exertion
      2. Dehydration, electrolyte imbalance
      3. Hypothyroidism
      4. ALS
      5. Medications—anticholinesterase drugs, clofibrate, diuretics
   B. Contractures
      1. Glycogenoses
      2. Lipidoses
   C. Myotonia
      1. Myotonic dystrophy
      2. Myotonia congenita
      3. Hyperkalemic periodic paralysis
   D. Tetany
      1. Hypocalcemia
      2. Hypomagnesemia
      3. Alkalosis

However, several potentially serious neuromuscular disorders may be associated with muscle pain and should be considered in patients who complain of myalgias.

Almost half of patients with immunologic *inflammatory myopathies* (polymyositis, dermatomyositis, and other collagen vascular diseases) complain of pain along with their muscle weakness. Elevated muscle enzymes, an abnormal EMG, and serological evidence of an immunologic disorder aid in establishing the diagnosis. Severe myalgias associated with influenza or coxsackie virus infection are more common but rarely are accompanied by weakness and are generally self-limited, benign syndromes. Rarely, patients develop fulminant symptoms with rhabdomyolysis.

The physician should always consider the diagnosis of polymyalgia rheumatica (PMR) in elderly patients complaining of pain, aching, and stiffness about the shoulder and hip girdle muscles. Morning stiffness and constitutional symptoms of weight loss, fever, and anorexia are common. An elevated sedimentation rate (ESR) (usually above 50 mm/hr) and prompt relief with corticosteroids support the diagnosis. As mentioned, temporal arteritis must be ruled out (see Arteritic Ischemic Optic Neuropathy, Chapter 14).

Acute denervating disorders may initially present with pain. In acute brachial neuritis (neuralgic amyotrophy) severe aching pain in one or both shoulders or arms is followed after a few days by wasting and weakness of the shoulder girdle muscles. Cases often follow trauma, infection, or recent immunization. Tingling in the extremities and back pain may herald the onset of Guillain-Barré syndrome. Ascending weakness, loss of reflexes and an elevated CSF protein help establish the diagnosis. In the syndrome of diabetic amyotrophy, severe pain often accompanies weakness and atrophy of the quadriceps muscle. Asymmetry and absent sensory impairment is characteristic. Other neuropathies associated with severe burning pain include those seen with alcoholism, arsenic, polyarteritis and porphyria.

Muscle cramps, or painful, involuntary muscle contractions, are experienced by almost everyone at some time and commonly occur after unaccustomed exercise. However, cramps may also be the initial manifestation of an anterior horn cell, peripheral nerve, neuromuscular junction or muscle disorder. Leg cramps are frequent in the early stages of motor neuron disease, but tend to subside as the disease progresses. Irritability of peripheral nerves in hypocalcemia and hypomagnesemia results in severe muscle spasms (tetany). Nerve irritability can be demonstrated by tapping over the facial nerve and observing facial twitching (Chvostek's sign) or by producing ischemia of an arm with a tourniquet and inducing spasm of the wrists and fingers (Trousseau's sign). Alkalosis due to hyperventilation, persistent vomiting, or hypokalemia may also produce tetany.

Complaints of cramping in a patient with myasthenia gravis should suggest an overdose of anticholinesterase medication. This situation occurs commonly after prednisone has been instituted and indicates that the immunosuppressive effect of the steroids has reduced the need for anticholinesterase drugs.

Exertional cramps, with or without myoglobinuria, suggest a disorder of glycogen or lipid metabolism. These disorders are described in the sections on diseases of muscle and disorders producing myoglobinuria. Several cramping disorders are characterized by myotonia, an abnormality in muscle membranes resulting in delayed relaxation. Myotonia can be elicited by percussing the thenar eminence or having the patient make a tight fist and observing him extend his fingers. Cramping and impaired relaxation is seen in myotonic dystrophy, myotonia congenita, and hyperkalemic periodic paralysis. Patients with hypothyroidism often complain of tightness in their muscles. Weakness and prolonged relaxation of deep tendon reflexes may be seen. An elevated CPK is characteristic, even in the absence of weakness and may provide an early clue to the diagnosis.

Several disorders affecting the central nervous system also produce abnormal muscle contractions. These include tetanus, strychnine poisoning, and the toxin from the bite of the black widow spider.

RHABDOMYOLYSIS/MYOGLOBINURIA (Table 10.7)[9]

Acute muscle cell destruction (rhabdomyolysis) may result from a variety of insults including extreme overexertion, trauma and toxins, and much less commonly from certain inherited and acquired neuromuscular disorders. The muscle cell breakdown releases myoglobin into the bloodstream which is rapidly filtered by the kidney, producing dark, reddish-brown urine.

Table 10.7 Rhabdomyolysis and Myoglobinuria

I. Exertion
   A. Unaccustomed exertion
   B. Prolonged seizures

II. Trauma or ischemia
   A. Crush injury
   B. Coma
   C. Arterial ischemia
   D. Surgery

III. Toxins
   A. Alcohol
   B. Medications—amphotericin, vincristine, chloroquine

IV. Metabolic disorders
   A. Glycogenoses
   B. Lipidoses
   C. Malignant hyperthermia
   D. Hypokalemia

V. Myopathies (including dystrophies)
   A. Infrequently with exertion

Acute renal failure from tubular necrosis may result from the excessive myoglobin challenge. Subsequent electrolyte imbalance (hyperkalemia, hypocalcemia) can produce life-threatening cardiac arrhythmias.

The finding of pigment in the urine (positive benzidine test) in the absence of red cells or evidence of hemolysis is characteristic of myoglobinuria. Specific antisera can also detect minute amounts of myoglobin. A strikingly elevated serum CPK is present in any patient with significant myoglobinuria.

Strenuous overexertion, as may be seen in army recruits who become dehydrated during forced exercise, is a common cause of rhabdomyolysis. Aching muscles are followed by fever, chills, nausea and vomiting. Extremities become swollen and tender and dark urine develops the next day.

Other common causes of rhabdomyolysis include status epilepticus, major injury to muscle due to electric shock, trauma, or surgery, embolic occlusions of major limb arteries, and prolonged coma, particularly if there is pressure-induced ischemia of a limb.

A number of toxins can produce muscle cell destruction, particularly alcohol but also amphotericin B, vincristine, chloroquine, barbiturates, delta amino caproic acid and plasmocid.

Patients with inherited glycogen (myophosphorylase, phosphofructokinase deficiency) and lipid metabolic defects frequently demonstrate exertional myoglobinuria. When exercised to the point where energy needs exceed supply, painful cramps (contractures) and cellular breakdown occur.

Malignant hyperthermia, a familial disorder characterized by fever, muscle rigidity, and rhabdomyolysis associated with general anesthesia, is seen in 1 in 14,000 general anesthetic procedures. Patients with certain known neuromuscular disorders (myotonic dystrophy, myotonia congenita, central core disease) appear to have an increased risk of this complication. The management of this disorder is outlined in an earlier section.

Although small amounts of myoglobin are readily detectable in the urine in a wide variety of myopathies using sensitive immunologic techniques, it is only rarely of clinical significance (urine is not dark). Most patients with neuromuscular disease do not exert themselves sufficiently to develop rhabdomyolysis.

Once the diagnosis of rhabdomyolysis and myoglobinuria has been established, careful attention to maintaining adequate blood volume and urine flow becomes important. Hypocalcemia, probably related to hyperphosphatemia from cellular breakdown, is common early in the course of rhabdomyolysis induced renal failure. Once urine flow is reestablished, however, hypercalcemia is common. Therefore, calcium salts should be given to patients in the oliguric phase only for life-threatening complications. Hyperkalemia due to cellular breakdown and renal dysfunction is also common and may require treatment (with calcium, sodium bicarbonate, glucose-insulin infusions, resins, or dialysis) when potassium levels approach dangerous levels.

RESPIRATORY COMPLICATIONS OF NEUROMUSCULAR DISEASE (Table 10.8)[8]

Patients with neuromuscular disorders are susceptible to respiratory complications for a variety of reasons. Weakness of the diaphragm, intercostal muscles and accessory muscles of respiration compromise ventilation. These patients demonstrate a restrictive patterns on pulmonary function testing with reduced tidal volumes and total lung capacities. In addition, they show poor inspiratory and expiratory pressures (Fig. 10.9). Bulbar dysfunction results in a poor cough and increases the risk of aspiration pneumonia. Progressive scoliosis secondary to paraspinal muscle weakness may contribute to a shrinking pulmonary reserve. Furthermore, a patient with limited movement of his extremities is susceptible to deep vein thrombosis and pulmonary embolism. Finally, occasional patients with peripheral nervous system disorders have accompanying central hypoventilation syndromes. All of these complications are more frequent as the neuromuscular disease advances, but respiratory insufficiency and failure may be the initial presentation of a neuromuscular process as well.

Respiratory depression is to be expected and anticipated in every patient with acute weakness. Symptoms of respiratory distress can be mild and non-specific, and include restlessness, irritability, and confusion. Arterial blood gases and pulmonary function tests (PFTs) should be closely monitored. Supplemental oxygen should be administered and intubation performed if carbon dioxide retention or respiratory muscle exhaustion occurs. When the vital capacity falls below 50 percent of normal (predicted = 25 cc/cm of height in men; 20 cc/cm height in women) and the disorder appears to be progressing, the patient should be considered for ventilatory support. If endotracheal intubation is performed, the breathing tube requires diligent care to prevent infection or tracheal mucosal erosion. Although acute neuromuscular weakness is frequently reversible, the patient often requires prolonged ventilatory support so a tracheostomy may be preferable.

Disorders that impair breathing function often cause swallowing dysfunction as well and nasogastric feedings may be necessary to prevent aspiration and insure adequate nutrition. The integrity of the swallowing mechanism

**Table 10.8 Pulmonary Complications of
Neuromuscular Disease**

Hypoventilation from muscular weakness
Loss of effective cough
Aspiration of oral contents
Pneumonia
Scoliosis
Inadequate respiratory drives
Thromboembolic disease from inactivity

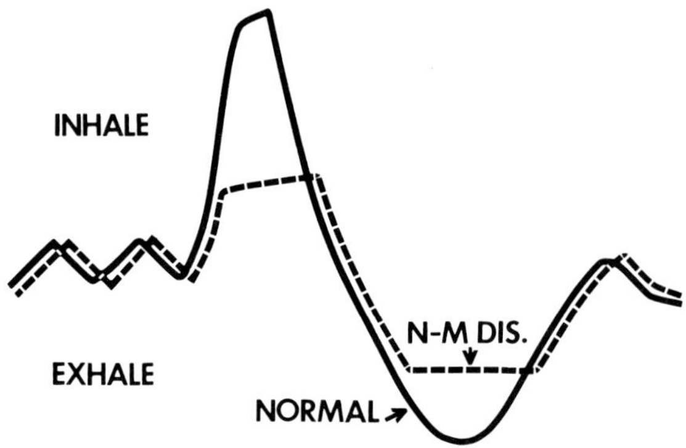

Fig. 10.9
Pulmonary Function Tests. Patients with neuromuscular disease should be closely monitored for numerous pulmonary abnormalities, which often begin insidiously yet can be life-threatening.

1. REDUCTION IN MAXIMAL INSPIRATORY AND EXPIRATORY PRESSURES

2. REDUCTION IN MAXIMAL BREATHING CAPACITY

3. REDUCTION IN VITAL CAPACITY

4. REDUCTION IN FLOW RATES, VERY LATE IN COURSE

in an intubated patient may be tested by having him swallow water colored with food dye, while suctioning through the endotracheal or tracheostomy tube.

Acute respiratory decompensation may result from disorders at every level of the neuromuscular system. Those disorders associated with profound weakness have already been described in the section on weakness. The disorders characterized by acute respiratory failure out of proportion to the amount of weakness include myotonic dystrophy, acid maltase deficiency, progressive external ophthalmoplegias and a variety of congenital and non-specific myopathies. Studies have indicated that these patients have a diminished central response to hypercarbia and/or hypoxia. That is, they may have the power to ventilate but not the reflex stimulation to do so.

Other patients with only mild neuromuscular weakness may develop acute respiratory failure due to selective or dominant diaphragmatic weakness. This condition has been noted with polio, brachial plexus neuropathies, GBS, and ALS. If diaphragmatic weakness is suspected, pulmonary functions should be obtained in both upright and supine positions, since the vital capacity will decrease considerably as the patient reclines. Phrenic pacing and curass ventilators have been used with variable success in patients with prominent diaphragm weakness.

Recurrent aspiration from chronic progressive dysphagia is a continual concern in patients with ALS, MG, oculopharyngeal dystrophy, myotonic dystrophy, adult forms of SMA and rarely with inflammatory myopathies. Chronic management of this difficult problem is detailed in the discussion of ALS. Maintaining nutrition while avoiding aspiration in a weakening patient requires constant attention and can be extremely frustrating.

Progressive scoliosis in a patient with a chronic neuromuscular disorder will further shrink already diminished respiratory reserve. A properly fitted wheelchair that maintains an erect spine and the use of a polypropylene thoracolumbar body jacket is helpful. When surgical fusion of the spine is considered, the physician must take into account the natural progression of the disease as well as the patient's level of disability. Few recommend surgery in Duchenne dystrophy, since the overall prognosis is so poor. On the other hand, patients with a static deficit (polio), or with slow progression (intermediate and juvenile onset SMAs) are better candidates for fusion. Careful attention to anesthetic complications and peri-operative respiratory therapy is critical in these patients because of their marginal respiratory reserve. In general, patients with vital capacities greater than 70 percent of normal tolerate surgery well. In patients with vital capacities below 30 percent of predicted, a period of post-operative mechanical ventilation should be anticipated.

In the patient with endstage neuromuscular disease, any further respiratory decompensation should quickly be assessed for potentially reversible causes. Infections and pulmonary emboli are treated if the quality of life is acceptable to the patient. Rarely, a patient with a severe neuromuscular disease requests mechanical ventilatory support, even if there is no prospect for future unassisted ventilation. Whenever possible, these issues should be addressed openly and honestly with the patient and his family in advance of impending respiratory failure, since momentary decisions can commit a patient and family to unanticipated suffering and expense. Assurance that the patient's comfort is of prime concern should be conveyed throughout the course of a progressive neuromuscular disease.

CARDIAC COMPLICATIONS OF NEUROMUSCULAR DISORDERS

Cardiac complications of neuromuscular disorders may be due to myocardial muscle involvement leading to impaired contractility, or to conduction system dysfunction, resulting in dysrhythmias or heart block. Cardiac dysfunction may also be due to autonomic involvement as seen in the Guillain-Barré syndrome.

Myocardial involvement is probably a constant feature in Duchenne muscular dystrophy (DUD) but is usually not detectable until the later stages. Tachyarrhthmias are common and sudden deaths have been reported, but congestive heart failure is not usual, perhaps because these boys are so limited in their activity. EKG abnormalities are seen in over two-thirds of patients. Tall R waves in the right precordial leads and deep Q waves in the left precordial and limb leads are characteristic. It has been suggested that selective myocardial muscle fibrosis of the left ventricle may account for these EKG changes. Digitalis has been used with limited success to treat the tachyarrhythmias and congestive failure in Duchenne dystrophy.

Minor EKG abnormalities have been described in other muscular dystrophies (Becker, facioscapulohumeral, limb girdle). These patients rarely have clinically significant cardiac complications except in some families with the Becker variety.

More than two-thirds of patients with myotonic muscular dystrophy (MYD) have EKG abnormalities, usually involving conduction blocks. Cardiac failure is not seen until late in the disease, but syncopal spells and cases of sudden death probably represent episodes of complete heart block. It has been our policy to carefully monitor MYD patients with yearly EKGs and to place demand pacemakers when progressive conduction defects are detected. In addition to high degree (2°, 3°) block, symptomatic sinus bradycardia may also be an indication for a pacemaker. In families where several members have documented conduction problems, His-bundle studies may be useful to diagnose preclinical disease. Certain drugs commonly used to treat the muscle myotonia (quinidine, procainamide, phenytoin) may depress cardiac conduction and should probably be avoided in patients with prolonged conduction intervals on EKG.

The heart may be involved in the inflammatory myopathies. Although EKG abnormalities, including arrhythmias and conduction disturbances have been reported in as many as half of patients, clinical symptomatology is rare. It has been suggested that the EKG changes fluctuate with the state of inflammatory activity in skeletal muscle, although autopsy studies have infrequently shown inflammatory changes in the myocardium.

Several disorders that produce progressive external ophthalmoplegia, particularly the Kearns-Sayre syndrome, have a high incidence of cardiac conduction defects. The conduction defects range from simple prolonged intraventricular conduction time through bundle branch block to complete AV block. In the Kearns-Sayre syndrome, up to 20 percent of cases have reportedly died from complete heart block. Demand pacing can be life sustaining.

EKG changes reflecting the fluctuations in serum potassium levels are common in the periodic paralyses. Rare cases of impaired cardiac contractility and rhythm disturbances have been described.

In the Guillain-Barré syndrome (GBS), autonomic dysfunction, including vasomotor instability and cardiac dysrhythmias is common. Sinus bradycardia, sinus tachycardia, paroxysmal atrial tachycardia, atrial flutter and fibrillation, ventricular tachycardia, and sinus arrest have all been noted. The time course of rhythm disturbances roughly correlates with that of neuromuscular severity. All patients with GBS should have continuous cardiac monitoring in the intensive care unit until they stabilize and begin to recover motor function.

INFECTIOUS COMPLICATIONS OF NEUROMUSCULAR DISEASES

Although pneumonia is more likely in patients with either bulbar dysfunction or respiratory muscle weakness, patients with myasthenia gravis, polymyositis, and dermatomyositis are at even greater risk because they are frequently treated with chronically administered corticosteroids or other immunosuppressive medications. Immunosuppressive therapy not only predisposes patients to infection but corticosteroids may also mask the usual signs of infection (i.e. fever, abdominal distension, etc). Common sites of infection include the urinary tract and lungs. Septicemia, peritonitis, and meningitis may also occur. Accordingly, the physician should have a high index of suspicion for subclinical infection in immunosuppressed patients who experience a sudden, unexplained deterioration. A thorough search for infection, including all appropriate cultures and radiologic investigations should be promptly undertaken.

ACKNOWLEDGEMENTS

The authors would like to thank Candace DeLapp for typing the manuscript and Julia Simon for preparing the illustrations. Our overall experience has been fostered by continuing support and encouragement from the Muscular Dystrophy Association.

REFERENCES

1. Adams, R.D., Victor, M.: Principles of Neurology, 2nd Ed. McGraw-Hill, Inc, 1981.
2. Brooke, M.H.: A Clinician's View of Neuromuscular Diseases. Baltimore, Williams and Wilkins, 1977.
3. Dubowitz, V., Brooke, M.H.: Muscle Biopsy: A Modern Approach. London, W. B. Saunders, 1973.
4. Haymaker, W., Woodhall, B.: Peripheral Nerve Injuries. Philadelphia, W. B. Saunders, 1953.
5. Johnson, E.W.: Practical Electromyography. Baltimore, Williams and Wilkins, 1980.
6. Layzer, R.B., Rowland, L.P.: Cramps. New Engl. J. Med. 285:31, 1971.
7. Mulder, D.W., ed.: The Diagnosis and Treatment of Amyotrophic Lateral Sclerosis. Boston, Houghton Mifflin, 1980.
8. Ringel, S.P., Carroll, J.E.: Respiratory Complications of Neuromuscular Disease. In Weiner, W.J., ed.: Respiratory Function in Neurologic Disease. New York, Futura, 1980.

9. Rowland, L.P., Penn, A.S.: Myoglobinuria. Med. Clin. N.A. 56:1233, 1972.
10. Vinken, P.J., Bruyn, G.W., Ringel, S.P., eds.: Diseases of Muscle, Parts I and II. Handbook of Clinical Neurology, Vols. 40 and 41, Amsterdam, North-Holland Publishing, 1979.

11
Drugs and Toxins Presenting as Neurological Disorders

John B. Sullivan, Jr., M.D.

DIAGNOSING DRUG OR POISON INDUCED NEUROLOGICAL DISORDER

The general physician may be confronted with a patient in the emergency room who has a suspected or known drug or poison ingestion presenting with a neurological syndrome. Various neurological manifestations can occur with drug intoxication and thus toxins should be considered in the differential diagnosis of a non-focal, diffuse neurological process, especially if the patient is comatose or manifests an organic brain syndrome. However, drugs or toxins do not usually present with a single well-defined syndrome. Also, drugs that are unrelated pharmacologically can produce a similar spectrum in overdose and usually do not produce focal clinical findings. Instead, the clinical spectrum of a drug overdose or poisoning usually involves multiple organ systems and the patient may present with varied and diffuse clinical manifestations.

History and physical exam usually provide some help in determining the etiology of a neurological disorder. In the case of an acute drug overdose, however, the history usually is unreliable. A patient may be unwilling to admit what was ingested in a suicide attempt, family or friends may not know what was ingested, or the patient may be comatose, too lethargic, or delerious and a factual history cannot be obtained. Conversely, concerning on chronic occupational or industrial exposures, the historical information about the workplace may be very beneficial in determining the etiology of the neurological disease. The physical examination along with clinical suspicion may be very helpful in determining whether a drug or toxin is the etiology of a neurological disorder. Also, the setting where the patient is found can provide diagnostic clues, an example being a patient found comatose in a burning room should be suspected of being poisoned with noxious gas inhalation such as carbon monoxide, hydrogen cyanide, hydrochloric acid and formaldehyde fumes. Also, more than one person may be involved if the toxin is from occupational exposure or is in a vapor, gas, or dust form.

Important points to remember when obtaining any history from or about the patient include: time of ingestion or exposure, how much was ingested, clinical status of the patient following the ingestion or exposure, any treatment rendered, and were multiple drugs involved.

Another important consideration in overdoses is that many drugs are absorbed slowly from the bowel and thus the patient's clinical status may change with time. A patient may be alert and tachycardic one minute and comatose, convulsing, and having cardiac arrhythmias the next minute. Observation of a poisoned patient is essential. Most serious overdoses can be managed with supportive cardiac and respiratory care and a few physiologic antagonist drugs.

POINTS TO CONSIDER ON PHYSICAL EXAM THAT INDICATE A DRUG OR TOXIN ETIOLOGY

1. Mental status—Lethargy, hyperalertness, confusional state, coma, delerium, or hallucinations, are often present.

2. Pupillary status—The pupils remain reactive in most drug ingestions and poisonings. However, narcotics and organophosphate insecticides will produce miotic pupils and anticholinergics may produce mydriatic pupils.

3. Myoclonus—Either spontaneous or elicited may indicate a metabolic or toxic etiology.

4. Oculomotor reflex changes—can be present or absent in drug overdoses.

5. Multiorgan system involvement—Changes in respiration, cardiac status, temperature, gastrointestinal motility, and muscle stretch reflexes.

6. Seizures—Many toxins cause both altered mental status and seizures.

SUMMARY OF PRINCIPLES FOR INITIAL CLINICAL EVALUATION

1. Drugs in different pharmacological groups may present with similar syndromes.

2. Drug overdoses or poisonings usually present a clinical syndrome that cannot be explained by a neuroanatomical lesion and involve various organ systems, not just the CNS or peripheral nerves.

3. The history is very unreliable in cases of intentional overdose and most non-intentional ingestions.

4. Drugs may have delayed action due to slow absorption or the production of a toxic metabolite. Prolonged observation is best if there is any doubt. A patient may be well at one moment and next succumb to respiratory difficulty.

5. Presentation of more than one person with a similar syndrome suggests a toxic or infectious etiology.

6. Important points to consider in the history are when did the ingestion occur, how much was ingested, has the patient received any treatment at home, what was the patient's clinical status after ingestion.

THE TOXICOLOGY LABORATORY AND CLINICAL TOXICOLOGY PHARMACOLOGY, POISON CENTER CONSULTANT

The general toxicology screen is overused and probably has very little place in managing an overdosed patient. The physician should become familiar with what the toxicology screen consists of before ordering it on a patient. Some labs are more sophisticated than others and will perform a variety of qualitative and quantitative analyses on both urine and blood. The general laboratory equipment for drug determination consists of gas-liquid chromatography, high pressure liquid chromatography, thin layer chromatography, and enzyme mediated immunological techniques. All of these systems have limitations. The sensitivity and specificity of the laboratory analysis is very important. An assay must not only be able to determine the difference between certain drugs and be able to specifically identify these drugs (specificity) without interference from other drugs but must be able to detect these drugs at certain low concentrations to make the assay valuable (sensitivity). A drug screen for a tricyclic antidepressant such as amitriptyline (Elavil) would not be useful if its sensitivity was very high and phenothiazines and antihistamines interfered with its detection.

Qualitative assays are as useful as quantitative assays in most cases. It is more important to know that the drug is present in a patient than to have an idea of the quantity present in the patient's plasma since most drug overdoses are managed according to the clinical status of the patient and not according to the drug plasma level. There are, though, some specific drugs where the plasma levels are very important to the care of the patient and will directly influence the treatment. These drugs are: salicylates, acetaminophen, theophylline, methanol, ethylene glycol, ethanol, phenobarbital, and phenytoin.

The physician should also know what specimens the lab requires to perform the drug screen—urine or blood. Some laboratories will do both acidic extraction and alkaline extraction of the submitted specimen in performing the assay; different drugs are detected in these two different procedures.

A medically sound approach to ordering laboratory drug screens would be for the physician to attempt to determine the class of drugs or toxins involved by history and physical examination and then order the appropriate laboratory screen to confirm the clinical suspicion. The physician should give the laboratory personnel an idea of what drug is suspected because this will enable a more thorough analysis for the particular drug or toxin. There is no good reason to save vomitus obtained from the patient for the laboratory. Almost all drugs can be assayed in urine or plasma. The only reason to save some gastric contents would be to detect phencyclidine (PCP) or ketamine if the plasma and urine analyses are negative and these drugs are suspected.

Heavy metal screens are usually performed on urine or blood depending on the metal. The physician should check with the lab performing metal analyses in order to assure that the specimen is properly collected in an appropriate container (such as a 24-hour urine specimen in a dilute nitric acid washed container) and labelled with the collection period.

Unless the physician practices in a major urban area or medical center the chance of having available clinical toxicology-pharmacology consultants is small. However, most areas of the United States and Canada are served by poison control centers that are able to consult with the physician by phone in an effort to provide up-to-date management information concerning drug overdoses and other poisonings. These poison centers serve both metropolitan and rural areas and usually have a medical director familiar with poison management and clinical pharmacology. The poison center number should be placed on the telephones in the emergency room and intensive care units.

SUMMARY OF PRINCIPLES FOR LABORATORY EVALUATION

1. Know what kind of drug screens your hospital can provide, what their limitations are, and what kind of specimens the laboratory requires.

2. Qualitative assays may be as helpful as quantitative assays.

3. For some drugs and toxins the quantitative analysis directly affects patient treatment: salicylates, acetaminophen, theophylline, methanol, ethylene glycol, ethanol, phenobarbital, and phenytoin.

4. Post your local or regional poison control center telephone number in your office, emergency room, and intensive care unit.

SEIZURES, COMA, REFLEX CHANGES

The clinician caring for a comatose patient with seizures and reflex changes should consider a drug overdose in the etiology of this syndrome. The most common drugs to consider are the tricyclic antidepressants, over-the-counter sympathomimetics, anticonvulsants, and phenothiazines. However, many other drugs and poisons can produce this syndrome. The physical examination and history of the ingestion can result in a drug differential. An electrocardiogram is often helpful along with other basic laboratory studies.

The common drug differential associated with the syndrome of seizures, altered consciousness, and reflex changes includes tricyclic antidepressants, phenothiazines, theophylline, caffeine, anticholinergics in both prescribed drugs and over-the-counter drugs, cocaine, amphetamines, carbamazepine (tegretol), phenytoin (dilantin), arsenic, strychnine, methaqualone, phencyclidine, narcotics, especially propoxyphene and meperidine, organophosphates, fluoracetate, clonidine, chronic lead toxicity, and lithium. Many of these drugs and toxins will be associated with other clinical toxicity such as cardiac dysrhythmias and acute agitation. Theophylline and caffeine in overdose can produce delerium, acute agitation, hyperreflexia, ventricular ectopy, and gastrointestinal bleeding. Tricyclic antidepressants include such drugs as amitriptyline (Elavil), doxepin (Sinequan), desipramine (Norpramine) and combinations of amitriptyline and a phenothiazine (Triavil). The tricyclic drugs are well known for producing coma, seizures, and cardiac dysrhythmias in overdose as well as hyperreflexia. Arsenic ingestion is associated with acute gastrointestinal irritation, seizures, and cardiac dysrhythmias as well as coma.[5,6]

The anticonvulsants phenytoin (Dilantin), carbamazepine (Tegretol), valproic acid (Depakene), and phenobarbital all produce altered states of consciousness in overdose. Phenytoin can produce nystagmus, nausea and vomiting, tremor, ataxia, coma, and seizures in overdose along with acute agitation, decerebrate rigidity, and some focal neurological signs such as hemiparesis.[12] Carbamazepine in overdose may result in coma, seizures, nystagmus, hyperreflexia, and EKG abnormalities with QRS prolongation.[15] Valporic acid overdoses result in lethargy and coma.[4] Phenobarbital in overdose is associated with coma and hyporeflexia but also can cause hypertonicity and hyperreflexia. Included in drugs of abuse should be methaqualone (Quaaludes) which can produce coma, hyperreflexia and seizures in overdose; phencyclidine which may produce coma, seizures, hyperreflexia, myoclonic activity, hypertension and tachycardia; and amphetamines and cocaine which can produce seizures, coma, and cardiac dysrhythmias.[8,10]

MOVEMENT DISORDERS

Movement disorders can occur with a variety of toxic ingestions and therapeutic doses of some drugs. Choreoathetosis, myoclonus, and orofacial dyskinesia can occur at therapeutic and toxic phenytoin levels.[12] Phenytoin is also associated with ataxia and nystagmus. Phenothiazines and butyrophenones (especially Haldol) are especially well known to cause dystonic reactions and oculogyric crises. Tricyclic antidepressants in overdose have been associated with myoclonus and choreoathetoid movements.[3] Lithium toxicity can result in tremors and heavy metals causing chronic poisoning (lead, mercury and arsenic) can cause ataxia, tremors, and peripheral neuropathy.[14] Carbamazepine (Tegretol) may cause nystagmus, ataxia, and myoclonus. Phenobarbital overdose can also produce myoclonus. Carbon monoxide induced demyelination and basal ganglia damage can produce incoordination and parkinsonism.[7,16]

METABOLIC CHANGES

Some poisons and drugs in addition to producing an altered state of consciousness along with other symptoms will result in a profound metabolic acidosis. The physician should be aware of a small number of drugs and toxins which produce a metabolic acidosis. These drugs and poisons may also result in coma and seizures in overdose. Salicylates, methanol, ethylene glycol, isoniazid, iron, ethanol, and paraldehyde may all produce a metabolic acidosis with a large anion gap. Salicylates, methanol, and ethylene glycol are the toxins usually involved. These three can produce seizures, confusional states, and coma. Isoniazid is usually associated with intense seizure activity in overdose as well as a profound metabolic acidosis. Toluene inhalation on a chronic basis may result in a renal tubular acidosis and an organic brain syndrome. The complications of coma include aspiration pneumonia and pressure neurosis involving skeletal muscles and cutaneous tissues which can result in rhabdomyolysis and myoglobinuria with the possibility of myoglobinuric renal failure. Rhabdomyolysis can also occur with intense seizure activity and myoclonus.

BEHAVIORAL DISORDERS, ORGANIC BRAIN SYNDROME, CONFUSIONAL STATES, DELERIUM

Drugs and other toxins are common causes of both acute and chronic organic brain syndromes, psychosis, delerium and hallucinations, confusional states, other behavioral and perceptional disorders. The most commonly involved drug in these cases is ethanol. Acute ethanol intoxication can be associated with slowed mentation and stupor or with hyperexcitable states, confusion, and violent behavior. Ethanol withdrawal following chronic abuse produces a syndrome of tremulousness, agitation, anxiety, hallucinations, delerium, and other autonomic nervous system manifestations (delerium tremens). Sedative-hypnotic withdrawal, such as from barbiturates or benzodiazepines, can produce a similar clinical picture.

Caffeine and theophylline toxicity can result in agitation, confusion, and delerium. These two drugs should be considered in a patient who is delerious, tachycardic, and hyperreflexic, who has experienced seizures and has GI bleeding. Caffeine is common in over-the-counter preparations for dieting and in "cold medicine."

Other over-the-counter (OTC) agents can result in an acute organic brain syndrome following overdose.[13] Most of these OTC drugs contain anti-histamines such as methapyrilene and pyrilamine and some contain scopolamine. Cimetidine (Tagamet), propranolol (Inderal), and metoprolol (Lopressor) can produce a confusional state in therapeutic doses, usually occurring upon the institution of therapy.

Phencyclidine (PCP, angel dust) and ketamine are similar anesthetic agents which can produce toxic psychosis, paranoia, and violent rage states with abuse. Phencyclidine intoxication can also result in seizures, hyperreflexia, tachycardia, hypertension, myoclonus, and nystagmus.[1] Due to the cutaneous anesthesia produced by both phencyclidine and ketamine, some patients may suffer a great deal of trauma without feeling pain. This trauma may also be self-inflicted.

Cocaine and amphetamine chronic abuse may result in a toxic psychosis, depression, hallucinatory activity, paranoia, perceptual difficulties, emotional lability, and extreme irritability.[8,10]

Phenytoin in both therapeutic and toxic plasma levels is associated with confusional states. Phenytoin plasma levels around 20 μg/ml (therapeutic 10–20 μg/ml) may cause drowsiness and decreased mental alertness. Phenytoin in overdose may cause acute agitation, delerium, hallucinations and combativeness.

Lithium toxicity (levels greater than 2 mEq/L) may result in an organic brain syndrome with delerium, agitation, and seizures.

Anticholinergic drugs such as tricyclic antidepressants and phenothiazines can result in delerium and hallucinations in overdose.[3]

Chronic heavy metal poisoning with mercury in both the organic and inorganic form, arsenic, and lead can produce an organic brain syndrome, psychosis, and behavioral disturbances.[9]

Carbon monoxide poisoning will result in acute confusion and disorientation. Damage to the basal ganglia along with demyelination of white matter can produce behavioral and motor disturbances.

Vapors of glue which include toluene may result in a chronic organic brain syndrome, ataxia and spasticity.

PARESTHESIA, MUSCLE WEAKNESS, PARALYSIS, NEUROPATHY

These neurological problems, when attributed to toxins, are usually due to heavy metals, organic solvents, organophosphate pesticides, or other hydrocarbon chemicals. The symptoms resulting from these toxins may be vague and include neuropsychiatric signs and symptoms such as headache, irritability, insomnia, memory difficulties, and in some cases, psychosis. It is sometimes difficult to make a diagnosis of hydrocarbon induced neuropathy because chronic exposure over several years' duration is usually required before symptomatology becomes obvious. Also, most of the exposures to these toxins is in industrial and work-place settings and other sources of neuropathy, such as trauma, can exist.

Organophosphate insecticides are widely employed in commercial and non-agricultural settings. These insecticides come as liquids and solids and have the common names of malathion, parathion, diazinon, disyston.[11] Organophosphate insecticides are found in hardware stores, supermarkets, and garden shops and they are commonly mixed with fertilizers. Another group of insecticides which has similar toxicity to organophosphates is the carbamates. This group is represented by the frequently used chemical Sevin and comes as a liquid or solid.

Both the organophosphates and carbamates interfere with acetylcholinesterase enzyme activity by binding to the enzyme. This binding inactivates the enzyme and allows acetylcholine to accumulate at parasympathetic nerve endings. The early signs and symptoms of poisoning from these agents are feelings of weakness, shortness of breath, abdominal cramping, vomiting, and diarrhea. Progression to increased salivation, muscle fasciculations, increased tracheobronchial secretions with pulmonary edema, miotic pupils, and bradycardia occur depending on the severity of toxicity. Coma, seizures, and cardiorespiratory arrest occur in severe cases.

Poisoning with organophosphate and carbamates may be acute or chronic. Acute toxicity overwhelms the acetylcholinesterase enzyme system in the body and allows initial receptor site stimulation by acetylcholine with eventual exhaustion of the receptors. The onset is usually rapid and if not treated early with atropine, the illness may be fatal. Chronic exposure to these insecticides may slowly deplete acetylcholinesterase and produce insidious symptomatology such as weakness, fatigue, insomnia, headache, and irritability. A person who has chronic acetylcholinesterase depletion may precipitate an overwhelming acute intoxication from further exposure to the insecticides and is at risk from amounts that would produce only mild or moderate toxicity in persons not chronically exposed.

Organophosphate symptomatology is divided into muscarinic and nicotinic signs. Muscarinic effects are salivation, diarrhea, vomiting, miosis, bradycardia, increased tracheobronchial secretions, and pulmonary edema. Nicotinic effects are muscle fasciculations and skeletal muscle paralysis. Atropine will reverse only the muscarinic effects by blocking muscarinic receptor sites where acetylcholine acts but will not block nicotinic receptor sites. Thus a patient who is adequately treated with atropine with reversal of muscarinic symptomatology may still suffer muscular weakness, skeletal muscle paralysis, and respiratory arrest. Another antidote, 2-PAM chloride (Protopam) is needed to reverse the nicotinic effects. Both atropine and 2-PAM should be employed in moderate to severe organophosphate poisoning. Massive doses of intravenous atropine are usually required early in the course of toxicity. One to two grams have been used over a 12 to 24 hour period.

Occasionally, organophosphates will produce mainly nicotinic symptomatology following exposure and the patient may have a perplexing muscular weakness and paralysis and normal CSF. Usually the exposure is insidious and there may be no history of organophosphate exposure at all. These patients are sometimes diagnosed as Guillan-Barré syndrome or ascending paralysis from an unknown cause. Clinical suspicion must exist to make the diagnosis. Organophosphate and carbamate toxicity can present as various other syndromes also: gastroenteritis, cerebrovascular accident with miotic pupils, hyperglycemic coma, or neuropsychiatric syndrome. Following a severe poisoning, it is not uncommon to have neurological and psychiatric sequela with feelings of depression, insomnia, vague somatic complaints, peripheral neuropathies, and personality disorders.

Heavy metal poisoning, especially chronic, is a well-known cause of peripheral neuropathies, psychiatric disorders, and central nervous system disturbances.[6,9] The most commonly involved heavy metals in poisonings are mercury, lead, and arsenic. The metals may be in their elemental state, as inorganic compounds such as mercuric chloride, arsenic trioxide, and lead oxide, or in organic combinations like methyl mercury, ethyl mercury or tetraethyl lead, as in gasoline.

Mercury poisoning can produce neurological disturbances in both acute and chronic poisoning. Elemental mercury is a vapor at room temperature and is well-absorbed through the respiratory tract. It can cause acute pneumonitis with pulmonary infiltrates, coma, seizures, tremors, peripheral neuropathies, and long-ranged psychiatric sequelae. The alkyl mercury compounds especially methyl mercury and ethyl mercury target the central nervous system for their toxicity and result in parasthesias, incoordination, coma, mental confusion, tremors, and neuropsychiatric problems. These alkyl mercury compounds are used as fungicidal agents. Acute inorganic mercury poisoning usually produces gastrointestinal disturbance as a first sign. Mercuric chloride ingestion can cause bloody vomiting and diarrhea with perforation of the intestines, renal failure, seizures, and coma.

Lead toxicity is always chronic. Inorganic lead found in old paints, car radiators and batteries, or in industrial settings is usually the source. Lead toxicity may present in both adults and children very insidiously following years of slow accumulation in bone and other tissues. Gastrointestinal upset with vague abdominal complaints is common. Sensory disorders of parasthesia, hyperasthesia, analgesia can occur. Anemia is usually present. Lead neuropathy tends to effect the extensor muscles most often. Encephalopathy can occur suddenly and has a poor prognosis.

Tetraethyl lead is the organic form seen in toxicity from gasoline vapor sniffing abuse. This results in a chronic syndrome of cerebellar signs, hallucinations, coma, agitation, personality changes, and peripheral neuropathies which are usually permanent.

Chronic arsenic poisoning may result in various neurologic disturbances ranging from coma to peripheral neuropathies. Hematologic changes may be present with anemia or leukemoid reactions. Acute arsenic toxicity may produce the same neurological syndrome but also includes severe gastrointestinal upset, coma, seizures, cardiac arrhythmias, and acute renal failure.

Other uncommonly encountered metals which produce central nervous system disturbances are thallium selenium and manganese. Thallium is especially interesting because it is employed as a rodenticide in many foreign countries but its use is no longer allowed in the United States. Thallium poisoning can cause hair loss, coma, cataracts, paralysis and peripheral neuropathy.

Treatment of the heavy metal poisonings is with chelators such as dimercaprol (BAL), calcium disodium EDTA, and d-penicillamine.[5]

Carbon monoxide poisoning can cause coma, seizures, and neurological damage through effects on cytochrome oxidase enzyme systems. Demyelination of white matter and anoxic damage to the basal ganglia occur resulting in parkinsonism, weakness, incoordination, ataxia, behavioral disturbances, and confusion.[16]

Isoniazid (INH) chronic administration can deplete pyridoxine[86] and result in peripheral neuropathies that are reversible by administration of the vitamin.

Chronic ethanol abuse may produce peripheral neuropathy through thiamine depletion. Carbon disulfide is an industrial solvent used in rubber and rayon industries. It produces tremor, polyneuritis, psychosis, lower extremity weakness, and paresthesias with chronic exposure. Extrapyramidal signs can also occur along with choreathetoid disorders following exposure to carbon disulfide.

The solvents n-hexane and n-butyl-ketone are metabolized to 2,5-hexanedione. Industrial workers chronically exposed to these solvents can develop peripheral neuropathies, cerebellar signs, and muscle weakness.[5]

Triorthocresyl phosphate (TOCP), cresyldiphenyl phosphate, and ortho-isoprophenyldiphenyl phosphate can produce neuromuscular paralysis.

Chlorinated hydrocarbon pesticides such as DDT, chlordane, endrin, and lindane may cause seizures, and tremors. 2,4-D (2,4-dichlorophenoxyacetic acid) and 2,4,5-T (2,4,5-trichlorophenoxyacetic acid) are chlorinated biphenyl herbicides that can produce intense tremors, polyneuritis, and muscular weakness following acute ingestion.[5] Table 11.1 lists common neurologic syndromes and the toxins that cause them.

Table 11.1 Drug and Toxins Causing Particular Neurologic Syndromes

Movement Disorders	Coma, Seizures, Reflex Changes	Confusion, Delerium, Behavioral Disorder, Organic Brain Syndrome	Metabolic Acidosis, Coma, Seizures	Muscle Weakness, Paralysis, Neuropathy, Paresthesias
Tricyclic anti-depressants	Tricyclic anti-depressants	Ethanol	Ethanol	Organophosphates
Phenothiazines	Phenothiazines	Phencyclidine	Methanol	Isoniazid
Butyrophenones	Lithium	Ketamine	Ethylene glycol	Ethanol-chronic
Carbamazepine	Theophylline	Phenytoin	Salicylates	Methyl mercury
Phenytoin	Caffeine	Amphetamines	Isoniazid	Tetraethyl lead
Chronic lead, mercury poisoning	Carbamazepine	Cocaine	Iron	Elemental mercury
Tetraethyl lead	Phenytoin	Sedative-hypnotic withdrawal	Toluene	Arsenic
Methyl mercury	Methaqualone	Ethanol withdrawal		Carbon disulfide
Inorganic lead	Phencyclidine	Caffeine		Butyl-ketone
Carbon monoxide	Narcotics	Theophylline		Hexane
Phenobarbital	Organophosphates	Antihistamines		2,4-D and 2,4,5-T
	Sodium monofluoracetate	Tricyclic antidepressants		TOCP
	Clonidine	Cimetidine		
	Arsenic-acute	Propranolol		
	Lead-chronic	Metoprolol		
	Cocaine	Lithium		
	Amphetamines	Chronic heavy metal poisoning		
	Valproic acid	Carbon monoxide		
		Cyanide		

BASIC PRINCIPLES OF MANAGEMENT

Management of any drug or poison ingestion is based primarily on the patient's clinical condition. Securing an airway is always a first priority, along with cardiovascular support. An intravenous line can be placed for administration of drugs as necessary. Any comatose patient where the etiology of the altered state of consciousness is not apparent should receive oxygen, a 50 cc, 50 percent dextrose in water IV bolus, and naloxone (Narcan) 0.8 mg (2 ampules) intravenously.

The initial evaluation of the poisoned patient in the emergency department must determine if the patient's life is in immediate danger and if there are associated illnesses or trauma. Pupillary status, level of consciousness, present or absence of bowel sounds, reflex status, presence or absence of myoclonus or seizures, vital signs and a rectal temperature should all be noted on the patient's chart. Subsequent evaluations should note changes in any of these parameters. A drug may be slowly absorbed from the small bowel and a patient's clinical condition can deteriorate rapidly so repeat examinations are as important as any treatment modality.

Associated illnesses and injuries may be missed if not considered. Absence of bowel sounds may indicate peritonitis or bowel obstruction. Patients who have ingested narcotics and anti-cholinergics are likely to have diminished or absent bowel sounds; however, absence of bowel sounds in a patient who has ingested a caustic like Drano, a heavy metal (zinc chloride, mercuric chloride) may indicate small bowel perforation.

A patient in shock following a suspected drug overdose should be resuscitated initially with intravenous crystalloids (normal saline or Ringer's Lactate). Hypotension secondary to a drug or poison ingestion may have various etiologies: [2]

1. Peripheral vascular pooling of blood due to vasodilation.

2. Myocardial depression through effects on contractility, stroke volume, heart rate and peripheral resistance.

3. Direct vascular endothelial effect with capillary endothelial leakage.

4. Direct effects on the GI tract causing volume loss.

If large volumes of intravenous fluid are being required to maintain adequate or low blood pressure then addition of a vasopressor such as dopamine (Intropin) or norepinephrine (Levophed) should be considered.

Cardiac monitoring should be instituted if necessary and a routine electrocardiogram obtained and checked for any abnormalities of the PR, QRS, or QT intervals which could occur with drugs such as tricyclic antidepressants, carbamazepine (Tegretol), or phenothiazines. Phenothiazines, tricyclic antidepressants, and chloral hydrate are also associated with ventricular ectopy.

The use of physiologic antagonists (antidotes) may be applicable in some cases. The commonly employed physiologic antagonists are:

1. Naloxone—Useful for narcotic overdoses and reverses CNS and respiratory depression. To reverse the effect of some narcotics such as propoxyphene (Darvon) and methadone, a large intravenous bolus of 2–4 mg (5–10 ampules) may be necessary. Naloxone is a pure antagonist and does not cause respiratory depression. Doses can be repeated as often as needed. Naloxone can be given intramuscularly, subcutaneously, or down an endotraceal tube if necessary.

2. Oxygen—Specifically used for carbon monoxide poisoning. One hundred percent O_2 will reduce the half-life of carboxyhemoglobin from 6 hours in room air to 30–60 minutes.

3. Cyanide Kit—(Lilly Co.) Contains amyl nitrite, sodium nitrite and sodium thiosulfate. Since hemoglobin in the oxidized state has a high affinity for cyanide, the production of methemoglobin by amyl and sodium nitrite aids in protecting the respiratory enzyme systems. The cyanmethemoglobin is detoxified by endogenous hepatic thiosulfate. Extra thiosulfate is included in the kit. The sodium nitrite is given first intravenously followed a few minutes later by the thiosulfate. The amyl nitrite is an inhalant to be used until the sodium nitrite is administered.

4. Atropine—Reverses the muscarinic (cholinergic) effects of organophosphate insecticides. Large doses may be needed intravenously to reverse the pulmonary edema and other effects of these insecticides. As much as 2 grams has been administered over a 24-hour period. Pralidoxime administration complements the action of atropine and should be given in all moderate to severe toxicities as early as possible. 2-PAM can be repeated every 6–8 hours as needed.

5. Methylene Blue—A non-enzymatic catalyst used to treat life-threatening methemoglobinemia induced by nitrites, nitrates, and other nitro containing compounds. Methylene blue is supplied as a 1 percent solution and is given intravenously to increase the activity of methemoglobin reductase enzymes.

Further management decisions include the use of gastric lavage or induced emesis with syrup of ipecac to help remove drug from the stomach and prevent further absorption. Inducement of emesis is contraindicated in a comatose patient, in the presence of seizures, in a patient who is semicomatose and who has no gag reflex, and in a patient who has ingested a caustic substance. The removal of drug or toxin already absorbed can be facilitated in some specific, limited cases by diuresis, hemodialysis, or hemoperfusion techniques. Consultation with a poison center or clinical toxicology consultant can be of benefit in determining which method may be useful.

SUMMARY OF MANAGEMENT PRINCIPLES

1. Airway support and maintenance.

2. Cardiovascular support and IV line.

3. Oxygen, glucose, naloxone for comatose patient.

4. Frequent vital signs check.

5. Check level of consciousness, pupillary status, reflexes, listen for bowel sounds, check for myoclonus.

6. Appropriate basic studies along with electrocardiogram.

7. Consider gastric lavage or emesis to remove drug remaining in the stomach.

8. Consider the use of a physiologic antagonist.

9. Hemodialysis, hemoperfusion, or diuresis may be useful in some specific instances.

REFERENCES

1. Aronow, R., Done, A.: Phencyclidine overdose: an emerging concept of management. JACEP, 7(2):56, 1978.
2. Benowitz, N., Rosenberg, J., Becker, C.: Cardiopulmonary catastrophes in drug overdose patients. Med. Clin. N. Am., 63(1):267, 1979.
3. Biggs, J., Spiker, D., Petit, J.: Tricyclic antidepressant overdoses—incidence of symptoms. JAMA, 238(2):135, 1977.
4. Browne, T.: Valproic acid. N. Engl. J. Med., 302(12):661, 1980.
5. Casarett & Doull, J.: The basic science of poisons. 2nd Ed. In Doull, J., Klaassen, C., Amdur, M., eds.: Toxicology. MacMillan Publishing Co., Inc., New York, 1975.
6. Chisolm, J.: Poisoning from heavy metals (mercury, lead, and cadmium). Pediatr. Ann., 9(12):28, 1980.
7. Garland, H., Pearce, J.: Neurological complications of carbon monoxide poisoning. Q. J. Med., 36(144):445, 1967.
8. Gay, G., Inaba, D., Sheppard, C.: Cocaine history, epidemiology, human pharmacology and treatment. Clin. Toxicol., 8(2):149, 1975.
9. Gerstner, H., Huff, J.: Selected case histories and epidemiologic examples of human mercury poisoning. Clin. Toxicol., 11(2):131, 1977.
10. Hart, J., Wallace, J.: The adverse effects of amphetamines. Clin. Toxicol., 8(2):179, 1975.
11. Hayes, W.: Toxicology of pesticides. In Hayes, W., ed.: Toxicology of Pesticides. William and Wilkins, Baltimore, 1975.
12. Mclellan, D., Swash, M.: Choreoathetosis and encephalopathy induced by phenytoin. Br. Med. J., 2:204, 1974.
13. Rumack, B., Peterson, R.: Poisoning. Ch. 30. In Kempe, C., Silver, H., O'Brien,

D., eds.: Current Pediatric Diagnosis and Treatment. Lange Medical Publications, Los Altos, 1980.
14. Saran, B., Gaind, R.: Lithium. Clin. Toxicol., 6(2):257, 1973.
15. Sullivan, J., Peterson, R., Rumack, B.: Acute carbamazepine toxicity resulting from overdose. Neurology, 31:621, 1981.
16. Winter, P., Miller, J.: Carbon monoxide poisoning. JAMA, 236(13):1502, 1976.

12

Acute Disorders of the Content of Consciousness

Bruce T. Volpe, M.D.
John J. Sidtis, Ph.D.

An acute change in mental status, a change in the content of consciousness, represents a disruption in the physiology of the brain. Since many of the disorders are reversible, rapid diagnosis is imperative (Table 12.1). Concepts that apply to general neurologic problems also apply to the diseases that cause acute changes in mental status. Thus cognitive disturbances result from physiologic injury that is either focal, multifocal, or diffuse.

For purposes of clinical analysis, this chapter details the symptoms and differential diagnosis of typical clinical disorders of orientation, language, and memory. It also includes an analysis of the hemi-inattention syndromes, the apraxias, and the global cognitive decline of the dementias. The discussion of each disorder includes additions to the standard clinical evaluation.

ORIENTATION DISORDERS

The mental status exam, the examination of the content of consciousness, begins with the assessment of the patient's orientation. If the patient is disoriented in time and space, then statements about memory and general

Table 12.1 Reversible Neurologic Disease Presenting as Acute Disorders of Content of Consciousness

---

I. Structural (Focal or multifocal):
    A. Subdural hematoma: global disorientation, with or without focal sensory motor signs
    B. Acute hydrocephalus: disorientation, memory loss, gait abnormalities
II. Metabolic (Major symptoms are global disorientation):
    A. Toxic drug or poison ingestion; drug withdrawal
    B. Sepsis
    C. Disorder of nutrients: O_2, glucose
    D. Disorder of electrolytes: Na, H_2O, Mg, Ca
    E. Seizures, partial complex: may have memory loss, aphasia, with or without focal sensory motor deficits

---

knowledge must be made with caution. A patient should be oriented in space and time; that is, know the date, month, and year, and know his present location. A patient should have the ability to concentrate on a given set of stimuli and not be distracted by other simultaneous stimuli. A patient should have the ability to sustain that concentration for at least 30 seconds.

The Symptoms Of Orientation Disorders

Confusional States

The patient may appear to have a psychiatric disorder, yet a reversible medical or neurological illness is often the cause of the disorder. Global orientation disorders (confusional states) occur in 5–10 percent of hospitalized medical or surgical patients, and the prevalence increases to 40 percent when geriatric patients are considered.[10]

Patients with global orientation disorders are awake but easily distracted, and often startled by extraneous occurrences in the environment. Patients with a mild disorder may not be grossly disoriented in time and space. If they are slightly disoriented, then their judgments of time (the day, month, year or season) will usually be disordered before their judgment of where they are. Patients with mild orientation disorders do not perceive, remember, or think with accustomed speed and clarity. This may also be exhibited by word finding difficulty, problems remembering names or recent events, lapses in performing ordinary tasks, and perceptual errors like mistaking the physician for an old friend. They cannot sustain attention on a single task for more than 30 seconds. For example, they cannot concentrate on the questions they are asked because they are distracted by the routine activity of the emergency ward or the hospital room. Their concentration wanders and they may have to be reminded repeatedly of the task or question at hand. They may repeat themselves over and over again. They may fall asleep, although they can be coaxed to respond by verbal questioning.

Delirious States

More severe disorders of orientation have been termed "delirium." Prominent symptoms of delirium include any or all of the symptoms described for the confusional states, with the addition of perceptual disorders like illusions and hallucinations. Visual hallucinations can be particularly vivid and complex. Confusional or delirious syndromes are not stable, and lucid periods may appear. The fluctuations, particularly early in the onset of symptoms, may increase during the evening. Confusion or delirium may be a manifestation of a disease process that may cause a progressive decline in the level of consciousness and coma.

The clinician needs to recognize two forms of delirium. The first is marked by the gradual reduction of alertness, withdrawal, muteness, and then a transition into lethargy, stupor, then coma. While the causes are several the clinician must be wary of reversible disease (Table 12.1). Subdurals or masses with increased intracranial pressure are common causes of withdrawal delirium. Uremia, pulmonary disease, and anoxia also produce withdrawal delirium.

The second form of delirium is marked by increasing excitement, hyperactivity, restlessness, and uninterrupted flow of incoherent speech, and then rapid transition to a withdrawn state. The prototypical metabolic etiology for hyperactive followed by hypoactive delirium is alcohol withdrawal—delirium tremens. Barbiturate withdrawal, acute liver necrosis and porphyria also cause an agitated delirium.

An example of a patient with an unusual toxic reaction to digitalis illustrates that the visual hallucinations can be complex and formed:

> A 66-year-old man was brought to the hospital because of confusion and disorientation. Two days before admission he experienced the appearance of friends who wore unusually bright colored clothes. The "friends" were not present, and represented a formed visual hallucination. The hallucinations appeared in all areas of the visual field. A month before, his digoxin dose had been increased to 0.375 mg twice daily to control congestive heart failure secondary to rheumatic heart disease. He also took furosemide and potassium supplement. Although he was actively hallucinating and, at times, disoriented, he was easily calmed and had no other neurologic deficit. Admission serum digoxin level was 6.5 ng/ml. The drug was withdrawn, and his hallucinations ceased when his serum digoxin level fell to 2.0 ng/ml.

The Differential Diagnosis Of Orientation Disorders

Global disorders of orientation demand consideration of a broad range of possibilities. The acute confusional/delirious state may signal a neurologic emergency. The most frequent causes of the confusional/delirious state include: toxic reaction to drugs, withdrawal from drugs, metabolic imbalance (particularly O_2 or glucose abnormalities), sepsis, or increased intracranial pressure. The many multifocal and diffuse (metabolic) causes of delirium are presented in Table 12.2.

The beginning of this section discussed the general features of global disorders of orientation and Table 12.2 enumerates the causes that must be considered. Other chapters in this book detail the orderly approach to the differential diagnosis of drug intoxication, metabolic imbalance infection, and intracranial space occupying lesions. Further discussion of the differential diagnosis of disoriented attention will focus on disorders of unknown cause: post-op and ICU delirium, and the psychiatric disorders of acute schizophrenic psychosis, affective disorder and conversion reactions.

Table 12.2 Multifocal and Diffuse Causes of Delirium

I. Drug intoxication or poison ingestion
  A. Alcohol, methanol, ethylene glycol, paraldehyde
  B. Sedatives: barbiturates, non-barbiturate hypnotics, tranquilizers, bromides, opiates
  C. Psychotropics: anticholinergics, tricyclics, lithium, LSD, mescaline, MAO inhibitors, amphetamines
  D. Other therapeutic drugs: penicillin, propranolol, digitalis, steroids, salicylates, cimetidene, L-DOPA
  E. Industrial poisons: carbon disulfide, organic phosphates, heavy metals, cyanide, insecticides, carbon monoxide
  F. Plants/mushrooms

II. Metabolic imbalance
  A. Hypoxia; decreased pO_2 and O_2 content, or poisoning with CO or CO_2.
  B. Ischemia; decreased blood supply
  C. Hypoglycemia/hyperglycemia
  D. Encephalopathy from failure of:
    1. Liver
    2. Kidneys (uremia)
    3. Lungs
    4. Pancreas (diabetes)
    5. Endocrine system
      a. Hyper/hypothyroid
      b. Addisons disease or Cushings syndrome
      c. Hypopituitarism
      d. Hypo/hyperparathyroidism
    6. Metabolic pathways (porphyria)
  E. Disorders of fluids/electrolytes
    1. H_2O, Na, Ca, Mg, PO_4 too high or too low
    2. Acidosis/alkalosis
  F. Nutritional
    1. B_{12} deficiency
    2. Niacin deficiency
    3. Pyridoxine deficiency
    4. Folic acid deficiency

III. Infections/Inflammation
  A. Systemic with fever
  B. Neurosyphilis (general paresis)
  C. Intracranial
    1. Meningitis
    2. Encephalitis
    3. Abscess
    4. Cerebral vasculitis

IV. Intracranial space-occupying lesions
  A. Tumor (especially frontal lobe)
  B. Subdural hematoma
  C. Hydrocephalus

V. Primary neuronal disorders
  A. Alzheimer's disease
  B. Pick's disease
  C. Huntington's disease

VI. Disorders of unknown cause
  A. "Post-op" or "ICU" delirium
  B. Thought disorders (acute schizophrenia)
  C. Affective disorders (manic-depressive illness)
  D. Factitious disorders: malingering
  E. Hysterical personality: dissociative and conversion reactions

Post-op and ICU Delirium

Post-operative delirium has been reported to occur in less than 1 percent of operated patients, but this low incidence may reflect a bias to evaluate extensively only the most florid delirious states. There are several medical complications which may contribute to post-op delirium. They are infection, hemorrhage with anemia, azotemia, or cardiac failure. Patients older than 60, or those with a history of alcoholism or acutely undergoing drug withdrawal frequently experience post-op delirium. Patients who have had open-heart surgery or orthopedic surgery have a somewhat greater chance of suffering post-op delirium.

Some studies have suggested that sensory deprivation of windowless ICUs with incessant irritating hums or beeps contribute to this delirium. The stimulation of clocks, calendars, and newspapers may help mildly confused patients re-orient. However, the clinician must be wary of metabolic or infectious causes of delirium, particularly when the delirium is persistent without lucid periods, or is continuous longer than a few days, or shows signs of progressing to stupor or coma.

The clinical picture for post-op or ICU delirium includes easy distractability, disorientation particularly for time, less often for space, poor perceptual processing, and slowed thinking. Many patients have insomnia. The patient may be quite agitated and actively hallucinating. Although these conditions are usually self-limited and resolve within a week, it must be emphasized that metabolic or infectious problems necessitate the appropriate treatment. Generally, the self-limited condition responds to sedatives.

Thought Disorders (Schizophrenia)

The differentiation of global disorders of attention due to neurologic causes from psychotic and affective disorders can be difficult. Confusional states and delirium are caused by multifocal or diffuse (toxic or metabolic) brain injury, and the temporal onset and course vary depending on the particular insult. Schizophrenia commonly occurs during adolescence and early adulthood. The disorder can either progress insidiously, or recur in acute episodes. The current operational criteria for the diagnosis of schizophrenia aid in distinguishing the difference between acute schizophrenic psychosis and an organic delirium;[8] some practical differential points follow.

A schizophrenic patient may exhibit delusions of being controlled from outside forces, and have the delusion of "thought broadcasting"; that is, others can know thoughts that are not explicitly expressed. If delusions occur in delirium, they are poorly organized, transient, and generally influenced by the concurrent hospital situation. The schizophrenic will often think in a bizarre or autistic manner, and a typical train of thought is often linked to a particular delusion. Delirious patients have difficulty following any train of thought.

The schizophrenic characteristically has a blunted affect, but the delirious patient, even in the hypoactive form, does not exhibit this tendency. Both types of patients can be withdrawn. In the hypoactive form the delirious patient may experience progressive withdrawal and become lethargic or stuporous. This decrease in the level of consciousness is different from the catatonic schizophrenic who remains alert, but displays waxy flexibility or catalepsy (vacant facial expression, pursed lips, maintaining a constant supine or sitting position). Also, delirious patients show fluctuations in the severity of their symptoms over the course of a day, that include lucid intervals; schizophrenics do not display such striking fluctuations.

Visual hallucinations are somewhat more common in delirium, and auditory hallucinations are more common in agitated psychotic episodes of schizophrenia. Also, in delirium the characteristics of the hallucinations or illusions tend to be the same from one delirious episode to the next. In schizophrenia, hallucinations or illusions are linked usually to a peculiar delusional system. The neurologic exam may be normal in both conditions; however, stereotyped motor activity like posturing (see catalepsy definition above) or grimacing suggest catatonia.

Affective Disorders

Differentiating between organic delirium and the major affective disorders in both manic and depressive phases can also be difficult. Past history of any similar illness is important information. Patients with affective disorders of the manic type can be easily distracted, confused, and have visual hallucinations. The disorientation of the delirious patient generally reflects a fearful agitation. Depressed patients can appear withdrawn, and have difficulty remembering names and events, but are usually oriented. Fluctuations in the degree of illness can occur in affective disorders, but rapid fluctuations, within hours and that include lucid intervals, favor a diagnosis of delirium. Also, in delirious patients the degree of disorientation often follows the deterioration of other spheres of cognition.

Factitious Disorders: Malingering

Voluntary malingering can present as a disorder of attention, particularly after head trauma. Patients with fluctuating levels of consciousness and disorientation who have had concussive head trauma must undergo prompt diagnostic maneuvers (see Chapter 9). However, when fluctuating levels of consciousness and disorientation are *not* accompanied by other defects in the neurologic exam, and are accompanied by defects in attention or memory, and a tendency to answer even the simplest questions incorrectly, voluntary malingering may be considered.

In addition to disorientation, the symptoms of voluntary malingering include peculiar memory defects, hallucinations, incoherent illogical thinking, inappropriate volatile affect. Patients with a factitious disorder may give an utterly incorrect, often ridiculous answer, although it is clear that the sense of the question was understood. While these patients say they are disoriented or that they are amnesic, their general behavior gives the distinct impression they are neither disoriented nor amnesic. In contrast to the schizophrenic who cannot sort out the appropriate concepts to answer a question, or a delirious patient who is disoriented and cannot concentrate or sustain attention, the patient with the factitious state appears to select purposely the approximate answer. Also, there are more inconsistencies in their histories as repeated to various examiners.

There is also usually a recognizable stressful event preceding the onset of symptoms. While stressful events can be elicited for any patient in the hospital, most people deal effectively with the stressful events of life. The patient with a factitious disorder often has a history of being completely incapacitated by stressful events, and this patient may depend on the constant, close assistance of others. A factitious disorder may be superimposed on other personality disorders, such as an hysterical personality with conversion or dissociative reactions or a sociopathic personality.

Dissociative/Conversion Reactions

The hysterical personality combines histrionic tendencies with dependency and seductiveness.[7] Dissociative phenomena occur in patients with hysterical personalities, and these phenomena are characterized by disorders of attention and memory. The patient with a dissociative reaction cannot remember the time, and quickly loses the information about his location. Another characteristic feature of the disorientation during a dissociative episode is the loss of personal identity. In an awake patient, the loss of personal identity almost always indicates a psychiatric disorder. This disorientation may take the form of a more extensive amnesia, particularly for events that occurred prior to some stressful event (retrograde amnesia).

A recent example of dissociative state occurred in a young woman who complained of numbness in the right hand after forearm and wrist trauma. Yet, on examination she had almost complete anaesthesia of the limbs on the opposite side. When confronted with this finding she replied insouciantly, "You did not ask about my left arm." Her indifference is a typical feature of a dissociative reaction.

Patients with conversion reactions commonly present with physical symptoms that include motor abnormalities—paralysis, tremors, gait disorders, choreiform movements, convulsive movements, even seizures. The motor abnormalities generally do not conform to the usual myotomal deficits that occur after physiologic damage to the neuraxis. For example, the gait disorders are characterized by lurching steps and frequent near falls. The tremors and chorea are highly organized and stereotyped. Conversion reaction seizures are usually characterized by wild thrashing gestures not rhythmic, clonic movements. The postictal period is characterized by resistance to limb movement or eye opening, and reasonable memory of the context of events during the seizure persists.

Sensory abnormalities, including blindness and double vision, are also common. A sensory loss that does not follow the distribution of a peripheral nerve or dermatome may indicate a conversion reaction. The differential diagnosis can be difficult when there is no dysfunction in the remainder of the neurologic exam, or the defect is transient. In the situation of a documented transient dysfunction, one must consider multiple sclerosis (see Chapter 8). Pain is another common form of conversion hysteria. The pain may affect any part of the body, and may present the most difficult differential diagnosis.

On the other hand, the examiner is urged to be cautious regarding the dismissal of signs or symptoms thought to reflect a non-physiologic deficit. There are several series of patients diagnosed as "hysterical" or as having a conversion reaction. When these patients were followed for some time, up to 30 percent were found to have focal, multifocal, or metabolic disease that explained their "factitious" symptoms.[13,14]

The Evaluation Of Orientation Disorders

It should be re-emphasized that global disorientation can be the first symptom of delirium that may, depending on the insult, progress to coma and death. Drug intoxication, drug withdrawal, sepsis, metabolic imbalance, increased intracranial pressure must be considered and treated. The clinician must rapidly consider the possibilities listed in Table 12.2, and use the appropriate laboratory aids to gather information.

The further evaluation of patients who are disoriented in time and space includes some special procedures.

The Electroencephalogram

Special laboratory aids in the diagnosis of global attention disorders include the EEG and the amytal interview. In acute toxic delirium from alcohol or sedative drugs, slow EEG activity predominates; in alcohol or barbiturate withdrawal, low voltage fast activity predominates. In other encephalopathies, for example with liver disease, slow EEG activity predominates. Focal EEG slowing may help diagnose a structural lesion, like a subdural. If the EEG is dominated by high voltage slow activity, or focal high voltage slow activity, in the disoriented patient; or if the EEG is dominated by low voltage fast activity in the agitated disoriented patient, then the likelihood of psychiatric disease recedes and multifocal or diffuse (metabolic) disorders should be considered.

The Amytal Interview

The amytal interview can be helpful in distinguishing among factitious disorientation, disorientation caused by psychiatric disease, and multifocal or metabolic disease. The amytal interview works best, however, when there is a suspected factitious or hysterical focal disorder of the cranial nerves or the sensorimotor components of the neuraxis (e.g., a paralyzed limb). Under these circumstances, important observations can be made regarding the function of the limb while the patient is under the influence of amytal. It is less reliable in evaluating disordered mental status; however, when used judiciously, it is safe and may provide diagnostic information.[4]

Sodium amobarbital is injected intravenously (about 25 mg/minute to a total dose of 150–300 mg) during a discussion of neutral topics. Patients with multifocal or metabolic disease will show immediate deterioration. In fact, signs that were not present in the neurologic exam (such as a hemiparesis) may appear. The effects are variable in psychiatric disease. There may be moments of lucidity in the schizophrenic, but generally there is no effect.

In factitious disorders, larger doses of amytal (up to 500 mg) are needed before any change in behavior occurs. The initial change is generally toward improvement. The clinician should be aware that personality disorders can be serious diseases and exact diagnosis and therapy should be determined with psychiatric consultation. Although amytal interviews are safe for diagnostic purposes, they should not be used repeatedly to remove or improve the symptoms.

Special Orientation Disorders: Defective Cognitive Control

Luria's extensive observations suggest that focal injury to the frontal lobes can present as a form of disordered attention.[9] This symptom is an inability to select from many possibilities. Once a selection is made, this symptom is characterized by an inability to sustain the concentration necessary to complete a task. Patients with frontal lobe lesions have difficulty organizing their attention and keeping it focused on a definite plan. They are easily distracted by irrelevant stimuli. They also may have problems initiating a plan of action, and there are many recorded instances of incoherent reasoning processes.

Since the cognitive disorders after frontal lobe injury can be subtle and affect personality, intellect, concentration, and initiative, we suggest the rubric of defective cognitive control as a shorthand to define a wide range of symptoms that may be present in patients with frontal lobe injury.

Symptoms of Frontal Lobe Injury

Patients with unilateral frontal lobe lesions will have contralateral motor disorders and often so-called primitive reflexes, such as a suck or snout. If the unilateral frontal lesion is left-sided, then there is often a language impairment that depends on the extent of the lesion. There may also be an apraxia of the left hand; that is, an inability to respond to verbal commands that require left hand activity (see section on the apraxias below). Patients with bilateral frontal lobe disease may not show dramatic cognitive defects, but they may display pronounced changes in personality, particularly if the lesion is mediobasal. The most common features are apathy, lack of concern over the consequences of any action, indifference, euphoria, jocularity and insouciance, irritability that can be explosive yet transient and inappropriateness that can be vulgar. Family members often describe the patient's behavior as childlike.

Evaluation of Frontal Lobe Injury

The physical examination of the patient with unilateral frontal lobe injury often reveals a contralateral hemiplegia; speech and language disorders occur if the dominant (left) hemisphere is injured. Various combinations of primitive reflexes may appear: grasping, suck or snout reflexes. There is a peculiar gait decompensation as well with bifrontal lesions. The patient takes short hesitant steps, and cannot easily execute postural adjustments. The posture is flexed. The gait has been described as "glue footed" because the patient displays inability to initiate the lifting and placing movement.

Vigilance tasks are said to be particularly sensitive in detecting patients with frontal lobe disorders. These tasks demand alternating movements with one hand or the other. In the fist-palm-side test the patient is instructed to hit the top of the table first with the fist, then the open palm, then the side of the hand. The examiner may have to demonstrate the task. The patient must continuously repeat that sequence and 15–20 seconds generally permits adequate assessment. Other coordination tasks require posturing of the hands in a fist alternating with a ring sign, that is, with index finger and thumb opposed to form a ring. Patients with dorsolateral frontal lobe dysfunction will have difficulty on these tasks.

SPEECH AND LANGUAGE DISORDERS

As a history is obtained and the patient's orientation and attentional capacity is evaluated, signs of speech and language disorders can also be noted. The first decision is to distinguish between dysarthria, which is a motor speech disorder, and aphasia, which encompasses a number of ideational components of both language expression and comprehension. In the acute phase of a neurological disease the accurate characterization of a speech or language dysfunction is important for the establishment of a clinical description consistent with other neurological findings. Careful description of language dysfunction can also be extremely useful in following the progression of the acute phase of an illness.

One of the most important characteristics of the neurology of language is its asymmetrical representation from the level of the thalamus to the cortex. In 95 to 98 percent of the right-handed population, language is lateralized to the left cerebral hemisphere. In nearly all right-handed individuals, then, pathology involving the left hemisphere, which is dominant for language, may produce an aphasia. In the left-handed and mixed-handed population, the hemispheric representation of language is different. For this group, 70 percent of the individuals have left hemisphere dominance for language, 15 percent have right hemisphere dominance, and 15 percent have language represented in both hemispheres.[12] Unlike right-handedness, which is a good predictor of the side of hemispheric dominance, left- or mixed-handedness should alert the clinician that language may be represented in either the left or right, or both hemispheres.

In addition to handedness, a second important characteristic in establishing hemispheric dominance is the presence or absence of left hemisphere damage early in life. Although there is no consensus on the definition of early, hemispheric damage that occurs prior to puberty can be characterized as such. The effect of an early left hemisphere lesion in both right- and left-handed groups is to increase in the tendency towards right hemisphere dominance or bilateral representation. In one series of 134 patients with definite clinical evidence of an early left hemisphere lesion, the right-handed group had the following composition: 81 percent were found to have a left hemisphere dominance and 7 percent had a bilateral language representation. The left- and mixed-handedness group consisted of 28 percent with left hemisphere dominance, 53 percent with right hemisphere dominance and 19 percent with a bilateral language representation.[12] Thus, handedness and early neurological history are both significant factors in establishing the etiology of an aphasia, and to a lesser extent, a dysarthria.

Symptoms Of Dysarthric Disorders

One recent classification of dysarthrias restricted the use of the term dysarthria to neurogenic motor disorders involving respiration, phonation, articulation, resonance and prosody, either in isolation, or in multiple combinations.[3] Although dysarthric speech can be characterized as slurred, thickened, indistinct, unclear or clumsy, the clinician should be aware that these descriptions emphasize the rhythm and pitch.

The Evaluation Of The Motor Aspects Of Speech

The first step in the assessment of speech quality should occur during the examiner's conversational speech with the patient. The patient should be encouraged to talk, so that the examiner can listen to the quality of the patient's spontaneous speech, observe the ease with which it is produced, and identify areas in which further testing is required. Since speech is a motor activity, the examiner should attend to specific characteristics of the function of the oropharyngeal and respiratory muscles. The evaluation of tone, power, and range of movements follows the examination of the peripheral motor system.

In addition to noting these characteristics of motor function, several characteristics of the sound pattern of speech should also be noted (Table 12.3).

In cases where the examiner wishes to examine speech more closely, especially with respect to articulation, this can be accomplished by having the patient carry out several repetitive non-verbal and verbal oral-motor activities. Non-verbal oral-motor acts require the controlled use of the articulatory musculature (e.g., protrude and retract the tongue movements from one side of the mouth to the other). These movements should be repeated for several seconds, and the examiner should note the degree of difficulty with which they are produced, the consistency of the motor activity, and possible declines in performance over several seconds of repetition. Similarly, verbal oral-motor activities require the patient to repeat a word or phrase for a several second period (e.g., ten-four, coast-to-coast, toy boat). As with the non-verbal repetitions, the examiner evaluates the patient's productions with respect to difficulty, consistency, and decline in performance. With both the verbal and non-verbal repetitions, the patient's speech should be characterized in terms of the characteristics of muscle function and voice quality listed above. Whereas the dysarthrias represent motor dysfunctions involving the mechanisms of speech production, the aphasias represent dysfunctions of language itself. The distinction between speech and language, which for the present purposes can be thought of as a distinction between motor output and ideation, is an important one, since dysarthric speech may obscure intact language functions. An appropriate evaluation of higher intellectual function, then, requires that the different levels

**Table 12.3 Clinical Features of the Motor
Aspects of Speech**

Phonation
Pitch changes
Loudness changes
Rhythm
Breathy voice
Harsh voice

of dysfunction involved in dysarthria and aphasia be accurately characterized.

Disordered Expression

One of the major features of language that allows for discrimination among
the types of aphasia is fluency. Non-fluent aphasia is marked by a decreased
output compared to the normal production rate of 100–150 words per minute. Spontaneous speech in such cases is often less than 10 words per minute,
and is produced with a notable increase in effort on the part of the patient.[1]
The sparseness of non-fluent speech can be seen in a shortening of phrase
length in conversational speech. Prepositions, articles, adverbs, and some
adjectives and verbs are deleted from spontaneous speech (telegraphic
speech). In severe cases of non-fluency, the patient's production may be
restricted to a verbal stereotype consisting of a single word or phrase. In
such instances, the patient may use the stereotype (e.g., "O.K.") to respond
to all questions.

Language production in the fluent aphasias is often in the normal range
of 100–150 words per minute. Articulation is normal and the production
process does not require abnormal effort on the part of the patient. The
fluent patient may utter phrases quite normally, but introduce an abnormally
long pause when a word finding difficulty occurs. This typically occurs when
a substantive word must be found. In instances when the correct word
cannot be found by the patient, a circumlocution consisting of a meaningless
description may be produced. In some instances, the absence of any substance to the fluent output has led to it being termed "empty" speech.

Paraphasias are often present in fluent aphasia. Several types of paraphasias occur. In literal paraphasias, an incorrect phoneme is substituted for
a correct one, so that a patient might call a "spoon" a "stoon." In verbal
paraphasias, an incorrect word is substituted for the intended word, so that
the "spoon" may be called a "fork." In neologism, a nonsense word is substituted for the intended word, so that the "spoon" might be called a "clib."
These paraphasias, unlike many word finding difficulties, are often produced
without any awareness of errors. Extended strings of paraphasic utterances
is referred to as jargon.

Disordered Repetition

Another characteristic important for discriminating among aphasic syndromes is repetition. The deficit may range from extremely impaired to
an almost automatic repetition of everything said to the patient. It should
also be noted that fluency does not mean that repetition will be intact. A
fluent aphasic's repetitions may be marred by paraphasic errors.

Word Finding Difficulty

Essentially all aphasic syndromes have a vocabulary restriction as a component. In the non-fluent aphasias, this restriction is observed as telegraphic speech. In the fluent aphasias, word finding difficulties tend to make the speech "empty."

Classification Of Aphasia

The major categories of aphasia are presented in Table 12.4, in which the dysfunctions are classified according to fluency, comprehension, and repetition. It is important to remember that vocabulary restrictions or word-finding difficulties are present in each of these categories. In all cases except anomic aphasia, which has been reported after both right and left hemisphere lesions, the critical anatomical areas are in the dominant (typically left) hemisphere. The classic lesions associated with each of these aphasias are presented in Table 12.5.

Broca's Aphasia

Referred to as motor or expressive aphasia, Broca's aphasia results from damage to the third frontal convolution of the left hemisphere. The fully developed syndrome requires destruction of deep subcortical white matter and anterior insula. Language production is effortful, and articulation is frequently impaired. Utterances use simple grammatical forms and short phrase lengths, and have thus been characterized as telegraphic or agrammatic. Comprehension is much less impaired than expression, and similarly, reading is more intact than is writing. Repetitions are marked by articulatory difficulties.

Table 12.4 Differential Diagnoses of Major Aphasic Syndromes Based on the Patient's Fluency, Comprehension and Repetition

Aphasic Syndrome	Language Characteristic		
	Fluent	Comprehension	Repetition
Broca's	No	Intact	Distorted articulation
Transcortical sensory	No	Impaired	Intact
Transcortical motor	No	Intact	Intact
Wernicke	Yes	Impaired	Paraphasias
Conduction	Yes	Intact	Literal paraphasias
Anomic	Yes	Variable	Intact
Global	No	Impaired	Absent

Table 12.5 Classic Lesion Sites of the Major Aphasic Syndromes. (In all instances except anomia, the lesions are in the dominant hemisphere.)

Aphasic Syndrome	Location of Lesion
Broca's	Third frontal convolution
Transcortical sensory	Watershed lesions
Transcortical motor	Frontal, anterior to Broca's area
Wernicke's	Posterior portion of superior temporal gyrus
Conduction	Arcuate fasciculus, deep supramarginal gyrus
Anomia	No specific location, typically dominant hemisphere
Global	Large lesion involving both anterior and posterior language areas

Transcortical Sensory Aphasia

An aphasia characterized by inability to initiate conversational speech, but these patients are able to repeat well what is said to them. This syndrome results from watershed infarctions in the left hemisphere. It is believed that such lesions isolate Broca's and Wernicke's areas from other sources of information in the brain, leaving repetition intact, but with severe comprehension deficits.

Transcortical Motor Aphasia

Results from lesions anterior to Broca's area and is similar to transcortical sensory aphasia in that repetition is intact but spontaneous speech is not initiated. Unlike transcortical sensory motor aphasia, however, comprehension is relatively intact in this disorder.

Wernicke's Aphasia

This is the result of a lesion of the posterior portion of the superior temporal gyrus in the left hemisphere, characterized by fluent production of speech with grossly normal rhythm, but comprehension is impaired. The content of speech is often described as "empty," with circumlocutions, word finding difficulties, and paraphasias. Repetitions contain paraphasic errors.

Conduction Aphasia

Characterized by fluent production and intact comprehension. Repetition is impaired by the intrusion of literal paraphasias. This syndrome is believed to result from a lesion of the arcuate fasciculus, a pathway that is thought to convey information from Wernicke's area to Broca's area.

Anomic Aphasia

Anomic aphasia is characterized by fluent production and repetition is generally intact. Comprehension is variable, such that in the extreme anomia, the patient's language is very much like that of a Wernicke's aphasic. In less severe instances, the dysfunction is restricted to problems with word finding, in the context of otherwise fluent and grammatical language. This syndrome is not the result of damage to a specific area; many areas, some in the non-dominant hemisphere, have been associated with this deficit.

Global Aphasia

Results in severely impaired output although the global aphasic is not typically mute. Repetition is absent, and comprehension is also severely impaired. This syndrome is the result of a large lesion affecting both anterior and posterior language areas.

Schizophrenic Language Versus Fluent Aphasia

Often, a communicative disorder is one of the most striking indications of a schizophrenic psychosis. At one end of the range of this disorder in schizophrenia, one may observe the ability to speak only after some resistance has been overcome (blocking), or even mutism, while at the other end, one may observe fluently produced sentences that are little more than a series of words unrelated to one another (word salad). Under some circumstances, especially when there are no other neurological findings, it may be difficult to discriminate between fluent aphasia and schizophrenic language, since the content of the communication in both disorders may be virtually meaningless. One important point to remember, however, is that in spite of a lack of substantive language content in both disorders, the aphasic will generally appear to be trying to communicate with the examiner, unlike the schizophrenic who may appear to have withdrawn from communication with the examiner by engaging in verbal play.

Gerson, Benson and Frazier analyzed the language output of schizophrenics and fluent aphasics, and were able to contrast the two groups along several characteristics of their language.[5] These contrasts are contained in Table 12.6. In response to open-ended questions, schizophrenics typically produced answers in excess of 100 words, and often much longer, and stopped when interrupted by the examiner. Fluent aphasics, on the other hand, typically produced much shorter answers, in the range of 20–30 words, and initiated their own pauses in anticipation of further questions from the examiner.

Fluent aphasics appeared to be more aware of their deficit than were the schizophrenics, and attempted to enlist the help of the examiner by pause and gesture, to make their efforts at communication successful. No such attempts were observed in the schizophrenic group. Paraphasias and

Table 12.6 Some Differential Characteristics of Schizophrenic and Fluent-Aphasia Language

Language Characteristic	Schizophrenic	Fluent-Aphasic
Length of response	Over 100 words	20–30 words
Awareness of deficit	Absent	Often present
Attempts to ensure communication	Absent	Present
Paraphasias, neologisms	Absent	Present
Vagueness of response	Due to attentional disturbance	Due to word finding difficulty, circumlocution
Content	Bizarre themes that are repeated	No persistent themes

(after Gerson, S.N., Benson, D.F., Frazier, S.H.: Diagnosis: schizophrenic versus posterior aphasia. Am. J. Psych., 134:966, 1977; with permission).

neologisms were observed in the language of all of the aphasics, but not in that of the schizophrenics. The vagueness of the patients' responses in the aphasic group was largely due to word finding difficulties and circumlocution, while in the schizophrenic group, it was due to an attentional disturbance that made the responses circumstantial, containing strings of loose associations. Finally, there were no persistent themes in the responses of aphasic patients. Schizophrenic patients, on the other hand, produced and repeated bizarre themes in their responses (Table 12.6).

The Evaluation Of The Aphasias

Conversational Speech

A significant part of the assessment of language expression and comprehension can be obtained from conversational and spontaneous speech while taking a history from the patient. It is important to note the characteristics of the patient's language production in response to open-ended questions such as: "What kind of work did you do before you became ill?," and "What happened to you to bring you to the hospital?"

In addition to characterizing conversational speech, it is important to more formally examine naming, repetition, comprehension, and writing. This can be done in the following way:

Confrontation Naming

A set of five common objects can be used (e.g., pen, keys, watch, comb, coin) for this test. Each item is presented singly, and the subject is asked to name it. The examiner should note whether the responses are quick (i.e., occur in less than five seconds) or slow (i.e., require more than five seconds). It is important to insure that the objects are presented to the intact visual field in cases where there is a visual field loss. If visual acuity is sufficiently impaired to preclude visual inspection of the objects, they can be presented to the patients tactually, realizing that manual manipulation is normally less efficient than visual inspection.

Responsive Naming

Unlike confrontation naming, which provides the referent to the patient, responsive naming requires more ideation on the part of the patient. The examiner can use a set of five questions in the following form: "What do you use to write with?" or "What do you use to tell time with?" If auditory comprehension is impaired, but reading comprehension has been spared, these questions can be presented in written form.

Auditory Comprehension

The examiner estimates the patient's auditory comprehension from the conversational exchanges that occurred when a history was taken. In patients for whom auditory comprehension is questionable, it is useful to evaluate this function both at the level of single words, and as described in the next section, the ability to follow commands. For word comprehension, the objects used for confrontation naming can be placed in front of the patient, again insuring that all of the objects are in an intact visual field. The examiner then asks the patient to "Point to the light" (or some other object).

Commands

Auditory comprehension can be further tested by requesting that the subject carry out a series of commands. Whereas the request to "Point to the comb" constitutes a one-step command, the request to "Point to the pen and then to the watch" constitutes a two-step command. The number of steps can be increased to five. It should be noted that in addition to testing auditory comprehension, this test also requires memory and attention.

Repetition

Repetition is an important function in the differential diagnosis of aphasia, and it should be tested at several levels. Five items in each of the following categories should be tested: easy words (e.g., pencil, chair, girl, ship, fence), hard words (e.g., wrist-watch, sassafras, Constantinople, emphasize, trigonometry), phrases (e.g., no ifs, ands, or buts; go to the store; if at first you don't succeed, try, try again; wait until April fifteenth; colorful flowers brighten the day).

Reading

Reading can be assessed by having the patient read a paragraph from a newspaper or magazine, and then provide the examiner with a paraphrase. If this cannot be done, then reading can be assessed at the level of word comprehension, by writing out the names of the objects used in confrontation naming. The patient is asked to read the word, then to point to the corresponding object. Finally, if the patient is unable to read words, single letters can be written out for the subject to read. The examiner can score the paragraph reading in terms of good or poor, and the word and letter reading in terms of the number of trials out of five correctly completed.

Writing

The writing assessment should begin by having the subject write his or her name and address. The sentence, "The quick brown fox jumps over the lazy dog" should then be presented visually for the subject to copy. If additional writing samples are needed for the evaluation, it is often useful to have the patient write a brief description of his or her home, or the hospital room. The important aspects of the writing are legibility, size, consistency, and the ease with which it is produced.

The careful characterization of the patient's conversational and spontaneous speech, along with the assessment of naming, repetition, comprehension and writing will allow the examiner to accurately identify the appropriate aphasic syndrome and infer the location of the lesion.

MEMORY

A patient with a specific memory problem, a so-called amnesic syndrome, is oriented, can sustain attention, and has generally intact cognitive function. However, cognitive function is limited by an inability to learn new information, particularly when the learning period is followed by some interfering task that prohibits constant rehearsal. For example, an amnesic patient may be told to remember the names of three unrelated objects. Typically, the amnesic can repeat the names without difficulty, yet, after five minutes of conversation, remembers none of the three objects. The amnesic's relatively normal cognitive function is limited also by an inability to recall the events immediately preceding the onset of the amnesia.

Disorders of memory can have an acute onset and brief duration as in transient global amnesia; or have an insidious onset and chronic duration, as in the dementias.

Disorders Of Memory

Anterograde Amnesia

This term defines an impairment in memory for events that occur after the onset of the disorder. The amnesic may be lost in new surroundings, and is unable to benefit from instruction. However, information about personal identity usually remains preserved. Activities such as grooming and social interaction are preserved.

Retrograde Amnesia

This term defines a loss of memories for particular events or objects or people in those events that occurred prior to the onset of amnesia. This memory loss may include only the few minutes prior to the brain injury, as with mild concussive closed head injury, or may extend for decades into the amnesic's past history, as in alcoholic Korsakoff's syndrome.

The Symptoms Of The Amnesic Syndrome

There are clinical characteristics common to amnesia even when caused by diverse pathophysiologic insults (Table 12.7).

Poor Free Recall

The inability to recall recent memories is the prime deficit in anterograde amnesia. Amnesic patients remember information for brief periods after exposure, and longer if allowed to rehearse, but they recall significantly less than normal after a few seconds of distraction. As mentioned, such patients usually fail to recall a single item from a list of three unrelated items after 5 minutes of distraction.

Intact Short Term Memory Capacity

The rate of forgetting in short-term memory differs among amnesias. However, short-term memory capacity, as measured by only a few seconds, like digit repetition span tests, is normal in patients with Korsakoff's syndrome, and those who had herpes encephalitis, or hypoxic ischemic injury.

Ability to Respond to Cues

Recognition cues have been shown to improve some amnesic's memories. After showing an object to an amnesic, recognition memory can be probed by asking the amnesic which of two objects he had been shown. If this is done several times for different objects, many amnesics will show better than chance performance.

Personal Identity Retained

Patients who have amnesic syndromes do not lose their senses of personal identity, they continue to know who they are. The clinician should consider the diagnosis of a factitious disorder or an hysterical personality disorder in a patient who is awake, alert, has intact language function, and who is complaining of the loss of personal identity. This condition, often called the Ganser State, usually has been recorded in prisoners. Also dissociative reactions in an hysterical patient may include the loss of personal identity.

Table 12.7 Causes of Amnesic Syndrome

I. Structural
    A. Tumors: midline, thalamic, third ventricle, with or without hydrocephalus
    B. Multiple strokes, particularly posterior circulation
    C. Subarachnoid hemorrhage
    D. Transient global amnesia
    E. Head trauma

II. Metabolic
    A. Wernicke-Korsakoff syndrome
    B. Hypoxia-ischemia (with coma after cardiac or respiratory arrest)
    C. Epilepsy, particularly temporal lobe

III. Infectious/Inflammatory
    A. Encephalitis, particularly Herpes simplex
    B. Vasculitis

Etiology

Focal Causes of the Amnesic Syndrome

Several pathophysiologic processes may cause amnesia. Structural causes include tumors, particularly midline deep tumors involving the thalamus and the third ventricle or the columns of the fornix with or without ventricular obstruction. Vascular pathology may cause permanent amnesic syndromes. The classically described patients have repeated episodes of posterior circulation stroke syndromes. Cerebrovascular accidents in this distribution are usually associated with progressive visual field loss.

There is a distinct syndrome of transient amnesia. Although the particular symptoms of transient global amnesia also include poor recall, intact short-term memory, these patients have little or no insight into their condition. They will repeatedly ask, "Why am I here, . . . How did I get here?" This condition rarely lasts more than 24 hours. Investigators suggest that the etiology of transient global amnesia involves temporary vascular insufficiency of the mesial temporal lobes. In the clinical situation, the patient with transient global amnesia may perform the typical motor acts in washing and preparing for work; even negotiate the transportation to work and then completely forget what the job requires.

A recent patient's history illustrates this point: A 53-year-old man who lived in Queens was shopping with his wife in the supermarket co-op some distance from their home. While picking an item off the shelf he turned to his wife and asked her what they were doing. She thought he was teasing. He finished shopping only with great prodding from her, and constant reminders of what he was sent to find. He paid for the groceries, but his lack of remembering had become alarming. He drove his wife home over a familiar, but not simple, route. At home she summoned an ambulance, and he was brought to the hospital where the diagnosis of transient global amnesia was made. His neurologic exam was normal except he could not remember unrelated objects and his digit span was 5 numbers. He could be cued to the appropriate date and place, but could not remember either after a minute or two. He spoke coherently and followed commands. He calculated with difficulty. He repeatedly asked the clinicians examining him why he was in the hospital, and what had happened. He had a normal CT scan, and some mild diffuse disorganization on EEG. Fifteen hours later, the memory defect had cleared.

Other focal structural causes of amnesia include subarachnoid hemorrhage, particularly from an aneurysm of the anterior communicating artery. This amnesic syndrome is infrequent and, according to some reports, is a transient condition. Chronic amnesic states after subarachnoid hemorrhages are reported but these cases are not well documented.

Diffuse Causes of the Amnesic Syndrome

Diffuse causes of the amnesic syndrome include head trauma, Wernicke-Korsakoff syndrome (thiamine deficiency), hypoxic-ischemic insult (after cardiac or respiratory arrest). Other diffuse causes of the amnesic syndrome include encephalitis, particularly Herpes simplex. Although neuropathologic changes are widespread after viral encephalitis, the temporal lobes show the major part of the injury. Finally, there are rare reports of a focal vasculitis (particularly of the thalamus) causing an amnesic syndrome.

An example of the permanent amnesic syndrome that can follow hypoxic-ischemic injury and cardiac arrest follows: A 42-year-old man was brought to the hospital complaining of chest pain, and soon thereafter had a cardiac arrest. During the arrest he was without pulse and respirations for less than 5 minutes, yet cardiac massage took 30 minutes to restore a stable pulse. Over the next 24 hours he was unresponsive to voice and made no response to noxious stimuli. By 48 hours his pupils were reactive and midposition, and late in the third hospital day he was awake, oriented to place, responded to command, and complained of difficulty seeing. The remainder of his hospital course was marked by steady improvement in cognitive function.

However, his severe anterograde amnesia persisted without much improvement. Two years later on examination of higher integrative functions, he was oriented and knew his birthdate and age. He had a digit span of six numbers, but remembered none of three unrelated objects after 5 minutes of distraction. He recognized friends and business partners but had difficulties remembering the identity of old clients. He recalled remote personal events antedating his injury, like the winner of college baseball games and the closing of several large real estate deals. His memory for the events immediately prior to his cardiac arrest was vague. He was unable to recall personal events, like taking his son to boarding school for the first time, and when reminded, he could not judge whether it was weeks or months ago. He recalled the seizure of the U.S. embassy in Iran, but forgot the Pope's visit to New York. He has not returned to work.

The Differential Diagnosis Of The Amnesic Syndrome

Focal or Diffuse Lesions

From the neuropathologic point of view structural damage to either the mesial temporal lobes, the mammillary bodies, or the connections to the medial and anterior nuclei of the thalamus, the fornix, or the cingulate gyrus is sufficient, although not necessary, to cause amnesia.

Amnesic syndromes after stroke, hypoxia-ischemia, subarachnoid hemorrhage, encephalitis, and trauma are distinguished by the acute onset and the dramatic change in behavior post-injury. These acute amnesic syndromes are to be differentiated from chronic forms of progressive memory loss. These later disorders often represent primary neurodegenerative disease and encompass all phases of cognitive process including attention, language, and mood (see Table 12.10 for a differential list, and section below on dementias for a discussion of pseudo-dementia and dementia).

Psychogenic Amnesia

The patient with a hysterical personality who has a dissociative or conversion reaction was discussed earlier in this chapter. Patients with this disorder are disoriented and may have a retrograde amnesia for the events prior to the stressful occurrence that precipitated the disorder. The memory deficit is characterized by inconsistent histories given to different examiners, and, often, a retained ability to learn new information. This disorder generally clears with treatment of the underlying personality disorder. The distinguishing feature includes the associated personality disorder.

There is another amnesic state that occurs without a discernable neuropathologic lesion. Ganser called it a hysterical twilight state characterized by peculiar defects in memory. Patients in this state answer even the simplest question incorrectly, but it is clear that the intent of the question was understood. For example, two plus two equals five. A distinguishing symptom in this state is the patient's loss of personal identity. Patients with amnesic syndromes after focal or diffuse injury generally maintain a knowledge of who they are. The EEG is generally normal in these instances of hysterical amnesia.

The Clinical Evaluation Of Disorders Of Memory

Confabulation Phenomena

There are some basic cautions in probing memory for the recent and remote past. Some amnesics have little insight into their memory loss, and they are said to confabulate; that is, fill in forgotten details with fabricated incidents. Korsakoff patients classically confabulate the details of recent past events, although an added diagnostic clue in Korsakoff's syndrome is the accompanying profound disorientation to time and place. Confabulations are generally too vivid and exaggerated for the examiner to miss; however, the examiner must seek another source to corroborate a patient's story. Also, the clinician must be sensitive to the patient's pre-morbid intellectual level. Job history, years of education, social exposure, and personal interests must be considered carefully in evaluating remote memory capacity. If important historical events are used to probe the remote past, then they should be tailored to the individual patient.

Evaluate Recent Memory

Perhaps the simplest evaluation of memory function is the new learning situation. The classical neurologic exam requires patients to learn three unrelated words and recall them some time later in the exam. Choose words that are semantically and phonemically unrelated, and make sure the interval between test and recall is filled with other tasks. Do not, for example, say "Remember these three unrelated objects: yellow rubber ball, turkey, 53 Broadway," then turn to tap the patient's reflexes. The tendency for some amnesics is to rehearse constantly. Interference, generally by conversation about some other aspect of the patient's problem or by giving the patient another mental task to do, is an important requirement of the evaluation.

Modality Specific Memory Loss

Other bedside tests of memory function probe verbal and visual memory. Tell the patient a story of several sentences and after a delay, ask the patient to tell everything he can remember. Probe visual memories by telling the patient to view a meaningless figure, and, after a delay, ask the patient to draw the figure as well as he can remember it. Other probes of visual memory require the patient to name a visually presented object. The patient watches the examiner hide the object, and after a delay period must find the object and/or name the objects hidden.

Remote Memories/Retrograde Amnesia

In the clinical situation remote memory can be tested by asking the patient for personal history. Other questions often include testing the patient's general knowledge of important dates or events in history.

Patients with head trauma generally have a retrograde memory loss. The extensive studies of Russell and Nathan show that retrograde amnesias (RA) are generally of shorter duration than the extent of anterograde amnesia (AA). For example, RA's of more than a few minutes are rare when the AA lasts only 24 hours. Additionally, RA may have a gradient so that the amnesia is most dense for the events immediately prior to the injury. The RA clears as the patient attempts to remember events that occurred in the more distant past. RA generally shrinks to include only a few moments prior to the injury.

Dense retrograde loss is unlikely in amnesia after posterior circulation stroke, subarachnoid hemorrhage, or hypoxic-ischemic injury. It is also unlikely in the early stage of Alzheimer's dementia, where personal remote memories remain intact.

Chronic and Progressive Memory Disorders

Chronic disorder of memory function is a common complaint that is often benign, and, while irritating to the patient, this memory loss does not alter life style. In fact, several investigators have collected data that suggests the performance on a series of memory tests of patients complaining of memory impairment correlated with severity of depression. The differential diagnosis of dementia and depression with pseudodementia is discussed later. This differential can be difficult becuse memory loss is often an initial complaint of patients with primary neuronal degenerative diseases.

SPECIAL DISORDERS: THE HEMI-INATTENTION SYNDROMES (Table 12.8)

Hemi-inattention syndromes range from mild disregard of sensory stimulation on one side of the body, to the inability to recognize one's own limbs, to the complete denial that a problem exists (anosagnosia). Hemi-inattention symptoms do not remain stable from day to day, and the deficits cannot be elicited as consistently as a pure sensory or motor deficit. In contrast to the patient with elementary loss of sensory or motor function, these patients are generally unaware of the extent of their deficit. The most subtle feature in this spectrum of disorders, the extinction phenomenon, can be uncovered with the technique of double simultaneous stimulation. When two sensory stimuli are delivered simultaneously, the side on which the stimulus is extinguished, or ignored, or misidentified suggests a lesion in the contralateral brain. Touch, pin prick, barognostic, vibratory, auditory, and visual information delivered as a single stimulation will not demonstrate the deficit.

Hemi-inattention syndromes are caused by acute posterior branch middle cerebral artery infarction, and by chronically progressive lesions (e.g., tumors or abscesses). The most florid symptoms rarely last more than a few weeks. It is often difficult during the acute period of the most conspicuous symptoms to distinguish inattention from the extent of elementary sensory loss. When the hemi-inattention wanes, generally over a couple of months, any residual defect will more clearly declare itself. However, complete clearing of the symptoms depends on the extent and nature of the lesion.[16]

Table 12.8 Clinical Features of the Hemi-Inattention Syndrome

Apparent failure of vision, sensory or motor function contralateral to brain lesion, so called "neglect," on double simultaneous stimulation.

Normal or near normal function when vision, sensory or motor function of the affected side is tested in isolation.

General orientation to space, time intact.

The Differential Diagnosis Of Hemi-Inattention Syndromes

Non-Dominant Parietal Lobe Lesions

Hemi-inattention syndromes are usually caused by lesions in the sensory association areas of the parietal lobe. Left hemisphere parietal lesions will cause hemi-inattention for the patient's right limbs and right sided visual space, but, as described in the previous section, inattention after left hemisphere injury is usually obscured by aphasia. Hemi-inattention syndromes are common after right parietal lobe damage.[2]

In patients with moderate to severe visual hemi-inattention syndromes, ordinary vision in the unimpaired field may be enough stimulation to cause an apparent visual field defect in the opposite field. One way to distinguish an elementary visual field loss from inattention is to examine the patient in a dimly lit room and have the patient identify a single light source. Patients with a homonymous hemianopsia will not see the light when it is flashed in the affected visual field. Patients with inattention will report seeing the light in all visual fields.

Double simultaneous stimulation (DSS) effectively uncovers the more subtle of cutaneous sensory hemi-inattention syndromes.[2] The technique can be performed simply at the bedside. Tactual stimulation should be applied to homologous areas on both sides of the body simultaneously. Visual stimulation should probe homologous areas of the right and left visual fields simultaneously. The stimulus that is not reported (extinguished) will be contralateral to the lesion.

Further evaluation includes simple drawing. Common figures like a clock are used because of the demand for symmetry about a vertical midline. Drawing a cube, a daisy or a house in perspective adds a degree of difficulty. Drawing a rough outline of the continental United States can be followed by having west coast, midwestern, and eastern cities placed appropriately on the map.

DISORDERS OF VOLUNTARY MOVEMENT

There is an acute disorder of cognitive function that has as its primary symptom a motor disorder, and the injury is not in the elementary motor pathways. These disorders are called the *apraxias*. They can be defined as an inability to perform a motor act, particularly to verbal command, that cannot be accounted for by weakness, sensory loss, incoordination, tremor, rigidity or spasticity, or adventitial movement. Patients with this disorder of movement are attentive and cooperative, and generally they demonstrate good comprehension.[6]

The Symptoms Of Apraxic Disorders

There have been arguments over the classes of gestural behavior that are disrupted in the apraxic disorders. For example, ideomotor apraxia has been defined as a disorder limited to single, simple gestures, and, while complex acts can be executed, the constituent elements are disturbed. With ideational apraxia, the patient cannot carry out complex gestures, in this disorder the constituent elements are executed correctly yet the logical sequence of these elements is disrupted. Motor activity is disordered by a sequencing problem. Ideomotor and ideational apraxia affect both limbs.

There are other forms of apraxia that affect one limb, or the face. In unilateral limb apraxia, the stimulus for the motor activity is a critical dimension. Patients with unilateral limb apraxia often have right hemiparesis and mild aphasia. They have difficulty moving the left limb to a verbal command. For example, to the command "Show me your left thumb," a patient may put his left hand behind his head, or in his pocket. They generally improve with imitation. For example, this same patient may be able to mimic the examiner when told to "Do what I do." Further, when these patients are observed acting in their hospital routines they may move the left (apraxic) limb normally. The buccofacial apraxias describe disordered voluntary movements of the face and tongue. In a manner similar to patients with unilateral limb apraxia who may move the apraxic limb normally in the context of environmental requirements, these patients chew, swallow, smile, and frown, generally without difficulty (Table 12.9).

A recent patient illustrates the salience of the verbal command: A 57-year-old accountant entered the hospital complaining that he could no longer use his calculator. He could understand the numbers, keep track of the rows and columns, and remember the reason for the calculation. He could see the keyboard. He said, "I cannot make my fingers hit the proper key." He went home from work where he had great difficulty opening his front door. His wife realized he could not understand everything that was said to him, and brought him to the hospital. On examination he was

Table 12.9 Clinical Features of the Apraxic Syndrome

The inability to act, particularly after verbal command.

Actions requiring unilateral or bilateral movement impaired. No primary motor dysfunction in the limb required to perform the task. Movements of face often spared. Actions requiring trunk movement often spared.

Mild to moderate aphasia often present.

alert and oriented. For the most part his speech was fluent and made sense, although there were neologisms. He understood commands but could not perform them. He displayed understanding by discussing the logical steps necessary to perform some of these commands. For example, he could name a toothbrush and toothpaste, could express the use of each, and the steps necessary to remove the cellophane wrapper from the brush and "apply the paste to the brush, and move the brush backwards and forwards while pressing it against my teeth," yet his attempt to perform this act was met with frustration. He never removed the toothbrush from the cellophane wrapper, but he unscrewed the toothpaste cap and applied the toothpaste to the wrong end of the brush and began to use the toothbrush as though it were a comb.

Perhaps the most striking (yet typical) example of the complexity of this disorder occurred when he was asked to name his reading spectacles. He said, without hesitation, that they were his reading glasses which perched on his nose and allowed him to read and to watch television. However, when handed the glasses and told to put them on, he could not. He also could not fold the bars and put them into the case. The examiner put the glasses in the case and then into the patient's pocket. The subject of discussion changed, and sometime later, as the examiner was about to leave, the patient picked up a newspaper. In the act of picking up the newspaper, he pulled his eyeglass case from his bathrobe pocket, extracted the glasses with ease from the case, and placed them appropriately on his face. Waving goodbye to the examiner, he settled down to read the newspaper! On CT scan he had an infarct in the left parietal lobe.

Anatomic Lesions Causing Apraxia

Cortical Lesions

Lesions in three cortical areas will produce apraxia. Lesions of the dominant left hemisphere usually in the vascular territory of the artery to the angular gyrus, cause the bilateral limb and buccofacial apraxias. These lesions of the inferior left parietal lobe often also produce aphasia.

More anterior left hemisphere lesions, particularly frontal lesions that cause non-fluent aphasia and right hemiparesis are associated with unilateral limb apraxias. The disruption of a pathway from the left to the right hemisphere has been postulated to cause unilateral apraxias. The apraxia in this particular instance can improve with imitation (based on miming the examiner's activity), and perhaps disappear with the handling of objects.

Callosal Lesions

The third type of lesion that causes apraxia destroys the corpus callosum and disconnects homologous cortical areas between left and right hemisphere. Tumors of the callosum are usually slow growing and rarely cause apraxia, but apraxic syndromes can occur after surgical removal.[15]

Differential Diagnosis Of The Apraxic Syndromes

Other conditions to consider in a patient who cannot perform commands to verbal instruction are aphasic disorders, attention disorders and memory disorders. Language or memory disorders should be revealed through testing along the lines suggested above. Patients with hemi-inattention syndromes and posterior parietal right hemisphere pathology may well have constructional difficulties or a dressing disorder. Constructional difficulties usually consist of a visual spatial defect so that the patient cannot reproduce models or draw cubes, clocks, maps, and other figures that require perception of a three-dimensional object. With dressing disorders, the patient might comb the hair on only one side of the head, or shave half the face, or put make up on only half the face. Similarly, the patient may have great difficulty appropriately orienting clothing. For example, turning a shirt haphazardly, the patient may place one arm (usually the right) in the sleeve and then stop, as if finished.

The Evaluation Of Apraxic Syndromes

A systematic approach starts with asking the patient to perform a motor activity. The examiner must be assured that the patient can understand the task and understands the components that must be moved. For example, "Show me your hand." The evaluation proceeds by increasing the abstraction and/or increasing the steps involved in the command. For example, "Show me how you would salute," or "Touch your right hand to your left shoulder while keeping your eyes closed."

Other forms of systematic evaluation include asking the patient how he would perform some activity like flipping a coin, or lighting a cigar. The task difficulty decreases with the introduction of the object. Presumably additional visual and proprioceptive cues facilitate performance. A list of typical buccofacial commands includes: stick out your tongue, drink through a straw, blow out a match. A typical list for limb commands include: "Show me your hand (finger), hammer a nail, comb your hair, brush your teeth, kick a football." And for whole body commands: "Stand up, turn around twice, bow, stand like a golfer."

DEMENTIAS

Dementia is a general term that refers to the progressive global decline of cognitive abilities. This decline eventually includes attention, memory, insight, and judgment. Affect is also altered, and personal and social behaviors deteriorate progressively with cognitive function. The onset and progression may be rapid or insidious, and the condition may result from a wide range of diseases. Because the presentation and progression of a dementia is not the same for all types of brain injury, it is more accurate to say dementias, a plural term, rather than dementia, a singular one. In the following section, the clinical presentation of several of the most frequent dementing diseases will be discussed, as will the problem of making the differential diagnosis of dementia versus pseudo-dementia.

Differential Diagnosis Of The Dementias

Cerebral Neuronal Atrophy

In diseases such as Alzheimer's disease and Pick's disease cerebral neuronal atrophy is the cause of dementia. Wells reviewed 222 cases of dementia from several published series and found that cerebral atrophy of unknown cause was the established diagnosis in 51 percent of this group. Vascular disease, alcoholism, and normal pressure hydrocephalus were the next most frequently established diagnoses, each with an incidence of less than 10 percent.[17]

In this most frequent of dementing diseases, the early signs are subtle, and the changes in cognitive function and affect may be similar to those seen in depression. In the earliest stages of the disease, the patient may seek medical help for vague psychosomatic complaints or minor illness. The patient typically maintains language skills at the conversational level, and normal social behavior early in the course. The decline in higher intellectual function is often first noted by a family member, friend, or business associate. The patient often will deny any cognitive impairment, and will attempt to conceal his or her deficits by attempting to change the subject on which a difficult question is based, or resisting further questioning. There is little or no insight into the nature or extent of the cognitive decline.

The patient, or more likely the patient's family, friends, or business associates, may complain of a marked increase in forgetfulness. Familiar and new names, appointments, the content of conversations, are frequently forgotten. Confusion may occur easily when the patient is faced with a moderately difficult task. When the patient tries to carry out a complex task, a single component may be carried out properly with the other parts confused or forgotten. Family members or business associates may note that the patient repeatedly asks the same question, forgetting both the answer and the fact that the question was asked. Orientation may be impaired, and the patient may become confused in familiar surroundings, lose his sense of direction, and become lost traveling to or from work or shopping.

The patient with early dementia often shows a decrease in initiative, some withdrawal from social situations, and decreased attentiveness to routine tasks and recreational pursuits. For example, checking accounts and bills may be ignored, even when the situation leads to problems with creditors and collection agencies. Patients may go through the motions of reading a newspaper or book without actually reading: questions about content will be responded to with vague answers or confabulation. Previously important forms of exercise or hobbies may be neglected.

Affect of the dementing patient is shallow and labile: minor events may trigger inappropriate tears or laughter. Family members with close contact with the patient often describe his or her behavior as childlike and overly dependent. This childlike quality to the behavior occurs not only in their affect, but in their judgment and critical thinking as well. The emotional and cognitive deficits tend to become greater later in the day.

In the more advanced stages of dementia due to cerebral atrophy, there is a further decline in cognitive function, especially memory. Other marked disorders in cortical function such as aphasia or apraxia may occur. There is a progressive loss of normal social behavior, and a decrease in personal hygiene. Patients may refuse to bathe, may clothe themselves in a bizarre fashion, or may be unable to dress themselves.

The progression of dementia in diseases of cerebral atrophy is generally slow, with no clear time of onset. However, in some instances, the onset may appear to be acute, especially in older patients, when there is a marked progression following febrile illness, a change in dose or new medication, or a significant alteration in the patient's personal or social environment. Such alterations are usually highly stressful: loss of a job, death of a spouse, withdrawal of family support. Often in such instances, a detailed history will reveal cognitive decline that predates the event that precipitated decompensation.

Multi-Infarct Dementia

This condition produces cognitive loss with an abrupt onset, which is accompanied by focal signs of the precipitating vascular event, and/or the residua from previous strokes. The progression of this dementia follows a stuttering course with stepwise declines. The characteristics of this dementia are typically much like those of the dementias due to cerebral atrophy, a fact that has led to the over-diagnosis of multi-infarct dementia. The history, and the signs and symptoms of vascular disease, rather than performance on mental status exams, should be used to distinguish multi-infarct dementia from the dementia in diseases such as Alzheimer's.

Normal Pressure Hydrocephalus

Normal pressure hydrocephalus typically presents with a triad of symptoms: gait disorder, cognitive decline, sphincter incontinence. The progression of this dementia may be similar to that of the dementia due to cerebral atrophy, but is typically more rapid.

In the early stages of this dementia, apathy and a loss of spontaneity are more striking than is the cognitive decline. The relatively mild cognitive decline is not as dramatic as the gait disorder. In the early stages of this disease, the abnormality has been characterized as a slowing rather than a loss of mental function. Because of the mental slowing, performance on neuropsychological tasks may be impaired, but this often reflects the long

time it takes patients to complete a task, rather than the complete inability
to do so.

Dementia Due to Intracranial Tumor

This is not a specific syndrome, but rather refers to the fact that changes
in cognition, personality and memory may occur with intracranial mass
lesions. Such changes in mental status frequently result from tumors involving the frontal and temporal lobes, fourth ventricle, and the corpus callosum.
Changes in mental status due to intracranial tumor may precede focal neurological signs, headache, or seizure.

Alcoholic Dementia

Alcoholic dementia is another non-specific syndrome that refers to changes
in personality and emotional control, and a decline in cognitive function,
especially memory. In most cases, these changes in mental status reflect
the Wernicke-Korsakoff's syndrome.

The Evaluation Of Dementia

The information necessary for establishing the diagnosis of dementia will
come from the patient's history, the history provided by family or associates,
and formal mental status testing. A significant portion of the information
about cognitive, social, and emotional changes in dementia will be obtained
from the history. Because of the demented patient's lack of insight and
tendency to confabulate early in the disease's progression, it is extremely
important to obtain separate histories from the patient, and from his or
her family or friends, whenever possible. When examined for orientation,
for example, the demented patient may provide a home address that is
20 or 30 years old. Such a response not only indicates disorientation, but
also suggests that remote memories are more intact than recent memories.

Several aspects of the general history are important in the evaluation
of dementia. The patient should be queried about possible changes in his
or her performance at work, home, and in other contexts such as social
groups and recreational activities. Have changes in attention, memory, and
initiative occurred? Has the patient become depressed, or emotionally labile? Have the patient's personal habits changed?

In addition to the history, the patient should be examined for orientation,
cognitive control, and memory. As described in the previous sections in
this chapter, the patient should be examined for orientation to person, time
and place. Cognitive control can be examined using tasks such as serial
sevens, repetition of the alphabet, etc. Memory should be tested for both
remote and recent forms. New learning should be tested by the recall of
three items after 5 minutes. If questions about the patient's language func-

tion arise during the exam, language should be evaluated using the previously described procedure.

Finally, it is generally useful to obtain a more formal evaluation of cognitive status by obtaining a formal neuropsychological examination of the patient. This will provide quantitative indices of verbal and non-verbal function in areas such as problem-solving and memory. In addition to demonstrating areas of impairment, and providing estimates of how the patient's performance on cognitive testing compares with the performance of others in the patient's age group, formal testing may also be useful in establishing whether the patient's deficits appear consistently across different tests of comparable function. The determination of consistency is often helpful in distinguishing between dementia and pseudodementia.

Dementia Versus Pseudodementia

Pseudodementia is a condition in which the changes in cognitive function and affect observed in dementia are mimicked by a functional psychiatric illness, commonly depression. The presentations of dementia and pseudodementia can be similar, and the diagnosis of pseudodementia is often made only after a patient makes an unexpected recovery or fails to progress. There are, however, several behavioral characteristics that are useful in differentiating between dementia and pseudodementia. The major points are summarized in Table 12.10.

Beginning with the history, the patient with pseudodementia will typically respond to open-ended questions in a coherent manner. They may provide

Table 12.10 Useful Characteristics in the Differential Diagnosis of Dementia versus Pseudodementia

Characteristic	Dementia	Pseudodementia
Source of complaint of cognitive decline	Noted by family, friends, or business associates	Noted by patient who describes dysfunction in detail
Compensation for deficits	Attempted	Not attempted
Response to content questions	Near-miss answers, patient attempts to hide disorder	"Don't know" answers, no attempt to hide disorder
Response to open-ended questions	Often coherent, accurate	Vague, rambling
Memory	Memory loss is a major finding; recent memory more impaired than remote memory	Memory loss is one of many complaints, recent and remote memory equally impaired
Neuropsychological profile	Consistent impairments across comparable tests	Inconsistent impairments across comparable tests.
Affect	Shallow and labile	Depressed, anxious
Previous psychiatric history	Uncommon	Common

a specific point of onset for their difficulties, accurately describe a temporal sequence of events in their history, and be logical about specific complaints. Although the patient may report lapses in attention and concentration, such lapses may not be evident in their responses to open-ended questions. As noted in the previous section, the demented patient will give a vague history, and usually attempt to hide cognitive deficits.

On higher intellectual function testing, patients with pseudodementia will frequently give negative responses: "I don't know" or "I can't remember." The patient may make little effort to think of the correct answer, and similarly, may make little effort to hide his or her dysfunction. The demented patient does not typically provide negative responses, but may produce "near miss" answers or confabulation. Further, although there may be an effort to hide cognitive deficits, the demented patient gives no evidence of insight into his or her problem. For example, when asked what brings him or her to the doctor, the demented patient may respond by claiming that the visit was for a routine exam for work, insurance purposes, or for some physical complaint.

Both patients with dementia and pseudodementia present with memory problems. A number of investigators, however, have noted that failing memory is rarely the chief complaint of patients with pseudodementia. In dementing illness, failing memory is typically the complaint of the relatives or associates of the demented patient. As with other aspects of the histories, patients with pseudodementias often provide great detail about their memory loss, demented patients do not. Pseudodementia typically presents with an equal loss of recent and remote memory, while in dementia recent memory is more impaired than remote memory.

On formal neuropsychological testing, the profile of the patient with pseudodementia may indicate inconsistent performance. Test scores may be low on one test of a particular function, but normal on another test of the same function. Demented patients, on the other hand, perform more consistently, showing comparable deficits on neuropsychological tests of comparable difficulty.

Affect may also aid in the differential diagnosis. Whereas both patients with dementia and pseudodementia may present with depression, patients with pseudodementia do not have the shallowness and lability of affect typically seen in demented patients. The patient with pseudodementia frequently shows signs of anxiety.

Other characteristics that have been suggested as useful in this differential diagnosis are the duration of illness prior to medical evaluation, and a personal or family history of psychiatric illness. In some series, patients with pseudodementia seek medical help much sooner than do patients with dementia. It has also been suggested that although a prior history of psychiatric illness is rare in dementia, it is common in pseudodementia. For a more detailed treatment of the differential between dementia and pseudodementia, see Wells and Nott and Fleminger.[11,18]

REFERENCES

1. Benson, D.F.: Aphasia Alexia and Agraphia. Churchill Livingstone, New York, 1979.
2. Critchley, M.: The Parietal Lobes. Edward Arnold and Company, London, 1953.
3. Darley, F.L., Aronson, A.E., Brown, J.R.: Motor Speech Disorders. W.B. Saunders Co., Philadelphia, 1975.
4. Dysken, M.W., Chang, S.S., Casper, R.C., Davis, J.M.: Barbiturate-facilitated interviewing. Biol. Psychol., 14: 421, 1979.
5. Gerson, S.N., Benson, D.F., Frazier, S.H.: Diagnosis: schizophrenic versus posterior aphasia. Am. J. Psych., 134: 966, 1977.
6. Geschwind, N.: The Apraxias: neural mechanisms of disorders of learned movement. American Scientist, 63: 188, 1975.
7. Lazare, A.: Conversion Symptoms. N. Engl. J. Med., 305: 745, 1981.
8. Lipowski, Z.J.: Delirium. Charles C. Thomas, Springfield, 1980, pp. 41–59.
9. Luria, A.S.: Higher Cortical Function in Man. 2nd Ed. Basic Books, Inc., New York, 1980, pp. 246–365.
10. McEvoy, J.P.: Organic brain syndromes. Ann. Int. Med., 95: 212, 1981.
11. Nott, P.N., Fleminger, J.J.: Presenile dementia: the difficulties of early diagnosis. Acta Psychiat. Scand., 51: 210, 1975.
12. Rasmussen, T., Milner, B.: The role of early left-brain injury in determining lateralization of cerebral speech functions. In Diamond, S.J., Blizard, D.A., eds., Evolution and Lateralization of the Brain. Ann. N.Y. Acad. Sci. 299: 355, 1977.
13. Slater, E.T.O., Glithero, E.: A follow-up of patients diagnosed as suffering from "hysteria." J. Psychosom. Res., 9: 9, 1965.
14. Slater, E.: Diagnosis of "Hysteria." Brit. Med. M., 1: 1395, 1965.
15. Volpe, B.T., Sidtis, J.J., Holtzman, J.D., Wilson, D.H., Gazzaniga, M.S.: Cortical mechanisms involved in praxis: observations following partial and complete section of the corpus callosum in man. Neurol. 32:645, 1982.
16. Weinstein, E.A., Friedland, R.P. (eds.): Hemi-inattention and hemisphere specialization. Advances in Neurology. Vol. 18. Raven Press, New York, 1977.
17. Wells, C.E.: Diagnostic evaluation and treatment in dementia. In Wells, C.E., ed.: Dementia. 2nd Ed., F.A. Davis, Philadelphia, 1977.
18. Wells, C.E.: Pseudodementia. Am. J. Psych., 136: 895, 1979.

13

Diagnosis and Treatment of Spinal Cord Compression and Acute Myelopathy

S. Clifford Schold, Jr., M.D.

INTRODUCTION

The spinal cord, which extends from the foramen magnum to approximately the level of the L_1 vertebra, transmits information between the brain and the periphery and mediates the sensation and motor activity of the body. The collection of lumbar and sacral roots, known as the cauda equina, extends to the bottom of the spinal canal at the level of the upper sacral vertebrae, and in this chapter these roots, technically a part of the peripheral nervous system, will be considered with the spinal cord. The entire cord is surrounded by the vertebrae which afford it protection but also limit its ability to tolerate deforming forces. The cord is also encircled by meninges, including the tough dura mater, and by a substantial epidural space, which normally contains only fat and venous networks.

Dysfunction of the spinal cord produces characteristic signs and symptoms precisely related to the location of the pathological process. Early diagnosis of reversible spinal cord disorders is essential to avoid permanent damage because structural damage is likely to resolve incompletely even if the underlying process is eradicated. Besides trauma, the spinal cord is susceptible to a wide variety of acute disturbances, including those of vascular, inflammatory, and neoplastic origin.

DIAGNOSTIC APPROACH

History

Patients with spinal cord disorders complain of some combination of pain, weakness, numbness or paresthesias, and autonomic symptoms. Motor or sensory symptoms are often worse or present only in the lower extremities, with involvement of the upper extremities dependent on a lesion extending into the cervical cord. The symptoms may be acute, subacute, or chronic, and the duration of symptoms provides a clue about their likely rate of progression, although precipitous deterioration can occur even in a patient whose symptoms have been quite indolent.

The nature and location of back pain associated with non-traumatic spinal cord disorders varies with the cause. Cord compression syndromes produce sharp pain commonly localized to the level of involvement. The pain may be radicular, following the course of affected root fibers, or it may even be referred and not associated with pain in the back. Occasionally, for example, pain from a thoracic cord lesion may mimic an acute abdominal crisis. The pain from spinal cord disorders is not from tissue damage in the cord itself, since the spinal cord, like the brain, is not pain-sensitive. Rather, distortion or destruction of surrounding pain-sensitive structures, such as the dura or vertebral bodies, produces pain. Pain can be considered a clue to localization, and, to some extent, its occurrence aids the physician in making an etiologic diagnosis.

Weakness of the lower extremities is generally a straightforward symptom, but patients may occasionally refer to it as "numbness" or clumsiness. Similarly, sensory symptoms are described in many ways, but numbness, deadness, or "pins and needles" are the most common complaints. The patient can often outline the area of diminished sensation quite accurately, and it is helpful to ask him to try to do that. He may define the dermatomal level for you. Urinary urgency or incontinence is the most frequent autonomic symptom in spinal cord disease. Rarely is fecal incontinence an early symptom. Erectile dysfunction may also be a prominent symptom in chronic spinal cord compression syndromes, so that elicitation of a history of recent sexual dysfunction from a patient with a suspected acute cord syndrome may be useful.

Physical Findings

The neurological abnormalities produced by spinal cord lesions reflect both the rostral-caudal level and the transverse area of involvement of the cord. The former is considerably more important since pathologic abnormalities may be located only at a single segmental level and recognition of that level will guide the work-up and treatment. The classical signs of spinal

Table 13.1 Physical Findings in a Fully Developed Spinal Cord Syndrome

Weakness, muscle atrophy, areflexia, and hypotonia at the level of the lesion.

Weakness, spasticity, hyperactive reflexes, and other pyramidal tract signs below the level of the lesion.

Loss of appreciation of all primary sensory modalities below the level of the lesion.

Loss of sphincter control.

cord lesions include an upper motor neuron pattern of dysfunction below the level of the lesion, lower motor neuron signs at the level of the lesion, and a sharp sensory "level" at the appropriate dermatome (Table 13.1). However, there are pitfalls with each of these signs, especially with an early, incomplete lesion.

Motor System

Classical lower motor neuron signs (i.e., weakness, atrophy, diminished reflexes, and hypotonia) are present at the level of a fully developed spinal cord lesion. Upper motor neuron signs (i.e., weakness, spasticity, extensor plantar response, and hypertonia) are present below the level of such a lesion. When present, this combination of upper and lower motor neuron signs permits precise localization of the spinal cord lesion. However, in the acute or subacute situation, neither spasticity nor atrophy have developed, and their absence is of no diagnostic value. Furthermore, since most spinal cord lesions occur in the thoracic cord (because of its length) and since lower motor neuron signs are practically undetectable in thoracic myotomes, the classical combination of motor findings is often absent even in the fully developed lesion. Also, because of the spinal-shock phenomenon, deep tendon reflexes below the level of the lesion may be paradoxically depressed in the early stages of a disease process. Ankle dorsiflexor, knee flexor, and hip flexor muscle groups are preferentially weakened by upper motor neuron lesions, and a screening examination should concentrate on them. A differential effect on lower abdominal muscles over upper abdominal muscles can be detected by asking the patient to raise his head from the supine position and observing the upward movement of the umbilicus (Beevor's sign).

Sensation

In a complete spinal cord syndrome, there is a sharp segmental level of diminished sensation to all modalities. Pin sensation is the most straightforward modality for testing, but one must remember that a pin level is usually 2–3 segments below the actual level of unilateral spinal cord involvement. Abnormalities of light touch, temperature, joint position and vibratory sensation will also give information about the spinal level, although joint position can only be tested in the extremities. It can be rewarding to examine vibratory sensation in detail, even on the trunk or the vertebrae, since sensory levels will sometimes only be detectable this way.

Spinal lesions are often incomplete, and, more often than one would think, they produce evidence of cord hemisection, leading to the classical Brown-Séquard syndrome. Since at the spinal cord level the posterior column fibers are uncrossed while the spinothalamic fibers are crossed, a functional hemisection of the cord will produce an ipsilateral loss of proprioception and a contralateral loss of pain and temperature sensation (Fig. 13.1). Ipsilateral

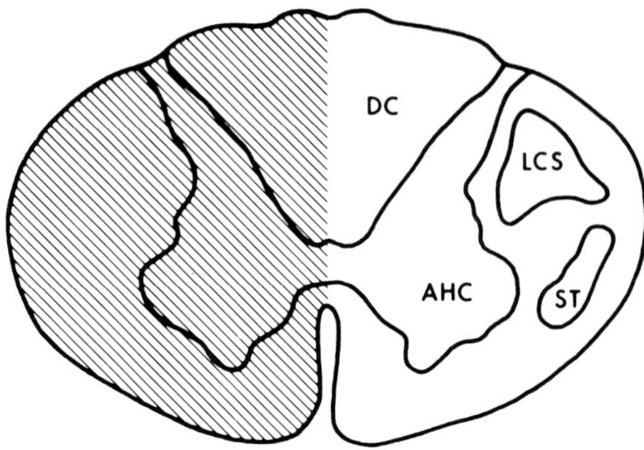

Fig. 13.1
This representation of a cross section of the spinal cord shows the effect of a cord hemisection (Brown-Séquard syndrome). The hatched area indicates the lesion. The tracts affected are the dorsal columns (DC), the lateral corticospinal tract (LCS), producing ipsilateral loss of proprioception and weakness below the level of the lesion, and the spinothalamic tract (ST), producing contralateral loss of pain and temperature sensation below the lesion. Damage to anterior horn cells (AHC) causes weakness and atrophy at the segmental level. Common causes of the Brown-Séquard syndrome include radiation myelopathy, infarction, and any subacute cord compression syndrome.

weakness is also a feature of the syndrome since the descending corticospinal fibers have already crossed. This is a characteristic pattern of spinal cord disease, and, when present, it eliminates the possibility of the responsible lesion being at other levels. As a minimum proprioception and appreciation of pin prick should be examined in both lower extremities of patients suspected of having spinal cord disease.

There are other pitfalls in the sensory examination of patients with spinal cord diseases. In early or incomplete lesions the sensory level is ill-defined and the degree of sensory loss may vary. One must appreciate the normal range of proprioception in the great toes, for example, to properly evaluate patients suspected of early cord lesions. One can also be fooled by finding a "stocking" pattern sensory loss in the lower extremities, implying a peripheral neuropathy, rather than a radicular pattern, which would suggest a cord or root lesion. A dermatomal level should descend ventrally, and the pattern should be reproducible anywhere in the dorsal-ventral axis. Finally, intrinsic lesions of the spinal cord commonly produce the phenomenon of "sacral sparing" because of the lamination of the ascending lateral spinothalamic tracts. Preserved sensation in the sacral dermatomes should not dissuade one from the diagnosis of a spinal cord lesion.

It is not necessary to commit to memory the whole dermatomal pattern of the human body, but it is useful to remember certain landmark levels. For example, C_6, C_7, and C_8 are represented in the thumb, middle finger, and little finger respectively. The nipple is at T_4, the umbilicus is at T_{10}, and the inguinal ligament is at L_1. In the lower extremities, the great toe is at L_5 and the lateral side of the foot is S_1. Also, the C_2 dermatome extends into the scalp and interfaces with the ophthalmic branch of the trigeminal nerve (there is no C_1 sensory root), and C_4 interfaces with T_2 at the clavicle.

Finally, the sensory examination is undoubtedly the most difficult part of the neurological examination. Techniques vary, patients are highly suggestible, and more attention is required to examine sensation. It is often a critical part of the examination, but subtle and inconsistent findings should not be over-interpreted.

Miscellaneous Signs

Other signs of spinal cord disease can be valuable. With compressive lesions, especially tumors and abscesses, there is frequently point tenderness over the affected vertebral spinous process, and sharp percussion of the spine will often localize the pathology. In patients with high cervical spine disease, percussion over the vertex of the skull will also often reproduce the neck pain. Rectal sphincter tone is often diminished in spinal cord lesions, and, again, one needs to have an appreciation of the acceptable normal range of sphincter tone. Mechanical signs, such as pain produced by elevating the extended leg, indicate spinal disease, especially conditions affecting the leptomeninges.

Diagnostic Tests

The definitive diagnostic test for suspected spinal cord disease is myelography. Various less invasive tests are frequently employed first in the evaluation of such patients, but in the acute situation urgent myelography may be indicated. The radiologist must be made aware of the diagnostic possibilities since his techniques will be affected. Specifically, if there is any suspicion of a complete block to the flow of contrast material, only a small amount (1–3 ml) is injected. If there is free flow the usual amount of dye is then injected and a more definitive study is undertaken. If there is a complete block, the upper level of the block must be defined (Fig. 13.2). To do this, a lateral C_1–C_2 puncture is made under fluoroscopic control, and contrast material is injected and allowed to gravitate to the level of the block. Myelography can be uncomfortable, but, in experienced hands, it is safe and it settles any questions about an obstructive lesion.

When possible, cerebrospinal fluid (CSF) obtained at the time of myelography should be sent for detailed analysis. Obstructive lesions commonly produce an elevated CSF protein concentration (sometimes exceeding 1 gm/ dl) below the block, but the fluid is usually normal otherwise. However, the possibilities of both microorganisms and tumor cells should be ruled out by examination of available CSF.

Plain radiograms of the spine can also be useful diagnostically. Metastatic tumors producing spinal cord compression will generally produce destructive lesions of the vertebral body. Abscesses may do the same, but infection more often involves the disc space or the epidural space sparing the vertebrae. Intradural tumors, such as meningiomas and neurofibromas, commonly produce radiographic abnormalities, such as widening of the spinal canal,

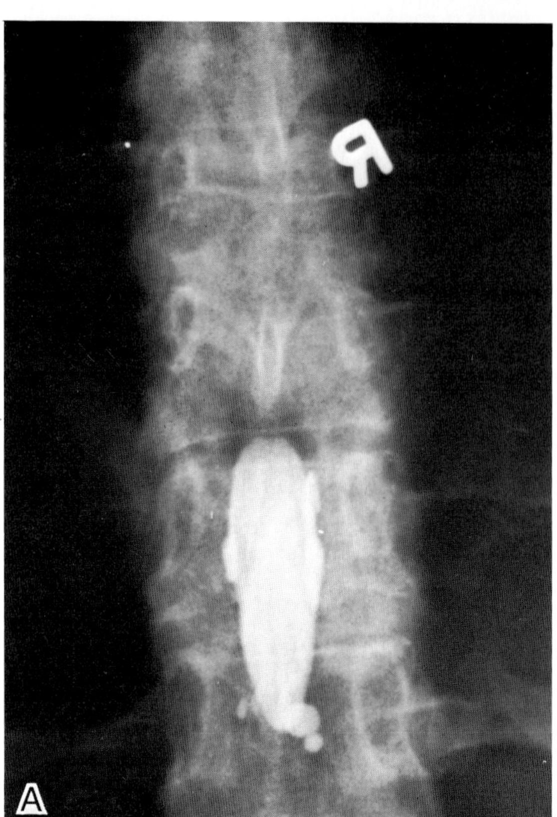

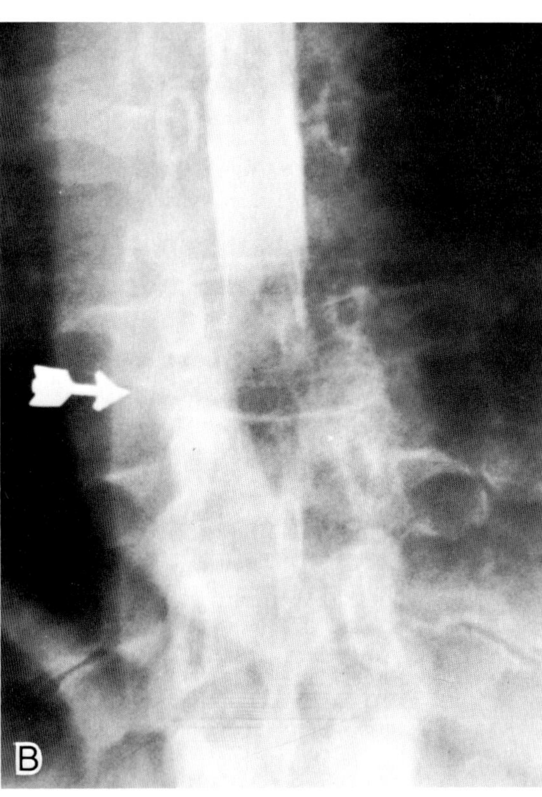

Fig. 13.2
Positive contrast myelogram in a patient with epidural spinal cord compression from metastatic cancer. (A) A complete block to the flow of contrast one vertebral segment below the vertebral body metastasis (the patient's head is at the top, and he is tilted head-down). (B) The contrast material has been injected at C_1–C_2. There is a complete block to the descending flow of contrast at the site of metastasis. In cases of complete block, if radiation therapy is to be used, it is imperative to define the full extent of the lesion by this method.

hyperostosis, or bone erosion. Of course, normal radiograms of the spine should not dissuade one from further investigation if a cord syndrome is suspected.

Computerized tomography (CT scan) of the spine is currently being evaluated in many medical centers for diagnosing spinal lesions. Myelography using a water soluble contrast material (metrizamide-Amipaque) and conventional X-ray technology shows excellent detail of spinal cord and nerve root anatomy. Combining metrizamide myelography with CT scan technology may further enhance our ability to visualize spinal lesions. However, the value and safety of metrizamide and CT scanning in the emergency setting has not been fully proven.

ACUTE SPINAL CORD COMPRESSION SYNDROMES

Conditions of diverse origin produce acute or subacute compression of the spinal cord. They have in common the potential for rapid neurological deterioration, abnormal myelograms, and the need for prompt therapeutic intervention.

Metastatic Epidural Neoplasm

Among the most common causes of an acute spinal cord syndrome is a metastatic epidural tumor. Such a lesion typically occurs in a patient with known systemic cancer, but it can be the first manifestation of a metastatic tumor. Any tumor that spreads to bone can produce this syndrome since the neurological abnormalities are almost always secondary to an expanding mass in the vertebral body compressing the spinal cord.[12] Lung and breast cancer, lymphoma, and carcinoma of the prostate are the most common offenders (Table 13.2).

Virtually all of these patients have back pain, often severe, at the time of their evaluation. The pain may have been present for days or even weeks before neurological symptoms have developed, but once these symptoms are present, progression can be rapid. In addition to the physical evidence of spinal cord dysfunction, there is often marked tenderness over the spinous process of the involved vertebra. Plain radiograms of the spine are abnormal in the vast majority of patients, showing destructive lesions of the vertebrae, but in the acute situation plain films may be unnecessary. The diagnosis is made definitively by myelogram, and, as discussed above, it is imperative that the radiologist know that a complete block is possible and that the techniques be adjusted accordingly. If a complete block is present and radiation is to be employed for therapy, both the upper and lower limits of the block must be defined to guide the radiotherapist. Once the diagnosis is established, or even before, if suspicion is high enough, corticosteroids, conventionally dexamethasone, are administered systemically. The optimal

**Table 13.2 Primary Tumors in 318 Cases
of Metastatic Epidural Spinal Cord
Compression**

Primary Tumor	Number of Cases (%)
Breast	69 (21.7)
Lung	41 (12.9)
Lymphoma/myeloma	38 (11.9)
Prostate	33 (10.4)
Kidney	20 (6.3)
Head and Neck	19 (6.0)
Bowel	15 (4.7)
Melanoma	13 (4.1)
Others	70 (22.0)

(from Gilbert, R.W., Kim, J.H., Posner, J.B.: Epidural spinal cord compression from metastatic tumor: diagnosis and treatment. Ann. Neurol., 3:40, 1978; and Greenberg, H.S., Kim, J.H., Posner, J.B.: Epidural spinal cord compression from metastatic tumor: result with a new treatment protocol. Ann. Neurol., 8:361, 1980; reprinted with permission.)

dose is unknown, but in many centers specializing in the treatment of cancer up to 100 mg of dexamethasone is given intravenously. This usually brings rapid relief of the pain, and it may improve neurological function substantially, but the effects are transient. More definitive oncolytic therapy, usually radiation, is then employed. Treatment success in this increasingly common clinical problem is directly related to the patient's clinical status at diagnosis. In one series, 75 percent of patients with this disease who were ambulatory at diagnosis remained ambulatory after therapy, compared to 45 percent of patients who were paraparetic and 5 percent of those who were paraplegic (Table 13.3).[10] Reported therapeutic results are generally better in surgically treated patients, undoubtedly because more favorable patients are operated on. Overall therapeutic success is much more strongly correlated with the patient's condition than with the choice of treatment. Accepted indications for surgical intervention in this disease include lack of a known primary tumor, deterioration despite maximum medical therapy, and recurrent epidural tumor after maximum radiation has been administered. In other circumstances, surgery can generally be avoided.

Spinal Epidural Abscess

Abscesses are important causes of compressive spinal cord syndromes because of their reversibility. Causes include bacterial, fungal, and parasitic infections. They are often associated with evidence of systemic infection,

Table 13.3 Therapeutic Results in Metastatic Epidural Spinal Cord Compression

Pretreatment Condition	Surgery + Radiation		Radiation Alone	
	Number Ambulatory / Number Treated (%)		Number Ambulatory / Number Treated (%)	
Ambulatory	14/22	(64)	46/58	(79)
Paraparetic	15/33	(45)	37/83	(45)
Paraplegic	1/10	(10)	1/29	(3)
Total	30/65	(46)	84/170	(49)

(from Gilbert, R.W., Kim, J.H., Posner, J.B.: Epidural spinal cord compression from metastatic tumor: diagnosis and treatment. Ann. Neurol., 3:40, 1978; reprinted with permission.)

but they may occur with no active systemic disease. The exact etiologic diagnosis can usually only be determined by culture of the aspirated material. Bacterial abscesses are most common, and Staphylococcus aureus is the most common organism. Many of these abscesses are associated with bacteremia, and, curiously, many are associated with recent mild, non-penetrating back injuries. Kaufman, et al [19] suggested that this association was due to the production of "devitalized" tissue by the injury. Other associations include any causes of bacteremia, including skin or subcutaneous infection, dental work, and endocarditis. An occasional patient will develop disc space infection following laminectomy. Infection may also be introduced into the epidural space by lumbar puncture through infected skin.

Most patients with epidural bacterial abscesses have back pain and generalized signs of infection, such as fever and leukocytosis. Often plain X-rays of the spine reveal disc space infection that may extend into the adjacent vertebral bodies. Normal X-rays, however, should not sway one from the diagnosis; in Kaufman's series nearly half of the patients had no abnormalities on plain X-rays of the spine. In these cases the infection is confined to the epidural space, usually posteriorly. The diagnosis of a compressive mass lesion is established by myelography and the CSF obtained during the myelogram should be examined and cultured since there may be concurrent bacterial meningitis (5/19 cases in Kaufman's series). Both definitive diagnosis and treatment are surgical, with post-operative antibiotic therapy essential. The prospect for recovery after surgical drainage is related both to the overall condition of the patient (e.g., older patients do worse) and to the degree of neurological disability at the time of surgery. As in other cord compressive syndromes, early diagnosis is vital if neurological function is to be preserved.

A variety of other microorganisms can infect the vertebral bodies and epidural space, especially in immunocompromised hosts. Echinococcus, brucellosis, actinomycosis, nocardiosis, cryptococcosis, blastomyocosis, and aspergillosis have all been reported to produce myelopathy by compression due to expansion of an epidural infection. Surgical drainage and culture are required to choose appropriate antibiotic therapy.

Patients with tuberculous spondylitis (Pott's disease) may develop myelopathy as the infection progresses.[11] Back pain is almost invariably present, and essentially all patients will have radiographic evidence of infection (Fig. 13.3). Evidence of systemic illness is less common, however, as the minority of patients are febrile, few have leukocytosis, and less than half have evidence of active tuberculosis at another site. This disease most often presents as a chronic, rather than an acute, neurological condition, although the myelopathy may progress rapidly. Treatment is surgical drainage and antituberculous chemotherapy.

Spinal Epidural Hematoma

A hematoma in the epidural space is another important cause of spinal cord compression. Many cases are spontaneous and idiopathic,[6] vascular malformations may be at fault in some cases, and systemic anti-coagulation has become an important cause of this syndrome in recent years.[14] Whatever the cause, patients present with sudden or rapidly progressive, localized back pain that soon develops into a spinal cord compression syndrome. The diagnosis can be suspected if the patient is on anticoagulants or, rarely, if there is a history of cutaneous angiomas,[8] but myelography is required. The treatment is surgical, and its success is related to the extent of disability when treatment is instituted.[23] Corticosteroids probably also protect the cord to some degree. Rarely, surgery may be contraindicated, and a relatively intact patient can be treated conservatively.[14]

Symptomatic spinal subdural hematoma may be produced by lumbar

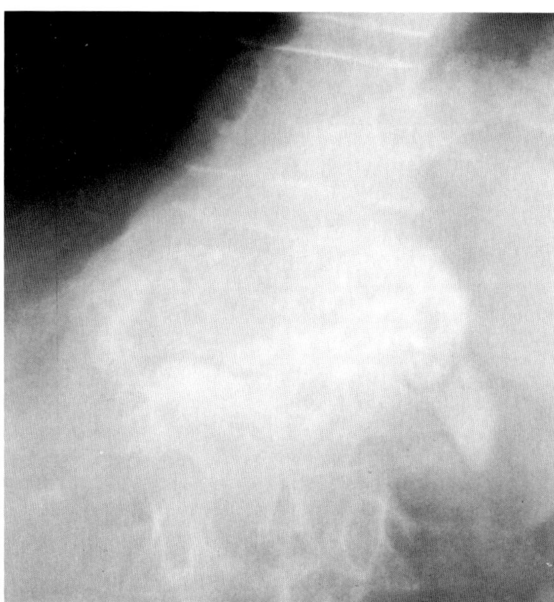

Fig. 13.3
Plain radiogram in a case of tuberculous spondylitis (Pott's disease). There is destruction and extensive calcification at T_{10-11}. There was an associated complete epidural block due to extension of the abscess.

puncture in thrombocytopenic patients.[7] Back pain and paraparesis develop within hours of the procedure in such cases. The role of surgical intervention is unclear, but it is clear that lumbar puncture should be performed very cautiously or not at all in patients with serious clotting deficiencies.

Herniated Disc

While the most common clinical syndromes produced by ruptured intervertebral discs are painful root syndromes, occasionally such lesions will produce acute myelopathies (Fig. 13.4). Herniated disc syndromes are most common in men in the fourth to sixth decades of life. Rupture of a thoracic disc produces pain in the back at the appropriate level, but root signs are minimal.[4] Paraparesis may be acute or subacute in onset. Herniation of a cervical disc usually at the C_6, C_7, or C_8 root levels, produces radicular pain and root signs and symptoms at the appropriate level. A midline disc may compress the spinal cord, especially in patients with congenitally nar-

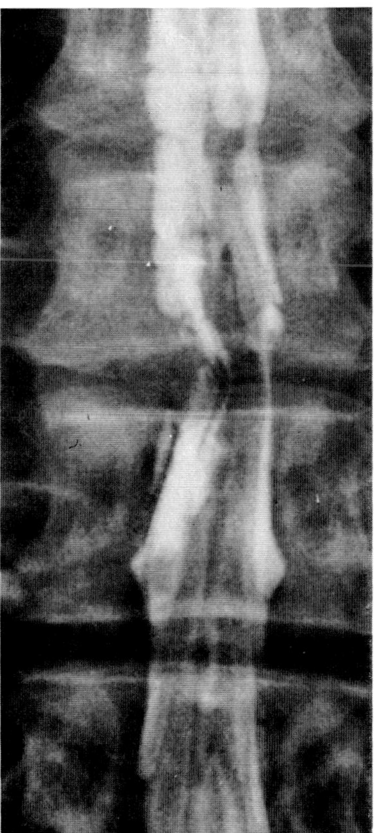

Fig. 13.4 Myelogram in a case of spinal cord compression produced by a herniated thoracic disc. The flow of contrast is interrupted by the disc, and the spinal cord is displaced.

row spinal canals.[26] If signs of cord compression are present, immediate surgical treatment of a ruptured disc is indicated.

Primary Spinal Cord Tumors

The most common intradural neoplasms affecting the spinal cord are meningioma, neurofibroma, hemangioblastoma, ependymoma, and astrocytoma. In most instances, these are relatively slow-growing tumors that produce insidiously progressive symptoms. Rarely, they may either present as a sudden acute cord syndrome, or sudden deterioration may punctuate a recent history of gradual cord dysfunction. This sudden deterioration is thought to be due to hemorrhage related to the tumor, and it occurs most often with ependymomas of the cauda equina.[24] The clinical picture may be confusing since subarachnoid blood can produce headache and altered mental status, obscuring the initial complaint of back pain. As in other acute spinal cord syndromes, myelography is required for diagnosis, and surgical resection is usually attempted. However, conventional pantopaque myelography should never be done when blood is present in the CSF. Blood and pantopaque combine to cause a high incidence of post-myelography arachnoiditis. The myelogram should be delayed until the blood has cleared or another contrast agent should be used.

ACUTE NON-COMPRESSIVE SPINAL CORD SYNDROMES

These conditions are distinguished from the compressive spinal cord syndromes because they are more often associated with normal or minimally abnormal myelograms and because neither urgent surgical nor radiotherapeutic intervention is indicated. However, many are treatable, and early diagnosis can be just as vital.

Acute Transverse Myelitis

Transverse myelitis, or myelopathy, refers to a symptom complex produced by a non-compressive, non-traumatic, complete transverse lesion of the spinal cord at any level. All motor and sensory functions below the level of the lesion are lost, and there may also be acute autonomic failure. Its known associations are extensive (Table 13.4), but in most cases it is not associated with any known underlying disease. Patients with the idiopathic condition present with a history of a few hours to a few days of initially patchy dysfunction, which rapidly progresses to a complete loss of function. There may be local pain, but pain is usually not a prominent complaint. It was present in 34 percent of 62 cases reviewed by Berman, et al [2] and in 35 percent of 52 patients in the series reported by Ropper and Poskanzer.[28] Physical findings depend on the level of the lesion, and there may be a "spinal shock" picture with flaccid paralysis initially.

**Table 13.4 Conditions Associated with Acute
Transverse Myelitis**

I. Infections
   A. Herpes zoster
   B. Bacterial meningitis
   C. Post-infectious and post-vaccination encephalomyelitis
   D. Syphilis
   E. Other virus infections
II. Vascular Conditions
   A. Aortic aneurysm
   B. Atherosclerotic infarction
   C. Abdominal aorta surgery
   D. Sickle cell disease
   E. Lupus erythematosus
   F. Periarteritis nodosa
   G. Arteriovenous malformation
III. Miscellaneous
   A. Therapeutic irradiation
   B. Multiple sclerosis
   C. Hematomyelia
   D. Acute necrotic myelopathy
IV. Toxins
   A. Intrathecal injections
      1. Chemotherapeutic agents
      2. Contrast media
      3. Anesthetics
   B. Arsenic

The diagnosis can be made only after a compressive lesion of the spinal cord has been ruled out by myelography, and the underlying cause must be pursued, although it is often elusive. The CSF is often abnormal with lymphocytic pleocytosis and mild elevation of the protein concentration. The prognosis for good functional recovery in those patient without known underlying disease is variable. In Berman's series, 22 of 59 patients (37 percent) had good recovery within 3 months of onset, and Lipton and Teasdall reported that one-third of a series of 29 adults with acute transverse myelopathy had good functional recovery.[21] Ropper and Poskanzer reported good or fair outcome in 28 of 48 patients (79 percent). They also found that the potential for recovery was inversely related to the initial rate of progression at the onset of the disease.[28] Corticosteroids are often used in this disease, but no controlled trial of their efficacy has been undertaken.

Radiation Myelopathy

Radiation myelopathy is becoming increasingly common as more success in the treatment of cancer is achieved. The typical patient has received radiation in a field encompassing the spinal cord at a level corresponding to the current symptoms at least 6 months before presentation.[20] The spinal cord will tolerate 4000–5000 rads in conventional fractions, but higher doses pose significant risk. Most commonly, the radiation has been at the upper

Table 13.5 The Clinical Distinction Between Radiation Myelopathy and Recurrent Neoplasm

	Radiation Myelopathy	Recurrent Tumor
Pain	Minimal	Prominent
Radiographic evidence of metastatic vertebral disease	Variable	Very common
Clinical transverse myelopathy	Present	Present
Progression of symptoms	Usually weeks or months	Often hours or days, but may be longer
Myelogram	Usually normal, cord may be swollen	Extradural block
CSF	Mild protein elevation, pleocytosis	Moderate to marked protein elevation, otherwise normal
Reversibility	Variable, but usually poor	Potentially reversible, but must be diagnosed early

thoracic level for Hodgkin's disease or lung cancer. Cervical levels produced by radiation for head and neck tumors and low thoracic or lumbar levels from abdominal irradiation also occur. The syndrome is usually painless and progressive over weeks. A benign syndrome of an isolated Lhermitte's sign (a shock-like sensation down the spine produced by neck flexion) occurs commonly during or shortly after radiation to the cervical cord. It is not accompanied by abnormal physical findings and has no prognostic importance. The diagnosis of radiation myelopathy cannot be made unless it is certain that the radiation encompassed the spinal cord level in question and unless a compressive lesion from the underlying malignancy has been ruled out. Myelography may show an enlarged cord, but it is usually normal, and the CSF protein concentration may be elevated. However, the diagnosis is difficult to establish with certainty in life. The principal consideration in the differential diagnosis is tumor (Table 13.5). The condition may arrest spontaneously before a complete transverse lesion develops. In other cases the administration of corticosteroids appears to have halted the progressive neurological picture. In most cases, however, treatment is ineffective and progression is inexorable.

Multiple Sclerosis

Multiple sclerosis (MS) is a common neurological illness with diverse signs and symptoms. A classical, although uncommon, early sign of MS is an acute transverse myelopathy. When combined with optic neuritis, this syndrome is known as neuromyelitis optica or Devic's disease. While some authors consider this complex a distinct clinical entity, most now consider it an MS variant. Neuromyelitis optica is significantly more common in Japan than in the United States.

Transverse myelitis in MS, with or without optic neuritis, produces a characteristic clinical picture. It is most common at thoracic levels and may be heralded by back pain. Numbness of the lower extremities ensues, followed in hours to days by weakness of the lower extremities and by urinary retention. In the early stages of the illness, the spinal level is ill-defined, and, in fact, there may be a zone of hyperesthesia (excessive or painful reaction to tactile stimuli) at the level of the lesion. As in other acute spinal cord lesions, upper motor neuron signs may not be present initially. Signs and symptoms may progress longitudinally, so that, for example, a patient with a thoracic level transverse myelitis may develop paresthesias and weakness in the hands as the lesion extends rostrally. While spinal cord signs and symptoms are common in MS, an acute myelopathy is an uncommon method of presentation of the illness, and a relatively small number of patients with acute transverse myelopathy subsequently develop typical MS. In Berman's series only 1 of 59 patients presenting with an acute unexplained myelopathy developed MS, while Ropper and Poskanzer reported that 7 of 52 patients (13 percent) with acute transverse myelopathy later developed typical MS.

The diagnosis cannot be established with certainty, and a mass lesion must be ruled out by myelography. However, even this can be confusing since an acute myelitis can produce a swollen spinal cord giving the impression of intrinsic tumor (Fig. 13.5). Surgery is occasionally required to establish the diagnosis. The CSF in acute transverse myelitis from MS may show an increase in numbers of inflammatory cells and an elevated protein concentration, but the glucose concentration is normal.

The course of the illness is unpredictable. In many cases complete recovery occurs over weeks or months. Others improve but are left with residual neurological dysfunction. A certain percentage of patients never improve. One cannot make a diagnosis of MS based on a single attack of transverse myelitis. Preceeding or subsequent attacks causing symptoms or signs at other levels of the neuraxis are required. There is no solid evidence that the prognosis for patients with MS who suffer an attack of transverse myelitis differs from that of other MS patients.

Post-Infectious Encephalomyelitis

Acute disseminated encephalomyelitis is an obscure illness that can follow exanthematous viral illnesses, vaccinations, or non-specific virus infections. Occasionally, this illness will preferentially or solely affect the spinal cord. Its course is highly variable, and the prognosis may range from permanent paraplegia to complete recovery.

Spinal Cord Infarction

The spinal cord is occasionally the site of an acute infarction.[15] This can occur in the setting of generalized atherosclerosis and thus pathogenetically is similar to acute cerebral infarction. It most commonly occurs at a mid

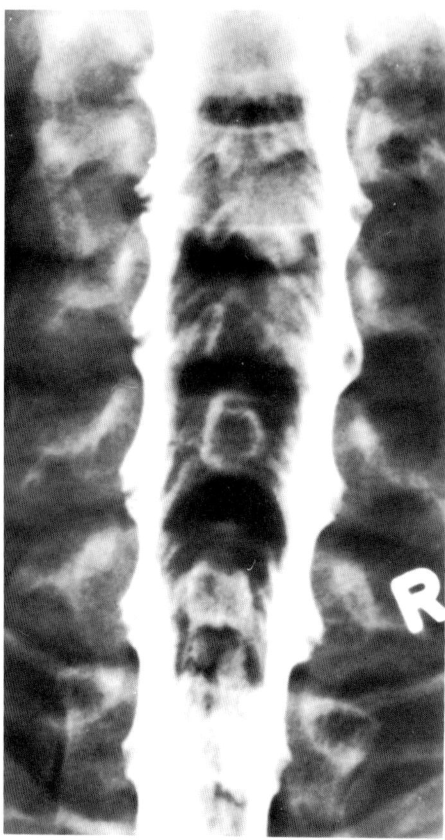

Fig. 13.5 Myelogram in a case of acute multiple sclerosis. The cervical spinal cord is abnormally widened. Biopsy was required to distinguish this lesion from intramedullary tumor.

to low thoracic cord level, frequently spares the posterior columns, and is usually irreversible. Both the myelogram and the CSF are normal. Even in the setting of known vascular disease and without clinical evidence of a compressive lesion, one should not be comfortable with the diagnosis of spinal cord infarction until myelography has been performed.

Infarction of the spinal cord also occurs in some other specific clinical settings. First, dissecting aneurysm of the aorta will sometimes compromise the anterior vascular supply of the cord. Sudden chest or thoracic back pain, an enlarged aortic shadow on chest X-ray, and diminished peripheral pulses are the common clinical findings, but the dissection can be painless. Second, abdominal aortic by-pass surgery will sometimes produce an acute spinal cord syndrome for similar reasons. In this circumstance, the patient will awaken from surgery paraplegic. Sickle cell disease has also been associated with spinal cord infarction.

Among the "collagen" diseases, disseminated lupus erythematosus will occasionally produce the clinical picture of acute transverse myelitis.[1] This usually occurs in patients with active and severe disease, but it may be a presenting feature of the illness. Its pathologic basis is presumably small vessel inflammation leading to ischemia and infarction. It can occur at any level of the cord and is clinically indistinguishable from idiopathic acute transverse myelitis, although the prospect for recovery is somewhat worse in lupus myelopathy. Only 4 of 26 patients reviewed by Andrianakos, et al [1] achieved functional recovery. However, of six patients treated with steroids within 24 hours of the onset of their myelopathy, two achieved functional recovery. In a number of reported patients, the CSF glucose concentration was depressed. Periarteritis nodosa has also been reported to produce an acute myelopathy.

Herpes Zoster Myelitis

Herpes zoster radiculitis, or "shingles," is a common and benign illness that produces its rash and neurological dysfunction in the distribution of a single nerve root, usually at a thoracic level. It is occasionally accompanied by evidence of spinal cord involvement at the same level, and it may produce the clinical picture of a fulminant transverse myelopathy. While this occurs most frequently in immunocompromised hosts, it can occur in otherwise normal individuals.[18] The diagnosis is not difficult since the clinical myelopathy usually begins after the appearance of the rash and the cord lesion is at the same segmental level. There is a lymphocytic pleocytosis in the CSF and the protein concentration may be elevated. The illness may progress with involvement of the spinal cord at higher levels and cerebral symptoms. It is important to consider the diagnosis of zoster myelitis in any immunosuppressed patient who develops zoster radiculitis because effective anti-viral therapy is now available.

Acute Spinal Cord Syndromes Following Intrathecal Injections

The injection of potent chemotherapeutic agents, especially methotrexate, intrathecally for the treatment or prevention of leptomeningeal neoplasm has produced an acute cord syndrome in some instances.[9] This complication may be associated with pain and other radicular symptoms during the injection, or it may develop a few hours after an uncomplicated procedure. Pain is usually prominent, and the clinical picture is otherwise indistinguishable from any acute transverse myelitis. Function may return over the next few hours or days, but in some cases paraplegia has been permanent. This complication has also been reported following intrathecal cytosine arabinoside.[3] If the lumbar puncture is unusually complicated or if the patient has pain or radicular symptoms during the injection, the procedure should be discontinued. The rare occurrence of complications following lumbar injection of this agent was one reason for the development of an in-dwelling subcutaneous reservoir for the intraventricular installation of chemotherapeutic agents.[27] There is also a very small incidence of paraplegia following spinal anesthesia.[5,13]

Hematomyelia

This refers to hemorrhage within the substance of the spinal cord. Trauma is the most common cause, but non-traumatic causes include intramedullary telangiectasis, venous angioma, and intramedullary neoplasm. It is clinically distinguished from most other forms of acute transverse myelopathy by its extremely abrupt onset.

MISCELLANEOUS ACUTE SPINAL CORD SYNDROMES

Subarachnoid Hemorrhage

Spontaneous subarachnoid hemorrhage may also produce an acute spinal cord syndrome.[25] In contrast to intracranial subarachnoid hemorrhage, aneurysm is a rare cause in the spinal cord. The most common underlying conditions are angiomas and tumors. Angiomas occur most often on the dorsal surface of the thoracic spinal cord. They may produce a chronic progressive myelopathy, but spontaneous hemorrhage may also be the first sign of the disease. Spinal subarachnoid hemorrhage produces sudden, severe pain at the site of bleeding, often in association with acute neurological dysfunction. The pain may spread rapidly to other sites, including the head, and multifocal signs may develop, including cranial nerve dysfunction and disturbance of consciousness. A clue to the correct diagnosis may be a bruit over the site of the angioma or an associated cutaneous angioma on the back, but these signs are only variably present, and myelography is required for diagnosis. The indications for surgical intervention are controversial.

Cervical Spondylosis

An occasional patient suffering from a chronic myelopathy from cervical spondylosis will experience an acute deterioration of the spinal cord syndrome. This is usually related to a hyperextension injury, which may be mild, and it classically produces a symmetrical central cord syndrome.[16] Physical findings in this condition mimic those of syringomyelia with preferential involvement of the crossing spinothalamic fibers producing dissociated sensory loss in a cape-like distribution. Involvement of other tracts is variable, although all are susceptible to injury in the chronically compressed cord. Immediate decompression is indicated if some function remains.

Acute Necrotic Myelopathy

This is a rare, ill-defined syndrome of widespread intramedullary necrosis of the spinal cord.[17] It differs from transverse myelitis in that the disturbance is not limited to a single spinal cord level. Inflammation is not present, and vascular lesions are inconsistent. Although in most instances there has been no associated systemic illness, a similar clinical syndrome has been reported in patients with underlying neoplasms.[22]

Toxins

The most common neurological complication of arsenic intoxication is a symmetrical polyneuropathy. Rarely, arsenic can produce an isolated myelopathy. Aortography with radio-opaque contrast media has caused myelopathy, presumably on a toxic basis.

CONCLUSION

The conditions discussed in this chapter have in common the potential for producing rapid and irreversible spinal cord dysfunction. Most are associated with back pain at the site of insult, and the clinical level of involvement can usually be determined by careful neurological examination, although in an early, incomplete lesion the exact level can be vague. Unless the clinical circumstances are unequivocal, myelography is required for diagnosis. The most common conditions producing acute compressive lesions of the spinal cord, including metastatic tumor, abscess, herniated disc, and epidural hematoma, require early intervention, either surgery or radiotherapy, to preserve neurological function. Early diagnosis is also important in the common non-compressive acute myelopathies since in many of them, including zoster myelitis and lupus vasculitis, effective treatment is available. Furthermore, accurate diagnosis of a non-compressive spinal cord lesion will usually eliminate the need for surgery. Corticosteroids have a role in most acute spinal cord syndromes, at least until the definitive diagnosis is established and specific therapy can be instituted.

ACKNOWLEDGEMENTS

The author expresses his appreciation to Dr. Dennis Osborne for providing the radiograms.

REFERENCES

1. Andrianakos, A.A., Duffy, J., Suzuki, M., Sharp, J.T.: Transverse myelopathy in systemic lupus erythematosus: report of three cases and review of the literature. Ann. Int. Med., 83:616, 1975.
2. Berman, M., Feldman, S., Alter, M., Zilber, N., Kahana, E.: Acute transverse myelitis: incidence and etiologic considerations. Neurology, 31:966, 1981.
3. Breuer, A.C., Pitman, S.W., Dawson, D.M., Schoene, W.C.: Paraparesis following intrathecal cytosine arabinoside. Cancer, 40:2817, 1977.
4. Carson, J., Gumbert, J., Jefferson, A.: Diagnosis and treatment of thoracic intervertebral disc protrusions. J. Neurol. Neurosurg. Psychiat., 34:68, 1971.
5. Case records of the Massachusetts General Hospital (case 42291). N. Engl. J. Med., 255:138, 1956.

6. Case records of the Massachusetts General Hospital (case 14–1982). N. Engl. J. Med., 306:855, 1982.
7. Edelson, R.N., Chernik, N.L., Posner, J.B.: Spinal subdural hematomas complicating lumbar puncture. Arch. Neurol., 31:134, 1974.
8. Foo, D., Chang, Y.C., Rossier, A.B.: Spontaneous cervical epidural hemorrhage, anterior cord syndrome, and familial vascular malformation: case report. Neurology, 30:308, 1980.
9. Gagliano, R.G., Costanzi, J.J.: Paraplegia following intrathecal methotrexate. Cancer, 37:1663, 1976.
10. Gilbert, R.W., Kim, J.H., Posner, J.B.: Epidural spinal cord compression from metastatic tumor: diagnosis and treatment. Ann. Neurol., 3:40, 1978.
11. Ginsburg, S., Gross, E., Feiring, E.H., Scheinberg, L.C.: The neurological complications of tuberculous spondylitis: Pott's paraplegia. Arch. Neurol., 16:265, 1967.
12. Greenberg, H.S., Kim, J.H., Posner, J.B.: Epidural spinal cord compression from metastatic tumor: results with a new treatment protocol. Ann. Neurol., 8:361, 1980.
13. Greene, N.M.: Neurological sequelae of spinal anesthesia. Anesthesiology, 22:682, 1961.
14. Harik, S.L., Raichle, M.E., Reis, D.J.: Spontaneously remitting spinal epidural hematoma in a patient on anticoagulants. N. Engl. J. Med., 284:1355, 1971.
15. Herrick, M.K., Mills, P.E., Jr.: Infarction of the spinal cord. Arch. Neurol., 24:228, 1971.
16. Hoff, J.T., Wilson, C.B.: The pathophysiology of cervical spondylotic radiculopathy and myelopathy. Clinical Neurosurgery, 24:474, 1976.
17. Hoffman, H.L.: Acute necrotic myelopathy. Brain, 78:377, 1955.
18. Hogan, E.L., Krigman, M.R.: Herpes zoster myelitis: evidence for viral invasion of the spinal cord. Arch. Neurol., 29:309, 1973.
19. Kaufman, D.M., Kaplan, J.G., Litman, N.: Infectious agents in spinal epidural abscesses. Neurology, 30:844, 1980.
20. Lambert, P.M.: Radiation myelopathy of the thoracic spinal cord in long term survivors treated with radical radiotherapy using conventional fractionation. Cancer, 41:1751, 1978.
21. Lipton, H.L., Teasdall, R.D.: Acute transverse myelopathy in adults. Arch. Neurol., 28:252, 1973.
22. Mancall, E.L., Rosales, R.K.: Necrotizing myelopathy associated with visceral carcinoma. Brain, 87:639, 1964.
23. McQuarrie, I.G.: Recovery from paraplegia caused by spontaneous spinal epidural hematoma. Neurology, 28:224, 1978.
24. Nassar, S.I., Correll, J.W.: Subarachnoid hemorrhage due to spinal cord tumors. Neurology, 18:87, 1968.
25. Odom, G.L.: Vascular lesions of the spinal cord: malformations, spinal subarachnoid and extradural hemorrhage. Clin. Neurosurg., 8:196, 1960.
26. Odom, G.L., Finney, W., Woodhall, B.: Cervical disc lesions. J. Am. Med. Assoc., 166:23, 1958.
27. Ratcheson, R.A., Ommaya, A.K.: Experience with the subcutaneous cerebrospinal fluid reservoir. N. Engl. J. Med., 279:1025, 1968.
28. Ropper, A.H., Poskanzer, D.C.: The prognosis of acute and subacute transverse myelopathy based on early signs and symptoms. Ann. Neurol., 4:51, 1978.

14

Neuro-Ophthalmologic Emergencies

Jonathan D. Trobe, M.D.

INTRODUCTION

The two most common symptoms of neuro-ophthalmologic emergencies are visual loss and diplopia.[3,8] You should be on the lookout for the principal emergent conditions that present with these symptoms, and learn the basic diagnostic features and tests that will enable you to single them out.

VISUAL LOSS

Acute and treatable non-traumatic visual loss may be caused by disease of the anterior part of the eye (cornea, sclera, anterior chamber, iris and lens), the posterior part of the eye (vitreous, retina, choroid and optic disc), and the retrobulbar visual pathway (optic nerve, chiasm, tract, lateral geniculate body, optic radiations and visual cortex) (Table 14.1).

Anterior Segment

Because the structures of the anterior eye are not of neural origin, visual loss associated with disease in this segment cannot be considered a true neuro-ophthalmologic emergency. But some familiarity with emergent diseases in this area is a necessary part of sophisticated triage. The principal considerations are keratitis and acute glaucoma. With few exceptions, both will present as "red eyes," and with pain, tearing, and photophobia. Other causes of red eyes rarely cause visual loss. Conjunctivitis, episcleritis, and inflammation of the ocular adnexal structures in front of the orbital septum, including the lid margins (blepharitis), sweat and meibomian glands (stye), lacrimal gland (dacryoadenitis), and lacrimal sac (dacryocystitis) produce discomfort but only disturb vision transiently when mucous debris covers the corneal surface. Blinking will clear up the blurred vision, except in

Table 14.1 Common Causes of Nontraumatic Acute Visual Loss

	Immediate Treatment	Non-immediate Treatment
Anterior segment of globe	Keratitis Acute glaucoma	Uveitis
Posterior segment of globe	Central retinal occlusion (<4 hours old)	Central retinal artery occlusion (>4 hours old)
	Arteritic ischemic optic neuropathy	Non-arteritic ischemic optic neuropathy
	Endophthalmitis	Choroiditis Retinitis
	Retinal detachment (macula attached)	Retinal detachment (macula detached) Vitreous hemorrhage Macular hemorrhage, edema, detachment
Retrobulbar	Orbital optic nerve compression *	Intracranial aneurysm
	Chiasmal compression **	Retrobulbar neuritis Occipital lobe arteriovenous malformation Occipital lobe stroke

* Cellulitis, hemorrhage, pseudotumor, hyperostotic lesions, meningeal carcinomatosis.
** Pituitary apoplexy, sinus mucocoele, cystic craniopharyngioma.

the rare case that a stye or other inflammatory mass deforms the globe. Anterior uveitis, or inflammation of the iris and ciliary body, may rarely cause visual loss if thick fibrinous debris occludes the anterior chamber and pupillary space. If uveitis is severe enough to elevate intraocular pressure, this condition may be difficult to distinguish from acute glaucoma or keratitis. Most cases are idiopathic, although granulomatous conditions such as sarcoidosis, lues, and herpes zoster may be causative. Treatment is urgent but not emergent, and consists of topical (and sometimes systemic) corticosteroids and topical cycloplegics.

Keratitis

Keratitis, or inflammation of the cornea, is generally accompanied by a foreign body sensation ("it feels like sand or gravel in my eye") unless the cornea is anesthetic (as in self-administered topical anesthetics, chronic Herpes simplex or Herpes zoster). Erosion of a portion of the epithelial surface can be diagnosed by observing a blurred reflection of a flashlight shined on the corneal apex. You may confirm a break in the epithelial surface by staining the cornea with fluorescein and observing with magnification and a cobalt blue light. A defect in the epithelium will fluoresce as green.

If corneal erosions are caused by foreign bodies, the patient will usually report that "something blew into my eye." Otherwise you should always suspect Herpes simplex keratitis. In its classic form, Herpes simplex keratitis will manifest a branching erosion ("dendrite"), but any configuration is possible. The history of a recent cold sore at the mucocutaneous (vermilion) border of the mouth is helpful but not necessary in making the diagnosis. Although immuno-virological tests are available, the diagnosis is essentially clinical: an acute corneal erosion occurring without a recent or remote history of trauma to the eye in a patient who has no signs of an abnormal "corneal milieu"—reduced tear production, lid laxity, a roughened palpebral conjunctival surface, or inturning lashes.

Presumed Herpes simplex keratitis is treated with anti-viral drugs, including trifluorothymidine (Viroptic), adenine arabinoside (Vira-A), and idoxuridine (Stoxil). Immediate treatment hastens recovery and may preclude spread of virus into the corneal stroma, with resultant scarring and permanent visual loss.

Corneal ulcers may also be caused by bacteria and fungi. They are most commonly encountered in immunocompromised patients, including alcoholics, the poorly nourished, those who have been treated for a prolonged period with topical corticosteroids, and after corneal trauma with fungus-contaminated plant material. Treatment consists of debridement and appropriate anti-microbials.

Acute Glaucoma

Acute glaucoma typically manifests a painful red eye with intense injection of the episcleral vessels adjacent to the cornea ("ciliary flush"). The extraordinarily high intraocular pressure causes the corneal endothelium to lose its ability to maintain deturgescence of the cornea. The cornea swells and vision becomes cloudy. If the swelling is sufficient to raise blebs on the corneal epithelium, the examiner may recognize a fine "bedewing" of the corneal light reflection. (This is a subtle sign and is easy to miss!) The high pressure may paralyze the iris sphincter and cause the pupil to be mid-dilated and unreactive to light.

This complex of symptoms and signs is often misinterpreted in emergency rooms. Patients may be in so much pain that they are nauseated and vomiting. They have often been admitted and worked up with mistaken diagnoses of "acute abdomen" or "intracranial bleeding."

Initial treatment of acute glaucoma consists of reducing the pressure with carbonic anhydrase inhibitors (acetazolamide (Diamox) and derivatives), oral osmotic agents (glycerin), and pilocarpine (to contract the sphincter and relieve congestion in the anterior chamber angle). The vast majority of cases of acute glaucoma are caused by closure of the anterior chamber angle. A special lens allows visualization of this structure in order to confirm the diagnosis. If the angle is closed, definitive therapy entails performing an iridectomy, or hole in the peripheral iris to allow aqueous fluid to flow from the posterior to the anterior chamber. This treatment is based on the concept that angle closure occurs when the iris obstructs aqueous flow around the pupil and then billows forward to occlude the outflow channels.

The iridectomy reestablishes a communication from inflow to outflow ports, restoring normal intraocular pressure if the outflow meshwork has not been permanently damaged. Early treatment is considered critical, both to eliminate vision-threatening elevated pressure and to preserve the outflow channels.

In the past, iridectomy was performed by surgical excision. Now the laser can be used to burn a hole in the iris.

Posterior Segment

Visual loss caused by disease of the posterior segment of the globe may be more difficult to diagnose because it requires careful ophthalmoscopy. Four conditions stand out as true emergencies: (1) central retinal artery occlusion (CRAO), (2) arteritic ischemic optic neuropathy (ION) in giant cell arteritis, (3) endophthalmitis, and (4) retinal detachment.

Central Retinal Artery Occlusion

Central retinal artery occlusion presents as painless and abrupt loss of vision. Visual loss may be described in any of a number of ways: blurring, dimming, greying, a curtain coming down or going up, or an enlarging blind spot. Visual loss may be total or confined to one sector of the field of vision. Although most often sudden, it may be preceded for 24 hours by transient dimming, or may evolve slowly over several hours.

Visual acuity will be subnormal in *almost* all cases. Occasionally the retina bearing the nerve fibers subserving central vision (acuity) will be spared, and the only evidence of visual dysfunction will be a focally contracted visual field. You may test visual field grossly with finger confrontation, but this will only identify large defects. Formal visual fields will be necessary for precise diagnosis.

The affected eye will usually show a relative afferent pupillary defect, sometimes called a "Marcus-Gunn" pupil (see section below on Examination of Patients with Acute Visual Loss). Fundus examination may be normal or changes will be very subtle if the infarction has just begun. This makes diagnosis very difficult. In fact, you will be misled into thinking the process is retrobulbar. Look carefully for one or more yellow-white intraluminal plaques, the calling-card of an embolus from the carotid artery or heart. Distal to the embolus, the retina will have a milky turbidity instead of the bright orange reflection of the underlying vascular choroid (Fig. 14.1). If the macular area is infarcted, it will show through as a "cherry red spot" because the retina is normally so thin in this area that the reflected color of the choroidal vessels is unaffected. Actually, the red color of the macula is enhanced by the surrounding retinal opacification. The entire retina need not be infarcted. The most vulnerable area appears to be the area bounded by the optic disc, macula and inferior and superior temporal retinal arteriole

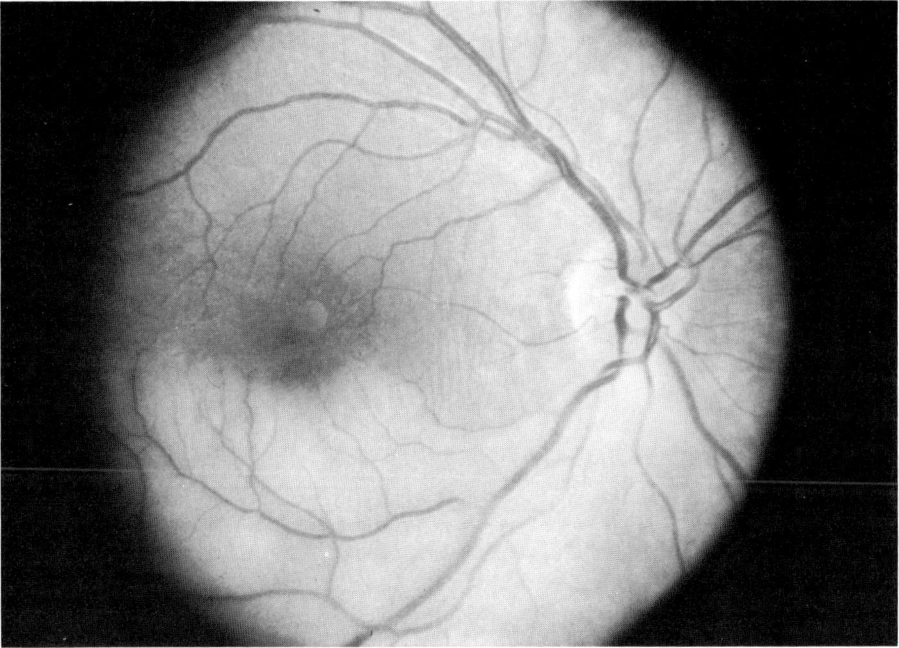

Fig. 14.1 Optic fundus of right eye in a patient with lower branch retinal arterial occlusion. Infarcted inferior retina appears milky white because underlying vascular choroid is obscured. To be effective, treatment must occur within 4 hours of onset.

arcades. Only one of the retinal arterioles may be selectively involved to produce a branch occlusion.

Emboli need not be present in CRAO; in fact they are the exception. Most often, CRAO occurs by blockage of the artery as it penetrates the scleral lamina in the optic nervehead. Whether this blockage is the result of in situ thrombosis or embolism is debated, for acute pathologic material has thus far been unavailable. But there is no doubt that essential hypertension is a frequent risk factor.

CRAO should be treated vigorously if symptoms are of recent onset, that is, of less than 2–4 hours duration. Within this interval, anecdotal reports have documented recovery of vision. Whether treatment was responsible for recovery or it occurred naturally is not known. A controlled clinical series dealing with this devastating problem has not been conducted.

Treatment is aimed at opening the clogged retinal vessels, and consists of reducing intraocular pressure in order to relieve external pressure, and attempting to dilate the retinal arterioles. The fastest (but very delicate) way to reduce intraocular pressure is to place a 27 gauge needle into the anterior chamber (paracentesis) and withdrawing 0.1 ml. of aqueous humor. Intravenous acetazolamide and osmotics have also been tried. Finally, the patient is given a paper bag to rebreathe expired CO_2, and thereby dilate cerebral vessels. Vasodilator agents, such as priscoline, have been injected retrobulbarly.

These heroic measures generally fail even if administered early. Yet the few reported "cures" propagate and justify the tradition of immediate treatment.

Patients who have suffered CRAO require a work-up to rule out embolic and hypercoagulable states, especially if normotensive. CRAO may rarely be caused by giant cell arteritis, a condition requiring immediate corticosteroid treatment to forestall involvement of the other eye (see below).

Arteritic Ischemic Optic Neuropathy

Another emergent cause of visual loss within the globe is arteritic ischemic optic neuropathy. The onset of loss of vision may be exactly like that experienced by patients having a CRAO except that in some cases both eyes will have become involved before the patient seeks medical attention. Ischemic optic neuropathy represents infarction in the ciliary circulation rather than in the retinal circulation. The retina will appear normal, all signs being confined to the nervehead and the area immediately adjacent to it. Examination will reveal subnormal acuity and field defects which correspond to the optic nerve fiber bundles that have been destroyed. An afferent pupillary defect will be present on the involved side; or, in the case of binocular involvement, on the side of the more damaged eye. A swollen nervehead will be evident on fundoscopy (Fig. 14.2). The swelling obscures the margin of the optic disc, and usually consists of dilated capillaries, white exudates (actually "dammed up" axoplasm), and flame-shaped hemorrhages. The swelling typically affects only a portion of the disc, implying segmental infarction. The remainder of the fundus examination is usually completely normal.

Arteritic ischemic optic neuropathy is most commonly found as part of giant cell arteritis (GCA), an idiopathic granulomatous arteritis of the elderly, affecting mainly the extracranial portion of blood vessels that supply the head.[2,5] But you must bear in mind that the arteritic form of ischemic optic neuropathy (ION) actually represents a very small fraction (less than 1 percent) of all cases of ION. The majority of cases are non-arteritic strokes probably caused by hypertensive intimal proliferation and occlusion. Non-arteritic ischemic optic neuropathy never strikes both eyes at the same time, although the second eye may become involved months to years later in 25–40 percent of cases. Because it is not treatable and not associated with active disease (except hypertension, which is rarely malignant), it is not considered an emergency.

But the arteritic form of ION is a true emergency. Untreated, it may progress in the involved eye and produce blindness in the uninvolved eye within days of onset of visual complaints.

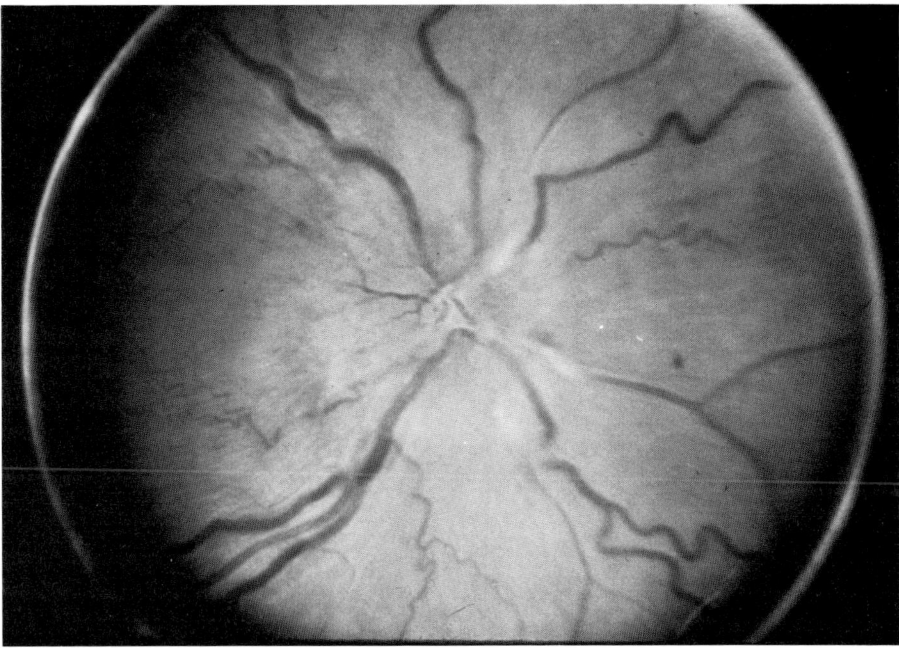

Fig. 14.2 Optic fundus of left eye in a patient with ischemic optic neuropathy. The optic nervehead is swollen with "constipated axoplasm" (white), dilated capillaries, and nerve fiber layer hemorrhages. The rest of the retina is normal. Vasculitis in giant cell arteritis produces this appearance, but a non-arteritic cause is far more frequent.

To consider the diagnosis of the arteritic form of ION (Fig. 14.3), you must have the typical eye findings of ION plus a history of either malaise, anorexia, fever, proximal muscle weakness and ache, and anemia (the "polymyalgia rheumatica" or PMR complex), or scalp tenderness, headache, jaw claudication (the GCA complex). The greater the number of positives from this list, the more likely the diagnosis. Be wary of the lack of specificity of many of these symptoms by themselves. Only in combination, and in the presence of a recent exacerbation do they add up to a presumption of GCA.

The clinical diagnosis is strengthened by finding an elevated sedimentation rate, but a normal sedimentation rate does not exclude the diagnosis. Although the Westergren method is favored, the traditional Wintrobe is adequate if the correction for hematocrit is used. The new Zeta method is acceptable as well. Be cautious in your interpretation of sedimentation rates, realizing that the normal value rises with age. A value between 30 and 50 (Westergren) in a 75-year-old is borderline. In bona fide cases of GCA, the sedimentation rate will be above 60, often over 100. Sedimentation rates are non-specific indicators of inflammation, and may be elevated by occult neoplasm or infection, inflammatory arthritis, or even atherosclerosis.

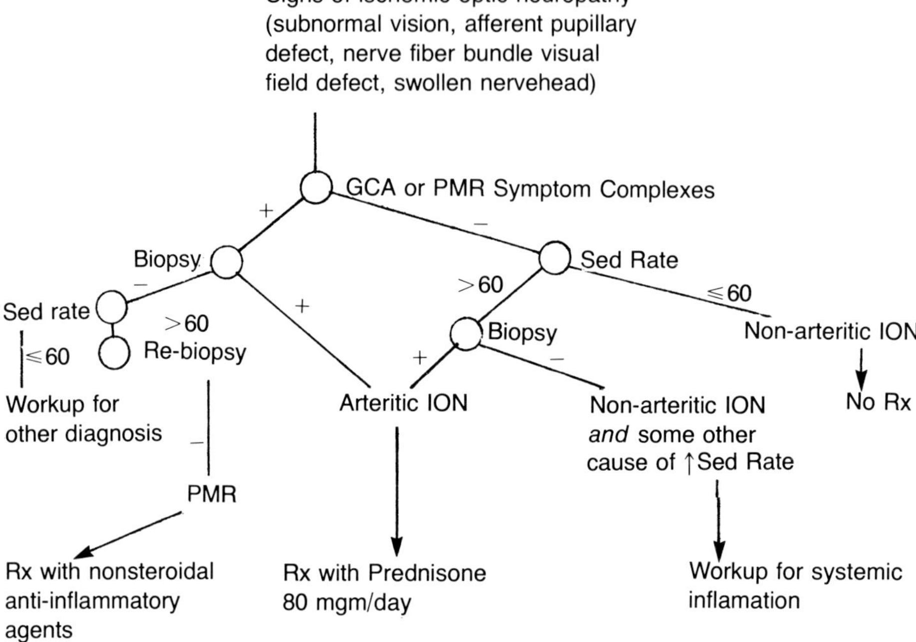

Fig. 14.3 Diagnosis of Arteritic Ischemic Optic Neuropathy.

Still, values over 60 in the appropriate setting are highly suggestive of GCA.

The diagnosis of GCA remains presumptive without pathologic verification. Even in iron-clad clinical cases, a temporal artery biopsy should be performed. Although some false negatives are reported from biopsy, these are rare with proper technique. You should biopsy a segment of the temporal artery (the most commonly involved accessible vessel) on the side ipsilateral to the affected eye. Sample at least 2 cm of vessel, performing multiple serial sections. Since at least 5 percent of GCA involves only one temporal artery, a negative biopsy on one side mandates a biopsy on the other side. A negative biopsy from both sides is incompatible with the diagnosis of GCA. Complications of biopsy are trivial.

The biopsy is necessary because non-arteritic ION is far more common than arteritic ION, and because the polymyalgia rheumatica (PMR) and GCA symptom complexes are often historically vague. Once you make the diagnosis, you are committed to long-term (at least 1 year) oral corticosteroid therapy with its attendant risks. The recommended initial dose regimen is prednisone 80 mgm per day in divided doses. Alternate-day regimens are less apt to produce side-effects but do not control the disease as well; these regimens are appropriate only for maintenance treatment. You should gauge the efficacy of therapy by the level of the sedimentation rate and the remission of non-ophthalmologic symptoms.

Fortunately for diagnosticians, when GCA produces a fixed deficit in vision, something will be visible in the fundus. If the retina and optic nerve head are normal in appearance, GCA is not at fault. In 95 percent of cases of GCA with visual loss, the target is the optic disc: arteritic ION. In the remaining 5 percent of cases, the retinal circulation is infarcted. Therefore, you need not and should not diagnose GCA in the presence of visual loss and a normal fundus. Of course, a patient complaining of transient (not fixed) visual loss may rarely be in the process of developing a disc or retinal stroke from GCA. Transient visual loss persisting beyond 48 hours is unlikely to be a stroke-in-evolution. For symptoms of more recent onset, be sure to inquire of PMR and GCA symptom complexes.

In the past, GCA was an underdiagnosed condition. But in recent years, physicians have become alert to this disease, to the point of overdiagnosing it! If vision loss has been averted in a few instances, it has been at the heavy cost of the complications of steroid therapy in cases without pathologic verification of the diagnosis.

Endophthalmitis.

Endophthalmitis is the term applied to suppurative (infectious) inflammation of the vitreous, uvea, and/or retina. It most commonly results from the introduction of bacteria or fungi into the eye at the time of intraocular surgery, from a septic corneal ulcer, or less commonly, from penetrating trauma ("exogenous endophthalmitis"). Rarely, pathogenic organisms may reach the retina or choroid by hematogenous routes, and establish a focal infection which spreads to involve the vitreous cavity ("endogenous endophthalmitis"). Hematogenously spread pathogens may be of all types, but candida albicans is the prime offender, coming from intravenous catheters or the bowel.

Patients complain of subacute blurring of vision in the affected eye. Pain is prominent only if the infection has spread to the outer coats of the eye ("panophthalmitis"). At that point, lids will be swollen, the conjunctiva injected, and the eye tender to the touch. But if only the vitreous cavity is infected, there may be no external signs. A layer of exudate may be seen at the bottom of the anterior chamber ("hypopyon"), consisting of organisms and neutrophilic debris. The view with the direct ophthalmoscope will be hazy or totally obscured by fluffy material in the vitreous cavity.

Diagnosis is made by aspirating the ocular cavities with a needle and syringe or with a special vitreous aspirating device. These maneuvers are performed under sterile conditions and high magnification. Treatment is urgent, and includes systemic, topical, and often intravitreal administration of appropriate antibiotics. Systemic and local steroids are sometimes added to reduce scarring within the visual axis. If medical treatment is not effective, it may be necessary to remove the infected vitreous surgically ("vitrectomy").

Retinal Detachment

Retinal detachment occurs when the neurosensory portion of the retina separates from the underlying pigment epithelium. Even in normal eyes, a potential space exists between these layers because the neurosensory layer derives embryologically from the inner portion of the optic vesicle, while the pigment epithelium derives from the outer portion.

The most frequent cause of a retinal detachment is the formation of a hole in the neurosensory retina, which allows fluid from the vitreous cavity to seep into the potential space and strip apart the two layers. As the retina becomes detached, the rods and cones are mechanically deformed and stimulated, giving the hallucination of sparkling flashes of light. Disconnected from the pigment epithelium, the rods and cones of the detached retina lose their ability to resolve images. If not reattached after several weeks, the receptors become nonviable.

Retinal holes usually result from local tugging by retracting vitreous, a process that occurs naturally with age, but prematurely in the eyes of those who have had intraocular inflammation, trauma, surgery, foreign body, or who have high myopia (nearsightedness). Retinal detachments caused by retinal holes ("rhegmatogenous detachments") will usually commence in the retinal periphery, anterior to the equator of the globe. This is because vitreous traction is greatest in this area. As the retina detaches, patients complain that a "curtain" has come over their sight from the side toward the center. If the retinal hole includes a crossing retinal blood vessel, the tear may damage the vessel and cause a brief vitreous hemorrhage. The patient sees this as a shower of floaters. Because the retina has no pain receptors, this whole process is painless.

Examination will reveal normal visual acuity if only the retinal periphery is detached. But the macula may soon detach as well, and, if so, the prognosis for good visual recovery is lessened dramatically. An abnormal visual field may be the only sign of disturbed vision. There will be no signs of inflammation in the anterior segment and the ophthalmoscopic view through the undilated pupil may be completely normal. A careful examination of the entire retina through a widely dilated pupil, however, would reveal a billowing detachment of the retina, and one or more tiny holes, usually in the far periphery, visible only after an exhaustive search.

Treatment depends upon the presence or absence of macular detachment. If the macula is not detached, patients must be placed at bed rest and operated upon immediately to forestall this development. If the macula is detached, surgery remains urgent, but need not be performed immediately. Surgery consists of sealing the hole with either diathermy (heat), cryopexy (cold), or laser photocoagulation, and with scleral indentation devices ("buckles"). Retinal detachments may rarely occur without retinal holes ("nonrhegmatogenous") when serous swelling results from tumor or inflammation of the choroid. Treatment is directed at the source of the swelling.

Retrobulbar

Retrobulbar visual loss is a frightening diagnostic problem, but rarely signals a treatable vision-threatening or life-threatening condition. However, there are some notable exceptions: acute compression of the optic nerve or chiasm.

Compressive Optic Neuropathy

This occurs acutely by soft tissue swelling at the orbital apex, by hyperostosis in the boney optic canal, or by intracranial masses.

In some patients with Graves' disease, the extraocular muscles become massively enlarged by lymphocytic and hyaluronic acid infiltration. Because their common origin at the orbital apex is a ring around the optic nerve, a panmyositis causes strangulation of the optic nerve, with interruption of axoplasmic flow. Patients will usually complain of transient blurring of vision for days to weeks beforehand, then suddenly develop a fixed visual deficit.

Patients with this type of visual loss always manifest the ocular adnexal signs of dysthyroidism, including lid retraction and lag, chemosis and conjunctival injection. Their eye movements will be reduced in amplitude and the eyes may actually become misaligned. The visual acuity in the affected eye will be subnormal and an afferent pupillary defect will be present on that side. The disc of the affected eye may be swollen, but it is usually normal.

To make the diagnosis, look for the signs of an optic neuropathy with or without a swollen disc and the soft tissue signs of Graves' ophthalmopathy. Computerized tomography of the orbits (CT) will reveal enlarged extraocular muscles, whose confluence at the orbital apex is often mistakenly interpreted as a tumor mass. Treatment is emergent and consists of either high-dose oral corticosteroids (prednisone 80–120 mg/day) or 2,000 rads X-ray to the two orbits. Steroids should be the first line of treatment; they frequently produce a dramatic reversal, and usually prevent further visual loss.

A similar process may occur in patients who do not have evidence of thyroid dysfunction.[7] These patients may have euthyroid Graves' disease (as evidenced by an autonomously functioning thyroid gland), orbital inflammatory pseudotumor (a lymphocytic infiltration), leukemia, or plasmacytoma. The treatment is as with dysthyroid optic neuropathy. In some cases the orbital apex compression of the optic nerve is by hyperostotic bone; visual loss may be very acute in metastatic prostate cancer or other osteoblastic metastases. Paget's disease, meningioma and fibrous dysplasia produce more chronic visual loss. Rapid compression of the optic nerve may result from orbital abscess, cyst or hemorrhage into a hemangioma. Treatment sometimes involves emergency orbital decompression.

Chiasmal Compression

The most common cause of acute chiasmal compression is pituitary apoplexy.[9] It represents hemorrhagic infarction of a pituitary adenoma with sudden expansion and pressure on adjacent structures, including the optic chiasm, and nerves, and the ocular motor nerves. In fact, the combination of acute visual loss and diplopia is most suggestive of this entity.

Visual acuity is typically subnormal in at least one eye; an afferent pupil defect is likely to be present. Visual fields will show a temporal hemianopic defect (aligned to the vertical fixational meridian) in at least one eye. Using finger confrontation, you must look for a marked difference in visual sensitivity between the nasal and temporal hemi-fields. Finding such a defect is strong evidence of chiasmal (or post-chiasmal) dysfunction.

In addition to their ophthalmic problems, patients with pituitary apoplexy are often febrile, hypotensive, and drowsy because of a sterile meningitis and hypopituitarism. They require immediate hospitalization, volume loading, and corticosteroid replacement. If radiologic studies confirm a sellar mass, transsphenoidal hypophysectomy should be performed as soon as the patient has been stabilized.

There are other, less frequent, causes of chiasmal compression, including ethmoid or sphenoid sinus mucocoele, and cystic craniopharyngioma, which may necessitate urgent transsphenoidal decompression. Supraclinoid carotid artery aneurysms may produce sudden visual loss but their propensity to rupture is low, so that treatment is generally not urgent.

Sudden compression of the post-chiasmal visual pathway is very rare. An arteriovenous malformation may bleed into the occipital lobe and adjacent meninges. Patients are operated, but not emergently.

Because it will be difficult to exclude a treatable cause of sudden retrobulbar visual loss, you should promptly refer all patients to an ophthalmologist, especially if you find (1) an afferent pupillary defect or (2) a hemianopic visual field defect. Patients with accompanying neurologic findings, including depressed consciousness, seizures, or motor or cerebellar signs, should be hospitalized and an ophthalmologic consultation obtained immediately.

Special Diagnostic Problems

Patients with transient visual loss and suspected malingering pose particular diagnostic problems.

Transient Visual Loss (Fig. 14.4)

Patients who complain that their vision in one or both eyes fades intermittently rarely constitute true emergencies. The vast majority of these patients have no active disease and no directly contributory findings on ophthalmologic examination. In the elderly and those with risk factors for arteriosclero-

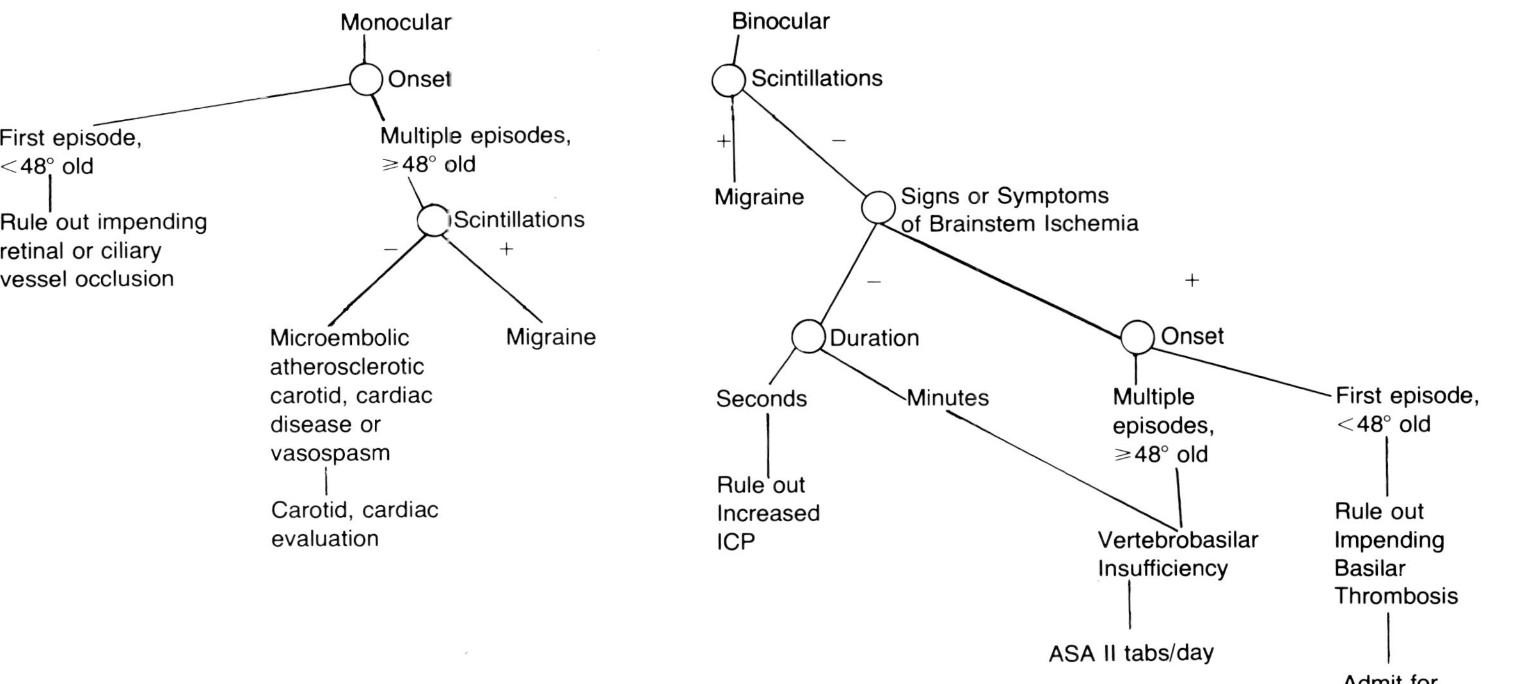

Fig. 14.4 Diagnosis of Transient Visual Loss.

sis, brief (lasting minutes) visual loss probably represents microembolism from atheromatous cervical carotid (monocular) or vertebrobasilar disease (binocular). Non-emergent carotid and cardiac evaluation is indicated if visual loss is monocular; if visual loss is binocular, carotid evaluation is not necessary.

In patients aged less than 40 years and those without arteriosclerotic risk factors, no cause is usually found for transient visual loss. If the symptom is homonymous (present in the fields of both eyes on the same side of visual space), and is accompanied by scintillations (flashing zig-zag, wavy lights, "heat waves" or colored sparkles), and followed by headache, it is almost certainly migraine. The problem is that many patients have non-classical presentations. Vasospasm is probably the underlying mechanism in most, but it is difficult to prove. In any case, no emergency exists.

A small proportion of patients with transient visual loss constitute true emergencies: those with impending stroke or increased intracranial pressure.

Impending Stroke

This may occur with occlusion of the ciliary or retinal circulation to the globe, that is, with ischemic optic neuropathy (ION) or central retinal artery occlusion (CRAO). Some 10 percent of cases of ION and CRAO are preceded by transient monocular blindness within the 48 hours before stroke. Look carefully at the fundus for the early signs of disc or retinal swelling. If negative, advise the patient to seek ophthalmologic attention at the moment that visual loss lasts longer than a few minutes.

Transient binocular visual loss may be part of an impending basilar artery thrombosis. If so, ischemic brainstem symptoms and signs should be present. Repeated and isolated binocular transient visual loss represents embolism from vertebrobasilar atheroma, cardiac valve disease, vasospasm, or occipital lobe arteriovenous malformation. These entities do not require emergent handling; they should be evaluated electively.

Increased Intracranial Pressure

Patients with papilledema may report that their vision in one or both eyes fades momentarily (lasting a second or less), especially when they quickly assume an upright body position. Vision is believed to be impaired by retinal ischemia resulting from the tightly-packed optic nerve head. These very short-lived "obscurations of vision" do not occur in any other condition, and should direct your examination to the optic discs. Papilledema will usually be unequivocal.

Feigned Visual Loss

Malingerers and hysterics frequently manifest acute visual loss. Sometimes they are difficult to identify, but some can be diagnosed by the following maneuvers.

Visual Acuity at Distance and Near Are Not Consistent

Feigners often read a line on the acuity chart perfectly well and then are totally unable to read the next lower (smaller) line. Patients with organic visual loss usually have a more gradual decline in acuity, missing the more difficult letters on the larger line and correctly identifying the easier letters on the smaller line.

Inappropriate Body Movements

Ask patients who feign complete blindness to appose their index fingers. Organically blind people use proprioceptive cues and are able to touch fingers slowly without mistakes. Those who feign blindness will flail their arms about spectacularly. The signature of the patient with feigned blindness will be extravagantly disordered, as against the relatively normal handwriting of the truly blind.

Those who pretend severe but subtotal visual loss will lurch about as they move, but manage to just avoid obstructions. The truly blind have learned to move cautiously.

Tunnel Visual Field

The tunnel visual field is pathognomonic of feigned visual loss. Ask the patient to fixate on your eye with the eye being tested (the other eye should be covered) at a meter's distance. Introduce the fingers of your hand from beyond the peripheral limits of the normal field, and ask the patient to signal first awareness of the moving fingers. Note where this occurs on nasal and temporal sides of the field of vision. If the boundary of the patient's field is markedly constricted compared to yours, then move back to a distance of 3 meters and repeat the same maneuver. If the patient's first awareness of the fingers occurs at the same point as before, you have defined a tunnel visual field constriction. Organic visual field constriction, as in CRAO, glaucoma or retinitis pigmentosa, would produce a funnel shape, enlarging with increasing test distance.

As helpful as these maneuvers are in sorting out functional from organic acute visual loss, it is best to always run through a standard set of tests before determining that visual loss is functional.

Steps In The Examination Of Patients With Acute Visual Loss

To identify conditions causing visual loss that require immediate treatment or referral, hone your examination to the following essentials:

History

How Recent Was the Visual Loss?

The more recent the onset, the more emergent the condition. CRAO lasting more than 5 hours, especially if not evolving, is unlikely to respond to treatment.

Is Visual Loss Static, Worsening, or Resolving?

A static course is most typical of stroke, worsening is most typical of infection, some types of inflammation, and retinal detachment; resolution implies inflammation or vitreous hemorrhage.

Is Visual Loss Monocular or Binocular?

Binocular visual loss, especially if concurrent, usually implies chiasmal or retrochiasmal visual pathway disease. Consecutive binocular visual loss (first one eye involved, then the other) is highly suggestive of cranial arteritis causing bilateral ischemic optic neuropathy.

Is the Visual Loss Scotomatous?

In other words, can the patient describe a discrete area of blurring within the field of vision? A central scotoma means macular or optic nerve disease, an altitudinal scotoma means optic nerve disease or retinal arteriolar occlusion, a bi-temporal defect means chiasmal disease and a homonymous hemianopic defect implies postchiasmal dysfunction, usually hemispheric.

Is There a History of Recent Intraocular Surgery, Corneal Ulcer, or Trauma (Including Foreign Body)?

A history of corneal ulcer leads to a suspicion of endophthalmitis. Recent intraocular surgery could have resulted in endophthalmitis, macular disease, or retinal detachment. Remember that endophthalmitis with bacterial pathogens usually occurs within 48 hours post-operatively, but fungal endophthalmitis may be delayed for weeks. Post-operative macular disease, commonly in the form of cystoid macular edema, may develop as long as 2 or 3 months after surgery. Retinal detachment typically occurs within the first year after intra-ocular surgery, but may occur even later.

Are There Any Other Symptoms Besides Visual Loss?

Ocular pain usually denotes anterior segment disease, but may occur with optic neuritis, chiasmal compression and even occipital (visual) cortex infarction by referral from trigeminal branches. Photophobia, tearing, swelling and redness suggest anterior segment ocular disease, while accompanying neurologic symptoms suggest intracranial involvement. The symptoms of polymyalgia rheumatica are often vague, but are helpful after you have noted the ophthalmic signs of either ION or CRAO. The recent history of light flashes and floaters helps to suggest retinal detachment.

Examination[4]

Visual Acuity

This is the cornerstone of the examination—you cannot neglect it. A distance (Snellen chart) acuity is most accurate. Always test monocularly, the right eye first, by convention. A near card test is adequate if held at the appropriate distance (14 inches from the eye), and if the patient is wearing the necessary optical correction (reading glasses or bifocals for those over age 40). Remember that in the Snellen acuity fraction, the numerator is the testing distance (usually 20 feet or 6 meters) and the denominator the smallest size optotype the patient is able to read with few mistakes (normal is "20"). Normal acuity does not mean normal visual function! Serious disease may be limited to the peripheral (non-acuity related) visual field, especially at the outset. That is why you should at least make an attempt to assess the field of vision.

Confrontation Visual Field

This is difficult to perform accurately, but can give gross localizing information if done correctly.

The best technique is to have the patient face you at a meter's distance, have him cover one (left) eye and look directly at your (left) eye with his open (right) eye. Present either one or two stationary fingers in one of the four quadrants of the visual field, about 10° from the horizontal and vertical meridians that pass through fixation. Ask the patient to identify how many fingers he sees in each quadrant tested sequentially. If he sees equally well in all quadrants, you have a very gross estimation that the peripheral field is intact. Repeat the procedure for the other eye. Record your confrontation field results by drawing two circles, dividing them into quadrants and indicating in which quadrants the patient could not count your fingers.

There are other, more sensitive, confrontation techniques, but they require a great deal of practice to be reliable.

Flashlight Exam

First look for obvious signs of inflammation, such as lid swelling, injection, corneal clouding, or pus in the anterior chamber. Next examine the pupils in very dim illumination with the patient fixating a distant object. You are checking first for anisocoria, a pathologic difference in resting pupil size, and a sign of a pupillo-efferent disorder (less than 1 mm difference in diameter may be physiologic). Next you look for an afferent pupillary disorder. Shine the light (it must be bright) directly into the right pupil, observe the reaction, and swing it across the nasal bridge to the other eye, and observe the reaction. Normally, if you have moved rapidly, there should be no change in the size of the already consensually-constricted left pupil. If the left pupil dilates, you have suggestive evidence of a left optic nerve lesion. If the left pupil constricts, you have suggestive evidence of a right optic nerve lesion. Swing the light back to the right eye and observe the pupil movement. If the pupil constricts, you have confirmed a left optic nerve lesion; if it dilates, you have confirmed a right optic nerve lesion.

Known as the swinging flashlight test, or Marcus-Gunn pupil test, this is one of the most valuable diagnostic maneuvers available to you. If repeated swings of the flashlight back and forth identify a consistent abnormality in pupillary dynamics, you have diagnosed either (1) a unilateral (ipsilateral) optic nerve lesion, (2) bilateral optic nerve lesions, worse on the side of the afferent pupillary defect, or (3) a severe retinal lesion on the ipsilateral side. Anterior segment diseases, including cataract, do not produce this abnormality; nor do post-chiasmal lesions.

Ophthalmoscopy

Holding the ophthalmoscope at a ⅓ meter's distance from the eye, note the red reflex. If absent, the ocular media are obscured by corneal, anterior chamber, lens or vitreous opacities. If the red reflex is present, you should be able to make out fundus details as you move closer. Examine the optic nervehead first for swelling, hemorrhages and exudates, a sign of either papillopathy (disease at the nervehead, including optic neuritis or ION), or papilledema (increased intracranial pressure). Look next at the macula for a cherry red spot (CRAO), then at the remaining visible retina. Remember that the retinal periphery can be adequately examined for detachment only with an indirect ophthalmoscope through a dilated pupil.

DIPLOPIA

Diplopia, or double vision, may signal life-threatening disease. But it is also a symptom of ocular or orbital disease with totally different clinical implications. Unless you are able to identify a pattern that clearly suggests an intracranial emergency, it is prudent to refer the patient to an ophthalmologist.

The eight diplopic syndromes and their associated emergent conditions (in parenthesis) are (Fig. 14.5):

1. Third nerve palsy (intracranial aneurysm) or transtentorial (uncal) herniation (see Chapter 4),

2. Sixth nerve palsy (increased intracranial pressure),

3. Fourth nerve palsy (hydrocephalus),

4. Unilateral ophthalmoplegia (pituitary apoplexy, cavernous sinus thrombosis),

5. Bilateral ophthalmoplegia (Guillain-Barré syndrome, myasthenia gravis, botulism),

6. Internuclear ophthalmoplegia (brainstem stroke, cerebellar hemorrhage),

7. Skew deviation (brainstem stroke, cerebellar hemorrhage),

8. Upgaze paresis (hydrocephalus).

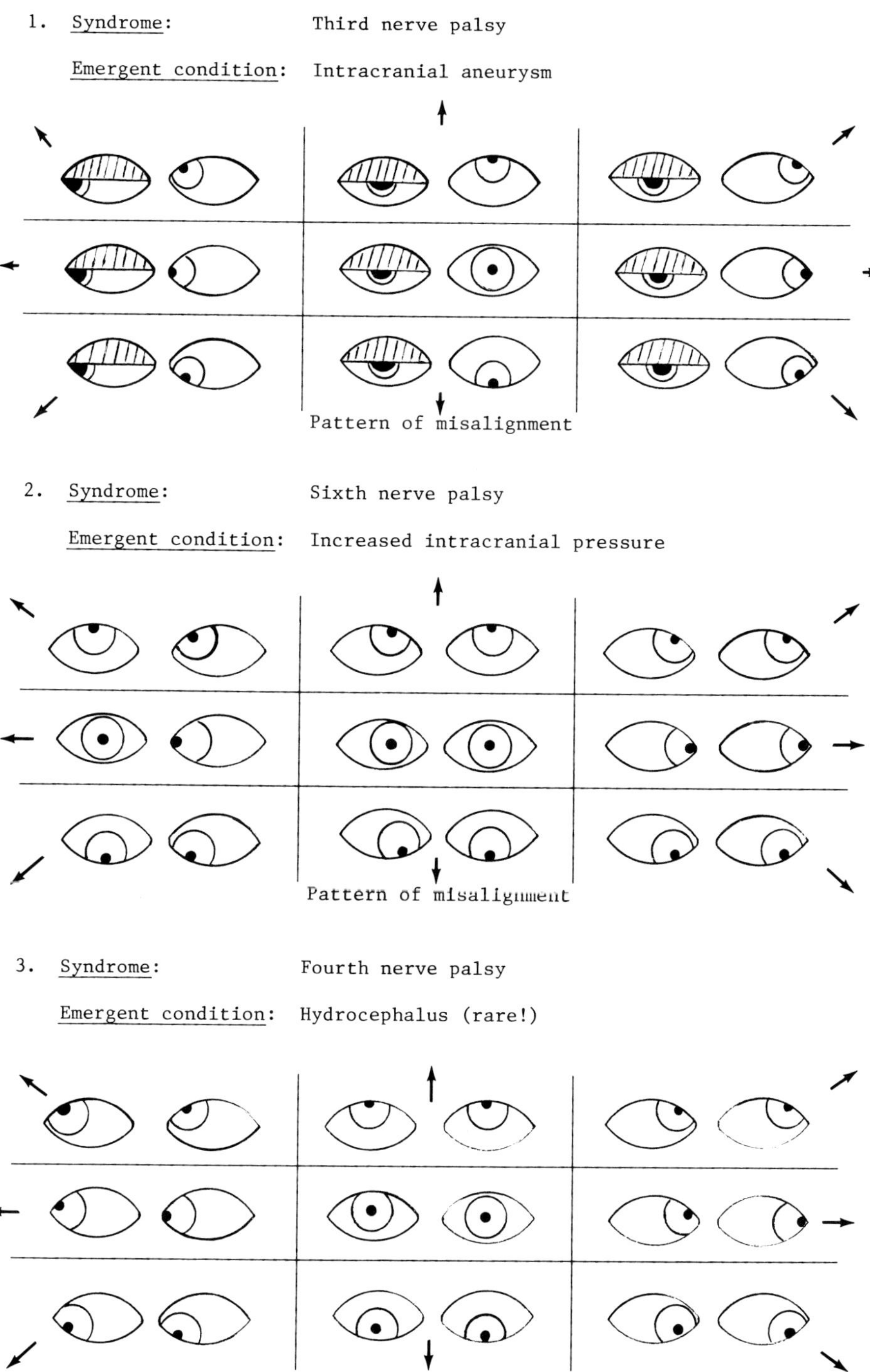

Fig. 14.5 Eight Diplopic Syndromes and Their Emergent Conditions.

4. <u>Syndrome</u>:   Unilateral ophthalmoplegia

   <u>Emergent conditions</u>:   Cavernous sinus thrombosis, pituitary apoplexy,
                               sphenoid sinus mucocoele

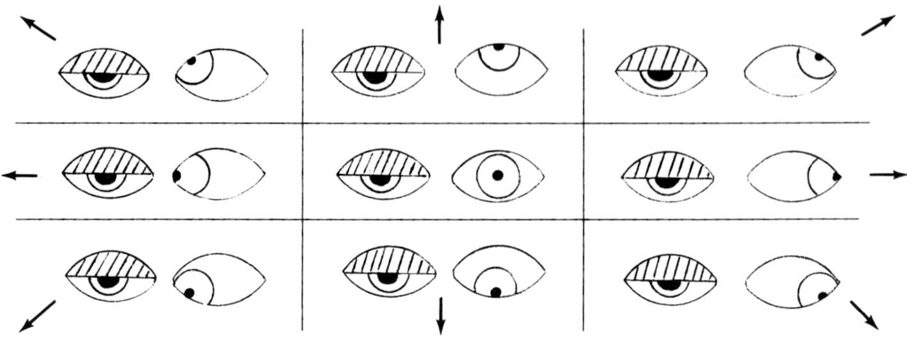

Pattern of misalignment

5. <u>Syndrome</u>:   Bilateral ophthalmoplegia

   <u>Emergent conditions</u>:   Guillain-Barre, myasthenia gravis, botulism

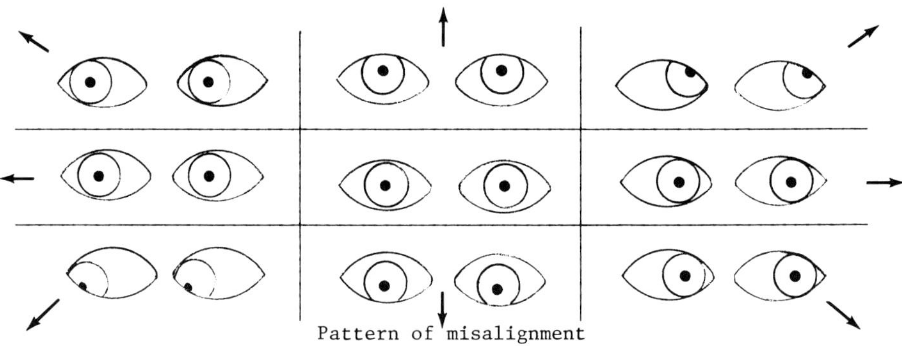

Pattern of misalignment

6. <u>Syndrome</u>:   Internuclear ophthalmoplegia

   <u>Emergent conditions</u>:   Brainstem stroke, cerebellar hemorrhage

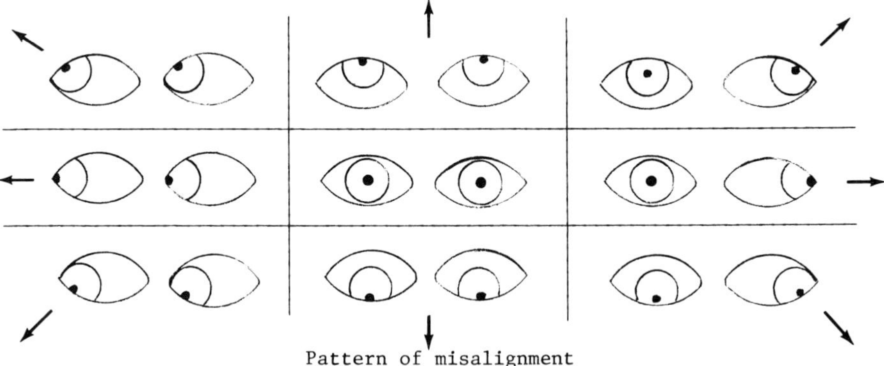

Pattern of misalignment

Fig. 14.5 *(continued)*

7. <u>Syndrome</u>: Skew deviation

    <u>Emergent conditions</u>: Brainstem stroke, cerebellar hemorrhage

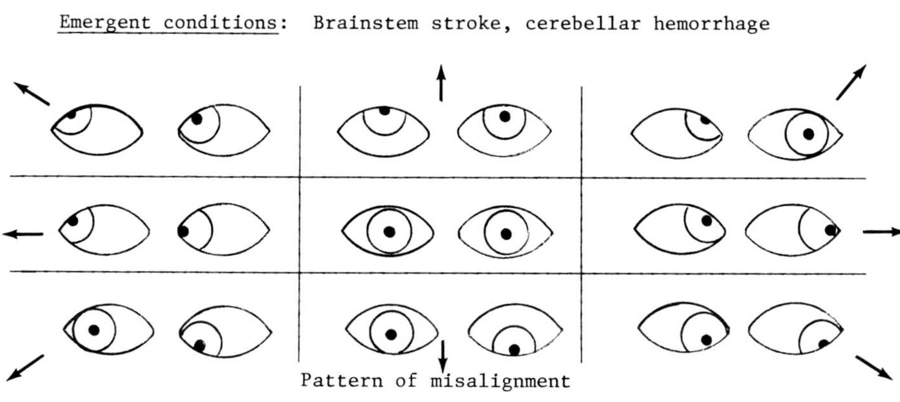

8. <u>Syndrome</u>: Upgaze paresis with convergence "nystagmus"

    <u>Emergent conditions</u>: Hydrocephalus, pinealoma, brainstem stroke

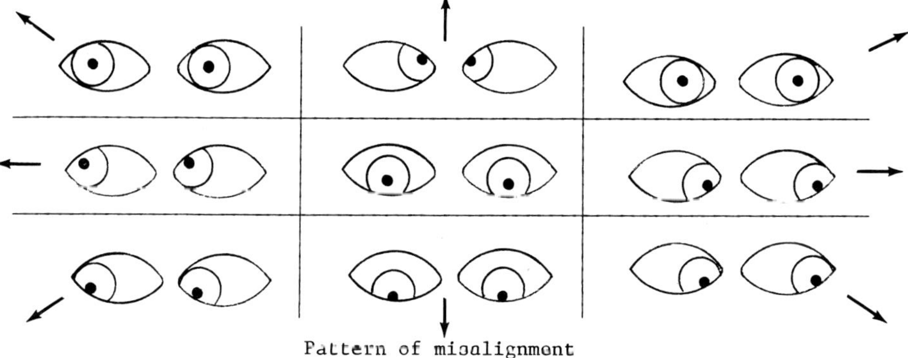

Fig. 14.5 *(continued)*

Emergent Diplopia[1,6]

Third Nerve Palsy

A small but important fraction of third nerve palsies is caused by aneurysmal compression. The intracranial aneurysm that most often presents with diplopia occurs at the junction of the internal carotid (IC) and posterior communicating arteries (PCA). Accounting for about 25 percent of all ruptured intracranial aneurysms, the IC-PCA aneurysms are distinctive in presenting more commonly with third cranial nerve palsy than with subarachnoid hemorrhage. Evidently the aneurysm first expands and compresses or bleeds into the substance of the oculomotor nerve; only with further rupture does blood spill into the subarachnoid space. It is critical to diagnose the aneurysm at the first stage, both because operative intervention is less hazardous and because a later hemorrhage may be fatal.

Intracavernous carotid aneurysms may also present with third nerve palsy. Equally often, however, they cause a complete unilateral ophthamoplegia (see below). Their treatment is not emergent because they rarely rupture.

Do not make the mistake of assuming third nerve palsies always signify intracranial aneurysm. At least 75 percent of isolated (no other neurological signs) oculomotor palsies in the elderly (aged greater than 60 years) are caused by microvascular infarction of the nerve, associated with hypertension, diabetes, and atherosclerosis. Fortunately, there is a convenient marker to separate these "non-surgical" third nerve palsies from those probably caused by aneurysmal (or rarely other) compression: the presence of pupillary paralysis. If the pupil is dilated and poorly reactive to light or a near stimulus, the chances are high that the third nerve palsy is caused by aneurysm. Similarly, a normal sized and normally reactive pupil virtually assures a non-surgical lesion. Therefore, the condition of the pupil determines the nature of the disposition. When a fixed (or poorly reactive) dilated pupil accompanies ptosis, reduced adduction, elevation and depression, aneurysm is the presumption, and urgent is the disposition.

Patients with expanding hemispheric masses or diffuse cerebral swelling may also have third nerve palsies. A fixed, dilated pupil is often the first sign. But transtentorial herniation is rarely incipient in the fully alert, ambulatory patient. It becomes a consideration only in the context of depressed consciousness. A corollary of this rule is that the fixed, dilated pupil which persists without ocular motility deficits or ptosis for more than 24 hours in an alert patient is unlikely to mean early third nerve palsy. More likely is that such patients have a peripheral cause for mydriasis—either an Adie's tonic (ciliary ganglionitis) pupil or contamination of the eye with an atropinic substance.

Sixth Nerve Palsy

Sixth nerve palsy is a common manifestation of either supratentorial or infratentorial masses causing increased intracranial pressure, or local compression of the nerve. Pressure displaces the brain stem downwards along the clivus, stretching and distorting the long basal portion of the sixth cranial nerve. You must check carefully for papilledema. Its absence virtually excludes increased intracranial pressure and means that the abduction palsy is caused by disease near or in the intracranial or orbital portion of the sixth nerve. Many cases of isolated sixth nerve palsy remain idiopathic and resolve within months.

Fourth Nerve Palsy

This syndrome produces the most difficult misalignment to diagnose. On the affected side, the eye will be higher, especially in the field of action of the superior oblique (depression in adduction). Ductions are often apparently full. Diplopia fields (see below) are useful in diagnosis. Fourth nerve palsies are rarely a sign of an emergent problem. They are most often caused by head trauma, by microvascular ischemia in diabetes or hypertension, or as decompensation of a congenital (and latent) paresis. However, they may reflect compression of the rostral and dorsal 4th ventricle, as by pinealoma, medulloblastoma, or ependymoma.

Unilateral Ophthalmoplegia

This syndrome is characterized by damage to cranial nerves 3, 4 and 6 on one side which often denotes a cavernous sinus lesion.

Mucormycosis is a potentially lethal infection caused by Phycomycetes fungi acting as opportunists in a compromised host. There are two principal syndromes, the systemic, seated in the lungs, and the nasal-sinus-orbital-cerebral. Patients with leukemia or lymphoma contract the former, while diabetics in poor control tend to be victims of the latter type.

The nasal-sinus-orbital-cerebral form usually presents as a unilateral ophthalmoplegia of rapid (less than one week) onset. The cavernous sinus has been invaded by fungi tracking along blood vessels and causing tissue necrosis and vessel thrombosis as they proceed. A tissue diagnosis is often available by examination of the nasal or palatal mucosa for black necrotic debris. Sinus radiographs may show clouding but normal films do not exclude the diagnosis. CT is typically non-contributory. The diagnosis must be presumptive, and must be made quickly. If untreated, the disease will kill within 2 weeks. Treatment consists of normalizing metabolic status, eliminating immunosuppressant medications, debridement of sinuses (maxillary, ethmoid, and sphenoid) and intravenous amphotericin B. With prompt therapy, survival is reported in 75 percent of cases.

Cavernous sinus thrombosis is generally the result of hematogenous spread from an infected source on the face, sinuses, orbit, middle ear, mouth, or neck. It may also rarely occur in the course of meningitis. Clinical signs include a unilateral ophthalmoplegia, partly, if not completely, caused by marked orbital soft tissue congestion—proptosis, swollen lids, and an injected conjunctiva. These signs may be difficult to differentiate from orbital cellulitis, but even this diagnosis is an emergency because it may lead to cavernous sinus thrombosis or meningitis. The presence of fever, lethargy, meningismus, or seizures demands the exclusion of cavernous sinus thrombosis or meningitis. Ptosis and pupillary mydriasis need not be present.

Often confused with cavernous sinus thrombosis is the carotid-cavernous fistula. Patients have usually suffered severe head trauma with basilar skull fracture, causing a rent in the intracavernous carotid. Some cases occur spontaneously, either as a blow-out of an arteriosclerotic intracavernous aneurysm or dural arteriovenous malformation. Congestive orbital signs may be quite dramatic with prolapsing conjunctival chemosis. Patients often complain of a cranial bruit synchronous with the heart beat. While the signs may be flamboyant and the symptoms bothersome, the condition is not life-threatening and may be approached without urgency.

Pituitary apoplexy, a cause of sudden chiasmal visual loss, may also produce a unilateral ophthalmoplegia if the infarcted gland swells laterally into the cavernous sinus instead of superiorly against the optic chiasm. Sudden compression of one cavernous sinus may also occur with breakthrough of a sphenoid sinus mucocoele. Treatment is transsphenoidal decompression.

Bilateral Ophthalmoplegia

Bilateral ophthalmoplegia usually implies peripheral nervous system disease (although rarely pituitary apoplexy may produce this syndrome). Three emergent conditions exist: Guillain-Barré syndrome, myasthenia gravis, and botulism.

Guillain-Barré Syndrome (GBS)

GBS is a diffuse sensorimotor (primarily motor) polyradiculoneuropathy commonly beginning in the lower extremities and ascending to involve the trunk and upper extremities. Cranial nerves may also become involved, and, in one variant (Fisher Syndrome), may be the most prominently affected. Diplopia results from bilateral but asymmetric ophthalmoplegia, often sparing both the lids and pupils. Diagnosis is assisted by finding elevated spinal fluid protein in the absence of a pleocytosis ("albumino-cytologic dissociation"). The emergency lies in the fact that patients may rapidly progress to respiratory paralysis and require immediate ventilatory support. Failure of bulbar muscles may precipitate aspiration of food.

Myasthenia Gravis

This often presents with transient but relapsing involvement of extraocular muscles and the levator palpebrae (causing ptosis). However, patients may develop a life-threatening "myasthenic crisis," especially during an illness, postoperatively, or after taking aminoglycoside drugs (such as gentamycin) which inhibit neuromuscular transmission. A patient in myasthenic crisis will typically have the sudden onset of bilateral ophthalmoplegia and ptosis; the deficits are likely to be quite asymmetric so that diplopia will result. Pupils are always spared in myasthenia. Look for coexistent bulbar and proximal extremity weakness. As with Guillain-Barré patients, myasthenics may require ventilatory support.

Botulism

Botulism is an acute poisoning from the toxin of Clostridium botulinum acquired from ingestion of inadequately cooked or defectively canned food. The toxin blocks conduction in cholinergic synapses. Symptoms begin within 5 to 50 hours after eating the contaminated food, and consist first of cramps, nausea, vomiting, diarrhea or constipation, lassitude and headaches. Soon afterwards, patients complain of swallowing difficulty, diplopia, dry mouth, and respiratory distress.

Examination reveals bilateral ophthalmoplegia of patchy type, ptosis, and dilated poorly reactive pupils (differentiating the condition from myasthenia gravis). Spinal fluid is characteristically normal, unlike that seen in Guillain-Barré. Treatment consists of administration of antitoxin and ventilatory support. (Further discussion of these three neuromuscular diseases is presented in Chapter 10.)

Inernuclear ophthalmoplegia

Caused by a lesion in the medial longitudinal fasciculus, this syndrome consists of reduced or slowed adduction on the ipsilateral eye and nystagmus in the contralateral eye. Although usually caused by intrinsic brainstem disease, (including an evolving brainstem stroke), it may also be seen in extrinsic compression, as in cerebellar hemorrhage. Other brainstem signs and symptoms are usually present.

Skew Deviation

This is a vertical misalignment of the eyes caused by a lesion of the supranuclear ocular motor pathways within the brainstem. Eye movements are usually of normal amplitude, although jerky pursuit movements and nystagmus may be seen. Lesions in the midbrain, pons, medulla and cerebellum have been associated with this abnormality of ocular alignment. It is not caused by a defect in a cranial nerve, but by a defect in the supranuclear ocular motor pathway. You will diagnose skew deviation when the vertical misalignment does not fit the characteristics of a third or fourth nerve palsy, of myasthenia gravis or restrictive ocular muscle conditions, and when other signs of brainstem compromise are present.

Upgaze Palsy

Patients with compression of the dorsal midbrain by aqueductal stenosis, pinealoma, or other causes of obstructive hydrocephalus will show a downward deviation of the eyes with deficient upgaze. In addition, the eyes may converge in attempted upgaze, producing momentary diplopia.

Non-Emergent Diplopia

Although diplopia may be a distress signal, often it is not. You should recognize the signs of non-emergent causes of double vision.

"Non-diplopia" Diplopia

Some patients (and physicians!) confuse other visual symptoms with double vision such as blurred or distorted vision in one eye, oscillopsia (illusory movement of the environment), scintillations, or floaters.

Monocular Diplopia

Ask the patient if the double vision persists with one or the other eye covered. If diplopia remains after either eye is closed, you must diagnose monocular diplopia, an optical aberration caused by early cataract or corneal disease.

Comitant Diplopia

Horizontal diplopia in which the two images are separated by the same distance in all fields of gaze ("comitant") is rarely caused by active or recent-onset neurologic disease. Instead, it is the result of a disturbance in alignment which has been latent since childhood and only recently become manifest. Why these latent comitant misalignments "break down" with time is not known.

Restrictive Diplopia

Diplopia may be the symptom of ocular misalignment that results from a myogenic rather than a neurogenic cause. Orbital inflammation, such as occurs in Graves' disease and in idiopathic (autoimmune) orbital pseudotumor, may produce scarring and contracture of extraocular muscles. Their reduced elasticity limits ocular movement. Orbital trauma may cause diplopia acutely, either by entrapment of the inferior rectus muscle in a floor fracture, by marked swelling, or by direct damage to muscles.

The ultimate confirmation of a restrictive extraocular myopathy comes from performing a forced duction test. After anesthetizing the conjunctiva (with topical 10 percent Cocaine), the insertion of the extraocular muscle is grasped with forceps and the eye moved in the direction of the reduced movement. If mechanically restricted, the eye will be limited in its excursion; if paretic because of a nerve or other nonrestrictive lesion, the eye will move normally. This is a test best reserved for the ophthalmologist. But be wary of diagnosing neurologic disease as the cause of diplopia in the presence of congestive orbital signs. Forced ductions may reveal a contractured muscle.

Steps In The Examination Of Patients With Diplopia

Ocular Versions

Ask the patient to follow your finger as you take him through the full range (right, left, up, down) of conjugate eye movements (versions). If the patient has a full amplitude of horizontal versions, the sclera will disappear into the canthi. In other words, a patient with normal versions should be able to "bury the whites of his eyes" with side gaze. It is more difficult to judge whether vertical versions are of normal amplitude. Upgaze diminishes with age but the patient should still be able to move the eyes at least 20°. Down gaze is not affected by age. Actually, it is more the difference in amplitude between the movements of two eyes that is diagnostic in patients with diplopia.

Ocular Ductions

If you observe a difference in amplitude of movement of one eye as compared to the other, test each eye separately while the other is covered (ductions). A reduced duction confirms your suspicion.

Diplopia Fields (Fig. 14.6)

In many cases of binocular diplopia, there will be no obvious reduction in versional amplitude because the deficits are small. In this circumstance, the most valuable maneuver is to plot a "diplopia field," using the patient's appreciation of the separation of the two images in different fields of gaze.

In a dimly-lit room, have the patient view a distant bright light at a distance of at least 3 meters (to avoid overlooking sixth nerve palsies). Ask him if he sees two lights. If not, either he does not have diplopia in straight ahead gaze, or he does not understand the instructions. To assist this communication, it sometimes helps to place a red filter over one eye so that one image appears white to the patient, the other appears red.

If the patient perceives two images, ask him to indicate their relative positions with his fingers. If the image seen with the right eye is displaced to the right, diplopia is called "uncrossed," and one eye is deviated inward. If the image seen with the right eye is displaced to the left, the diplopia is called "crossed," and one eye is deviated outward.

Now move the patient's head to the left so that his eyes are in right gaze. Have him indicate the positions of the two images. Repeat this maneuver for the four eccentric gaze positions. The gaze position of the greatest separation of images is the most critical. The lateral image always belongs to the affected eye; the muscle responsible for its movement into that field of gaze is either paretic or restricted in its function. For example, if the

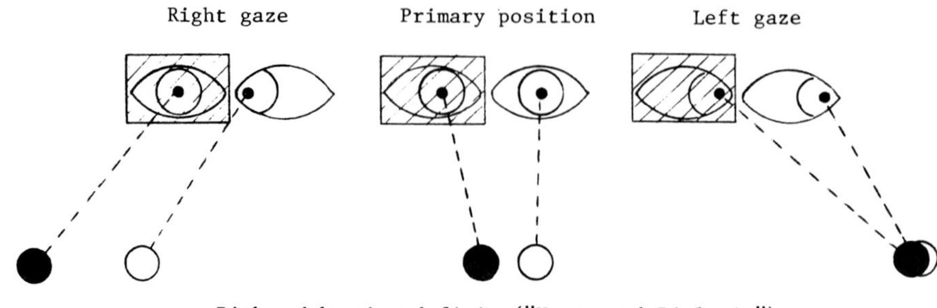

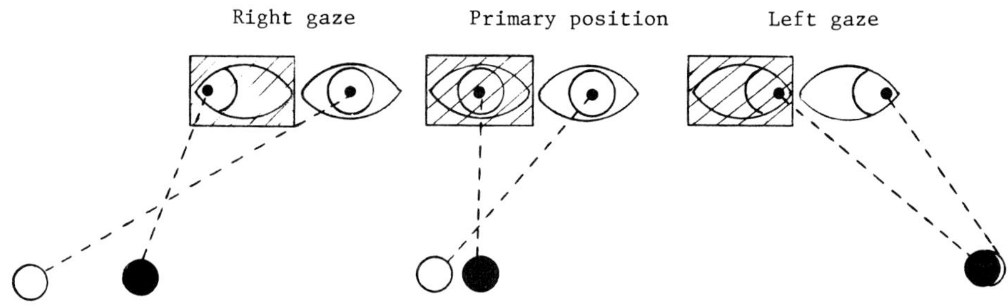

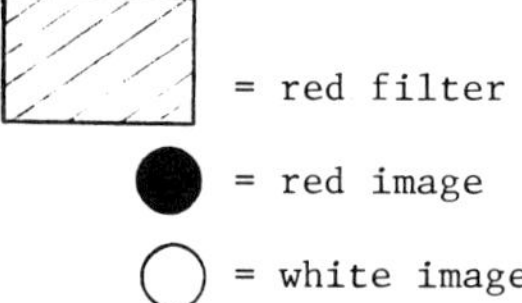

Fig. 14.6 The Diplopia Field Test.

patient describes uncrossed diplopia with greatest image separation in the right gaze, then the right lateral rectus is either weak or restricted (Fig. 14.6a). If diplopia is crossed and greatest separation of images occurs in right gaze, then the left medial rectus is paretic or restricted in its duction (Fig. 14.6b).

In vertical diplopia with greatest separation of images in up gaze, the higher image belongs to the affected eye, whose elevators (superior rectus and/or inferior oblique) are weak or restricted. In vertical diplopia with greatest image separation in down gaze, the lower image belongs to the affected eye, whose depressors (inferior rectus or superior oblique) are paretic or restricted.

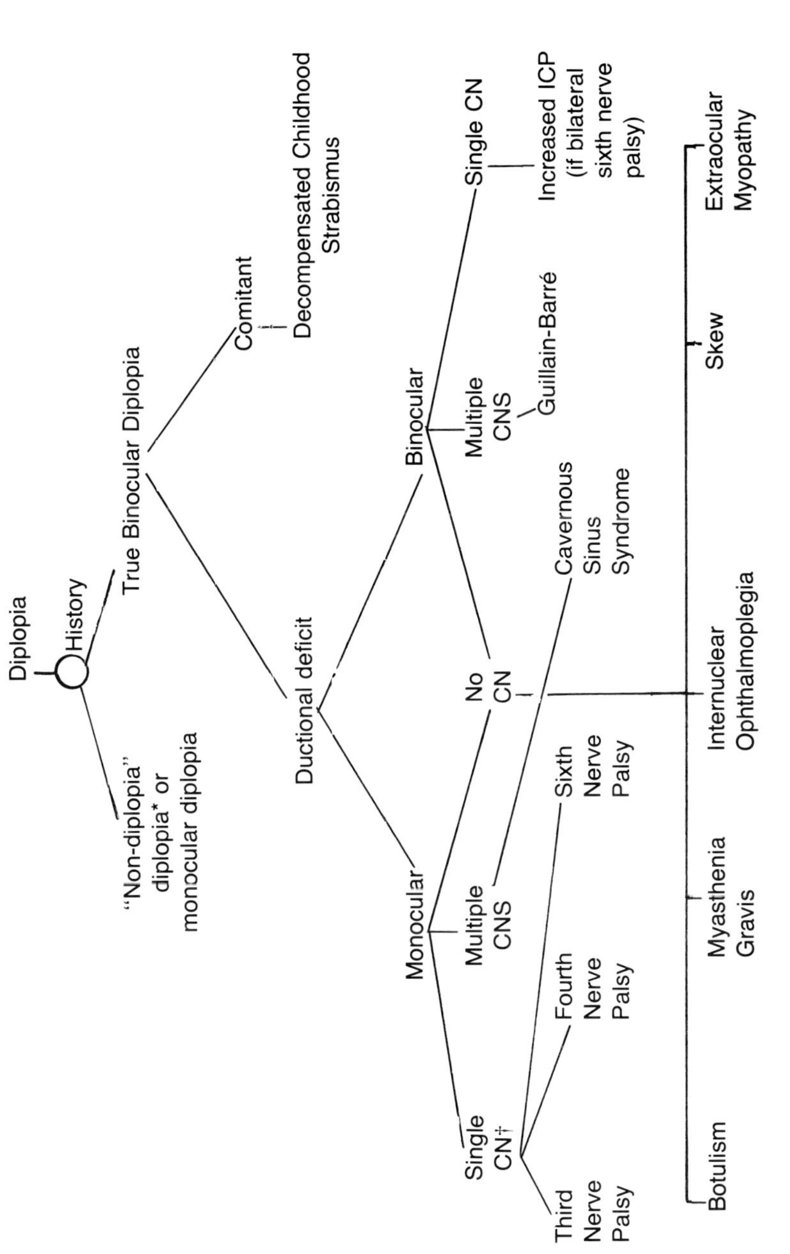

*Blurred vision, oscillopsia, floaters.
†Cranial Nerve

Fig. 14.7 Diagnosis of Diplopia.

Diagnosing the Diplopia Syndrome (Fig. 14.7)

Once you have determined in which field of action the reduced eye movement is present, consider which muscle is active in that domain. Now ask yourself if the findings are explainable by weakness of a single ocular motor cranial nerve (3, 4, or 6) on one side. If not, is the deficiency caused by involvement of more than one cranial nerve on one side (unilateral ophthalmoplegia)? This would suggest cavernous sinus involvement.

If you believe that motility is impaired on both sides, is it due to impairment of a single cranial nerve or many? Involvement of a single nerve on both sides is most common in bilateral sixth nerve palsies associated with increased intracranial pressure. Impairment of multiple cranial nerves on both sides suggests Guillain-Barré.

If the motility findings do not obey a cranial nerve pattern, regardless of whether the deficit is unilateral or bilateral, you are dealing either with (1) botulism, (2) myasthenia gravis, (3) internuclear ophthalmoplegia, (4) skew deviation, or (5) a restrictive extraocular muscle condition. Using the information you have been given, you should be able to make the distinction among these entities.

REFERENCES

1. Cogan, D.G.: Neurology of the Ocular Muscles. Charles C. Thomas, Springfield, 1956. (A succinct and well-written short text, considered a classic.)
2. Cullen, J.F., Coleiro, J.A.: Ophthalmic complications of giant cell arteritis. Surv. Ophthalmol., 20:247, 1976. (The best source for ophthalmic signs in this disease.)
3. Duane, T.D., Ed.: Clinical Ophthalmology. Harper & Row, Philadelphia, 1981. (This is the most up-to-date reference for clinical problems of all kinds.)
4. Glaser, J.S.: Neuro-Ophthalmology. Harper & Row, Philadelphia, 1981. (The best short reference book for all neuro-ophthalmic diseases.)
5. Goodman, B.W.: Temporal arteritis. Amer. J. Med., 67:839, 1979. (The most comprehensive recent article on the subject.)
6. Rush, J.A., Younge, B.R.: Paralysis of cranial nerves III, IV and VI. Cause and prognosis in 1000 cases. Arch. Ophthalmol., 99:76, 1981.
7. Trobe, J.D., Glaser, J.S., LaFlamme, P.: Dysthyroid optic neuropathy. The clinical course and rationale for management. Arch. Ophthalmol., 96:1199, 1978.
8. Walsh, F.B., Hoyt, W.F.: Clinical Neuro-ophthalmology. Williams & Wilkins, Baltimore, 1978. (A prodigious (three volumes) collection of facts—the most comprehensive reference in this field.)
9. Weisberg, L.A.: Pituitary apoplexy. Am. J. Med., 63:109, 1977. (A good summary.)

15

Multiple Sclerosis

Jack S. Burks, M.D.
David S. Thompson, M.D.

INTRODUCTION

Although multiple sclerosis is one of the most common neurologic diseases
in the United States, most health care professionals feel inadequate to care
for the numerous problems encountered by the MS patient. The MS patient
presents a challenge even to the most sophisticated physician. Since MS
can affect any area of the central nervous system, symptoms are so varied
as to often be confusing when the patient presents in the emergency room.
To ensure appropriate treatment, the diagnosis of MS must first be confirmed. Once a diagnosis has been confirmed, the most difficult problems
are deciding if the symptoms are secondary to (1) an acute exacerbation,
(2) another medical problem, or (3) a worsening of a previous exacerbation
secondary to factors such as stress or fatigue. In this chapter, we hope to
prepare the physician to better treat the problems encountered with the
MS patient.

DEFINITION

Multiple sclerosis is characterized by destruction of multiple areas of central
nervous system myelin. Symptoms of MS depend on the location of these
myelin plaques. The severity and range of symptoms vary widely. Some
of the more common symptoms of MS include decreased vision, weakness,
ataxia, paresthesias, diplopia, bowel/bladder and sexual dysfunction.

The vast majority of multiple sclerosis patients have symptoms which
occur in "attacks" or exacerbations followed by remissions. To classify a
patient as having definite MS, the following criteria need to be met: (1) a
relapsing/remitting course with at least two episodes separated by 1 month
or a step-wise progression over 6 months, (2) neurological signs indicating
central nervous system demyelination at two or more sites within the central

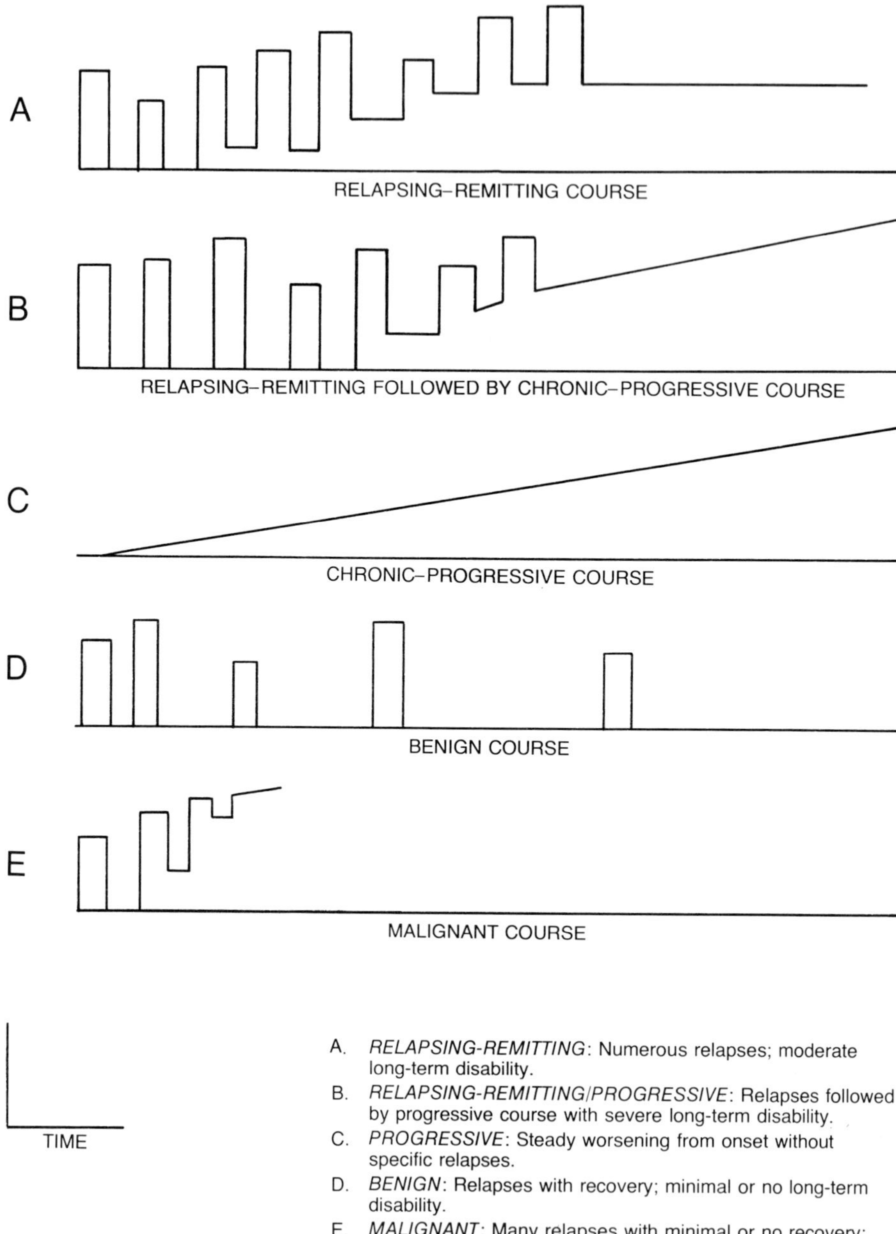

Fig. 15.1 Courses of multiple sclerosis. (Adapted from McAlpine, D., Lumsden, C.E., Acheson, E.D.: Multiple Sclerosis—a reappraisal. Churchill Livingstone, Edinburgh, 1972; with permission.)

nervous system, (3) age of onset between the ages of 10 and 50, and (4) no better explanation for the symptoms.[2]

An exacerbation of MS is defined as a period of worsening or new neurologic symptoms lasting for at least 24 to 48 hours.[2] Therefore, a patient who has decreased vision while playing tennis, which resolves within a few hours (Uhthoff's syndrome), is not considered to be having an exacerbation.

The relapsing/remitting form of the disease usually has an onset between the ages of 20 and 40. Many patients who have the onset of symptoms in the relapsing/remitting form in young adulthood may have less frequent exacerbations in their forties and fifties. However, they may experience a slowly progressive deterioration as they become older.

About 10 percent of MS patients have a slowly progressive course from the initial presenting symptom (i.e., they do not experience exacerbations). The symptoms often start in the lower extremities with a spastic paraparesis between the ages of 30 to 50.

Another group of patients have a benign course. The benign form is defined as an MS patient who has minimal or no disability many years after the onset of their first symptoms. The incidence of benign MS is hard to assess since an accurate diagnosis may be difficult without pathological confirmation.

A rare form of MS is the malignant form. These patients experience a rapidly progressive deterioration with severe incapacitation or death within months to a few years after the onset of their disease (Fig. 15.1).[14]

PROGNOSIS

The natural course of the disease for any given patient is difficult to assess since there is so much individual variability. Some patients who have numerous attacks initially, will continue to have minimal or no disability. Other patients who have had just a few attacks, will not recover from those attacks. However, there are certain guidelines which are useful. First, patients with minimal or no disability 5 years after the onset of their symptoms tend to have a more benign course throughout their life. Patients with primarily sensory, brainstem, or visual symptoms tend to have less long-term disability than patients with primarily pyramidal tract dysfunction, ataxia or bowel and bladder dysfunction.

For an individual exacerbation, approximately two-thirds of the patients will improve spontaneously. The degree of recovery is inversely proportional to the duration of symptoms. In other words, patients whose symptoms are short-lived tend to have more complete recovery. The longer the attack persists, the less likely the patient will recover completely.[9]

In the early course of the disease, the "average" patient will have a relapse within 2 years of the onset of the disease. The possibility of further exacerbation decreases if the patient is exacerbation-free for over 3 years.

The long-term prognosis for an individual patient is difficult to assess. In general, one-third of MS patients have a benign course. Another third of patients have moderate disability. The remaining third have a severe disability. A Mayo Clinic study demonstrated that 50 percent of patients who survived for 29 years after the disease onset, maintained the ability to walk.[15]

The average duration of the illness from onset of symptoms to death is between 25 and 35 years for most patients. Therefore, MS is not a fatal disease in the usual sense. Deaths are most often due to infections, such as pneumonia, urinary tract infections, or complications of decubitus ulcers.

EPIDEMIOLOGY

A number of epidemiologic observations have been noted in groups with a higher incidence of MS. These factors include where one has lived during the childhood years, race, educational level, socio-economic status and genetic make-up. To be more specific, multiple sclerosis is more common in temperate climates. Epidemiologists have shown that this high incidence of multiple sclerosis in temperate climates is carried with persons if they move as an adult to a low-incidence area, such as a tropical climate.[8] MS is a disease that is less often seen in Blacks and Orientals than in the Caucasion populations. An explanation of the racial imbalance resides in possible immune regulatory abnormalities which are genetically determined.[17] MS is approximately 10 times more common in family members of MS patients as compared to the normal population.[8] Again, this indicates a genetic predisposition, but there is no evidence for a specific Mendelian pattern of inheritance.

ETIOLOGY OF MULTIPLE SCLEROSIS

There are three major theories for the cause of multiple sclerosis. The first is the allergic or hyper-immune theory which states that subsets of lymphocytes are somehow sensitized to the body's myelin, and therefore, destroy the myelin. Antibody has also been implicated in the destructive process.

The second theory is the viral suppression theory that states a virus infection suppresses the immune system. While the immune system is suppressed, the virus destroys the myelin.

The third theory is a multi-factorial theory involving (1) a genetic predisposition, (2) an environmental exposure to an agent such as a virus, (3) the age of exposure to this virus or other environmental agents and (4) an abnormal immune regulatory response. A latent virus infection of oligodendroglial

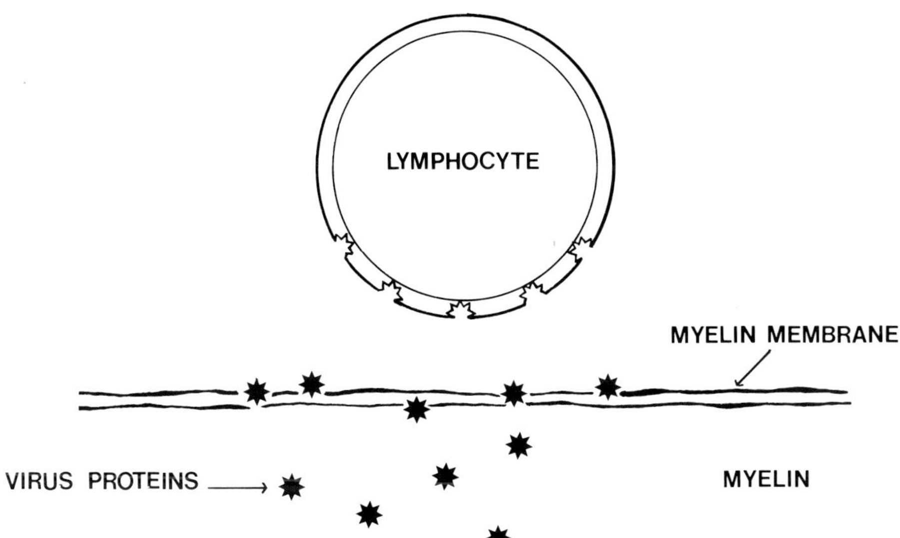

Fig. 15.2 An illustration depicting a viral induced immunopathologic mechanism of demyelination in MS. Viral antigens are expressed on myelin membranes. Lymphocytes with virus receptors acquired by being previously sensitized to the virus, attach to and destroy the virus, which is still part of the meylin membrane. In the process, the myelin membrane or oligodendroglial cell is damaged or destroyed.

cells (myelin-producing cells) occurs in childhood. Later, possibly years later, the virus is activated by factors which are unknown, but may include temperature elevation, infection, trauma, emotional stress, and allergies. When the virus is activated, it is released from the cell by budding off cell membranes. In the process of budding off cell membranes, the immune system (lymphocyte mediated) which has been previously sensitized to the virus, "sees" the virus on the cell membrane and destroys the virus and the cell membrane (Fig. 15.2). This viral induced, immunopathologic process causes the myelin destruction.

The mechanism of a remission is also not well understood. Part of the recovery or remission may be related to resolving edema and inflammatory response around the acute lesion. Re-myelination may also play a role in the recovery process.[6]

DIFFERENTIAL DIAGNOSIS

In the emergency room, problems possibly related to multiple sclerosis should be divided into two groups. The first group are patients who present with neurologic problems where multiple sclerosis arises in the differential diagnosis. The second group are patients who have a diagnosis of multiple sclerosis and are presenting with new symptoms or an exacerbation of previous symptoms.

For the patient who has neurologic symptoms for which multiple sclerosis is in the differential diagnosis, it is important to obtain a detailed medical history with particular attention to any history of previous neurologic problems. On examination, it is important to try to localize more than one area of central nervous system involvement before a diagnosis of MS is seriously considered.

Even with evidence of "multiple lesions in time and space," other neurologic conditions should be considered. Cervical spondylosis may be especially difficult to differentiate from MS when there is cord compression with bilateral pyramidal tract signs. Also, cervical spondylosis may cause vertebrobasilar insufficiency with intermittent brain stem signs. Usually, cervical spondylosis is an illness of the older adult population, while MS tends to be a disease of patients under the age of 40.

Spinal cord angiomatous malformations may often be associated with attacks and remissions of neurologic dysfunction, which may mimic multiple sclerosis. However, symptoms from an AVM are usually confined to one level of the spinal cord.

Tumors may be confused with multiple sclerosis, especially in certain locations. For example, foramen magnum tumors have an unusual ability to cause step-wise progression of symptoms with unusual patterns of extremity weakness. Parasagittal meningiomas may present with a spastic paraparesis. Cerebellar cyst and midline tumors often give confusing and intermittent neurologic signs.

Myelopathies associated with vitamin deficiency, diabetes, or toxins such as triorthocresylphosphate may mimic MS but can be distinguished by the history and specific laboratory tests. The various forms of transverse myelitis can usually be distinguished because the spinal cord involvement is limited to one level.

Collagen vascular disease may be very difficult to distinguish from multiple sclerosis, especially in young women with systemic lupus erythematosus presenting with neurologic signs. Amyotrophic lateral sclerosis (ALS) causing motor neuron dysfunction usually can be distinguished from MS because of the lack of sensory involvement and the prominent muscle wasting and fasciculations in ALS.

In young people, vascular disorders may present with intermittent symptoms. Embolic infarcts, especially from the heart can give multifocal signs and symptoms of neurologic dysfunction. Therefore, a thorough cardiac exam should be performed.

Classical migraine headaches are sometimes confused with multiple sclerosis when focal neurologic signs and symptoms are a prominent feature of the prodromal period. In the early course of migraine headaches, the prodromal period may be followed by only a mild headache or no headache. However, in classical migraine headaches, the symptoms resolve quickly.

The migraine headache patient should have a normal neurologic examination within a few hours after the onset of symptoms. MS patients develop symptoms more slowly and the symptoms resolve much more slowly.

Rarely, difficulty arises in distinguishing MS from hereditary spinocerebellar degenerations and olivopontocerebellar degeneration. Most of these illnesses are progressive in nature and a family history may be obtained of similar illnesses. In addition, the progressive form of MS typically involves primarily the spinal cord without major cerebellar symptoms or signs.

Progressive multifocal leukoencephalopathy, a disease usually associated with lymphoma and immune deficiency states, consists of multifocal lesions within the white matter. These patients usually have dementia and a relatively rapid progressive course over 6 to 18 months in addition to their multifocal neurologic signs.

In the setting of a history of alcohol abuse and signs of pontine dysfunction, the diagnosis of central pontine myelinolysis, which may be associated with low sodium, should be considered in the differential diagnosis of multiple sclerosis.

Drug intoxication is unlikely to be mistaken for multiple sclerosis due to change in mental status associated with drugs. Intravenous amphetamine abuse with subsequent vasculitis may present with multifocal signs.

Another problem that may arise in the emergency room involves the patient with a seizure. Could the seizure patient have multiple sclerosis? Seizures occur more frequently in multiple sclerosis patients than in the general population. An estimated 1 to 4 percent of MS patients have seizures. However, a seizure presenting as the initial symptom in multiple sclerosis is very unlikely.

Other conditions which should be considered in the differential diagnosis of multiple sclerosis are included in Tables 15.1 and 15.2.[20]

When a known multiple sclerosis patient enters the emergency room with neurologic complaints, the differential diagnosis is still important. One cannot automatically conclude that the new symptom is an exacerbation of multiple sclerosis. For example, emotional and physical stress factors can play a major role in a subjective worsening of symptoms. The degree of objective neurologic involvement should be documented and compared to previous neurological examinations.

The MS patient's symptoms may not be related to multiple sclerosis, but may be related to medications. Common medications taken by MS patients include anti-spasticity medications, anticholinergics, and anti-convulsants. All of these have potential toxicity. Therefore, it is imperative to take a comprehensive drug history. A blood and urine toxin screen may be worthwhile in some circumstances.

Infections are very common in the debilitated multiple sclerosis patient. Often, during infections, patients will experience an increase in their multiple sclerosis symptoms. Pneumonia and urinary tract infections are two of the most common medical complications.

Table 15.1 Differential Diagnosis of MS

Major Causes of Disease	Specific Disease Considerations
Congenital malformations	Platybasia Syringomyelia Arnold-Chiari malformation Vertebral malformation Brain stem angioma
Hereditary	Hereditary ataxias Adrenal leukodystrophy
Inborn errors of metabolism	Wilson's disease
Vascular	Thrombosis Cerebral infarction Brain stem infarction Cerebral vascular insufficiency
Nutritional	B_{12} deficiency (subacute combined degeneration)
Neoplastic disorders	Pontine glioma Acoustic neurinoma Spinal cord tumors, especially at foramen magnum Metastatic disease
Bony mechanical entrapment	Cervical spondylosis a) Radiculopathy b) Cord compression c) Arterial compression
Infection and inflammation	CNS syphilis Arachnoiditis Subacute sclerosing panencephalitis (SSPE) Progressive rubella panencephalitis Progressive multifocal leukoencephalopathy
Postvaccinal and postinfectious syndromes	Postinfectious encephalomyelitis Postvaccinal encephalomyelitis Guillain-Barré syndrome Acute transverse myelitis
Autoimmune diseases	Systemic lupus erythematosus (SLE) Polyarteritis nodosa Temporal arteritis
Intoxication	Triorthocresylphosphate Alcoholism
Unknown	Amyotrophic lateral sclerosis (ALS) Primary lateral sclerosis Leber's optic atrophy Sporadic Schilder's disease Subacute necrotizing myelitis
Functional syndromes	May be present to some degree in all patients; occasionally such symptoms may be secondary to CNS dysfunction

(from U.S. Veterans Administration: Multiple Sclerosis: guidelines for diagnosis and management. Neurology service, pub. 1B 11–70, 1980; reprinted with permission.)

Table 15.2 Differential Diagnosis of Spinal Cord MS

  I Related to bone and joint pathology
   A. Cervical spondylosis (root entrapment, cord compression, vertebrobasilar insufficiency)
   B. Median herniation of cervical disc
   C. Odontoid process abnormalities
   D. Basilar impression
   E. Arnold-Chiari malformation
   F. Vertebral malformations, e.g., spina bifida or Klippel-Feil with associated cervical spinal
      cord abnormalities
 II Tumor
   A. Meningioma
   B. Neurofibroma (neurolemmoma)
   C. Glioma
   D. Granuloma
   E. Metastasis
   F. Congenital extradural cyst
   G. Chordoma
   H. Cholesteatoma
    I. Multiple myeloma
   J. Lymphoma
   K. Arteriovenous malformation
III Metabolic or toxic
   A. Subacute combined degeneration (vitamin B_{12} deficiency)
   B. Toxic (anticholinesterases, triorthocresylphosphate (TOCP))
   C. Diabetic myelopathy
 IV Transverse myelitis
   A. "Viral" myelitis
   B. Syphilis (Erb's spastic paraparesis)
   C. Arachnoiditis
      1. postinfectious
      2. postirritant
   D. Remote effect of cancer
   E. Idiopathic
  V Collagen diseases
   A. Polyarteritis
   B. Lupus erythematosus
 VI Motor neuron disease

(from U.S. Veterans Administration: Multiple Sclerosis: guidelines for diagnosis and management. Neurology service, pub. 1B 11–70, 1980; reprinted with permission.)

SIGNS, SYMPTOMS AND TREATMENT OF MS EXACERBATIONS

The following discussion of signs and symptoms in MS exacerbations is based on the assumption that the patient has "clinically definite" multiple sclerosis as defined in the introduction, and that extraneous factors such as fever and adverse reaction to medication have been excluded. Because of the multiplicity of white matter lesions, which may occur in multiple sclerosis, there is a natural tendency to ascribe all neurological signs and symptoms to the patient's multiple sclerosis. However, certain signs and symptoms are extremely rare in MS and others form common patterns. While MS symptoms and signs may develop insidiously over a period of days or weeks, a significant number can develop abruptly. In a study of 212 patients by McAlpine, 39 percent developed their symptoms in a period of minutes to hours.[14] In addition to the insidiously waxing and waning course so commonly associated with multiple sclerosis, paroxysmal symptoms lasting seconds to minutes may also occur. While not classified as "exacerbations," they are important to recognize because of their treatment potential.

GENERAL PRINCIPLES OF MANAGEMENT

As with most chronic diseases, an individual will be better able to physically and emotionally cope with future disability if he follows a few basic principles of health maintenance. These include a daily exercise program, adequate rest, well-balanced meals, and particularly in MS, an avoidance of unnecessary physical and emotional stress.

A daily exercise program is essential, not only for maintaining muscle function, but also in reducing the common symptom of fatigue. MS patients should have a baseline physical therapy evaluation which should be updated regularly to reflect the patient's current physical condition. In addition to exercise, rest is also important in combating fatigue. Patients should be encouraged to budget their energy and to take brief rests of 15 to 30 minutes when they note the onset of fatigue rather than taking specific rest periods throughout the day. Because of the common observation of MS patients that they have more energy in the morning and greater fatigue in mid-afternoon, patients should try to do most of their strenuous activity, such as cleaning and shopping, in the morning.

There have been no studies which have convincingly shown that a particular vitamin, absence or presence of a particular food substance, or a specific diet are of benefit for MS. Therefore, we recommend the patient follow a well-balanced diet with emphasis on maintaining ideal body weight.

Previous studies have reported an adverse effect of physical stress on MS.[9] Fever or elevated ambient temperature have also been observed to have a transient adverse effect on MS symptoms. For example, the patient presenting with an upper respiratory infection and quadriparesis may experience a prompt resolution of symptoms with reduction of fever. Physicians have incorporated this observation in a diagnostic hot bath test to produce transient neurological symptoms from clinically "quiet" lesions in a patient suspected of having MS.[11]

An MS exacerbation, or relapse, is defined as the development of new symptoms or signs, or significant worsening of old symptoms over a period of 24 to 48 hours. More subtle fluctuations in a fixed symptom are more likely secondary to physical or emotional stress. Because of the real and potential side effects of some of the various symptomatic treatments to be discussed, the physician should make every effort to determine that the patient is, in fact, having an exacerbation of his disease rather than a natural fluctuation in its course. As discussed in more detail in the section on diagnostic tests, CSF myelin basic protein assay, evoked potentials and CT scan may aid in making this distinction.

The fluctuating course of the disease, particularly natural remissions, should be taken into account when evaluating the efficacy of symptomatic treatment. A final consideration is the placebo response which was well documented in a cooperative study of ACTH versus placebo where 75 percent of patients in the placebo group were felt to improve during the study.[18] This placebo response may account for the numerous claims of "cures" from a variety of treatment modalities.

STEROID TREATMENT

Because of the inflammatory response with associated edema shown pathologically in acute MS plaques, steroids in various forms have been a mainstay of treatment of MS exacerbations. However, other than the previously mentioned cooperative study of ACTH versus placebo, no large study has compared various steroid preparations in the treatment of MS exacerbations. For that reason, the choice of a particular steroid preparation is largely a matter of physician preference and patient convenience.

In the cooperative study, ACTH was found to shorten exacerbations of acute optic neuritis and pyramidal, brainstem, and bladder dysfunction. ACTH was found to be of no significant benefit for exacerbations consisting of either sensory or cerebellar dysfunction.

The long-term course of the disease has not been shown to be altered by steroids. The patient should understand that the primary purpose of the steroid therapy is to shorten the duration of the exacerbation. Steroid therapy should always be supplemented with appropriate rest and physiotherapy. Prescribing steroids for more than 2 or 3 weeks has not been proved useful.

ACTH and prednisone are the two most common steroid preparations used in treating exacerbations. An acceptable regimen for ACTH is 40 units subcutaneous or intramuscularly, b.i.d. for 3 to 5 days, 30 units b.i.d. for 3 days, 20 units b.i.d. for 3 days, 10 units b.i.d. for 3 days, and 5 units b.i.d. for 3 days. Prior to the initiation of therapy, all patients should have baseline serum electrolytes, serum glucose, weight, vital signs, and appropriate screening to exclude concomitant infection. These parameters should be monitored during the course of therapy in individuals with underlying medical disorders.

Adverse reactions of short-term steroids include hypokalemia, fluid retention, nausea, insomnia, menstrual irregularities, hypertension, diaphoresis and mental alterations, most commonly depression and euphoria. Patients with diabetes, hypertension or mental illness should be monitored more closely. The prophylactic use of potassium supplement (20 to 40 mEq daily), non-constipating antacids, and a low salt diet should be considered for patients on ACTH therapy. If possible, patients contemplating elective surgery should postpone surgery until after their course of ACTH, because of delayed wound healing. Because of the potential of adrenal insufficiency and the lack of evidence that prolonged ACTH therapy is of benefit, there is no indication for prolonging therapy beyond that recommended above.

Prednisone and other steroids are alternate forms of therapy, and in many cases are more convenient for the patient because of their oral route of administration. An appropriate regimen for prednisone consists of 80 mg each morning for 3 days followed by taper by 20 mg every fourth day. The guidelines recommended for ACTH on patient selection, adverse reactions, and prophylactic measures should be followed.

WEAKNESS AND SPASTICITY

Perhaps one of the most common symptom complexes in MS involve the pyramidal system. While this may present dramatically with the acute development of paralysis, a significant number of patients may present with the non-specific complaint of easy fatiguability with prolonged ambulation or "clumsiness" of gait. Even in this group, however, evidence of upper motor neuron dysfunction consisting of increased muscle tone, hyperreflexia, and extensor plantar responses is commonly found. These latter signs can fluctuate dramatically over a period of hours or days. A pattern of spastic paraparesis with relatively symmetric weakness is most commonly described in various MS series.[9] This is frequently associated with bladder dysfunction and impairment of vibratory sensation in the lower extremities. As mentioned earlier, exacerbations of weakness may be shortened through the use of either ACTH or steroids.

An unusual and confusing finding in the upper extremities consists of diminished reflexes and occasional atrophy of the hand musculature, resembling a lower motor neuron lesion. These findings have been ascribed by past investigators to involvement of the posterior root component of the reflex arc and to direct involvement of the anterior horn cell by an MS plaque.

In addition to paresis, a patient's complaint of "weakness" may also represent changes in the degree of spasticity, cerebellar or sensory ataxia, elevated temperature, or depression.

The neurologic examination will distinguish between increased spasticity versus increased weakness. Other terms used by patients to describe their spasticity include "stiffness," "spasms," and "cramping."

In evaluating the need for treatment, remember that patients with mild spasticity, particularly in the legs, may require this spasticity for ambulation. Medical therapy is usually not indicated for mild spasticity, though physio-therapy may be of benefit. Individuals with greater degrees of spasticity usually require both physio-therapy and medication.[22]

The three medications most commonly used for spasticity include baclofen (Lioresal), dantrolene sodium (Dantrium), and diazepam (Valium). Baclofen is particularly effective in treating flexor and extensor spasms. Because of its proposed action at the spinal cord level, less sedation is noted with baclofen than with diazepam. In our experience, baclofen has been the most effective drug with fewer side effects in treating spasticity. A recommended trial of therapy would consist of 10 mg at bedtime for 3 days, 10 mg b.i.d. for 3 days, 10 mg t.i.d. for 3 days, 10 mg q.i.d. for 3 days increased to a maximum dosage of 20 mg q.i.d. Adverse reactions include transient nausea, drowsiness, fatigue, dizziness, and confusion. With reduction in the patient's spasticity, patients will occasionally complain of increased weakness. This can usually be managed by lowering the drug dose. Because of reports in the literature of hallucinations following abrupt withdrawal, baclofen should be tapered by 10 to 20 mg daily if therapy is to be discontinued.

Dantrolene sodium is felt to act on the muscle directly. It has been re-ported in some series to be particularly effective in reducing clonus. Because of reports in the literature documenting hepatic toxicity, patients should have CBC and liver function tests at appropriate intervals while on therapy. Other adverse reactions include transient drowsiness, dizziness, weakness, fatigue and diarrhea. In our experience, increased weakness has been a major limiting factor in giving this drug to ambulatory patients. Initiation of therapy consists of 25 mg daily, which can then be increased by 25 to 50 mg increments every 4 to 7 days to a total of 100 mg q.i.d. However, we have found that patients rarely tolerate more than 100 mg per day.

Diazepam was one of the earliest drugs used in the treatment of spasticity. Doses of 10 to 40 mg daily in divided doses may be effective in reducing spasticity, but carry the side effect of significant sedation and depression when used in larger doses.

Physical therapy, including passive range of motion and stretching exercises (at a minimum), should supplement treatment of a patient's spasticity. Patients who have spasticity which is resistant to medical therapy and con-servative physical therapy may benefit from an evaluation by a physician specialized in nerve and motor point blocks.

OPTIC NEUROPATHIES

Development of either optic or retrobulbar neuritis is one of the most fright-ening and dramatic symptoms in MS. Symptoms usually develop over a period of days and initially consist of retro-orbital pain (which is increased with eye movement), photophobia, and blurred vision (which the patient may accurately describe as a "central blind spot"). An additional complaint of the patient may be that colors are "washed out," reflecting diminished red/green color acuity. Because of the central scotoma, visual acuity may be markedly impaired. However, complete blindness is rare.

In acute optic neuritis the disc frequently appears hyperemic and disc margins are indistinct with occasional hemorrhages noted (Fig. 15.3). This can be distinguished from papilledema because optic neuritis impairs visual acuity, whereas acute papilledema does not affect acuity. With retrobulbar neuritis, the optic disc acutely may appear normal. However, optic pallor, particularly along the temporal margin, can be noted in the convalescent stages. The finding of optic pallor is not specific because of the natural variability in disc color. In particular, pale discs can be noted in myopia.

"Blurring" of vision may not always represent optic neuritis. Other causes include diplopia, nystagmus, or adverse reactions to medications. A final cause of visual blurring is Uhthoff's phenomenon. This consists of transient visual blurring following exertion or rise in body temperature in an individual who has experienced previous optic neuritis.

An exacerbation of optic neuritis or retrobulbar neuritis may be shortened with a course of steroid therapy. The doses of ACTH or prednisone have been discussed previously. Because of impaired visual acuity, lack of depth

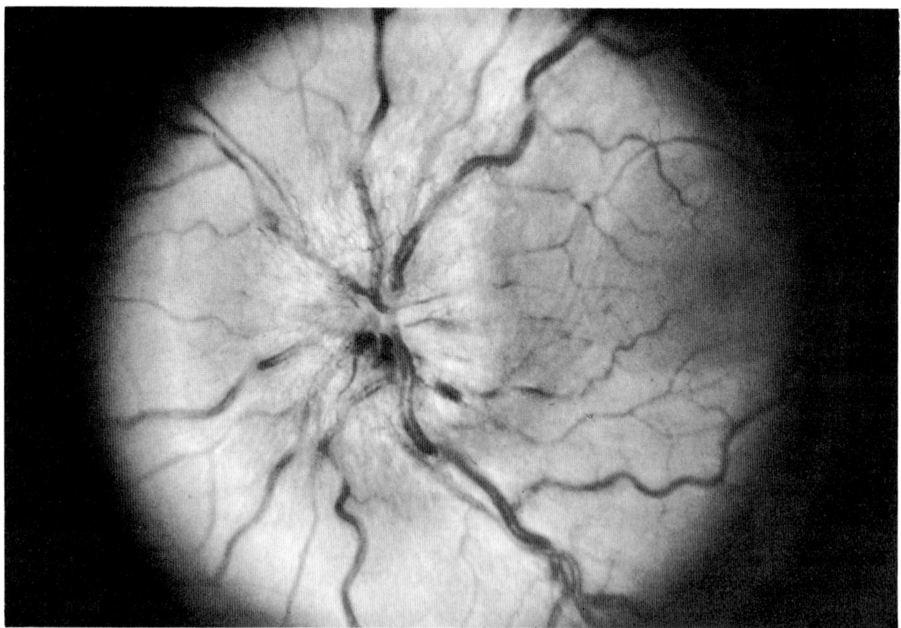

Fig. 15.3 Funduscopic photograph of patient with acute optic neuritis. Note the hyperemic elevated indistinct disc margin. (Photograph courtesy of Dr. Bruce Wilson)

perception and impaired color acuity (particularly for red and green), patients should be discouraged from driving during their exacerbation.

SENSORY DYSFUNCTION

A relative paucity of findings in an MS individual with various sensory complaints is common. This discrepancy has often resulted in a diagnosis of hysteria or anxiety neurosis with referral of the patient to a psychiatrist. Of all the MS symptoms, sensory symptoms are the most diverse. In addition to the more common complaints of "pins and needles" and "numbness," the patient may complain of excessive sensitivity (hyperpathia), pruritis, burning, "swelling" of the affected limb, and, least commonly, pain. A band-like sensation at the uppermost extent of the sensory involvement is common.

The sensory dysfunction is most commonly symmetric and tends to involve the trunk and lower extremities more often than the upper extremities. Vibratory sensation is often impaired out of proportion to other modalities. In individuals with intact vibratory and pin sensation, 2 point discrimination may be the most sensitive indication of neurological dysfunction.

An unusual sensory phenomena originally felt to be pathonomonic of multiple sclerosis is Lhermitte's sign. This is described by the patient as a tingling sensation or "electric shock," which radiates down the spine and/or into the legs and/or arms with flexion of the head. More recent studies have shown that this may also occur in other disease entities such as cervical spondylosis and cervical spinal cord tumors.

The sensory symptoms of "numbness" and "pins and needles" have proven refractory to medical treatment. However, patients with dysesthesia, hyperpathia, and Lhermitte's sign may benefit from treatment with carbamazepine (Tegretol) or phenytoin (Dilantin). Tegretol is usually more effective, but requires regular CBC and liver function test because of potential toxicity. The dosages of both medications are the same as those employed in treating seizure disorders, specifically 400 to 1,200 mg of carbamazepine and 200 to 400 mg of phenytoin each day. Both drugs have the advantage that serum levels are available which may help identify the appropriate dose for an individual patient. When sensory symptoms occur in isolation, there is no indication for steroid therapy.

BRAINSTEM DYSFUNCTION

Disturbances of eye movement are the most common brainstem finding in multiple sclerosis. These include nystagmus, internuclear ophthalmoplegia and isolated extraoccular muscle weakness. The nystagmus most commonly is horizontal. However, rotatory and "jelly-like" nystagmus have also been described. The type of nystagmus is not usually helpful in localization of the lesion within the brainstem. Internuclear ophthalmoplegia follows a lesion of the medial longitudinal fasciculus and consists of paralysis of ipsilateral adduction and horizontal nystagmus of the contralateral eye with lateral gaze (Fig. 15.4). Of the three extraocular nerves, symptoms referable to the VIth nerve are most common, followed by the IIIrd nerve with the IVth nerve being rarely involved.

Brainstem findings may be initially confusing to the emergency room physician. Isolated facial weakness in MS is most commonly of the peripheral type and taste may be intact. An eye patch is important to prevent corneal damage from incomplete eye closure. MS is the most common cause of tic douloureux in young adults. The symptom complex of vertigo, nausea and vomiting is a common one in MS and is difficult to distinguish from acute labyrinthitis. Hearing loss is exceptionally rare in multiple sclerosis as is isolated tongue weakness. Dysarthria and dysphagia are usually a mixed disorder involving cerebellar, brainstem and corticospinal tract dysfunction.

An exacerbation of diplopia or internuclear ophthalmoplegia, particularly when occurring with other brainstem signs and symptoms, may be shortened with a course of steroids. Isolated diplopia is reported in many large series to be a short-lived symptom and to have an excellent prognosis without steroid therapy. An alternating eyepatch should be employed for the comfort of the patient and to improve the patient's mobility and coordination.

Vertigo with associated nausea is a particularly distressing symptom for the patient and can be difficult to distinguish from acute labyrinthitis. Because of the positional component to the vertigo, many patients have already placed themselves on bedrest at the time of presentation. Patients may

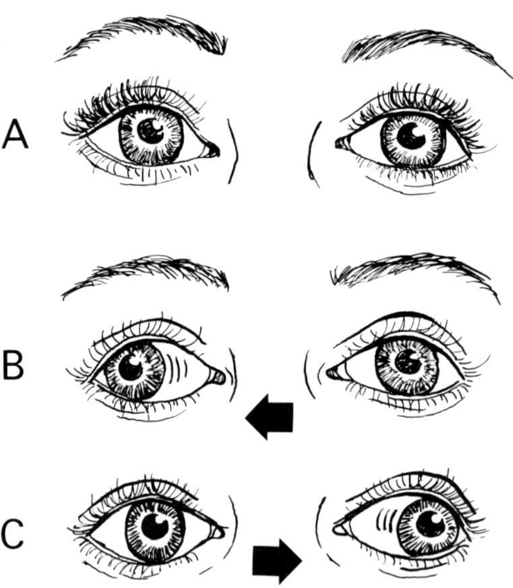

Fig. 15.4
Bilateral internuclear ophthalmoplegia. (A) The patient has been directed to look straight ahead. (B) The patient is looking to the right. Note the paralysis of left eye adduction and horizontal nystagmus in the right abducting eye (left internuclear ophthalmoplegia). (C) The patient is looking to the left. Note the paralysis of right eye adduction and horizontal nystagmus in the left abducting eye (right internuclear ophthalmoplegia).

note some reduction in intensity of the vertigo from meclizine HCl (Antivert) in dosages of 12.5 to 25 mg t.i.d. For individuals with associated nausea and vomiting, prochlorperazine (Compazine) or trimethobenzamide HCl (Tigan) suppositories supplemented with increased fluid intake may be of benefit. Individuals with protracted nausea and vomiting should be admitted to the hospital for parenteral therapy.

ATAXIA AND TREMOR

Ataxia represents one of the most debilitating symptoms of MS. This symptom is frequently associated with weakness which further incapacitates the patient. The intensity of this symptom can range from mild intention tremor to truncal ataxia to gross chorea-like movements. Though cerebellar involvement usually presents insidiously, it may present as paroxysmal attacks (see below).

Ataxia and tremor have also been one of the most resistant symptom complexes to effective treatment. Patients with significant ataxia should be evaluated by a physiatrist, physical therapist and occupational therapist to determine whether the patient may benefit from extremity weight cuffs, cervical collar, and balance exercises. Because of the significant effect of stress or anxiety on any movement disorder, a few patients may benefit from bio-feedback and self hypnosis therapy. Medical therapy with propranolol (Inderal) in doses of 80 to 160 mg daily is worth trying, but results are usually disappointing.

BOWEL AND BLADDER DYSFUNCTION

The most common bladder dysfunction in MS consists of a spastic neurogenic bladder, usually associated with urinary frequency, urgency and urge incontinence. Often a neurogenic bladder has been previously misdiagnosed and treated as a recurrent urinary tract infection. Given that both entities occur commonly in MS, the patient should have a urological evaluation including a urinalysis, cystometrogram, cystoscopy, and IVP to further delineate the problem. Recent urological studies have shown that the distinction between a flaccid and a spastic bladder cannot be made on the basis of history alone.[1] Therefore, proper treatment is very difficult without urodynamic testing.

Patients presenting with urinary symptoms should have a urinalysis to exclude infection. In addition to appropriate antibiotic therapy for an infection, a concerted effort should be made to reduce the patient's fever because of many patients' marked sensitivity to temperature. If a urinary tract infection is not present, a urological evaluation is still indicated.

Bowel incontinence is much less common than bladder incontinence in MS. A more common bowel finding is constipation. Constipation is frequently found in individuals with significant pyramidal tract involvement and secondary inactivity. Medications may also add to the problem of constipation.

The common symptom of constipation can usually be managed effectively with adequate ingestion of bran or psyllium hydrophilic mucilloid (Metamucil) in conjunction with increased fluid intake. Specific stool softeners are rarely indicated and their use on a chronic basis should be discouraged.

PAROXYSMAL SYMPTOMS

Seizures, secondary to multiple sclerosis have been reported in 1 to 4 percent of patients in large series.[13] The seizures may be generalized or focal and cannot be clinically distinguished from the idiopathic variety. Tonic seizures represent an unusual seizure disorder and are felt to be of spinal cord or brainstem origin.[12] Clinically, they are characterized by painful, unilateral tonic spasms without associated clonus, lasting seconds and without alteration of consciousness. The patient's posture during such an episode consists of flexion at the elbow and wrist and extension of the leg with inversion of the foot. The episodes can be precipitated by sensory stimulation or voluntary movement. The EEG is normal during the episodes which can occur 15 to 30 times a day. Carbamazepine (Tegretol), and less commonly phenytoin (Dilantin), in the doses outlined in the section on sensory symptoms, may be effective in treating tonic seizures.

Paroxysms of dysarthria and ataxia lasting seconds and occurring several times during the day for a period of weeks to months have also been described in multiple sclerosis.[19] Though the EEG is normal in such episodes, these individuals may also respond to anticonvulsants.

MENTAL AND PSYCHOLOGICAL IMPAIRMENT

The occurrence of cognitive impairment in isolation of other neurological symptoms is rare in MS. Though acute confusional states have been described, an MS patient presenting with confusion or alteration of memory should prompt a search for other etiologies such as medication effect and other toxic/metabolic etiologies. Past studies have documented that cognitive impairment can occur in MS (e.g., memory deficits, concentration difficulties), but seems to be a function of duration of disease.[16]

Though euphoria has been said to be common in MS, subsequent studies have shown that depression is much more prevalent. In our experience, euphoria has frequently been associated with mental impairment. The euphoric patient may also be depressed. In addition to the vegetative signs of insomnia, apathy and decreased appetite, depression may also accentuate existing MS symptoms. Recent studies have shown that emotional stress can intensify MS symptoms. Therefore, every patient should be questioned as to the possible relationships between current symptoms and recent stress or depression.

Because multiple sclerosis affects primarily young adults in the prime of life and because of the chronic uncertainty of the disease regarding future symptoms, psychological adjustment to the disease is a very distressing problem for the patient. For patients having difficulty adjusting to the disease, psychological support groups should be encouraged. The education of the family regarding the disease process and family support groups should not be overlooked. Social service and vocational rehabilitation referrals can be extremely useful in selected patients. Through the use of patient and family education, support groups and the various social agencies, the difficulties encountered by the patient, particularly in the early stages of the disease, can be lessened.

The diverse nature of many MS symptoms, and in particular sensory symptoms, often leads to an incorrect diagnosis of hysteria or anxiety. As mentioned in earlier sections of this text, all symptoms, *particularly* in MS, should be treated as genuine and based on organic causes.

Because of the adverse effect of emotional stress on physical symptoms in MS, many patients benefit from various stress management techniques, including self-relaxation, yoga, hypnosis, and specific stress-management classes. The chronic use of minor tranquilizers is frequently the easiest course for both the physician and the patient, but should be discouraged. Antidepressants should be combined with counseling in the treatment of depression. The adverse effect of many antidepressants on MS symptoms, particularly bowel and bladder, do not justify their use in many MS patients.

DIAGNOSTIC TESTS

The past decade has seen the development and application of several new tests, which are helpful in supporting a clinical diagnosis of multiple sclerosis and in assessing disease activity. These tests include evoked potentials, CT scan, cerebrospinal fluid oligoclonal banding, myelin basic protein assay, and IgG index. These tests are used only to support a clinical diagnosis of MS and none of the tests are specific for MS.

Evoked potentials are a group of physiologic tests based on the observation that loss of myelin slows nerve conduction time. The test carries the significant advantage of being noninvasive and carrying no risk to the patient. The visual evoked potential (VEP) or visual evoked response (VER) is obtained by having an individual stare at a checkerboard screen while a series of evoked electrical waves are then recorded from EEG scalp electrodes over the occipital visual cortex. With the advent of microcomputers, the small evoked potential signals can be extracted from the ongoing higher amplitude brain wave activity (EEG). A reproduceable wave occurs normally at approximately 100 msec (i.e., the "P100" wave).

In an individual who has had previous optic neuritis with subsequent loss of myelin, the conduction time of this "P100" wave is delayed to 120 msec, or more. In acute optic neuritis, the "P100" wave is also frequently of lower amplitude because of impaired visual acuity (Fig. 15.5). With resolution of the retrobulbar or optic neuritis and concomitant improvement in visual acuity, the amplitude returns once again to normal. However, the latency remains delayed indefinitely in 95 percent of patients.

Evoked potentials testing can be particularly helpful in trying to document more than one area of CNS involvement. For example, in an individual who has experienced an episode of paraparesis with no other past neurologic symptoms, an abnormal VEP is compatible with a clinically silent demyelinative lesion and supports the diagnosis of multiple sclerosis on the basis of "lesions disseminated in space."

In addition to the visual pathway, the brainstem auditory, and central sensory pathways can be evaluated with evoked responses.[3] Brainstem auditory evoked potentials are elicited through a set of headphones which deliver

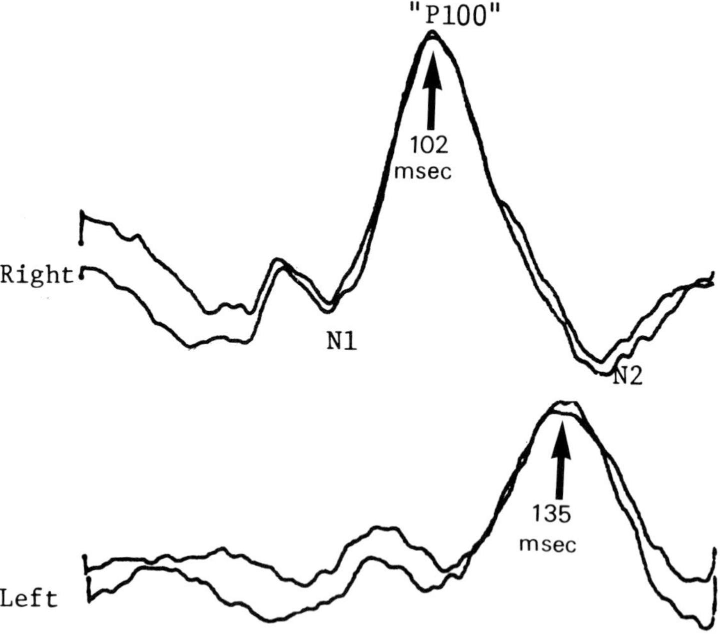

Fig. 15.5 Visual evoked potentials in an individual with acute left optic neuritis. Compared to the normal "P100" wave in the right eye, note the delayed latency and decreased amplitude of the wave (arrow) in the left eye.

a series of "clicks" to the auditory nerve. Six waves of short latency (less than 10 msec) can be recorded from scalp electrodes and represent ascending pathways within the brainstem. Somatosensory evoked potentials are obtained through electrical stimulation of either the median nerve in the arm or peroneal nerve in the leg. Evoked potential signals are then recorded from electrodes placed over the brachial plexus, cervical spine, and sensory cortex.

Through the use of the complete battery of evoked potentials (visual, brainstem auditory and somatosensory), anatomic sites which are frequently involved in MS can be physiologically evaluated. In addition to supporting a diagnosis of multiple sclerosis, abnormal evoked potentials are also helpful in evaluating acute exacerbations of the disease, particularly if previous evoked potentials are available for comparison.

The CT scan has revolutionized many areas of medicine. This test has also found an application in acute exacerbations of multiple sclerosis.[5] During acute exacerbations of their disease, MS patients may have enhancement of white matter plaques following injection of contrast (Fig. 15.6). While not pathonomonic of MS, this CT scan abnormality provides supportive evidence of an acute exacerbation. There is frequently a poor correlation between the site of the enhancing lesion(s) on CT scan and the patient's clinical signs and symptoms. With resolution of the exacerbation, enhancement of the CT lesion resolves. However, a low density white matter lesion may persist.

With the advent of nuclear magnetic resonance scanning, physicians may be able to more accurately delineate white matter plaques in MS.[21] This technique differentiates between gray and white matter more accurately than CT scan and has the additional benefit of being able to define smaller lesions than CT scan.

Another new development in diagnostic tests in MS involves the analysis of spinal fluid. An elevated ratio of CSF gamma globulin (IgG) to CSF total protein has been used as supportive evidence of MS in an individual with compatible signs and symptoms. However, this test is non-specific and is abnormal in only 75 percent of patients with clinically definite MS.

Spinal fluid oligoclonal banding is a newer test which detects qualitative abnormalities in IgG even when the IgG level is normal.[10] For this test, an electrophoresis of spinal fluid is performed. In the IgG region of the gel, normally a homogenous pattern or one IgG band is seen. In up to 95 percent of MS patients, two or more oligoclonal bands in this region have been noted (Fig. 15.7). This abnormal banding pattern has also been reported in both viral and bacterial CNS infections, carcinomatous meningitis, syphilis, and lupus erythematosus. Although oligoclonal banding may be helpful in supporting the diagnosis of MS, it is not helpful in assessing either the severity or the activity of the disease. The number and intensity of the bands usually remain unchanged during the lifetime of the MS patient regardless of disease course.

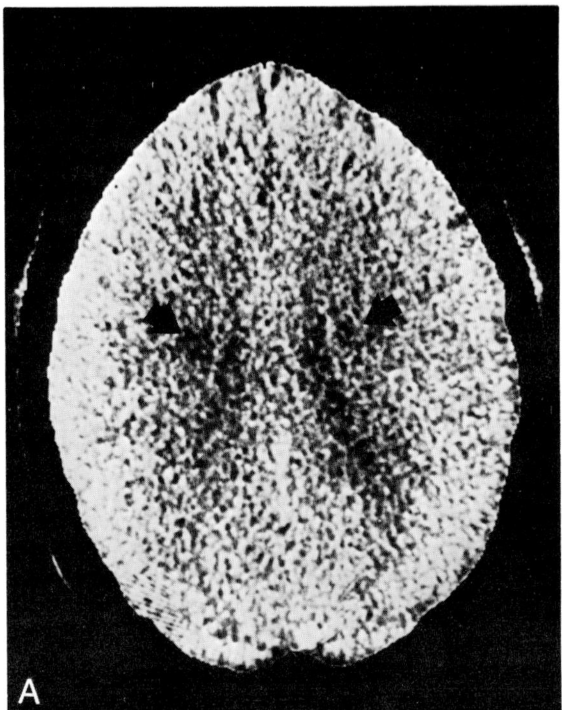

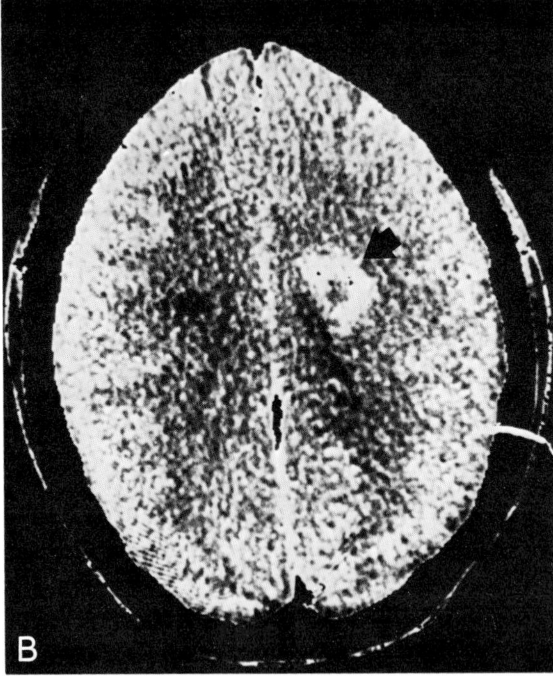

Fig. 15.6
(A) CT Scan prior to contrast administration. Bilateral periventricular low density lesions are noted (arrows). (B) CT scan following contrast administration. The right periventricular low density lesion noted without contrast now enhances following contrast (arrow). This finding is consistent with an acute MS plaque.

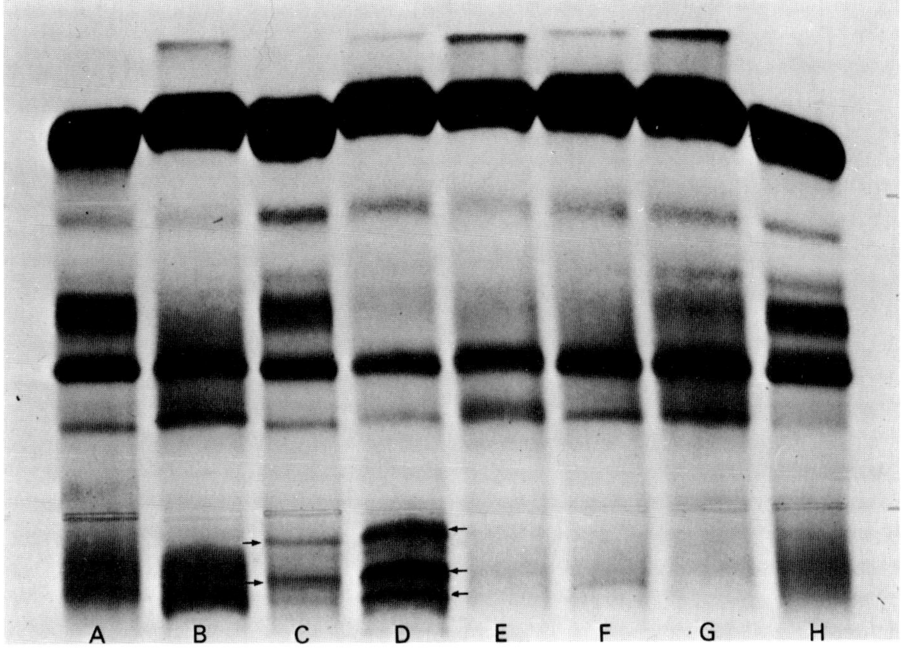

Fig. 15.7 Spinal fluid electropheresis on agarose gel. Note the oligoclonal banding (arrows) in patients C & D compared to normal patients, A, B, E, F, G, and H.

Cerebrospinal fluid IgG index represents a formula which indirectly evaluates the integrity of the blood brain barrier and provides indirect evidence of intrinsic CNS IgG production.[7] The formula requires that both CSF and serum IGg and albumin concentrations be determined. The equation consists of:

$$\frac{\text{CSF IgG} \times 10^3}{\text{serum IgG}} \bigg/ \frac{\text{CSF albumin} \times 10^3}{\text{serum albumin}}$$

Abnormally high serum IgG concentrations can elevate the CSF IgG concentration. The CSF/serum IgG ratio corrects for this potential error. The CSF/serum albumin ratio is a means of evaluating blood brain barrier integrity. The IgG index has been found to be elevated (greater than 0.65), in 75 to 95 percent of MS individuals.

Spinal fluid myelin basic protein assay is most useful in assessing disease activity.[4] Myelin basic protein (MBP) is a major component of myelin, which has been found to be present in abnormally high concentrations in the spinal fluid of individuals sustaining acute demyelination from various causes. It is not specific for MS, but is specific for myelin breakdown.

Normally, little or no myelin basic protein is found in spinal fluid. Therefore, the degree of elevation of MBP indicates the degree of demyelination. In MS exacerbations, MBP may be markedly elevated coincident with the development of clinical signs and symptoms. A gradual fall over a period of weeks to normal levels parallels the resolution of signs and symptoms. In summary, this test may be helpful in differentiating an acute exacerbation from fluctuation in the course of a previous lesion.

CONCLUSION

The most important points in this chapter for general physicians to consider are:

1. MS is a common neurologic disease, especially in the young adult Caucasian population.

2. The etiology of MS is most likely related to a complex interaction of a genetically determined immune regulatory defect and an environmental exposure, possibly a virus.

3. Multiple sclerosis symptoms are diverse because the lesions are so variable in their duration and CNS location.

4. MS symptoms, especially sensory symptoms, are often misdiagnosed as hysteria, anxiety, or other psychiatric conditions.

5. Recently developed diagnostic tests may be very helpful in supporting a clinical diagnosis of multiple sclerosis.

6. Acute exacerbations of MS need to be differentiated from natural fluctuations in the disease course or worsening of symptoms secondary to medical problems such as medications or infection.

7. Most MS patients will improve spontaneously after an acute exacerbation.

8. Steroids may shorten an exacerbation, especially visual or motor disturbances, but they do not alter the long-term prognosis for the disease.

9. Determination of a spastic versus a flaccid bladder is very difficult by history alone, and urodynamic testing is important in the proper management of bladder problems.

10. General health maintenance such as exercise and rest, well-balanced meals and avoidance of stress are important in the long-term adjustment of the MS patient.

11. The psycho-social adjustment of the MS patient is as important as the medical management of specific symptoms.

12. MS is not usually a fatal disease, and most MS patients die from complications of infections.

REFERENCES

1. Blavis, J.G.: Management of bladder dysfunction in multiple sclerosis. Neurology, 30(2):12, 1980.
2. Brown, J.R., Beebe, G.W., Kurtzke, J.F., et. al.: The design of clinical studies to assess therapeutic efficacy in multiple sclerosis. Neurology, 29:3, 1979.
3. Chiappa, K.H.: Pattern shift visual, brainstem auditory and short latency somatosensory evoked potentials in multiple sclerosis. Neurology, 30(2):110, 1980.
4. Cohen, S.R., Herndon, R.M., McKhann, G.M.: Myelin basic protein in cerebrospinal fluid as an indicator of active demyelination. Arch. Neurol., 33:384, 1976.
5. Harding, A.E., Radue, E.W., Whitley, A.M.: Contrast enhanced lesions on computerized tomography in multiple sclerosis.: J. Neurol., Neurosurg., Psychiatry, 41:754, 1978.
6. Herndon, R.M., Weiner, L.P., Price, D., et. al.: Regeneration of oligodendroglia during recovery from demyelinating disease. Science, 195:693, 1977.
7. Hershey, L.A., Trotter, J.L.: The use and abuse of the cerebrospinal fluid IgG profile in the adult: a practical evaluation. Ann. Neurol., 8:426, 1980.
8. Kurland, L.T.: The epidemiologic characteristics of multiple sclerosis. p.63. In Vinken, P.J., Bruyn, G.W. Ed.: Handbook of Clin. Neurol. Vol. 9, American Elsevier Co., New York, 1970.
9. Kurtzke, J.F. Clinical manifestations of multiple sclerosis, p.161. In Vinken, P.J., Bruyn, G.W., ed.: Handbook of Clin. Neurol. Vol. 9, American Elsevier Co., New York, 1970.
10. Johnson, K.P., Arrigo, S.C., Nelson, B.J., et. al.: Agarose electrophoresis of cerebrospinal fluid in multiple sclerosis.: Neurology, 27:273, 1977.
11. Malhutra, A.S., Goren, H.: The hot bath test in the diagnosis of multiple sclerosis.: JAMA, 246:1113, 1981.
12. Matthews, W.B.: Tonic seizures in disseminated sclerosis.: Brain, 81:193, 1958.
13. Matthews, W.B.: Paroxysmal symptoms in multiple sclerosis.: J. Neurol., Neurosurg., Psychiatry, 38:617, 1975.
14. McAlpine, D., Lumsden, C.E., Acheson, E.D.: Multiple sclerosis—a reappraisal. Churchill Livingston, Edinburgh, 1972.
15. Percy, A.K., Kurland, L.T., Nobrega, F.T., et. al.: Multiple sclerosis in Rochester, Minnesota—a 60 year appraisal. Trans. Amer. Neurol. Assoc., 93:264, 1968.
16. Peyser, J.M., Edwards, K.R., Poser, C.M., et. al.: Cognitive function in patients with multiple sclerosis.: Arch. Neurol., 37:577, 1980.
17. Prineas, J.W.: The etiology and pathogenesis of multiple sclerosis. p.107. In Vinken, P.J., Bruyn, G.W., ed.: Handbook of Clin. Neurol. Vol. 9, American Elsevier Co., New York, 1970.
18. Rose, A.S., Schumacher, G.A., Kurtzke, J.F., et. al.: Cooperative study in the evaluation of therapy in multiple sclerosis; ACTH vs. placebo—final report. Neurology, 20:1, 1970.
19. Twomey, J.A., Espir, M.L.: Paroxysmal symptoms as the first manifestation of multiple sclerosis.: J. Neurol., Neurosurg., Psychiatry, 43:296, 1980.

20. U.S. Veterans Administration.: Multiple sclerosis: guidelines for diagnosis and management. Neurology service, pub. 1B 11–70, 1980.
21. Young, I.R., Hall, A.S., Pallis, C.A., et. al.: Nuclear magnetic resonance imaging of the brain in multiple sclerosis. Lancet, 2:1063, 1981.
22. Young, R.R., Delwaide, P.J.: Drug therapy—Spasticity: N. Engl. J. Med., 304(1):28 and 304(2):96, 1981.

16

Neurologic Emergencies of Children

Chester J. Minarcik, Jr., M.D.

INTRODUCTION

The infant or child with a neurologic problem is more likely to present in the local emergency room than in the office of a pediatric neurologist. Diseases of the nervous system and diseases secondarily affecting the nervous system are very common. Various estimates of the prevalence of neurologic disease in infancy and childhood suggest that 20 to 50 percent of children admitted to pediatric hospital beds have neurologic disorders as primary or secondary diagnoses.

This chapter highlights the special problems and considerations facing the physician providing initial care for neurologic problems in the pediatric age range. Pathophysiologic and therapeutic insights that differ from the comparable situation in adults will be discussed to allow the primary care physician to address critical differences in infants and children. Helpful "hints" in the examination as well as in the interpretation of pediatric signs and symptoms will be given. Many of the specific disorders will be dealt with in greater depth in other chapters of the book; uniquely pediatric aspects will be emphasized here. The reader is directed to the index for additional information.

Encompassing specific issues in the care of the infant or child with a neurologic emergency are two very obvious yet often forgotten principles. The first is the necessary reminder that children, particularly small children, are not miniaturized adults. Physiologically they may differ radically. Even though this reminder may not be required for most physicians, iatrogenic complications which are the result of physiologically inappropriate management still occur frequently.

Principle number two is that the differential diagnosis for a given clinical presentation will be modified by the age of the patient. Coma and seizures resulting from an inherited metabolic disorder will be a reasonable entry

387

**Table 16.1 Common Neurologic Emergencies in Infants and
Children**

Category	Specific Entity
Infections	Meningitis Encephalitis Brain abscess
Infection related	Reye's syndrome Acute cerebellar ataxia Guillain-Barré syndrome

Toxins	Accidental ingestions
	Non-intentional overdose
	    Salicylates
	    Anticholinergics
	Intentional overdose
	Environmental exposure
	    pesticides
	    lead

Vascular disease	Traumatic subdural hematoma Spontaneous subarachnoid hemorrhage Moya-Moya disease Homocystinuria

Metabolic disease	Inherited metabolic disorders
	    Urea cycle abnormalities
	    Aminoacidurias
	    Organic acidurias
	    Glycogenoses
	    Lipid storage diseases

Trauma	Accidental Non-accidental
Epilepsy	Status epilepticus Post-ictal states

on the differential diagnosis for the young infant but not the teenager who
was previously normal. Meningitis will be a common consideration in the
youngest patients, somewhat less so in older patients, but never totally ex-
cludable from the differential. Non-accidental trauma to the brain may occur
without other external evidence of trauma or a history thereof. The physician
should always be aware of this.

As in the adult, there will always be a certain group of conditions resulting
in neurologic emergencies that will be seen repeatedly. These common
entities should be well understood diseases for the physicians likely to encounter them. A listing of the most common problems is given in Table
16.1.

THE NEUROLOGIC EXAM AND DECISION MAKING IN INFANTS AND CHILDREN

The identification or suspicion of acute neurologic disease often raises additional problems for the primary physician. Many generalist physicians remain uncomfortable evaluating neurologic disease in both the young and

the old. Almost every physician finds the neurologic exam more difficult to perform in young patients. Even when it may be performed adequately, its interpretation is more complex. The younger the patient, the greater is the complexity. It is widely appreciated that the immature brain is more plastic than the mature one, yet how much more so? This is a critical factor in designing therapy appropriate for the pediatric patient. It dictates how far rescuscitative procedures should be carried. It accounts for the reacquisition of speech following destruction of the primary language areas in the brain. It additionally accounts for the difficulty in applying traditional brain death criteria to young children.

The primary goals of management in neurologic emergencies are outlined in Chapter 1. Respiration and cardiovascular integrity must be maintained to preserve organ function (in this instance the brain) while decisions are being made. The pathophysiology of injury and recovery is essentially the same in the mature brain as in the immature.

Basic emergency care requires the consideration of additional factors. Failure to apply specific pediatric principles may result in significant iatrogenic complications. Intubation must be performed with the proper sized endotracheal tube. Improper tube size can cause damage to the larynx or trachea as well as resulting in ineffective ventilation. Whereas the older child's neck is hyperextended for intubation (like the adult), small infants should be intubated in the supine position without hyperextension. The non-intubating hand is placed behind the neck to stabilize the head and move the larynx and trachea into a position in which intubation can be accomplished with ease. Intubation is almost always successful in children, making emergency tracheotomy rarely necessary. If epiglottitis is suspected (clinically or with the aid of a lateral neck X-ray), intubation should be performed in an operating room or other area where trained personnel can perform emergency tracheotomy if intubation fails.

Volume expansion requires particular attention to measurements. The smaller the infant or child, the more easily that child can suffer from fluid mismanagement. In some small infants a precarious balance is kept between hypovolemia and cardiac failure, neither of which is advantageous for adequate brain function. Calculations for routine fluids and volume expanders should be made using body weight or surface area. Detailed information about fluid and electrolyte requirements in normal and special circumstances may be found in any standard textbook of pediatric medicine.

STRUCTURAL VERSUS NON-STRUCTURAL: THE SIGNIFICANCE OF FOCAL FINDINGS

No other topic confuses physicians whose neurologic experience has been with adults (rather than children) more than this. The classic neurologic exam rests upon the knowledge that the organization of the brain allows for the localization of function and dysfunction. Focal dysfunction is expected to cause focal findings on examination. Again, however, in the case of children, we must first apply the "younger, the less likely" rule.

The younger the child, the less likely is a given focal finding indicative of an isolated, focal lesion. This is not to say that a focal finding will not point to a specific area of dysfunction. This is true at all ages. It is truer to say that "focal" really means "multifocal" in the infant or young child. The focal finding becomes a manifestation of a diffuse process. By keeping this principle clearly in mind, one will tend to remember the necessary enjoinder.

This is not to say that focal (and presumably structural) abnormalities are not to be pursued with diagnostic vigor! When the computerized tomographic scan is negative in the child with a focal finding, however, the physician should be led to investigate diffuse, non-structural etiologies as well as considering whether additional structural studies such as angiography should be performed.

DECISION MAKING IN ACUTE PEDIATRIC NEUROLOGIC DISEASE

The speed and precision with which a physician analyzes and takes action on an acute neurologic problem in an infant or child is a reflection of the ease with which the physician can interrelate general pediatrics with general neurology. This may not be as complex as it might at first seem. If the symptoms and signs are exclusively neurologic, the physician should try to think first as a neurologist would think, and secondarily as a pediatrician would think. Conversely, if systemic (non-neurologic) signs and symptoms predominate, the physician would attempt to think first as a pediatrician and then as a neurologist. In this manner the likely diseases or disorders responsible for the clinical situation will come to mind first.

A second aid in decision making is the recognition that common diseases occur commonly. The unconscious child undergoing a seizure will have a toxic ingestion as the etiology far more often than argininosuccinicaciduria (which could present in the same manner). Likewise, approximately 50 percent of patients presenting with seizures will not be found to have an identifiable etiology.

Common diseases nevertheless present in variant ways. The variety often seems limitless. Textbook descriptions of clinical or pathologic entities are not often seen apart from the textbook (though the majority of the symptoms and signs may fit the description perfectly, some unusual feature may perplex the physician). The clinician's major value as a diagnostician lies in the ability to appreciate and recognize the variability with which a disease process is manifested in a given individual.

THE NEUROLOGIC EXAMINATION IN INFANTS AND CHILDREN

To be appropriate, the standard neurologic examination must be modified in numerous ways when applied to the immature brain. A detailed knowledge of the normal maturation of the functions of the nervous system is essential. A standard text in child development will give details on the age-specific milestones in motor, cognitive, and social spheres. The major textbooks in pediatric neurology should be consulted for a full description of the examination of infants and small children.[12,13] It must be recalled that assessment of function in small children (even in "well" children) must often rely upon parents' reports without verification by the physician. In the acutely ill child (as in the adult) much of this information will be available only by history.

Careful attention to history may help give the physician information about etiology. Developmental delay will regularly accompany many inherited metabolic disorders that also can have acute presentations as coma (hyperammonemia), seizures (phenylketonuria, argininosuccinicaciduria), or ataxia (Hartnup's disease). The incoordinated toddler not yet walking as steadily as you would expect (perhaps suggesting developmental delay) who presents with increased intracranial pressure should have an emergency computerized tomographic scan to rule out the possibility of a posterior fossa mass lesion explaining both symptoms.

Assessment of cranial nerve function in young infants who are not acutely ill often requires perseverance and ingenuity. Fortunately, this problem is greater in the healthy appearing infant that the acutely ill one. The abnormalities of cranial nerves characteristic of coma and herniation syndromes are found in infants and children as well as in adults. One common pediatric problem which might be expected to complicate the assessment of oculomotor function is pre-existent strabismus. Here again, the history may clarify the nature of the unusual findings.

The motor examination is less difficult. Paralysis will be detected but more subtle weakness may be difficult to assess because of incomplete cooperation. The normal variability in tone seems greater in infants and children than in adults. Here one must be careful to separate tone (assessed when the muscles are at rest) from strength (assessed when the muscles are fully contracted). Reflexes are elicited in the same manner as in adults. It may be easier to elicit the Achilles reflex by striking your finger held on the sole of the partially dorsiflexed foot than in the traditional manner.

A controversy over the interpretation of "toe signs" has existed in the literature for an extended period of time. The argument involves the expected movement of the great toe in infants under 1 year of age. The examiner should expect that appropriate testing for the response, with care given to avoid both the grasp and withdrawal responses, will demonstrate a bilateral flexor response in the normal infant. The infant must be awake (extensor responses may occur at all ages during sleep) in a supine position with the head in the midline throughout the test. The lateral aspect of the foot is stroked gently and the initial movement of the great toe observed. The lateral aspect of the foot is preferred to avoid the grasp and withdrawal responses. In this manner flexor and extensor responses may be distinguished. A small percentage of the youngest infants will have transient bilateral extensor responses without demonstrable dysfunction, but this is not the rule. Unilateral extensor responses should always be interpreted as abnormal (if the test is performed correctly). Demonstration of extensor toe responses must alert the examiner to search diligently for other evidence of upper motor neuron dysfunction in the corticospinal tracts. However, isolated extensor responses should not be overinterpreted.

The sensory examination cannot be completed in detail until the child is approximately 5 years old. Those sensory responses required for interpretation of the exam in the comatose or semi-comatose infant or child, however, are not confusing. Remember that the difficulty in the interpretation of the sensory examination in the child is largely a matter of the child's understanding of the task involved and the consistency with which responses are made. Sensory inputs producing motor or behavioral responses that the examiner can interpret will not cause this problem.

If a mental status examination is to be performed as part of the evaluation, care must be taken to consider the age of the child in asking pertinent questions. Recognition of parents, siblings, familiar toys or objects is often the only available measure of orientation of alertness.

SPECIAL PEDIATRIC CONSIDERATIONS IN THE USE AND INTERPRETATION OF LABORATORY TESTS

Among the variety of tests available for the assessment of acute neurologic problems, the lumbar puncture is the one which is most readily available. As in adults, the lumbar puncture should be delayed if increased intracranial pressure is suspected (particularly if a mass lesion is suggested by the history and physical exam) unless meningitis is likely. If meningitis is the expected diagnosis, prompt sampling of the spinal fluid for analysis and culture should be done so that treatment can be instituted immediately.

The technique for lumbar puncture differs little from the technique in adults. A shorter needle (1½ inches in infants, 2½ inches in children) is used. Most often a 22 guage is the most desirable. A stylet must always be used. Local anesthesia is not required in infants and toddlers. Restraint is a requirement for a safe and accurate procedure, and is best accomplished with one or two helpers. Pressure measurements are important in spite of a crying, uncomfortable patient. Often, with the spinal needle in place, part of the restraint can be relaxed to allow the patient to rest quietly for a minute, giving a more valid pressure reading.

Computerized tomography of the brain is the most useful test in the delineation of normal and abnormal brain structure. Unless there is some specific contraindication, scans should be done in both the uncontrasted and contrasted mode. Newer, rapid scanners allow for much higher quality scans in infants and children. If sedation is judged necessary for the performance of this or any other test, its effect on the level of consciousness and clinical exam must be weighed in light of the importance of the information to be gained. In infants with open fontanels consideration may be given to the performance of an ultrasound examination through the fontanels. This is most helpful in the assessment of ventricular size, the identification of intraventricular blood, and the localization of mass lesions. Subtle changes in brain density, diffuse edema, and similar abnormalities are not as well seen on the ultrasound exam and should be evaluated with computerized tomography. Because of the relative newness of ultrasound technology applied to the examination of the brain, most physicians presently follow ultrasound examinations with a computerized tomogram when an abnormality is identified. This practice may change significantly with increased experience.

The computerized tomogram has almost completely replaced the angiogram and pneumoencephalogram in the emergency evaluation of neurologic disease. At times an angiogram or air study will be required at a later date for more specific information about the intracranial vasculature or flow through the ventricular system. Presumed arteriovenous malformations, angiomatous tumors, or certain congenital malformations might necessitate these studies. Most often additional specialist physicians are involved by the time these studies are considered and the acute situation controlled satisfactorily.

Accurate interpretation of the pediatric electroencephalogram is often beyond the expected skills even of the well-trained adult neurologist. When used in the setting of an acute neurologic emergency, the electroencephalogram may provide helpful diagnostic or confirmatory information. Telephone transmitted EEG is not recommended in any situation and is likely to cause performance and interpretation difficulties in the acute situation. A trained technologist and encephalographer will be required to assist the physician in a thorough investigation of the electrical activity of the brain. Table 16.2 lists some acute neurologic conditions in which the EEG may be of help in sorting out the differential diagnosis.

INCREASED INTRACRANIAL PRESSURE[1]

Increased intracranial pressure in infants and children is manifest primarily in alterations in level of consciousness, cranial nerve dysfunction, papilledema, and signs specific to the particular etiology (focal neurologic or associated systemic findings). Findings may be delayed if the process is rela-

Table 16.2 Electroencephalographic Findings in Acute Neurologic Diseases

EEG Finding	Clinical Correlates
Persistant ictal discharges	Status epilepticus Obtundation (spike-wave stupor)
Periodic lateralized epileptiform discharges	Acute hemispheral disease Acute lead poisoning Epilepsia partialis continua
Periodic complexes	Herpes simplex encephalitis Acute viral encephalitis Jacob-Creutzfeld disease Hepatic encephalopathy Subacute sclerosing panencephalitis
Focal slowing	Tumors of the hemispheres Abscess Acute vascular occlusion Post-ictal states (focal seizures) Migraine (acutely)
Intermittent rhythmic slow waves (FIRDA)	Midline structural disorders Seizures Metabolic disorders
Normal findings	Conversion reactions (hysteria) Breath holding spells (post-episode)
Lateralized suppression of activity	Subdural fluid collections Acute vascular occlusions

tively chronic since the skull is not closed in infants and the cranial sutures may be split in older children, allowing for expansion of intracranial contents. In infants, disproportionate or excessive head growth is therefore a common manifestation of processes that would cause more overt evidence of increased intracranial pressure in older children. When the increase in pressure is rapid these compensating mechanisms are easily overcome and clinical signs appear. A full discussion of the management of increased intracranial pressure is found earlier in the book (see Chapter 4).

Table 16.3 lists common causes of increased intracranial pressure in children. Although the table lists a variety of etiologies, it should be appreciated that there are very few mechanisms for increased pressure: increased blood volume, cerebral edema, increased cerebrospinal fluid, and mass lesions.

REYE'S SYNDROME

One of the frequently encountered causes of increased intracranial pressure in children is Reye's Syndrome. The following case illustrates a typical presentation.

A previously healthy two-year-old arrives comatose in the emergency room. Respirations are rapid. Cranial nerve function is intact, but only posturing is seen in response to pain. You are given the history that the child

Table 16.3 Common Causes of Increased Intracranial Pressure in Infants and Children

I. Hydrocephalus

II. Intracranial hemorrhage
   A. Intraventricular or intraparenchymal bleeding
   B. Subarachnoid hemorrhage
   C. Subdural hematoma
   D. Cerebral contusion

III. Mass lesions
   A. Tumors
   B. Abscesses

IV. Infections
   A. Meningitis
   B. Encephalitis
   C. Subdural Empyema

V. Cranial trauma

VI. Venous sinus occlusion

VII. Diffuse cerebral edema
   A. Hypoxic-ischemic encephalopathy
   B. Lead encephalopathy
   C. Systemic diseases
   D. Metabolic causes (hyponatremia)
   E. Hypertensive encephalopathy

VIII. Benign increased intracranial pressure (pseudotumor cerebri)
   A. Endocrine related
   B. Vitamin A
   C. Steroids
   D. Naladixic acid
   E. Systemic diseases
   F. Infectious diseases (especially mastoiditis with lateral sinus thrombosis)

was recovering from varicella when vomiting began followed by a decreased level of consciousness. This occurred over a period of 24 hours. Apart from the neurologic findings the examination reveals an enlarged liver and healing varicella lesions. There is no history of toxic ingestion although the child had received aspirin, acetaminophen, and diphenhydramine during the acute phase of his varicella.

Laboratory studies yield the following pertinent abnormal values: ammonia—640; SGOT—210; bilirubin—0.6; WBC—7000 (with a normal differential); screen for toxic substances—negative; prothrombin time—20.6 with a control of 12.4 seconds. While awaiting the laboratory results, the patient begins to have spontaneous decerebrate posturing, sluggish pupillary reactions, and irregular respirations. You intubate the patient, provide controlled hyperventilation, and plan more aggressive management.

The diagnosis is Reye's Syndrome (acute encephalopathy and fatty degeneration of the liver). First described in 1963, it is a severe but self-limited disease of children with a rare case appearing in young adults. The disease most commonly appears while recovering from a viral illness such as influenza or varicella. The incidence of mild forms is uncertain; more severe forms are readily identified because of the need for prompt medical attention.

Clinical Observations

Clinical observations show a step-wise progression for the disease, at times with amazing rapidity, corresponding to the magnitude of alteration in consciousness. A period of agitation and irritability generally precedes deeper coma. The depth of coma is characterized in the usual fashion with the usual attention to cranial nerve function, responses to stimuli, spontaneous movements and posturing. Numerous classifications have been devised. The one devised by Lovejoy is used widely and divides the illness into five stages.[7] The likelihood of survival decreases directly with the depth of coma. Rapid progression to coma, early seizures, and coagulopathy appear to increase the risk for a poor prognosis.

Initial Laboratory Investigation

Initial laboratory investigation is outlined in Table 16.4 and should be considered part of the emergency management. Correctable abnormalities (hypoglycemia, hypophosphatemia, hypoxia, acidosis) should be corrected. It is not generally believed that reduction of the ammonia through dialysis, exchange transfusion, or neomycin enemas is of significant benefit to the patient although adequate studies have not been performed.

Table 16.4 Reye's Syndrome—Initial Laboratory Investigation

Basic Tests	Ancillary Tests	Tests for Neurophysiologic Monitoring
Glucose	Lactate	EEG
SGOT/SGPT	Pyruvate	
NH$_3$	Amino acids	Brainstem auditory
Electrolytes	Serum free fatty	evoked potentials
Phosphate	acids	Somatosensory
Osmolality	Lumbar puncture*	evoked potentials
Prothrombin time		
PTT		
Bilirubin		
BUN		
Creatinine		
Blood gases		
pH		
Toxicology screen		

*While the lumbar puncture has been done safely in many patients with Reye's Syndrome, the presence of increased intracranial pressure is a relative hazard and needs to be taken into account. Treatment with mannitol just prior to the lumbar puncture may increase the safety but does not eliminate the risk.

Pathophysiology and Natural History

The pathophysiology and natural history of the entity are important to consider. Reye's Syndrome occurs more commonly in the winter (perhaps related to predisposing viral illnesses). Year to year variation in total number of cases is quite marked. Minor epidemics occur periodically. Males and females are affected equally. More patients are in the 6–11 year age bracket than any other 5 year period. To date, more cases have occurred in rural and suburban areas than urban ones. Caucasian patients predominate. The association with viral illnesses is clear although the mechanism undefined. Reports linking the appearance of the disease with the administration of aspirin, phenothiazines, and other medication are suggestive but far from conclusive. Jamacian vomiting sickness, a somewhat related disorder, is produced by a known toxin, hypoglycin, from the unripe fruit of the Akee tree. Reye's-like illnesses have been seen in rare circumstances in conjunction with valproic acid administration. Metabolic disorders with hyperammonemia (urea cycle abnormalities) may also produce similar clinical pictures and are a major diagnostic possibility in patients with "recurrent Reye's Syndrome."

Untreated severe cases have an associated mortality as high as 80 percent. Overall mortality with aggressive therapy should not exceed 20 percent. Uncontrolled elevated intracranial pressure is the usual life threatening situation although coagulopathy and multisystem organ failure occur. Treated or untreated, the disease tends to last from 2 to 5 days. Complications from the acute phase may cause protracted symptoms of major proportion.

Treatment

Treatment is outlined in Table 16.5 as an early management flow chart for patients with confirmed disease. Earlier protocols frequently emphasized exchange transfusion or dialysis as part of the routine management. These procedures have not been shown to alter outcome when compared with aggressive management not including these procedures. Whereas exchange transfusion may be necessary to correct a significant coagulopathy, or dialysis for unresponsive hyperkalemia, the routine use of these procedures cannot be recommended.

SEIZURES, EPILEPSY, AND RELATED PAROXYSMAL DISORDERS

General information about seizures and their primary evaluation is found in an earlier chapter (see Chapter 6). The reader is referred to that discussion for etiologic considerations, classification of clinical seizures, laboratory tests, and standard therapy.

Table 16.5 Reye's Syndrome—Early Management Flow Chart

Lethargic or Stuporous (stage 1,2)			Comatose (stages 3,4)		
Intracranial Pressure	Supportive Care	Metabolic	Intracranial Pressure	Supportive Care	Metabolic
Alert Pediatric Intensive Care Unit of Possible Transfer of Patient			Arrange Transport to Pediatric Intensive Care Unit Immediately		
If rapidly progressive symptoms or deeply stuporous	NG tube Foley catheter	Maintain serum glucose	Intracranial pressure monitor	Arterial line	Maintain previous support
Mannitol 0.5–1.0 g/kg to serum osmolality 320–330 mOsm/L	Large vessel IV Monitor respiration heart rate	Maintain serum phosphate	Elevate head of bed 30°	Intubation–controlled ventilation	
		Monitor coagulation give vitamin K	Decrease noxious stimuli	Induce paralysis prn (Pavulon)	
Elevate head of bed 30°		Oxygen	Avoid jugular distension		
Sedation to decrease agitation (Morphine) (barbiturates)			Mannitol or other osmotic agents		
Avoid noxious stimuli			Barbiturate coma		

Neonatal Seizures

Neonatal seizures represent a conceptually distinct entity from other seizures. Most often associated with significant underlying central nervous system dysfunction, such as birth asphyxia, morbidity and mortality are high. Principles pertaining to the treatment and prognosis of seizures in older infants and children are quite different than those for the neonatal period. Neonatal seizures are classified exclusively by clinical manifestations (Table 16.6) and are dominated by "subtle" or "fragmentary" types. Etiologies are listed in Table 16.7. The diagnosis or elimination of treatable causes is the first task in the management of neonatal seizures. An outline for the evaluation and management of seizures in this population can be found in Table 16.8.

The unique nature of neonatal seizures makes the usual therapeutic deci-

Table 16.6 Neonatal Seizures—Clinical Types

Multifocal clonic
Myoclonic (rare, and indicative of a poor outcome)
Unifocal clonic
Tonic (must be distinguished from posturing responses)
Subtle (chewing, bicycling, nystagmus, sucking, apnea,
and many others, often difficult to separate from
normal behavior)

sions more complex. If a reversible etiology is not found, some form of specific anticonvulsant therapy is ordinarily given. Most neonatal seizures are relatively short-lived, continuing for several days (appearing intermittently during those days) whether or not medication has been given effectively. This natural history is most compatible with the understanding that the usual etiology is "metabolic" (including hypoxic-ischemic encephalopathy, the most common cause) in nature and behavior. With the resolution of the primary phase of the insult to the brain, the likelihood for further seizures is reduced. This had led to the recent practice of discontinuing anticonvulsants in those infants with neonatal seizures whose seizures were due to an acute process (e.g., asphyxia, hypocalcemia) and who are seizure free and neurologically normal when they leave the nursery. Additionally, an etiology not expected to produce continued or recurrent seizures is necessary. Infants with persistent seizures or neurologic abnormalities are candidates for continued anticonvulsant therapy.

In spite of the trend to discontinue medication early, some investigators feel that there is the potential for the seizures themselves to do damage to the developing nervous system. Such damage has been reported in animal models but is uncertain in humans. Such a concern, however, leads to the aggressive management of the seizures as they occur.

Special problems in the use of anticonvulsants in the newborn period

**Table 16.7 Neonatal Seizures—
Etiologies**

Perinatal asphyxia
Congenital anomalies of the brain
Intracranial hemorrhage
Intracranial infection
Hypoglycemia
Hypocalcemia
Hypomagnesemia
Drug withdrawal
Sepsis
Pyridoxine deficiency or dependency
Bilirubin toxicity (kernicterus)
Inherited metabolic disorders

**Table 16.8 Flow Diagram for the Initial Investigation and
Management of Neonatal Seizures**

	Clinical seizures suspected	
Initial Management	Later Management
Observe seizures to classify them	Institute anticonvulsant therapy (phenobarbital 20 mg/kg)
Draw blood for metabolic studies	Obtain electroencephalogram (pyridoxine should be given during EEG monitoring)
Give intravenous glucose	Computerized tomogram of the brain or ultrasound examination
Give calcium during EKG monitoring	Specific treatment for neonatal narcotic withdrawal when diagnosis documented
Give intravenous or intramuscular magnesium	Additional blood studies for unusual causes or inherited metabolic diseases
Give pyridoxine (50–100 mg) during EEG monitoring	

are well known. Phenobarbital, given in a loading dose of 20 mg/kg may yield therapeutic blood levels for several days. Maintenance doses should not be started immediately, but only after the blood level has begun to fall. Additional doses may be given in response to the change in blood level rather than on a routine basis. Drowsiness, an expected side effect from phenobarbital, often is difficult to assess in light of pre-existent encephalopathy. Phenytoin (Dilantin) presents a variety of pharmacologic problems which makes rational use difficult at this age. Side effects from phenytoin toxicity (except cardiac disturbances from severe toxicity) are virtually impossible to detect in the newborn. Since the active (unbound) fraction of the drug causes both the therapeutic and toxic effects, the ability to measure the unbound fraction would provide the best means for following the blood level. Normally 10 percent of the total amount of phenytoin present in the blood exists in the unbound form. In neonates unbound fractions as high as 50 percent have been found. A total level of seven micrograms per milliliter with binding of 50 percent is equivalent to a total level of 35 with the normal binding of 10 percent. The combined unpredictability of the binding and inability to detect clinical evidence of toxicity make for a complex clinical situation.

Diazepam (Valium) and paraldehyde have been widely used to abort single prolonged seizures and as adjuncts to phenobarbital and phenytoin. Other anticonvulsants, including carbamazepine, valproic acid, primidone, and ethosuximide, have been used less and inadequately investigated. Acetazolamide (Diamox) has been used in the newborn period for the treatment of hydrocephalus secondary to intraventricular hemorrhage but has not been investigated as an anticonvulsant in this situation.

Febrile Seizures

Febrile seizures, while not generally a medical emergency, are a common reason for a frightened parent to appear in the emergency room with an ill child. When the febrile seizure occurs in a neurologically and developmentally normal child between the ages of 6 months and 6 years, and when that seizure is brief (less than 20 minutes), non-focal, and clearly associated with a fever, the episode may be considered a benign febrile seizure. A search for other etiologies, including metabolic disturbances and meningitis, should be unrevealing. Such benign febrile seizures carry a low risk for subsequent epilepsy (approximately a 2 percent incidence in that population) unless complicated or non-febrile seizures occur in the future. Presently, treatment or prophylaxis is not considered necessary unless several episodes have occurred. In those situations in which treatment is desired, phenobarbital and valproic acid have been demonstrated to be effective in preventing recurrences; phenytoin and carbamazepine have not been effective. In Europe, rectal diazepam (Valium) is popular for acute prophylaxis. What is not clear in any of the data on patients with febrile seizures is whether prophylaxis alters the incidence of later epilepsy. Clinical judgment weighing the potential risks against the potential benefits must be exercised.

Breath Holding Spells

Breath holding spells, or reflex anoxic seizures, often present a diagnostic dilemma. The primary care physician is the person most likely to be consulted in this situation. Typically an infant or toddler will have episodes characterized by a involuntary holding of the breath in expiration (voluntary breath holding almost invariably occurs in inspiration). Most often the child becomes pale and unconscious, with no detectable heartbeat or pulse. If the episode continues for more than 10 to 20 seconds, tonic stiffening and even clonic jerks may occur. A clinically generalized seizure observed in this manner is the direct result of cardiac asystole and a loss of cerebral perfusion. When the cardiac rhythm is re-established, cerebral perfusion resumes and the episode terminates. Although most episodes are followed by a prompt return to normal, a small percentage will have a relatively brief "post-ictal" period.[6]

In other forms, cyanosis rather than pallor may be present. A profound bradycardia is detected rather than asystole. Chest wall movement may be detected but effective air exchange does not take place. Anoxic seizures are less common in this form of breath holding spell.

Although quite frightening to parents, particularly when the spells occur often, reassurance is appropriate. The episodes are benign and eventually cease. A small percentage of children will have typical vagal syncopal episodes in later years. Quite typically a positive family history for breath holding spells or syncope is obtained. Treatment is generally unnecessary, although vagolytic agents will block the response in the classical pallid form. Very small doses of atropine may be given orally (0.01 mg/kg) with careful attention to the development of signs of anticholinergic toxicity (dry mouth, decreased urination, tachycardia).

The evaluation necessary is quite limited, the diagnosis being most often made on clinical grounds. When further confirmation of the spells is desired, or when the episodes are atypical, an electroencephalogram will be of value. The optimal situation would be to record the EEG as a clinical episode occurs. This can often be accomplished using a provocative vagal stimulus. Ocular compression (bilaterally, for 10 seconds) will produce a clinical spell in at least 50 percent of the children with the pallid form. Fewer positive responses are obtained in the cyanotic form. The EEG changes are quite typical and confirm the diagnosis. High voltage delta slowing is seen diffusely followed by a period of severe attenuation of all EEG activity. During this phase, usually corresponding to the period of asystole, the EEG is very nearly isoelectric. A resumption of high voltage slowing (when systole is resumed) is usually followed within 10 seconds by a return to normal or near normal EEG rhythms. When a typical spell is not recorded in this manner judgment is made purely on clinical grounds.

The Lennox-Gastaut Syndrome

The Lennox-Gastaut Syndrome, a loosely defined syndrome, occurs in children who are generally mentally retarded and have difficulty controlling seizures of the myoclonic, atonic, tonic, and absence types. The EEG shows "slow spike and slow wave." In addition to their typical seizure types, these patients may have rather prolonged episodes of less well-defined seizure activity with altered consciousness. Individual seizures may be difficult to recognize during these periods, which may last from several minutes to many hours. These episodes are similar to other clinical situations which have been described as "petit mal status" or "spike-wave stupor." Most of these episodes will resolve spontaneously. Attempts have been made with varying success to abort the episodes with intravenous diazepam. Overaggressive therapy may cause additional difficulty assessing a patient whose primary manifestation may be alteration of consciousness. Adjustment of the patient's routine anticonvulsants is frequently necessary.

CEREBROVASCULAR DISEASES

Beyond the neonatal period, cerebrovascular disease in infants and children is most often the result of trauma. Isolated head trauma and head trauma accompanying multiple trauma may result in subdural and subarachnoid hemorrhages, cerebral contusions, and intraparenchymal hemorrhage. Nontraumatic etiologies exist as well. Major vessel occlusion, arteritis, aneurysms, arterio-venous malformations, and others are seen in children as well as adults.

A six-year-old child presents to the emergency room in coma. No focal signs are present but nuchal rigidity is demonstrated. The child had been well previously. No history of toxic exposure is obtained. No rashes or other systemic manifestations are detected. A computerized tomographic scanner is not available in your town. Because of the possibility of bacterial meningitis, a lumbar puncture is performed. The opening pressure is 280 mm water. Bloody fluid with a hematocrit of 17 percent is collected.

Subarachnoid hemorrhage presents in this fashion. When trauma is the etiology, a cerebral contusion is often present. The spontaneous subarachnoid hemorrhage, unlike the one associated with trauma, leads the investigator searching for an etiology. Arterio-venous malformations are more common than aneurysms in young people, yet both occur. Rarely would an angiogram be necessary acutely; indeed, it might be dangerous in that situation. Computerized tomography may demonstrate the etiology and can be performed safely during the acute phase. Initial treatment must be directed toward reducing the likelihood of rebleeding. Excessive stimulation must be avoided. Straining during coughing and defecation need to be reduced. Blood pressure, which may increase acutely, must be controlled adequately. Return to activity should occur slowly. If necessary, sedation should be used to prevent excessive agitation or activity during the highest risk period for rebleeding.

Occlusive vascular disease is also seen in the pediatric population.[8] Specific diseases may predispose to vascular occlusion. Homocystinuria, sickle cell disease, cyanotic congenital heart disease, hyperviscoscity syndrome in newborns, and leukemia with an extremely high white blood cell count have all been recognized as etiologic. An extremely rare condition is Moya-Moya disease, in which repeated vascular occlusions occur. Collateral circulation develops with a network of small blood vessels that appear on angiography as a "puff of smoke." The term Moya-Moya refers to that appearance. Diagnosis is by arteriography of the cerebral vessels.

The classical traumatic vascular syndromes (epidural and subdural hematomas, contusions, intraparenchymal hematomas) are not significantly different in children than in adults. The reader is referred to the appropriate chapter for further information (see Chapter 9).

In the newborn period, intraventricular hemorrhages in premature infants are the result of bleeding in the subependymal germinal matrix. More limited hemorrhages will be confined to the subependymal area without an intraventricular component. The etiology of such hemorrhages is incompletely understood. Factors such as hypoxia, acidosis, altered cerebral blood flow, transfusions, shock, volume expansion, and bicarbonate administration have all been proposed. Term infants more typically have bleeding into the choroid plexus with or without extension into the ventricles. Asphyxia is the usual etiology. It is extremely important to remember that some of these infants will not present clinically until the end of the first or beginning of the second week of life. Seizures and encephalopathy are the usual clinical features.

A final reminder cannot be overemphasized. Subdural hematoma in infancy without an obvious etiology (known trauma) requires the physician to consider intentional injury (child abuse) until proven otherwise. Shearing of the bridging veins can occur from vigorous shaking as well as the more traditional acceleration-deceleration injuries. Social service agencies should be enlisted immediately and attention given to state laws for the reporting of such injuries.

COMPLEX HEADACHES IN CHILDHOOD[5]

As in adults, the ultimate question facing the physician is "are these headaches the result of a significant intracranial process that needs intervention?" The availability of computerized tomography has made it possible to obtain such an answer easily whenever it is judged necessary. Unfortunately, the evaluation of headaches is one of the areas in which computerized tomography has been abused. It would be very easy to scan each individual with severe or unusual headaches, and to be reassured that no obvious structural cause exists. Even if one restricts scanning to patients with headaches and neurologic findings, one would eventually screen many children with nothing but migraine. Selecting patients with headaches for further study is always easier if one has the opportunity to follow such patients for a reasonable period of time.

In the emergency room the physician rarely has this luxury. Decisions are made on the best available information to insure that serious causes are identified or excluded. In general, these causes, (including hydrocephalus, tumors, hematomas, vascular malformations, and abscesses) are best identified with computerized tomography. When the physician is seriously considering these possibilities, concern about overutilization of the scanner may be saved for discussions in the doctors' lounge.

The headaches presenting the greatest diagnostic difficulties in children are the complex vascular headaches. All of the various forms of complicated migraine occur in children as well as in adults. Hemiplegic, ophthalmoplegic, aphasic, and basilar artery migraine may be seen. The first occurrence often prompts a trip to the emergency room, especially when a family history of similar episodes is absent. Other manifestations, including loss of consciousness, vertigo, visual loss, dysarthria, and sensory loss, may also be encountered. Since the differential diagnosis for these episodes includes most of the major intracranial catastrophes, the evaluation should be designed to give the most information as rapidly as possible. A negative evaluation with a full return to normal often leads the physician to make the diagnosis of complicated migraine. Repeated episodes may help confirm this diagnosis, although seizures and vascular malformations may also present with intermittent symptomatology.

Vascular headaches occur in additional circumstances including fever, anoxia, post-ictal states, hypertension, and nasal vasomotor congestion. Central nervous system stimulants, nitroglycerin, nitrates and nitrites also may cause similar episodes.

Once serious causes have been ruled out, the physician will direct attention to treating the episode. Often, large doses of narcotic analgesics will be required to ameliorate the pain. These drugs, as well as benzodiazepines, may also help to reduce anxiety and promote sleep. For milder headaches, or when neurologic findings are the sole manifestation, aspirin may be given.

Prophylaxis should be considered when the episodes are frequent or interfere with functioning. There is some concern in giving ergots to patients with complicated migraine and possibly causing further vasospasm. This should be considered carefully before prescribing. Prophylaxis has also been successful using phenobarbital, phenytoin, and propranolol.

COMPLICATIONS OF ACUTE INFECTIONS [2]

Numerous complications may occur following, or in association with, serious infections of the nervous system. A full discussion is available elsewhere in this book. The reader should be familiar with those details as they pertain to children. Several special circumstances deserve further emphasis.

In children with cyanotic congenital heart disease, the possibility of an intracranial abscess should be considered whenever neurologic signs appear. These abscesses may be multiple, confounding the clinical picture. Computerized scanning is the best available test for identifying an organized brain abscess. Electroencephalography is a very sensitive means for identifying abscesses but provides no means for identifying etiology or even distinguishing an abscess from certain other mass lesions. Nevertheless, it is extremely sensitive and at times will suggest additional focal areas of concern.

Complications following bacterial meningitis are common in infants and children. Seizures, intellectual compromise, motor deficits, coordination difficulties and hearing loss are the expected ones. It is not uncommon for small extra-axial fluid collections to be present in Hemophilus influenza meningitis. In general, these effusions do not require treatment and can be followed conservatively. Long-term complications from the presence of these fluid collections are not expected.

Venous sinus thrombosis may accompany sepsis and meningitis but is also seen in the context of fever and dehydration. Extravasation of blood often accompanies the thrombosis. Focal cerebral signs (seizures, paresis) are common when an isolated cortical vein is thrombosed, whereas more profound focal signs and depression of consciousness accompany major sinus thrombosis.

NEUROMUSCULAR DISEASES[4]

Neuromuscular diseases are not a common cause of neurologic crisis in the pediatric population. When they do occur they can often be anticipated and managed appropriately. Respiratory failure accompanying anterior horn cell disease (Werdnig-Hoffman) or the cardiomyopathy seen in certain congenital myopathies are examples of emergencies that should be anticipated. Little is necessary in the acute evaluation of acute neuromuscular disease apart from the history and clinical examination. Since cardio-respiratory manifestations are the most common emergencies, evaluation of pulmonary function (blood gases, pulmonary function tests) and cardiac function (EKG, echocardiogram) will be necessary. Support measures will include cardiotrophic drugs, mechanical ventilation, and pulmonary toilet.

In the newborn period, congenital neuromuscular diseases (neonatal myotonic dystrophy and congenital myopathies) may cause apnea and respiratory failure. Transient neonatal myasthenia gravis will also cause weakness and concomitant respiratory difficulties.

Transient Neonatal Myasthenia Gravis

Transient neonatal myasthenia gravis is a self-limited disease of some infants born to mothers with myasthenia gravis. It is thought to be due to the transplacental passage of antiacetylcholine antibodies. When the clinical syndrome is suspected, edrophonium (Tensilon) 0.15 mg/kg may be given as a test dose intravenously. It is helpful to give a similar quantity of saline as well, and for the physician evaluating the clinical response to be unaware as to which is being administered. Infants with the syndrome typically worsen over the first several days and then gradually improve over the next few weeks. Respiratory support may be necessary. Drugs increasing the availability of acetylcholine may be necessary but this requirement is quite variable. Breast feeding does not produce or prolong symptoms.

Neonatal Myotonic Dystrophy

Neonatal myotonic dystrophy also occurs in certain infants whose mothers have typical myotonic dystrophy. The severity of the mother's disease (as in transient neonatal myasthenia) does not predict the severity of disease in the child. Polyhydramnios and abnormalities of labor are common. Hypotonia, arthrogryposis, weakness, decreased tendon reflexes, and bulbar problems may all be present at birth. Additional findings are facial weakness, diaphragmatic paralysis, congenital cataracts, decreased peristalsis, and EKG abnormalities. Myotonia may be demonstrated on the electromyogram but is never present clinically. Muscle biopsy demonstrates maturational arrest, indicating the onset of the process prior to 28 weeks gestation. Creatinine phosphokinase (CPK) is normal.

Infantile Botulism

Infantile botulism is a disease distinct from the usual form of adult botulism. In infants symptoms are caused by the absorption of toxin formed in the lumen of the intestine rather than by the ingestion of pre-formed toxin. The disease should be suspected in infants presenting with constipation, poor feeding, weakness, weak cry, and respiratory difficulties. Findings of diffuse lower motor neuron weakness will be evident on exam. Ptosis, uncommon in weakness from systemic illness, is common. Attention must be given to the prevention of superinfection (pneumonia), aspiration, and respiratory failure.

Apart from the clinical findings, the disease may be confirmed by the identification of C. botulinum organisms or toxin from the gut. The electromyogram shows brief, small, abundant motor unit action potentials with an incremental response. This finding is virtually diagnostic of botulism when the diagnosis is in doubt.

Treatment consists of respiratory support and avoidance of complications. Antibiotics are given to prevent further growth of the organisms (unlike typical adult food-borne botulism in which antibiotics do nothing to pre-formed toxin).

Patients with neuromuscular diseases in general are particularly susceptible to the effects of skeletal muscle relaxants and to the neuromuscular side effects of aminoglycoside antibiotics. Malignant hyperthermia is also more commonly seen in this patient population.

ACUTE METABOLIC DISEASES IN INFANCY

The effects of metabolic disease on the individual are quite variable, with a spectrum from the absence of identifiable clinical disease to death in early infancy. In general, the symptoms likely to be seen in patients with acute neurologic disease on a metabolic basis are coma and seizures. Since these clinical findings are the most commonly seen in all of acute neurology, metabolic causes may not always be first on the list of differential diagnostic possibilities.

Quite often it is the laboratory abnormalities that lead the physician to suspect metabolic disease. Whereas transient metabolic derangements (electrolyte abnormalities, hypoglycemia, hypocalcemia) will be ruled out or confirmed early, inherited metabolic disease may only be suggested by the

**Table 16.9 Some Inherited Metabolic Diseases
for which Specific Treatment is
Possible**

Galactosemia
von Gierke's glycogenosis
Lactic acidosis
Maple syrup urine disease
Methylmalonic acidemia
Isovaleric acidemia
Propionic acidemia
Pyridoxine deficiency
Phenylketonuria

initial evaluation. There are certain tests that constitute an excellent "emergency" screen for inherited metabolic disease. Those tests are serum glucose, ketones, ammonia and pH plus urine sugar and ketones. More elaborate tests such as serum and urine amino and organic acids may be important to perform later but are virtually never available on an emergency basis. Abnormalities of the basic tests listed above will detect most abnormalities of carbohydrate and protein metabolism. Disorders of carbohydrate metabolism generally cause some combination of glycosuria, hypoglycemia, ketosis, and metabolic acidosis. Aminoacidopathies are often reflected as hypoglycemia, ketosis, metabolic acidosis, respiratory alkalosis, and hyperammonemia.

The identification of inherited metabolic disorders is important because successful treatment is available for many of them. Early treatment can prevent neurologic sequelae. Table 16.9 lists a variety of such disorders for which treatment is available.

In addition to supportive care, treatment consists of correcting the acid-base status, selective avoidance of any responsible nutrients, chemical supplimentation (glucose, pyridoxine, vitamin B_{12}), and, in seriously ill children, exchange transfusion or dialysis.

In young infants with serious neurologic symptoms or signs, the physician should keep the possibility of metabolic disease in mind. A few simple laboratory tests often provide the basis for decisions about fuller investigations; these screening tests may not be abnormal apart from the acute situation.

ACUTE ATAXIA IN CHILDHOOD[14]

Ataxia (cerebellar incoordination) may present acutely, insidiously, or be present statically on a neurodevelopmental basis. All children are somewhat ataxic as they learn to walk, reflecting the rather immaturely developed cerebellum. Complete functional maturity of the cerebellum is not reached until young adulthood (loosely corresponding to the development of athletic prowess). When the appearance of ataxia is acute, a relative neurologic emergency exists. The evaluation of the patient must proceed in consideration of the likely etiologies. Table 16.10 lists the common causes.

Because acute ataxia in children may indicate a posterior fossa mass lesion, lumbar puncture should be delayed until a definitive study, usually computerized tomography, is obtained. This is a critical management decision since an injudicious lumbar puncture could result in a central herniation syndrome. In general, these patients do not appear to have bacterial meningitis, so an emergency lumbar puncture is not necessary. When papilledema or a hemiparesis is found, a posterior fossa mass becomes even more likely.

Symptoms co-existing with ataxia in patients with posterior fossa masses are most often the result of impaired flow of cerebrospinal fluid. Hydrocephalus with increased intracranial pressure may result from direct compression of the ventricular system by the mass or compression secondary to edema. Sudden changes in clinical findings are often the result of acute hydrocephalus or hemorrhage. In younger children and infants where an open fontanel is present or the sutures easily split, these findings may be delayed and an enlarging head found. In older children headache, vomiting, irritability, restlessness, and papilledema are commonly seen.

It is important, although sometimes difficult, to distinguish between cerebellar ataxia and vertigo. This is most difficult in the very young child. At times there is a significant overlap in symptoms and signs (nystagmus, vomiting, incoordination). The identification of true vertigo shifts the differential diagnosis towards peripheral causes: benign paroxysmal vertigo, labyrinthi-

Table 16.10 Common Causes of Acute Ataxia in Childhood

Mass Lesions	Primary cerebellar tumors
	medulloblastoma
	ependymoma
	astrocytoma
	Brain stem tumors (gliomas)
	Abscesses
	Posterior fossa subdurals
Infectious/Post-Infectious	Measles
	Mumps
	Varicella
	Rubella
	Enterovirus
	Epstein-Barr virus
Traumatic	Cerebellar contusion
	Posterior fossa subdurals
	Vestibular damage
Toxins	Alcohol
	Phenytoin
	Sedative-hypnotics
Metabolic	Hartnup's disease
	Maple syrup urine disease
	Argininosuccinicaciduria
Miscellaneous	Conversion reaction
	Acute cerebellar ataxia syndrome of childhood

tis, intoxication. Vestibular dysfunction on a traumatic basis is also common.[15]

Testing relies upon both structural and functional assessments. The computerized tomogram will generally provide the necessary structural information. Calorics, electronystagmography, somatosensory and auditory evoked potentials and routine electroencephalography should also be considered. These are generally not part of the emergency evaluation.

BRAIN DEATH DETERMINATION IN INFANTS AND CHILDREN

It must be recognized that brain death is the same at all ages: total cessation of whole brain function in an irreversible clinical situation. The complicating factor in small infants and young children is identifying an irreversible state. Our comments about the plasticity of the immature brain come home never more hauntingly than in this situation. We are far less eager to declare an infant brain dead, even when the clinical criteria are fully met, for fear of failing to recognize a potentially reversible situation. This fear is appropriate. The immature brain has remarkable recuperative powers.

Some have been concerned that failure to declare a patient brain dead may cause a loss of the opportunity to do so. This is not the case. Brain dead patients have *no* brain function and do not recover function. Waiting an additional day or two will not change the clinical situation apart from making it clearer.

Confirmatory tests are more confusing. The criteria for electrocerebral silence (isoelectric EEG) do not pertain to children under age five.[10] The studies done to verify EEG findings in patients with brain death were not done in infants and young children. The EEG, therefore, should not be used as a criterion for brain death in this situation. Indeed, clinical criteria (not EEG criteria) are the basis for the Uniform Brain Death Act and the overwhelming majority of state laws pertaining to brain death determination.

REFERENCES

1. Bell, W.E., McCormick, W.E.: Increased Intracranial Pressure in Children. 2nd Ed. W.B. Saunders Co., Philadelphia, 1978.
2. Bell, W.E., McCormick, W.E.: Neurologic Infections in Children. 2nd Ed. W.B. Saunders Co., Philadelphia, 1981.
3. Cartlidge, N.E.F., Sharo, D.A.: Head Injury. W.B. Saunders Co., Philadelphia, 1981.
4. Dubowitz, V.: Muscle Disorders in Childhood. W.B. Saunders Co., Philadelphia, 1978.
5. Friedman, A.P.: Headache. p. 1. In Baker, A.B., Baker, L.H., eds.: Clinical Neurology. Vol. II. Harper & Row, Philadelphia, 1979.

6. Gastaut, H.: A physiopathogenic study of reflex anoxic cerebral seizures in children (syncopes, sobbing spasms and breath-holding spells). p. 257. In Kellaway, P., Petersen, I., eds.: Clinical Electroencephalography of Children. Grune & Stratton, New York, 1968.

7. Lovejoy, F., Smith, A., Bresnan, M., et. al.: Clinical Staging in Reye's Syndrome. Am. J. Dis. Child, 128:36, 1974.

8. Mastri, A.R., Silverstein, P.M., Gold, L., Eselius, E.P.: Multiple progressive intracranial arterial occlusions, Stroke, 4:380, 1973.

9. National Institutes of Health Consensus Development Conference Summary. Febrile Seizures, Vol. 3, Number 2, 1980.

10. Niedermeyer, E., da Silva, F.L.: Electroencephalography. Urban & Schwarzenberg, Baltimore, 1982.

11. Plum, F., Posner, J.B.: The Diagnosis of Stupor and Coma. 3rd Ed. F.A. Davis, Philadelphia, 1980.

12. Swaiman, K.E., Wright, F.S., eds.: The Practice of Pediatric Neurology. C.V. Mosby Co., St. Louis, 1975.

13. Volpe, J.: Neurology of the Newborn. W.B. Saunders Co., Philadelphia, 1981.

14. Weiss, S., Carter, S.: Course and Prognosis of Acute Cerebellar Ataxia in Children. Neurology, 9:711, 1959.

15. Wolfson, R.J., Silverstein, H., Marlowe, F.I., Keels, E.W.: Vertigo. Clinical Symposia (Ciba), 33(6), 1981.

17

Acute Management of Severe Brain Anoxia

John J. Caronna, M.D.

INTRODUCTION

The Brain Requires A Constant Supply Of Oxygen To Meet Energy Demands

Under normal circumstances, 90 percent of the cerebral energy needed to maintain ionic gradients across cell membranes and to transmit nervous impulses is derived from the oxidation of glucose. The brain does not store oxygen and therefore can survive for only a few minutes if its oxygen supply is reduced below critical levels.

Non-oxidative Glucose Metabolism Cannot Meet Brain Energy Demands

During anoxia, cerebral aerobic metabolism falls and glycolysis, the anaerobic degradation of glucose to lactate and pyruvate, is accelerated. The energy produced by glycolysis under circumstances of anoxia is only a fraction of the brain's needs and clinical symptoms and electroencephalographic (EEG) abnormalities appear.

During acute total anoxia, as occurs in sudden decompression of an aircraft at high altitudes, consciousness is lost within 15 seconds. The effects of anoxia on the EEG parallel the effects on consciousness. The human EEG slows when there is arterial hypoxemia (PaO_2 35 mmHg or less), or when cerebral blood flow (CBF) is reduced to 40 percent of normal. The EEG becomes isoelectric ("flat") when cerebral venous PO_2 reaches 20 mmHg or after about 18 seconds of total anoxia.[3]

DEFINITIONS AND DESIGNATIONS OF FOUR TYPES OF ANOXIA

Human anoxia is a complex state of decreased oxygen availability, systemic acidosis, hypercapnia, and eventual ischemia. Therefore, the term as used here includes all forms of inadequate delivery of oxygen to the brain, namely, hypoxemia, ischemia, and circulatory arrest. The various forms of anoxia are anoxic, anemic, histotoxic, and stagnant (ischemic). These categories are best used to describe experimental anoxic states produced under laboratory conditions and have limited application to the clinical situation in which hypoxia and ischemia overlap. Nevertheless categorical distinctions aid the analysis of the pathophysiology of clinical anoxic syndromes (Table 17.1).

Anoxic Anoxia

Anoxic anoxia implies a reduced arterial partial pressure of oxygen such as might occur whenever oxygen is deficient in the environment or when the exchange of oxygen from the atmosphere to the pulmonary capillary is impaired.

Decreased availability of oxygen in the atmosphere occurs at high altitudes and when oxygen is displaced in an inhaled gas mixture by smoke or by other gases, as in anesthetic or industrial accidents.

At sea level, hemoglobin is normally 95–98 percent saturated. Hemoglobin saturation does not begin to fall below 90 percent until altitudes of 10,000 feet or more are attained. The first important physiologic effect of hypoxia occurs at about 5,000 feet when night vision becomes impaired. At 10,000 feet, dyspnea appears and mental concentration becomes difficult. Headache, restlessness, and bradycardia or reflex syncope may appear. Above 15,000 feet irritability, euphoria, impaired memory and judgment, cyanosis, and muscular incoordination occur. The most extreme type of anoxic anoxia occurs during sudden atmospheric decompression at an altitude of more than 37,000 feet. In primates, such profound hypoxia results in rapid unconsciousness followed within minutes by cardiovascular collapse and death.

Failure to exchange oxygen between environmental air and alveolar capillaries can occur because of paralysis of respiratory muscles; acute airway

Table 17.1 Types of Anoxia

---

1. Anoxic anoxia = Decreased oxygen in the environment or impaired oxygen exchange from atmosphere to pulmonary capillary.
    Example = Lung disease
2. Anemic anoxia = Decreased transport of oxygen to tissues.
    Example = Severe anemia
3. Histotoxic anoxia = Metabolic block causes tissue asphyxia.
    Example = Cyanide poisoning
4. Stagnant (Ischemic) anoxia = Decreased blood flow from lungs to tissues.
    Example = Cardiac arrest

---

obstruction, as in aspiration of food or attempted suidicide by hanging; pulmonary disease such as pneumonia, pulmonary edema, drowning or emphysema; or with heart disease when pathological shunting allows venous blood to bypass the pulmonary circulation.

In general, normotensive anoxic anoxia is tolerated well. Compensation for cerebral oxygen deprivation occurs primarily by an increase in CBF; delivery of glucose and removal of metabolic wastes are unimparied. Evidence from animal experiments indicates that as long as the brain is perfused by an adequate blood flow, a decrease of PaO_2 to as low as 15 mmHg can be sustained for up to 30 minutes. In these hypoxemic experiments, cerebral parenchymal lactic acidosis was prominent, but concentrations of adenosine triphosphate (ATP), adenosine diphosphate (ADP), and adenosine monophosphate (AMP) remained essentially normal. The cerebral hypoxia that occurred during short-term normotensive anoxemia was reversible and did not lead to permanent cell damage.

When anoxic anoxia is severe or prolonged, secondary depression of the myocardium supervenes and the resulting fall in blood pressure leads to severe disturbances in cerebral energy state. Cardiovascular depression accounts at least partially for the high rates of death and brain damage that follow clinical cases of asphyxia.

The pre-terminal cardiovascular collapse caused by anoxia is not due to weakness of the hypoxic heart muscle; hypoxia may even potentiate the contractile strength of the heart. In a series of experiments, isolated dog hearts, as well as hearts beating *in situ*, did not fail acutely as long as PaO_2 was above 15 mmHg; when the arterial oxygen tension fell below this level, the hearts quickly ceased to beat. Hearts chronically maintained at PaO_2 between 40 and 15 mmHg accumulated fluid in muscle fibers (myocardial edema) and became less distensible. It is likely that hypoxia causes cardiovascular collapse acutely by means of reflexes from the carotid artery territory which induced bradycardia, increased arterial resistance, and augmented venomotor tonus. The critical level of carotid arterial PO_2 at which bradycardia and severe cardiac failure occurred in dogs varies between 45 and 15 mmHg.[1]

Anemic Anoxia

In anemic anoxia, the oxygen tension within the respiratory system is normal, but the oxygenation of hemoglobin is insufficient to allow adequate levels of oxygen in tissues. Acute hemorrhage, chronic anemia, and carbon monoxide poisoning are most commonly responsible.

Anemia increases CBF in man, suggesting that the oxygen supply to brain is maintained by a homeostatic increase in CBF. Patients with pernicious anemia and hemoglobin values of 7g or less were found to have increased CBF but decreased cerebral oxygen and glucose consumption, as well as reduced cerebral venous oxygen tension. The decrease in jugular venous oxygen tension probably reflected a similar decrease in cerebral tissue PO_2, which resulted in cerebral parenchymal acidosis with arteriolar dilatation and increased CBF. The metabolic regulation of CBF in anemic anoxia therefore appears to be similar to that in anoxic anoxia. In these patients there was no correlation between the degree of anemia and cerebral oxygen consumption or between EEG changes and measured cerebral metabolic functions. There was a good correlation, however, between severity of neurologic state and cerebral oxygen consumption. The depressed cerebral oxygen consumption reflected permanent neurological damage since it did not increase to normal when therapy reversed the anemia. It is impossible to determine whether cerebral injury in these cases was the effect of prolonged anemic anoxia or deficiency of vitamin B_{12}.

Hemodilution can increase CBF before cerebral tissue hypoxia occurs. In experimental dilutional anemia in rats, researchers found four-fold to five-fold increases in CBF when cerebral oxygen consumption and cerebral venous PO_2 remained constant. The unchanged venous PO_2 suggests that a change in tissue PO_2 did not occur, and therefore there was no cerebral hypoxia to signal for increased CBF. Blood viscosity, therefore, may have an important role in the maintenance of cerebral homeostasis during dilutional anemic anoxia.

In carbon monoxide poisoning, the oxygen-binding capacity of the blood is reduced but the viscosity is unchanged. Carbon monoxide intoxication is not exclusively an anemic anoxia since its adverse effects also result from interference with release of oxygen to the tissue; the presence of carboxyhemoglobin causes a shift of the oxyhemoglobin dissociation curve to the left, increasing the oxygen affinity of the remaining hemoglobin. In awake human subjects, a significant increase in CBF was observed at a carboxyhemoglobin concentration of only 20 percent. During carbon monoxide exposure, PaO_2 remained constant but jugular venous PO_2 decreased, suggesting that impaired delivery of oxygen caused cerebral tissue hypoxia.

The neuropathological findings in cases of lethal carbon monoxide intoxication are noteworthy because of their anatomic location. The major lesions, instead of affecting cerebral cortex, have been found in the basal ganglia, particularly the caudate, putamen, and globus pallidus and in the central white matter. Although it is tempting to ascribe the restricted topography of the cerebral injury to a purely anoxic insult without interruption of cerebral circulation, clinical experience dictates otherwise. Lesions typical of carbon monoxide intoxication have been described following anoxia of any type.

Histotoxic Anoxia

Except for carbon monoxide and the cyanides, no clinically important agent produces histotoxic anoxia. Cyanides are among the most rapidly acting poisons known. When inhaled, absorption is so rapid that death may be almost instantaneous. Oral doses act more slowly; as the blood cyanide level increases, there is headache, nausea, dyspnea, circulatory collapse, seizures, unconsciousness, and death within minutes to 1 hour. Cyanides combine with iron-containing enzymes such as neuronal cytochrome oxidase and catalase. Hydrogen and electron-transport are blocked, energy-releasing mechanisms cease, and death occurs from tissue asphyxia. Because the metabolic block is in the tissues rather than the blood, hemoglobin remains saturated with oxygen and cyanosis is not observed until apnea occurs.

Most experimental studies of brain damage caused by intoxication with cyanide compounds have not excluded the adverse effects of apnea, hypotension, and seizures. In the rat, normotensive histotoxic anoxia produced only damage to cerebral white matter and damage to neurons did not occur unless cerebral perfusion declined. Therefore, in the rat, hypoxic neuronal damage of a purely histotoxic type does not exist.

Stagnant (Ischemic) Anoxia

Ischemic anoxia occurs when CBF is insufficient to meet cerebral oxygen demands. Localized ischemia is a consequence of thrombotic or embolic occlusion of a cerebral artery and the result is a cerebral infarct or stroke, but cerebrovascular disease will not be discussed here.

Generalized brain ischemia is most commonly a consequence of systemic circulatory collapse due to cardiac arrhythmia or standstill, and the result is a spectrum of neurological disorders. Ischemic anoxia often follows a period of anoxic, anemic, or histotoxic anoxia that leads to cardiovascular failure. Neurological consequences are more severe than those of the uncomplicated anoxias, perhaps because, in ischemia, delivery of glucose as well as oxygen is diminished, as is removal of metabolic waste products.

NEUROPATHOLOGICAL FEATURES OF CLINICAL ISCHEMIC-ANOXIA (CARDIAC ARREST)[1]

Pathological changes in the central nervous system after cardiac arrest depend mainly upon the degree and duration of ischemic-anoxia. Many factors, however, can modify the distribution and severity of cerebral infarcts: the proportion between the period of true circulatory arrest with complete cerebral ischemia, and the preceding and succeeding periods of hypotension with maintained but reduced cerebral perfusion; the degree of systemic hypoxemia and hypoglycemia; and the cerebral energy requirements. For example, states of reduced cerebral energy requirements, such as deep anesthesia and hypothermia, have prevented brain damage during a variety of ischemic insults. By contrast, hypermetabolic states, such as status epilepticus leading to cardiac arrest, may predispose the cerebral cortex to ischemic damage. (Table 17.2)

Table 17.2 Factors Which Affect Severity of Cerebral Damage after Cardiac Arrest

   I. Degree of circulatory arrest
      A. Complete collapse
      B. Hypotension
  II. Duration of circulatory arrest
 III. Cerebral energy requirements
      A. Reduced
          1. Coma
          2. Anesthesia
          3. Hypothermia
      B. Increased
          1. Epileptic seizures
          2. Hyperthermia
 IV. Other factors
      A. Unfavorable
          1. Preexisting cerebrovascular disease
          2. Hypoxemia
          3. Hyperglycemia
          4. Hyperosmolarity
      B. Favorable
          1. Unknown

Neuropathological lesions usually can be grouped into one of several categories, although there may be overlap in individual cases.

Focal CNS Injury (Table 17.3)

Injury to Neurons in Vulnerable Areas

In cases of brief anoxia, ischemic cell death is limited to those neurons most sensitive to anoxia. The neurons of the hippocampus and cerebellum are the cells most frequently damaged in anoxia. Such hippocampal and cerebellar lesions may be responsible for amnesia and ataxia after cardiac arrest, but often produce no clinical deficits.

Anoxic Leukoencephalopathy [4]

Focal injury of cerebral white matter, often of delayed onset, has been reported following all types of anoxic-ischemic insults. The pathological lesions are restricted primarily to the deep white matter of the parietal and occipital lobes.

The clinical syndrome of anoxic leukoencephalopathy is distinctive: days to weeks after apparent recovery from ischemic-anoxia, patients suffer progressive neurological deterioration and either die or remain comatose. Delayed anoxic deterioration follows no more than two out of each thousand cardiac arrests and is not predictable by the type of anoxic-ischemic insult or the preceding clinical course.

Table 17.3 Focal Infarcts Following Global Anoxic-Ischemia

I. Border zone infarction—between major arteries
  A. Cerebral cortex
  B. Cerebellar cortex
  C. Spinal cord
II. End zone infarction—distal field of arteries with collateral circulation
  A. Basal ganglia
    1. Caudate
    2. Putamen
    3. Globus pallidus

Infarction in Border Zones

A period of circulatory arrest preceded or followed by appreciable periods of hypotension often leads to ischemic alterations concentrated in the border zones or distal fields between the major cerebral and spinal arteries. When border zone infarcts occur in the cerebral cortex, ischemic necrosis following profound hypotension is most severe in the parieto-occipital regions where the territories of the anterior, middle, and posterior cerebral arteries meet. The cerebral cortex commonly is affected bilaterally, or unilaterally if there is atherosclerotic compromise of the vessels to one hemisphere.

Cortical border zone infarcts often are hemorrhagic because of re-perfusion when blood pressure is restored. Border zone infarction and diffuse cortical necrosis may co-exist.

Within the spinal cord there are border zones between the anterior spinal artery and the segmental arteries from the aorta. Severe hypotension or disruption of the segmental arteries causes infarction of the spinal cord in the costo-cervical and the lower thoracolumbar regions. The thoracic cord usually is involved at the border zone between the anterior spinal artery and the artery of Adamkiewicz.

Infarction in End Zones

Within the cerebral hemispheres there are end arteries such as the lenticulostriate branches of the middle cerebral arteries. Under normal circumstances brain tissue nourished by these arteries does not have a collateral supply from anastomones with other arteries. Severe hypotension may result in end zone infarcts in the basal ganglia. At autopsy after ischemic anoxia necrotic areas can include the caudate, putamen, globus pallidus and substantia nigra. Lesions in these structures may be responsible for the clinical movement disorders, including the Parkinsonian syndrome, that are observed in cardiac arrest survivors.

The border zone and end zone hypotheses together best explain the focal neurological deficits observed in patients resuscitated after cardiac arrest. However, the topography and severity of cerebral infarcts cannot be predicted from clinical estimates of the efficacy and duration of resuscitative efforts.

Diffuse CNS Injury

Prolonged cardiac arrest causes widespread death of neurons. Certain groups of neurons are vulnerable to even moderate degrees of anoxia: pyramidal cells in Somner's sector of the hippocampus, Purkinje cells of the cerebellum, and pyramidal cells of the third and fifth layers of the cerebral cortex. More severe degrees of anoxia affect neurons in the amygdala, lateral putamen, caudate, lateral geniculate, thalamus, substantia nigra, and inferior colliculus. Hypothalamic neurons usually are spared. Profound anoxia affects even the brainstem nuclei including the locus ceruleus, the vestibular, trigeminal, dorsal vagal, and hypoglossal nuclei, as well as pontine neurons. By contrast, the medullary olives and the cuneatus and gracilis nuclei are resistant to anoxic ischemic injury in adults, but are more vulnerable in children.

CLINICAL NEUROLOGICAL SYNDROMES CAUSED BY ISCHEMIC ANOXIA (TABLE 17.4)

> ***PRINCIPLE 1:*** Cardiac arrest may be considered to cause both "metabolic" (largely reversible) and "structural" (largely irreversible) damage to the CNS.

Milder degrees of cerebral ischemic anoxia result in a syndrome that has the clinical features of a transient metabolic encephalopathy. Consciousness may be only mildly disordered, and coma, if present, lasts only a few hours, usually less than twelve (Table 17.4I). On awakening, these patients do not demonstrate focal, motor, or sensory deficits but may have intellectual deficits (confusion and anterograde amnesia). Recovery is rapid and usually complete so that these patients can resume their previous occupations. Rare patients suffer delayed neurological deterioration due to necrosis of CNS myelin (leukoencephalopathy).[4]

> ***PRINCIPLE 2:*** Patients with more severe or prolonged systemic ischemic anoxia suffer stroke-like infarcts in specific areas of the brain.

Patients in this group (Table 17.4II) have suffered more severe degrees of cerebral ischemic-anoxia than the group described above. By contrast, these patients are usually in coma for 12 hours or more, and upon regaining consciousness, manifest lasting focal or multifocal motor, sensory, and intellectual deficits. Recovery occurs slowly over weeks to months and often is

Table 17.4 Neurological Syndromes Following Severe Brain Anoxia

I. Return to consciousness < 12 hours
  A. Pathology: No damage or scattered ischemic neurons
  B. Clinical: Transient confusion often followed by anterograde amnesia
  C. Outcome: Rapid, complete recovery; delayed anoxic leukoencephalopathy (rare)
II. Unconsciousness >12 hours
  A. Cerebral syndrome
    1. Pathology: Focal or multifocal infarcts of cortex, especially in boundary zones and end zones
    2. Clinical: Amnesia and dementia
      Bibrachial paresis or quadriparesis sparing the face
      Cortical blindness or visual agnosia
      Also may occur: ataxia, seizures, myoclonus, parkinsonism
    3. Outcome: Slow, often incomplete recovery
  B. Spinal cord syndrome (may occur in isolation or accompany cerebral syndrome)
    1. Pathology: Focal or multifocal infarcts of spinal cord
    2. Clinical: Flaccid areflexic paralysis of lower limbs
      Urinary retention
      Loss of pain and temperature sense
      Preserved touch and position sense
    3. Outcome: No or incomplete recovery
III. No recovery of consciousness
  A. Destruction of hemispheres alone
    1. Pathology: Laminar necrosis of cortex (neocortical death)
    2. Clinical: Persistent vegetative state (akinetic mutism)
    3. Outcome: Prolonged survival in vegetative state
  B. Brain death
    1. Pathology: Necrosis of cortex + brainstem ± spinal cord
    2. Clinical: No evidence of cortical activity, no brainstem reflexes, reflexes of purely spinal origin may persist
    3. Systemic death within days to weeks

incomplete so that many patients remain dependent on others for daily needs.

Among the focal signs manifest in this group of patients are partial or complete cortical blindness, paresis of both arms and quadriparesis. Cortical blindness is usually transient and probably results from disproportionate ischemia in the arterial border zones of both occipital lobes. Bilateral infarction of the cerebral motor cortex in the border zone between the anterior and middle cerebral arteries may be responsible for the bibrachial paresis, sparing the face and legs, which is sometimes seen following cardiac arrest.

> ***PRINCIPLE 3:*** The border zone and end zone hypotheses explain the presence of focal subcortical or spinal cord infarcts when the "more vulnerable" cerebral cortex is spared.

The spinal cord is more resistent to transient ischemia than more rostral parts of the central nervous system. Nevertheless, cases of spinal cord infarction, without evidence of cerebral injury, occur (Table 17.4II). Necrosis of the central structures of the spinal cord can occur in critical border zones at the periphery of the territory supplied by a main contributory vessel.

> ***PRINCIPLE 4:***   Some patients who never regain consciousness (awareness of self and environment), regain wakefulness (eye opening) after cardiac arrest.

A third group of resuscitated patients (Table 17.4III) with more widespread destruction of brain either remain hospitalized in a vegetative state (VS) or die a neurological death. Some patients with severe irreversible brain damage who survive for more than a few days regain eye opening, sleep-awake cycles, spontaneous roving eye movements, and other reflex activities at brainstem and spinal cord levels but remain in a functionally decorticate state of wakefulness without awareness.[7] This vegetative state is distinct from the sleep-like condition of coma. In certain extreme cases, prolonged survival for weeks or months in a vegetative state has been associated with an isoelectric EEG. Detailed neuropathological analysis of two such cases indicated that the hemispheres had been destroyed while vital brainstem and spinal structures remained intact. This neuropathological condition has been called neocortical or cerebral death and must be distinguished from *total* cerebral *and* brainstem destruction (brain death). In our experience, neocortical death has occurred most often in cases of cardiac arrest superimposed upon a cerebral hypermetabolic state induced by generalized motor seizures.

CLINICAL CRITERIA OF BRAIN DEATH

Several committees and reviewers have proposed clinical criteria for brain death (see Plum and Posner 1980 for review).[13] Representative criteria are outlined in Table 17.5. In essence, brain death may be diagnosed when there is no discernible evidence of either cerebral hemispheral or brainstem function, for an extended period, usually 12 hours or more, and when the loss of brain function is the result of structural and not of reversible metabolic disease. The clinical examination for brain death includes attention to cerebral hemisphere function and brainstem reflexes, as well as laboratory tests.

Coma Of Established Cause

The cerebral lesion must be structural, bearing in mind that an initially metabolic insult, as occurs in prolonged anoxia, also can lead to irreversible structural damage. Any possibility that the patient has suffered from drug poisoning, or that hypothermia or an electrolyte abnormality is contributing to the depth of coma, must be excluded by appropriate laboratory tests. The patient should have no clinical evidence of cerebral function or brainstem reflexes for a period of at least 12 hours with no demonstrable improvement whatsoever. This period of observation must be extended to 24 or more hours or until negative toxicology screen results are obtained, if drug overdosage is a possibility. The period of observation may be shortened

Table 17.5 Brain Death Criteria
(Adapted from the By-Laws of The New York Hospital)

Determination of brain death shall be made in accordance with the mandatory criteria listed below. All observations, tests and findings shall be recorded in the patient's chart. Supplementary criteria may be used at the physician's discretion.

Mandatory Criteria

I. Coma of established cause
   A. No potentially anesthetizing amounts of either toxins or therapeutic drugs can be present. Hypothermia below 30°C or other physiological abnormalities must be corrected to the extent medically possible.
   B. Irreversible structural disease or a known and irreversible endogenous metabolic cause due to organ failure must be present.
   C. A twelve-hour period of no brain function must have elapsed.
II. No cerebral function
   No behavioral or reflex response involving structures above the cervical spinal cord can be elicited by noxious stimuli delivered anywhere in the body.
III. No brainstem reflexes
   A. The pupils must be fixed to light.
   B. No corneal reflexes can be present.
   C. There must be no response to icewater caloric (50 ml in each ear).
   D. No spontaneous respirations must occur during apneic oxygenation for a period sufficient to maximally stimulate breathing.
NOTE: The circulation may be intact and purely spinal cord reflexes may be retained.

Supplementary Criteria

The twelve hour period of observation may be shortened to as little as 6 hours in cases of established irreversible structural damage provided that the mandatory clinical criteria are confirmed by one or more of the supplementary criteria.

I. An EEG for 30 minutes at maximal gain reflects absence of cerebral electrical activity.
II. Brainstem auditory evoked responses reflect absence of function in vital brainstem structures.
III. No cerebral circulation present on angiographic examination.

(These criteria are included with permission of the New York Hospital-Cornell Medical Center. Neither the author nor the hospital represents that these guidelines are or will continue to be acceptable under the laws of any particular state or will be applicable for every case.)

to as little as 6 hours if, for example, a competent neurosurgeon explores a head wound and finds the brain transected, or if one or more of the supplementary tests (Table 17.5) confirms the absence of cerebral circulation and/or electrical activity.

No Cerebral Function

The patient's supraorbital ridges, sternum and each extremity should receive noxious stimulation. There must be no appropriate response to stimulation: the patient must not rouse, groan, grimace, withdraw the head or limbs from an applied stimulus, or attempt to push away the examiner's hand. Reflex responses such as decerebrate extension or decorticate flexion of the limbs, which are mediated by subcortical but supraspinal cord pathways, are not permitted. The spinal cord may be intact, therefore rudimentary reflex responses such as muscle stretch reflexes, plantar flexion, plantar withdrawal (triple flexion), abdominal reflexes, and tonic neck reflexes, all of which depend upon functions of the spinal cord, may be preserved.

No Brainstem Reflexes

The pupils must be fixed to light stimulation. The pupils may be either widely dilated (as may happen when a dopamine infusion is necessary to maintain the circulation) or mid-dilated, but stimulation with an intensely bright light must fail to yield any evidence of pupillary constriction.

The corneal blink reflex must be absent when the tip of a cotton applicator is applied forcefully to either cornea.

The oculocephalic (doll's eyes) and oculovestibular (ice water caloric) responses both must be absent. The oculovestibular response is elicited by irrigating each tympanic membrane with 50 ml of ice water for 30 to 45 seconds and observing whether there is any movement of the eyes toward the side of the tympanic irrigation. There should be no ocular movement during 3 minutes of observation after ice water has been injected.

The patient must be apneic and not recover spontaneous ventilatory function after the respirator has been turned off to allow arterial PCO_2 ($PaCO_2$) to attain a level high enough to maximally stimulate respiratory drive. Evidence indicates that the threshold for respiratory stimulation may approach a $PaCO_2$ of 60 mmHg in patients with brain damage and that the rate of rise of $PaCO_2$ during respiratory arrest is approximately 3 mmHg/min. The duration of respiratory arrest needed to allow $PaCO_2$ to reach or exceed 60 mmHg is not constant and will vary depending on the level of $PaCO_2$ prior to the onset of apnea. Therefore, to confirm absolute apnea, blood gas monitoring is required to verify either normocapnia, prior to beginning apnea for 10 minutes, or, if a patient is hypocapnic, $PaCO_2$ in excess of 60 mmHg at the end of apnea. No absolute period of apnea sufficient to establish brain death can be recommended in the absence of blood gas determinations.

The respirator should be disconnected according to the following procedure: All patients are mechanically ventilated with 100 percent oxygen for 10 minutes before the start of apnea. The electrocardiogram is monitored continuously and the blood pressures measured intermittently before and during apnea. An arterial blood sample is drawn and analyzed for pH, PaO_2, and $PaCO_2$ before beginning apnea so that hypoxemia may be detected. Caution is advised when hypoxemia exists in individuals being mechanically ventilated with high concentrations of oxygen, since apneic oxygenation may worsen this abnormality. The respirator then is disconnected and 100 percent oxygen at a rate of 6 L/min is administered via endotracheal tube. The reservoir bag must be observed for signs of spontaneous respiratory activity. Arterial blood samples for pH, PaO_2 and $PaCO_2$ should be drawn at the end of 10 minutes, more in apneic patients. Patients who breathe should be replaced on mechanical ventilation.

The circulation may still be functioning normally. If all the above criteria are met, the presence of a normal blood pressure does not indicate a recoverable brain.

When the above conditions have been fulfilled, a physician can certify that death has occurred.

The clinical diagnosis of brain death generally is not difficult, nor likely to be in error, if the criteria outlined in Table 17.5 are rigorously followed. The validity of the clinical criteria for diagnosing brain death (independent of supplementary tests) has been confirmed by several published series both in the U.S.A. and the U.K.[6] Nevertheless, recovery after supposed brain death has been alleged in patients who were thought to be brain dead but, in fact, were not. Review of such cases has revealed that in each instance the clinical criteria were not satisfied. There has not been, so far as we know, a single reported case in which the criteria of brain death were met and the patient survived.

In our own series of 500 patients in coma, not due to trauma or drug intoxications, there were 14 patients who met the clinical criteria for brain death. In no case was ventilation discontinued, yet all suffered cardiac arrest within hours to 28 days after the diagnosis.[8]

Supplementary Tests

It is our view that the clinical criteria are reliable and so conservative that, when properly applied, they will never lead to the diagnosis of death in a patient who might survive. Therefore, there is no need for confirmatory tests when all the clinical conditions for diagnosis of brain death have been fulfilled. Nevertheless, the diagnosis of brain death carries a heavy responsibility, and some medical centers have found it useful to employ supplementary tests to provide verifiable support to the clinical evaluation or to shorten the period of observation.

Although brain death is a common occurrence and has gained wide acceptance among physicians, many laymen, and indeed some physicians, are not fully confident about the accuracy of the diagnosis of brain death. This anxiety can only be dispelled by more extensive clinical experience and continued discussion by members of the fields of medicine, law, philosophy and theology of the questions generated by new medical technologies.

A PROSPECTIVE STUDY OF ANOXIC COMA

As part of a cooperative study to define more accurately clinical factors that predict outcome in non-traumatic coma, we conducted serial neurological examination on 210 adult patients in coma following an episode of hypoxia-ischemia and followed them for one year.[8]

The study was conducted on patients in coma caused by cardiac arrest, primary respiratory arrest followed by circulatory collapse, or profound hypotension who were admitted to the hospital and who were in coma for at least 6 hours after resuscitation. Coma was defined as a sleep-like state of unarousable unresponsiveness without evidence of awareness of self or the environment.

Neurological condition at admission was judged by evaluating cerebral and brainstem function on physical examination aided by appropriate radiological and other investigations. Nearly all patients were seen within 6 to 12 hours of the onset of coma and followed at regular intervals thereafter until death or until 1 year after cardiac arrest.

Four levels of recovery were defined: *Good outcome* implied the ability to achieve independence in daily living. *Severe disability* implied that patients regained cognition but depended on others for daily support. *Vegetative state* meant that the patient was awake, but unaware. *No recovery* implied persistent coma to death.

Of the 210 comatose patients only 12 percent achieved independence in daily life (good outcome) within the first year; the remainder either died while still in coma (58 percent), never improved beyond the vegetative state (20 percent), or regained consciousness but remained severely disabled (10 percent).

Analysis of early clinical signs permitted the patients to be separated into groups having a relatively good or a poor prognosis. At admission (Fig. 17.1), the absence of any two of pupillary, corneal or motor responses identified 66 patients with a poor prognosis, only one of whom subsequently improved even to a level of severe disability. The presence of any motor response to pain in the remaining 144 patients identified 99 subjects, 22 of whom achieved a good outcome.

One day after admission, there were 166 survivors. In this group, the absence of any two among spontaneous eye movements, pupillary responses, or corneal responses identified 39 patients with a poor prognosis, none of whom ever regained consciousness. By contrast, the presence of any motor response, normal spontaneous eye movements, or normal ice water caloric

ANY 2 REACTIVE? PUPILS CORNEALS MOTOR	NUMBER OF PATIENTS	BEST ONE-YEAR RECOVERY		
		No. Recov. Veg. State	Sev. Disab.	Mod. Disab. Good Recov.
MOTOR PRESENT? — Yes →	99	62%	16%	22%
No — No →	45	84%	7%	9%
→	66	98%	2%	0%

Fig. 17.1 Association of neurologic signs at admission with best one-year recovery (210 patients).

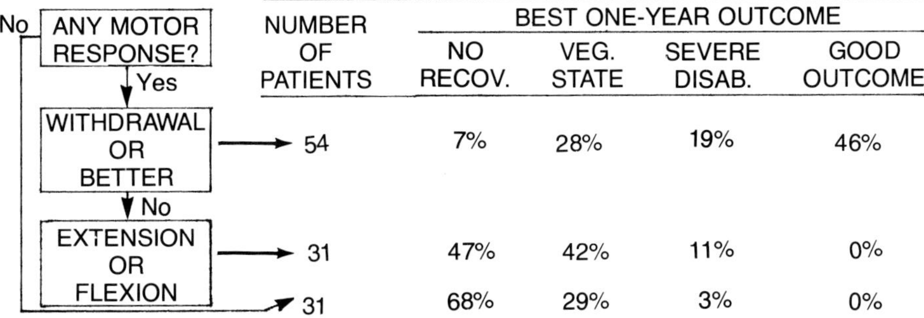

Fig. 17.2 Association of neurologic signs after three days with best one-year recovery (123 patients).

responses (nystagmus), in the remaining patients, identified 93 subjects, 24 of whom achieved a good outcome.

At three days, 123 patients survived (Fig. 17.2), in whom the absence of any motor response or the persistence of only a reflex response identified 69 patients, none of whom achieved a good outcome. The presence of withdrawal or better (purposive motor responses) identified 54 patients, almost one-half of whom achieved a good outcome.

This analysis implies that recovery from hypoxic-ischemic coma is closely associated with clinical features of brain dysfunction. In addition, this investigation has suggested a mechanism for identifying patients with relatively poor and relatively good prognoses.

ELECTROCUTION AND LIGHTNING INJURIES[5,10,20]

Deaths from electrical injuries constitute less than 1 percent of accidental fatalities in North America and Europe. Ninety percent (90 percent) of fatal electrocutions are due to technical, that is man-made, currents, and only 10 percent due to atmospheric electricity, namely lightning strikes.

> **PRINCIPLE 1:** The chief factor which determines the pathophysiological effects of electricity is not the voltage of the installation with which the victim has contact, but the current strength or amperage.

Electrophysiology (Voltage, Resistance, And Amperage)

A volt is the unit of electromotive force. Low voltage currents up to about 100 volts are not of pathophysiological importance. However, 60 volt currents have resulted in death. By contrast, high voltage sources of 50,000 volts or more need not result in fatalities. Perhaps up to 70 percent of fatalities result from medium voltage injury (200–250 volts). Current flow is increased by grounding, as occurs in common household accidents with electrical appliances as the source and with the victim grounded in water. In the United States, domestic fatalities account for one-third of a total of some one thousand lethal electrical accidents per year.

Resistance, measured in ohms, is the deciding factor in the amount of current passing through any substance. Ohm's Law states that the current in amperes is equal to the voltage divided by the resistance in ohms (A=v/o). In human tissue, resistance is highest in the skin and subcutaneous fat. For example, calloused, dry skin can have a resistance of up to one million ohms. Thin, moist skin can have a resistance of one thousand ohms or less. Resistance is low in muscle and brain (1,000–2,000 ohms) and higher in bone (4,000–10,000 ohms). If skin resistance is lowered by moisture, for example, then a 110 volt current can produce fatal ventricular fibrillation.

> **PRINCIPLE 2:** The effect of current on the human body depends upon three factors:
>
> 1. Current strength
> 2. Current duration
> 3. Current pathway through the body.

Current is expressed in amperes and depends upon voltage and resistance according to Ohm's Law. Therefore the operative current strength in any accident is never certain but can only be estimated from measurement of voltage and resistance.

The duration of contact may be longer in accidents due to low tension currents than in high tension accidents. In high tension accidents the duration of current flow is very short due to the automatic disconnection (safety cut-out) features of such installations.

In the event of contact with low tension currents, the circuit is not interrupted and the victim may not be able to withdraw because of tetanic muscle contraction. The resultant action of the current may last for seconds or even minutes.

Current passes through tissues by the shortest path along the points of contact. There is a direct effect of current on organs, so that it is important to establish the pathway followed by the current through the body. Current passage across the heart and brain is particularly dangerous. The passage of a current across the heart may disturb the coordinated action of the individual muscle fibers and produce a flaccid state, with asystole or with fibrillations of individual muscle fibers. Respiratory arrest and asphyxia may result from either passage of current through the brainstem or from tetanic contraction of respiratory muscles. Death from lightning probably is of cerebral origin in a majority of cases due to entry of the current into the head and brain. The current route in these cases is from scalp, across brain, to hand or foot.

In non-fatal electrical accidents, the current pathway can be determined by questioning the victim and bystanders, or if necessary by examining the skin for burns at the sites of entry and exit. At the point of entry, a high resistance converts electrical energy to heat, which can be intense enough to cause necrosis of skin or bone. In cases of electrical injury with hand to hand passage of current, the high mortality (up to 60 percent depending upon the amount of current) is due to involvement of the cervical spinal cord between C_4-C_8 segments causing respiratory muscle paralysis or tetanic contraction. In hand to foot current passage, fatalities are much fewer (up to 20 percent).

Acute Syndromes Of Electrical Injury

The clinical features of acute life threatening electrical injuries depend upon whether the central nervous system or the cardiorespiratory system is affected.

The Central Nervous System Syndrome

When loss of consciousness occurs, the sequence of events afterwards is similar to what is observed following closed head trauma. Loss of consciousness may be associated with seizures, myoclonic jerks, apnea, paralysis, and followed by agitation, confusion, and amnesia. When consciousness is regained, headache and psychoneurotic symptoms remain, similar to those encountered in post-concussion patients.

Respiratory arrest may complicate electrical injury. By this term we mean a sustained arrest of respiration persisting after the flow of the shock current has ceased. There is evidence that this effect is produced only if the current pathway includes the brainstem. Passage of current through the hemispheres alone does not produce persistent apnea. In fact, electroconvulsive therapy, in which a current of several hundred milliamperes is passed between the temples of a human patient for one or two seconds, rarely arrests respiration beyond the period of current flow.

Respiratory arrest may occur if a person in contact with a current source is unable to let go. This happens because the forearm muscles are put into sustained contraction by the flowing current, and, because of flexor muscle preponderance over extensors, the grip is tightened. If the current pathway includes the chest, and if the current is of sufficient magnitude, the chest muscles may be involved in this reaction, resulting in a complete arrest of breathing lasting for the duration of the current. If the current is maintained for several minutes, respiration may not start again spontaneously once the current has been discontinued.

Cardiac Arrest Syndrome

An electric current passing through the heart may produce ventricular fibrillation or asystole. The treatment for this syndrome is external cardiac massage (see below).

Resuscitation Of The Electrical Trauma Victim

The importance of considering the pathway taken through the body by an electrical current has been noted above. If the current pathway includes the brainstem, respiration can be arrested, and if it includes the heart, circulatory arrest can occur. Sometimes both respiration and circulation can be arrested. In these cases standard cardiac arrest procedures should be employed. However, no large series of resuscitated patients exists from which one can describe neurological outcome.

ANOXIC ENCEPHALOPATHY DUE TO DROWNING AND NEAR-DROWNING [9,11,12]

Drowning is one of the major causes of death in childhood, accounting for approximately 10 percent of accidental deaths. Young children, often under the age of 5 years, and usually male, are the major victims. The site of most near-drowning and drowning accidents in the United States is a home swimming pool. Therefore cases of freshwater drowning are more common than those in saltwater.

Dry Versus Wet Drownings

In approximately 10 to 15 percent of drowning cases water is not inhaled into the lungs because of the presence of severe laryngospasm. Death by asphyxia in such cases of "dry drowning" is due to upper airway obstruction. In 85 to 90 percent of drowning accidents, however, water is present in the victim's pulmonary alveoli and can cause persistent hypoxemia and a progressive decline in pulmonary function following resuscitation.

Freshwater Versus Saltwater Drowning

Freshwater Drowning

Death from drowning in freshwater results from acute asphyxia complicated by the inhalation of water. Freshwater is hypotonic to blood and therefore passes from the pulmonary alveoli into the pulmonary capillaries. The movement of fluid from the lungs to the circulation causes surfactant to be washed out of the lung. Loss of surfactant results in decreased lung compliance or "stiff lung". Anoxia, hypercapnia, and acidosis result. In addition, aspiration of fluids, debris, and bacteria can result in bronchospasm, laryngospasm, bacterial pneumonitis, pulmonary edema, and hypoxemia-induced respiratory distress syndrome. Pneumothorax and pneumomediastinum can occur as complications of resuscitation efforts.

The systemic complications of freshwater drowning include hypervolemia, hemolysis, hemodilution, hyponatremia, and hypoproteinemia. Cardiac arrest or arrhythmia is a common terminal event.

Saltwater Drowning

Inhaled saltwater is highly irritating to the alveolar membrane because of its hypertonicity. As a result of damage to pulmonary capillaries, pulmonary edema and hemorrhage develop. In addition to its irritating effect, the hypertonic solution induces a transudate from the plasma into the alveoli further increasing the pulmonary edema. If a large amount of fluid leaves the vascular space, the victim may develop hemoconcentration, hypotension, and finally hypovolemic shock.

Clinical Features Of Near-Drowning In Salt Or Freshwater

Near-drowning victims have a similar clinical picture regardless of whether immersion took place in fresh or saltwater. Pulmonary edema, in some series, has occurred with equal frequency in seawater and poolwater near-drownings. Electrolyte problems tend to be mild because only small amounts of seawater and freshwater enter the circulation. Acute tubular necrosis and/or myoglobinemia have been associated with oliguria. Hemolysis has been observed in freshwater near-drownings but not in those in seawater.

Hypoxia is the primary problem in near-drowning. The central nervous system (CNS) damage in near-drowning is caused primarily by hypoxemia and ischemia before rescue and resuscitation. However, further CNS insult occurs after resuscitation, due to persisting pulmonary dysfunction.

Treatment And Prognosis

There is evidence that survival is higher after immersion in seawater than after freshwater near-drowning, provided the water is not extremely cold. Nevertheless whether or not a resuscitated person will suffer brain damage is crucial to the management of drowning and near-drowning victims.

Several studies by pediatricians have found that the neurologic outlook for the post-immersion child is very good. The combined data indicate that any child who survives a serious near-drowning incident (that is regains spontaneous respirations after on-site cardiopulmonary resuscitation, CPR) has better than a 90 percent chance of being neurologically normal. The prognosis for children who are still apneic, with or without a spontaneous pulse, when they reach an intensive care unit is different. A California series noted that every near-drowning patient still requiring CPR in the emergency room developed permanent brain damage. A study from Florida reported that children who were conscious on admission survived; by contrast, all comatose children with unreactive pupils died.

Failure to resume spontaneous breathing following rescue site resuscitation, provided body temperature has not been lowered significantly, is at present the only reliable guide to a poor outcome (death or brain damage) following near-drowning. Additional studies are required to define prognosis accurately and to identify prognostic indicants. Regardless of estimates of prognosis, it seems justified to begin intensive hospital-based life support on all near-drowning victims and to maintain such efforts until they are rendered unnecessary by either recovery or death (brain or systemic).

TREATMENT OF ACUTE BRAIN ANOXIA

Cardiopulmonary Resuscitation

Closed chest compression for cardiopulmonary resuscitation (CPR) is an effective therapeutic modality in the management of sudden cardiac arrest. Many patients who previously would have died of acute brain anoxic ischemia before reaching the hospital now survive because of CPR initiated by bystanders or paramedics. Unfortunately many who survive do not recover consciousness. In some cases CPR may not have generated a flow of blood sufficient to maintain the viability of the brain. The search for more effective methods of CPR has led to new insights into the basic physiology of closed chest massage.

Traditional CPR Explanation

CPR produces blood flow by direct cardiac compression, that is, the heart acts as a pump.

The current explanation for the therapeutic efficacy of CPR is that closed chest massage compresses the heart between the sternum and the backbone. During compression, it is thought, the mitral valve closes and sternal pressure transmitted to the left ventricle ejects blood into the aorta.

Recent observations do not support this traditional explanation and indicate that cardiac compression is not the sole or even the most frequent mechanism for forward blood flow during CPR.[17] For example, in the presence of a flail chest caused by multiple rib fractures, sternal compression leads to direct cardiac compression and CPR should be maximally effective. Yet under such "ideal" circumstances CPR has failed to generate an effective peripheral blood pressure. Furthermore during cardiac arrest in man, two-dimensional echocardiographic studies have shown first, that the mitral valve remains open and incompetent during sternal compression, and second, that the pulmonary artery and the atria, rather than the ventricles, are compressed.[21] These observations in arrested human hearts during CPR challenge the compression mechanism of CPR.

New Explanation

The lung is a blood reservoir from which blood is expressed through a passive heart during CPR.[2]

From these clinical observations and experimental results, many cardiologists have concluded that an increase in intrathoracic pressure, not direct cardiac compression, is the most important factor in CPR. According to this model, blood is squeezed during chest compression from the pulmonary circulation through the left heart and into the systemic circulation. Therefore a number of maneuvers (chest compression, cough, positive pressure ventilation, abdominal binding, and Valsalva's maneuver) will produce a rise in intrathoracic pressure and maintain peripheral blood flow.

Throughout the period of CPR, according to this model, cyclic rises and falls in intrathoracic pressure lead to peripheral blood flow. In order for peripheral blood flow to occur there must be an intrathoracic reservoir from which blood emanates. Studies indicate that the lungs are the thoracic reservoir from which blood flows through the left heart, which is a passive conduit, and then into the peripheral arterial bed.

Blood returns to the lungs from the periphery when the elevated intrathoracic pressure falls below the extrathoracic venous pressure between compressions. Extrathoracic venous pressure is high because of forward flow from the arteries to extrathoracic veins. With the fall in intrathoracic pressure, blood flows from these high pressure veins into the now low pressure central veins, right heart, and pulmonary circulation. The fall in intrathoracic pressure also may be accompanied by retrograde arterial flow. During cyclical periods of low intrathoracic pressure, the right heart serves as a passive conduit for the movement of blood from the veins into the lung's vascular bed.

Knowledge of the mechanisms described above suggests ways to optimize peripheral blood flow during CPR. For example, it is known that repetitive coughing can maintain consciousness in patients with ventricular fibrillation. Therefore one method to maintain brain perfusion during a witnessed cardiac arrest is to utilize voluntary coughing as long as the patient is conscious.

Abdominal binding or compression during CPR can increase peripheral blood flow by augmenting the increase in intrathoracic pressure from chest compression. Intrathoracic pressure also can be increased by using simultaneous mechanical ventilation to augment positive intrathoracic pressure during chest compression and to produce negative intrathoracic pressure during the period of relaxation.

The results of initial animal experiments using the new CPR are encouraging. In dogs, brain blood flow was 3 to 4 times greater during new CPR (simultaneous chest compression and ventilation, with abdominal binding) than during conventional CPR. At best cerebral blood flow still was less than 40 percent of normal control values (normal, spontaneously beating heart). During CPR, flow to the heart and kidneys was very low for both conventional and new CPR, suggesting that there was almost no perfusion of organs within the compressed thoraco-abdominal cavity.

At the present time, the new CPR cannot be recommended for clinical use. Clinical trials are needed to establish the efficacy and define the risk-benefit characteristics of experimental CPR. Nevertheless it is certain that in whole or in part these new approaches will find clinical application in the area of cardiopulmonary resuscitation. One hopes that the result will be a reduction in the number of brain damaged survivors of ischemic anoxia.

Attempts To Modify Ischemic Anoxic Brain Damage Post-Resuscitation

> ***PRINCIPLE 1:*** Prevent further anoxia by treating extracranial complications.[18]

The clinical management of patients in coma following cardiac arrest involves the prevention of further anoxia. Adequate cerebral circulation should be restored immediately by the elimination of both hypotension and severe hypertension. If either medullary depression or injury to the chest wall prevents adequate ventilation a mechanical ventilator must be employed. Controlled ventilation via endotracheal tube should maintain arterial PO_2 > 100 mmHg, arterial PCO_2 at 25–35 mmHg, and arterial pH between 7.3 and 7.6. Prolonged controlled hyperventilation does not increase survival following brain anoxia. Acid-base and electrolyte abnormalities should be corrected and any seizures controlled. Seizures and or myoclonus occur in 20 to 30 percent of comatose post-arrest patients. Control of seizures is essential to minimize cerebral metabolic demands during the post-arrest state. Phenytoin, followed if necessary by phenobarbitol, is the drug of choice to maintain control of seizures. Diazepam may be administered intermittently to stop major motor seizures while "loading doses" of phenytoin or phenobarbitol are being administered.

Normothermia should be maintained. Hyperthermia increases cerebral metabolism and edema, and if it occurs, must be corrected by cooling and the use of appropriate drugs to prevent shivering and vasoconstriction.

Increased intracranial pressure (ICP) cannot be recognized reliably by clinical means without direct measurements by ventricular catheter or subdural balloon. Such monitoring is indicated in cases of coma following head injury or certain types of encephalopathy, but is used uncommonly in cardiac arrest cases.

Beyond basic measures to restore homeostasis, no other uniformly satisfactory methods of treatment have been implemented. Empirical attempts to reduce ICP and control the development of cerebral edema following ischemic anoxia have not been successful. The administration of corticosteroids and dehydrating agents and anesthetics, and the application of hypothermia and controlled hyperventilation, have not improved the prognosis of anoxic coma.

The beneficial effects of corticosteroids are best documented for brain tumors and least documented for ischemic stroke and trauma. In stroke and ischemic anoxia the extent of cerebral edema is approximately proportional to the amount of brain infarcted. Thus, if the amount of brain injury is negligible, the degree of brain swelling will be correspondingly small. By contrast, if virtually all of the hemispheral substance is infarcted, the resultant swelling may be great enough to cause herniation and death. In the latter instance, therapy aimed at reducing cerebral edema, even if effective, hardly can be expected to produce neurological recovery.

Primary Insult Versus Secondary Events In The Production Of Anoxic Brain Damage

It is probable that neuronal cell damage occurring after cardiac arrest is determined mainly by the severity of the ischemic anoxia before resuscitation.[19] Recent observations however suggest that the ultimate tissue damage may result at least in part from post ischemic events which add a secondary insult to the primary event.[14]

There now is evidence that the brain glucose concentration at the onset of cerebral ischemia may be one of a number of variables that affect the severity of ischemic brain damage.

> ***HYPOTHESIS:*** Anaerobic metabolism of glucose by hypoxic brain tissue leads to lactic acidosis and increased cell damage.

Several researchers observed that starved animals made a better recovery than fed animals following transient ischemic anoxia. It now is postulated that excessive anaerobic metabolism of glucose during ischemic anoxia produced a severe cerebral lactic acidosis that precipitated edema and cell deaths. These results seem to explain the paradoxical finding that experimental animals made a better recovery following complete, rather than severe incomplete, ischemia. A continued supply of glucose to severely hypoxic tissue may enhance tissue lactic acidosis and contribute to cell damage.

> ***HYPOTHESIS:*** The formation of noxious substances such as prostaglandins, free radicals, and other substances, may damage neurons.

During ischemia, energy depletion is associated with a marked rise in the tissue content of free fatty acids (FFA), including arachnidonic acid. Following recirculation FFA gradually returns to normal. The oxidative metabolism of arachidonic acid gives rise to the formation of prostaglandins and related substances. There is suggestive evidence that such events contribute to cell damage and that post-ischemic damage is ameliorated if fatty acid cyclooxygenase is inhibited by indomethacin.

In normal brain, CBF is closely coupled to cerebral metabolism ($CMRO_2$). The effects of transient ischemia on CBF and $CMRO_2$ or CMR glucose are complex. In humans, CBF and $CMRO_2$ are 50 percent of normal at 2–6 hours after cardiac arrest, and rise to near normal values by 60 hours. In such patients, $CMRO_2$ is more depressed than CBF. These results suggest that decreased metabolic activity may be only one of several factors affecting vascular tone. Release of vasoactive amines, formation of vasoactive products of arachidonic acid metabolism (see above), and disturbances of calcium ion homeostasis in cerebrovascular smooth muscle, may contribute to post-ischemic vasoconstriction.[15,16]

What remains is to determine the role of the above factors in the productions of ischemic neuronal damage and then to determine whether modification can improve the clinical outcome of cardiac arrest.

Additional Treatments Of Uncertain Value

Several therapies, singly or in combination, have been applied to post-cardiac arrest patients. Treatments include moderate hypertension, normovolemic hemodilution with plasma substitutes, and heparinization. Whether these agents improve brain reperfusion is uncertain, and their risk/benefit ratio has not been determined.

Barbiturates are among the most promising of post-anoxic therapeutic agents. Barbiturates are known to reduce cerebral metabolic rate, CBF, and edema formation, and to suppress seizure activity. Other possible mechanisms of barbiturate action that have not yet been proven include "scavenging" chemical free radicals evolved during ischemia, altering metabolic pathways from "energy" to "synthesis" tasks, and suppressing catecholamine induced hypermetabolism.

Thus far, barbiturates have only ameliorated focal, not global, ischemia. Barbiturates reduce ischemic anoxic brain damage only by depressing cellular activity and metabolic rate. Therefore they are effective only against incomplete focal ischemia, but not against the complete ischemia of cardiac arrest, when there is no metabolism.

At the present time barbiturate anesthesia appears to be justified only for protection against anticipated brain ischemia during neurosurgical procedures and to control ICP in cases of head injury or Reye's syndrome. At the present time, the administration of barbiturates in anesthestic doses is not without risk and the general use of these agents to treat resuscitated patients cannot be recommended.[18]

CONCLUSION

Brain damage after ischemic anoxia is mainly the result of the initial insult and partially of post-resuscitation events. The mainstay of present therapy is the restoration of circulatory, respiratory and metabolic homeostasis and the prevention of further anoxia. Several potentially useful pharmacologic therapies exist, but as yet, cannot be recommended for use outside controlled clinical studies.

ACKNOWLEDGEMENTS

Supported by contract NS-42328 and grant NS-03346 from the National Institute of Neurological and Communicative Disorders and Stroke, of the United States Public Health Service.

REFERENCES

1. Caronna, J.J.: Diagnosis, prognosis and treatment of hypoxic coma. p. 1. In Fahn, S., Davis, J.N., Rowland, L.P., eds.: Advances in Neurology. Vol 26. Raven Press, New York, 1979.
2. Chandra, N., Rudikoff, M., Weisfeldt, M.L.: Simultaneous chest compression and ventilation at high airway pressure during cardiopulmonary resuscitation. Lancet, 1:175, 1980.
3. Cohen, M.M.: Clinical aspects of cerebral anoxia. p. 39. In Vinken, P.J. and Bruyn, G.W., eds.: Handbook of Clinical Neurology. Vol 25. North Holland Publishing Co., Amsterdam, 1976.
4. Ginsberg, M.D.: Delayed neurological deterioration following hypoxia. p. 21. In Fahn, S., Davis, J.N., Rowland, L.P., eds.: Advances in Neurology, Vol. 26. Raven Press, New York, 1979.
5. Golde, R.H., Lee, W.R.: Death by lightning. Proc. IEE, 123:1163, 1976.
6. Jennett, W.B., Gleave, J., Wilson, P.: Brain death in three neurosurgical units. Brit. Med. J., 282:533, 1981.
7. Jennett, W.B., Plum, F.: The persistent vegetative state: a syndrome in search of a name. Lancet, 1:734, 1972.
8. Levy, D.E., Bates, D., Caronna, J.J. et. al.: Prognosis in non-traumatic coma. Ann. Int. Med., 94:293, 1981.
9. Modell, J.H.: Pathophysiology and Treatment of Drowning and Near-Drowning. Charles C. Thomas, Springfield, Ill., 1971.
10. Panse, F.: Electrical trauma. p. 683. In Vinken, P.J., Bruyn, G.W., eds.: Handbook of Clinical Neurology. Vol. 3. North Holland Publishing Co., Amsterdam, 1975.
11. Pearn, J.H., Bart, R.D., Yamaoka, R.: Neurologic sequelae after childhood near-drowning: a total population study from Hawaii. Pediatrics, 64:187, 1979.
12. Peterson, B.: Morbidity of childhood near-drowning. Pediatrics, 59:364, 1977.

13. Plum, F. and Posner, J.B.: The Diagnosis of Stupor and Coma. 3rd Ed. F.A. Davis Co., Philadelphia, 1980.
14. Pulsinelli, W.A., Brierley, J.B., Plum, F.: Temporal profile of neuronal damage in a model of transient forebrain ischemia. Ann. Neurol., 11:491, 1982.
15. Pulsinelli, W.A., Levy, D.E., Duffy, R.E.: Regional cerebral blood flow and glucose metabolism following transient forebrain ischemia. Ann. Neurol., 11:499, 1982.
16. Rehncrona, S., Siesjö, B.K.: Metabolic and physiologic changes in acute brain failure. p. 11. In Genvik, A., Safar, P., eds.: Brain Failure and Resuscitation. Churchill Livingstone, New York, 1981.
17. Rudikoff, M.T., Maughan, W.L., Effron, M., et. al.: Mechanisms of blood flow during cardiopulmonary resuscitation. Circulation, 61:345, 1980.
18. Safar, P.: Resuscitation after brain ischemia. p. 155. In Grenvik, A. Safar, P., eds.: Brain Failure and Resuscitation. Churchill Livingstone, New York, 1981.
19. Siesjö, B.K., Plum, F.: Pathophysiology of anoxic brain damage. p. 319. In Gaull, G.E., ed.: Biology of Brain Dysfunction. Vol. 1. Plenum, New York, 1972.
20. Silversides, J.: Effects of electrical shock on the nervous system. p. 940. In Sering, E.H., ed.: Injuries of the Brain and Spinal Cord. Springer, New York, 1974.
21. Werner, J.A., Greene, H.L., Janko, C., et. al.: Visualization of cardiac valve motion in man during external chest compression using two-dimensional echocardiography: implications regarding the mechanisms of blood flow. Circulation, 63:1417, 1981.

18

Evaluation and Management of Severe Headache

K.M.A. Welch, M.D.C.H.B., M.R.C.P.

INTRODUCTION

This subject is approached from the viewpoint of the physician meeting, for the first time, in the office or emergency room, a patient who presents with the acute onset of headache. The first procedure is, of course, diagnosis. The physician can only approach the diagnosis of acute headache with an intimate knowledge of the differential diagnosis of acute headache. With this in mind, a searching and precise history supported by physical examination can categorize the headache in the majority of cases. If this discipline is adopted, only in the minority of cases do the appropriate supporting laboratory examinations reveal an unconsidered diagnosis.

GENERAL APPROACH TO THE DIAGNOSIS OF EMERGENT HEADACHE

As with every emergent problem, the clinician must approach the patient who has the prime complaint of headache armed with knowledge and experience of the problem. Experience is a variable and cannot be obtained from reading books. Knowledge is based on learning and experience. What then does the general physician need to know about the problems of acute headache? Actually, only a limited portion of the copious literature contributed by authorities on the mechanism and management of headache will be of help to the general physician faced in an emergency setting with the problem of diagnosing the cause of acute headache. In this situation the general physician is likely to be more experienced than many authorities on the subject who practice for the most part in headache clinics attended by patients with chronic recurrent migraine or tension headache. Such experts are less frequently challenged with a differential diagnosis of life-threatening headache such as the general physician or internist often faces.

The information on the mechanisms of headache required by the emergency clinician is relatively brief and straight-forward. Firstly, Table 18.1 which lists the pain sensitive intracranial and extracranial structures, should be reviewed. Note that, for the most part, all pericranial structures are pain sensitive and that the pain sensitive intracranial structures are largely also extracerebral.

The nerve pathways involved are also relatively uncomplicated. Briefly, pain is appreciated via the three divisions of the trigeminal nerve (V), the glossopharyngeal nerve (IX), the vagus (X) and the upper three cervical nerves (C_{1-3}). Intracranial problems above the tentorium refer pain to the eye, forehead and temples because the pain sensitive intracranial structures in this compartment are supplied by branches of the first division of cranial nerve V. Conversely, pain from infratentorial problems is referred to the occipital and neck area, because structures in this compartment are supplied by IX, X and C_{1-3}. However, because of the descending sensory nucleus of V, infratentorial disturbances can cause pain to be referred to the frontal area and vice versa. The site of pain appreciation from pericranial structures is dependent on the anatomical site of the involved structure. Pain in structures of the anterior half of the cranium is sensed by the three divisions of V, and structures of the posterior half of the cranium by C_{1-3}.

At this time, many researchers are attempting to identify more precisely the neurotransmitter systems involved in the pain pathways of the head and neck. For example, recent papers have explored the distribution of peptidergic and serotonergic neurons to extracranial and intracranial struc-

Table 18.1 Headache

I. Pain sensitive intracranial structures
   A. Venous sinuses
   B. Cortical veins
   C. Circle of Willis
   D. Proximal anterior and middle cerebral arteries
   E. Dura of anterior and posterior fossa
   F. Cranial nerves V, IX, and X

II. Insensitive structures
   A. Bones
   B. Pia, arachnoid and dura
   C. Brain parenchyma
   D. Ependyma
   E. Choroid plexus

III. Sensitive extracranial structures
   A. Skin
   B. Muscles
   C. Orbit
   D. Mucus membranes of sinuses
   E. External and middle ear
   F. Teeth
   G. Arteries

tures. However, such information is not yet of critical significance to the diagnostician.

From the point of view of differential diagnosis, key points involving pain are:

1. Chemical, metabolic and mechanical (such as dilation of vessels or displacement of structures) stimuli will induce pain.

2. Supratentorial and infratentorial structures have a separate neurogenic supply which may aid in pain localization.

3. Referred pain is common so that, for example, a patient with cervical spondylosis may present with a frontal headache.

Probably the most important information needed by the diagnostician is a general knowledge of headache classification and a differential diagnosis of the headache types.[2,3,6] This information is summarized in Table 18.2. Lists of headache classification in textbooks on headache or neurology are

Table 18.2 Varieties of Headache

I. Non-vascular headache—intracranial origin
  A. Meningeal irritation
    1. Subarachnoid hemorrhage
    2. Meningitis
    3. Encephalitis
    4. Post-pneumoencephalographic reaction
  B. Displacement of intracranial structures
    1. Space-occupying lesions
      a. Tumor
      b. Hematoma
      c. Abscess
    2. Increased intracranial pressure
      a. Non-communicating hydrocephalus
      b. Communicating hydrocephalus
      c. Venous sinus thrombosis
      d. Raised venous pressure
      e. Cerebral edema
        I. Cerebral infarction
        II. Malignant hypertension
        III. Hypocalcemia
        IV. Adrenal corticosteroids
        V. Addison's disease
        VI. Benign intracranial hypertension
          A. Hormonal causes
          B. Hypervitaminosis A
      f. Acute pressor reactions
        I. Acute nephritis, pheochromocytoma
        II. Tyramine ingestion by patients taking MAO inhibitors
      g. Early morning headache of hypertension
    3. Reduced intracranial pressure
      a. Following lumbar puncture

(continued)

Table 18.2 (*continued*)

II. Non-vascular headache—extracranial origin
    A. Muscle contraction headache
        1. Secondary to other factors, as in eyestrain, imbalance of bite, cervical spondylosis
        2. Primary muscle overaction (tension headache)
        3. Neck and occipital pain from whiplash injury
        4. Muscle contraction (tension) headache of post-traumatic anxiety state
    B. Cranial nerve disorders
        1. Compression or inflammation of cranial nerves (e.g., postherpetic neuralgia)
        2. Trigeminal neuralgia
        3. Glossopharyngeal (and vagal) neuralgia—Treatment with carbamazepine
    C. Local cranial disorders
        1. Expanding lesion within cranial bone
        2. Inflammation of cranium of scalp
    D. Referred pain
        1. Eyes (e.g., increased intraocular pressure, inflammation)
        2. Ears, nose and throat, as in sinusitis, nasopharyngeal carcinoma
        3. Teeth (e.g., root abscess)
        4. Neck (e.g., cervical spondylosis)
        5. Tempero mandibular joint strain
III. Non-vascular headache—psychogenic
    A. Depressive, delusional, conversion or hypochondriacal state
IV. Vascular—non-migrainous
    A. Simple intracranial vasodilatation
        1. Toxic—hangover, infections, CO_2 poisoning
        2. Metabolic—hypoxia, hypoglycemia, hypercapnia
        3. Vasodilator drugs—histamine, nitrites
        4. Post-convulsive
    B. Cerebral ischemia
        1. Thrombo-embolism
        2. Transient ischemic attack
        3. Arteriovenous malformation (AVM)
        4. Dilation of intracranial aneurysm
    C. Post-traumatic headaches
V. Vascular—migrainous type
    A. Common migraine
    B. Complicated migraine
        1. Classical
        2. Hemiplegic
        3. Familial
        4. Vertebro-basilar
        5. Ophthalmoplegic
        6. Ophthalmic
        7. Meningeal
        8. Equivalents
    C. Cluster headache
VI. Incompletely classified
    A. Cough headache
    B. Orgasmic cephalalgia

---

as legion as the causes themselves. This classification does not presume to be an improvement over others but simply reflects the approach of this author to the diagnostic problem. Naturally, it reflects also certain prejudices that this author holds, namely, that common migraine and muscle contraction headaches are organic diseases, that it is important to differentiate vascular from non-vascular headaches as far as possible and that complicated migraine is a potentially serious disease whose diagnosis frequently overlaps with other cerebrovascular diseases whose serious import is more established. This author acknowledges the drawback that, in a number of the clinical conditions classified as vascular, the mechanism of the headache may not be precisely defined, although it is generally accepted that the vascular component is an important one. Also, the sub-division of headache into "vascular" or "non-vascular" does imply a certain faith that the description of the headache reflects the mechanism; but that is not always the case! The most obvious example is common migraine, which, although thought to be vascular in origin, may not have a throbbing pulsatile quality but may be experienced as a constant aching pain. However, in that case, there are often other historical features and examination findings that lead to a correct diagnosis.

The other departure of this classification from that generally accepted is the inclusion of classical migraine in the complicated migraine group. This is because classical migraine is complicated by a neurological deficit and because in practice there is frequently no sharp distinction between the prodrome and the headache phase. Furthermore, experience shows that classical migraine may be the presenting complex of symptoms and signs that indicate the presence of a number of structural lesions in the brain, particularly an arteriovenous malformation (AVM). Therefore, classical migraine should be designated as complicated if for no other reason than to alert the diagnostician to the potentially serious differential diagnosis of complicated migraine. To reiterate, classical migraine should not be treated with anything other than the utmost suspicion of an underlying structural cerebral lesion.

At first glance, the long lists in Table 18.2 look ominous. However, it is unnecessary to learn these lists parrot-fashion. The table should be used simply to increase awareness that headache can be associated with any number of clinical conditions and it may accordingly be the presenting complaint. This comes as no surprise, since headache is the most prevalent neurologic symptom associated with any disease. For the most part, many of the diagnoses listed will become obvious to the experienced general physician as the history and examination of the patient progresses. However, the diagnostic crunch comes when the clinician is faced solely with the historical features of the headache in the presence of a normal examination. This is a challenge to the diagnostician and can indeed provoke a good deal of anxiety. Nonetheless, it is also a situation which provides an exciting intellectual exercise, and at no time is the art of the clinical diagnostician more in evidence.

KEY QUESTIONS IN THE HISTORY

The key questions to be asked of the patient with the presenting complaint of headache are: "How long have you had it?"; "What do you think it is due to?"; "Where is it?"; and "What is it like?". The responses to these four questions alone can take the clinician a long way towards making a firm diagnosis. Therefore, let us separately analyse each one of these questions for their diagnostic significance in the order in which they are asked and see why they are preferably asked in such order.

How Long Have You Had The Headache?

The response to this question may tell you immediately whether: (1) the patient is suffering from a chronic headache of 25 years duration which has suddenly become worse (e.g., muscle contraction headache), or (2) whether the patient has a chronic paroxysmal headache (e.g., migraine) in attacks occuring weekly over the past 25 years, or (3) whether the patient has the headache for the first time.

This question can also provide information on the time of headache onset. For example, a headache of onset 5 to 6 weeks before the consultation, with increasing severity may imply raised intracranial pressure perhaps due to a neoplasm. Alternatively, the headache onset may have been a few hours prior to consultation and in the middle of the night. Awakening with headache usually indicates organicity and may occur in such conditions as cluster headache, migraine, hypertension or cerebral neoplasia. A question posed early in the interview which provides information on onset, duration and frequency of headache can in the emergency setting relieve the clinician's anxiety or increase alertness to the life threatening potential of the headache.

What Do You Think The Headache Is Due To?

This question can provide much immediate insight into the cause of the headache. For example, the response that it is in some way due to sexual intercourse because the headache came on during the act of making love will alert the physician to the possibility of subarachnoid hemorrhage. Conversely, the reply "It's because all those people at work are pointing their pencils at me," should immediately alert the physician to the possibility of a paranoid psychosis and headache of psychogenic or conversion origin.

To elicit the precipitating factors of the headache can be most valuable in directing the course of the rest of the interview. Key points following along this line of questioning include the possible precipitation of the headache by activity, straining, blood pressure increase and sudden head turning, all of which may indicate raised intracranial pressure. Any relation to stress, fatigue, concentration, social problems, excitement, hunger, attitude, chocolate and use of the contraceptive pill or estrogens may indicate a migrainous syndrome. A history of fever or the ingestion of exogenous toxins, caffeine, alcohol, tobacco and nitrates suggests headache of chemical, toxic or metabolic origin. The features of psychogenic headache will be discussed in later paragraphs.

To ask the patient what he thinks his headache is due to is to run the risk of a response such as, "That's what I'm paying you to tell me." Nevertheless, at the worst, opening oneself up for such embarassing retorts may produce great insight into the psychologic status of the patient.

Where Is The Headache?

In answer to this question, the clinician is also occasionally subjected to sarcastic retorts such as "Where do you think it is, in my knee?" This kind of response again will provide insight into the psychological make-up of the patient and attitude to the examining clinician. Such a response is not infrequent in patients with headache of non-serious nature. Alternatively, however, patients with psychogenic headache may describe their problem in excrutiating detail.

Serious organic headache due to mischievous events occuring infratentorially will most often be localized to the occipital region. The frontal region is usually involved if the problem is supratentorial. Remember however, that pain from infratentorial structures may be referred to frontal regions and vice versa. Structural lesions obstructing the CSF circulation in the infratentorial ventricular system also can produce frontal headache pain secondary to hydrocephalus of the lateral ventricles.

A hemicranial localization of the pain may suggest migraine and a severe pulsatile retro-orbital pain, either an ophthalmic artery aneurysm or cluster headache. Chronic pain experienced over the vertex or in a hat band distribution around the head may suggest muscle contraction headache.

Other points to consider concerning the localization of the headache include: (1) Initially a unilateral headache is frequently on the same side as the lesion when due to a mass and ipsilateral or contralateral when vascular. (2) When headache presents unilaterally and progresses over time to become bilateral (usually bi-frontotemporal) this may be due to the effect of a mass and progressively increasing intracranial pressure. (3) Lesions that cause traction on the falx or midline structures may cause pain in one or the other eye. (4) Cerebellopontine angle tumors produce pain behind the ear and lesions involving the lateral sinus result in pain deep in the ear. (5) Carotid or middle cerebral artery occlusion may cause pain in the same side of the head or behind or above the eye, basilar occulsion at the back of the head or the forehead and unilateral vertebral occlusion may produce pain behind the ear.

What Is The Headache Like?

This question provides information on the character and severity of the headache. For the most part the severity of the headache is a subjective response and not overly helpful in diagnostic terms. Nevertheless, information on increasing or decreasing severity is most valuable.

The character of the headache is important. Headache of a throbbing, pulsatile nature is highly indicative of vascular origin. Sharp lancinating or ice pick-like pains may also be of vascular origin and when localized behind the eye for example, may suggest cluster headache. Similar sharp lancinating pain in the face however, may be indicative of trigeminal neuralgia thus demonstrating the importance of localizing the headache. A steady pain is less likely to be vascular in origin except, as explained earlier, in the case of the common migraine. A steady pain of increasing severity over weeks may indicate intracranial pressure elevation. Another characteristic feature of intracranial pressure is the bursting nature of headache enhanced by activities such as bending, stooping, coughing, defecation and sexual intercourse. A constant vice-like gripping pain or a dull pressure pain may indicate muscle contraction headache.

Associated Symptoms

After having completed these four major lines of questioning the diagnostician is now in the position to ask pertinent questions concerning symptoms that are specifically associated with each headache type to aid in the refinement of the diagnosis. Questioning should be directed broadly towards defining symptoms associated with the central nervous system pathology, systemic pathology or both.

Visual Symptomatology

Visual symptomatology is relatively frequent in migraine and may occur as a prodrome to the headache (e.g., scintillating phenomena, teichopsia, hemianopic field defect, scotoma, and photophobia). Rapid and progressive impairment of vision, particularly associated with a centrocaecal scotoma may be seen in association with headaches and papilledema due to a mass or raised intracranial pressure of other cause. Amaurosis fugax occurs in association with vascular headache due to extracranial cerebrovascular disease and persistent visual field defects are a serious complication in patients with temporal arteritis. Other visual symptoms of potentially serious significance include diplopia (particularly when it is persistent). The elicitation of visual symptoms is of key importance in the differential diagnosis of acute headache.

Vomiting

Vomiting is a potentially serious symptom and when witnessed is usually most helpful in confirming organicity. Vomiting frequently accompanies a severe migraine headache and if it alleviates the headache can be a diagnostic feature of this condition. On the other hand, projectile vomiting associated with headache may indicate raised intracranial pressure. In the above instances, vomiting is related to central nervous system abnormality, but equally it can be a symptom of those systemic conditions likely to be associated with headache, such as fever, toxic influences, allergic reactions, sun stroke, etc.

Motor and Sensory Symptoms

When associated with headache, symptoms of motor or sensory disturbance (the former including paresis, paralysis or ataxia) may indicate structural lesions and should always be regarded as of serious import. The duration, severity and frequency of these symptoms should be established. A paroxysmal occurrence of such symptoms usually indicates that the associated headache is vascular in origin (see Complicated Migraine below).

Head and Neck Structures

Direct questions should be asked about soreness, tenderness and stiffness of the head and neck structures. The vascular headache of temporal arteritis may be associated with soreness and tenderness over one temple. Local tenderness may be a symptom of sinusitis. Neck stiffness and soreness may be an early sign of meningeal irritation or rarely herniation of the cerebellar tonsils.

Occular Symptoms

Occular symptoms frequently associated with head pain include photophobia during migraine, lacrimation during cluster headache and acute red eye and headache in acute glaucoma.

Nasal Symptomatology

Nasal symptomatology includes the nasal stuffiness associated with vascular headache of migraine type, particularly cluster headache. A nasal drip also may be associated with cluster headache (secondary to lacrimation) or sinusitis.

Other Central Nervous System Symptomatology

Other central nervous system symptomatology such as lack of energy, sleeplessness, dizziness, restlessness, lethargy, anxiety and episodes of hyperventilation, although important to elicit, are less helpful in defining the diagnosis. A history of impaired consciousness usually portends a headache of serious nature.

The symptoms associated with systemic causes of headache are wide reaching in scope and therefore any interview should include a searching inquiry into all of the systems. In particular any question of exposure to infections or presence of fever is important.

PAST AND FAMILY HISTORY

The past medical history is frequently helpful. The patient may have had frequent visits to emergency rooms with the same headache complaint or may even be a familiar customer in your own emergency room. In these cases, a life-threatening cause of headache is improbable and a diagnosis of migraine, muscle contraction or psychogenic headache will become more likely. In these same cases, there may be a history of numerous hospitalizations and repeated neurological evaluations which have resulted in an undefined cause for the complaint. These same patients may be on long term prophylactic medications for headache. All too frequently, they may present with headache in the expectation of a narcotic shot based on expectations from previous hospitalizations.

Nevertheless, serious organic causes for headache may be revealed by past history. For example, a patient with new onset of headache suggesting raised intracranial pressure may have had a previous craniotomy with removal of a meningioma and now most likely has a recurrence of the tumor. The importance of extensive questioning into the past history is obvious.

The family history is probably of the greatest significance in the diagnosis of migraine. A family history is positive in 60 percent of cases, usually in the parent. In familial hemiplegic migraine, history of headache and identical neurological deficit may be obtained in members of the same family.

KEY POINTS IN THE GENERAL CLINICAL EXAM

The importance of painstaking history cannot be overstressed because frequently at the end of the clinical exam the physician is left solely with the historical features to make the diagnosis of headache. This also means that in a number of instances (e.g., migraine, muscle contraction headache) the diagnosis can be made prior to the exam. There is a strong tendency, therefore, to curtail the examination. This should be resisted at all costs. A negative examination is as important to the diagnosis of migraine as is a positive exam to the diagnosis of neoplasm. Actually, there are always positive findings to be made in the examination of a patient with headache, even if only the response of the patients to their pain.

Behavioral Reaction

The behavioral reaction of the patient to the pain will be observed by the clinician even before taking the history. A record of this response is important in view of the subjective nature of pain but is complicated by differences in pain threshold between individuals. A patient who complains of severe headache yet is sitting up brightly discussing it usually has a less serious reason for the pain than the patient in a darkened room who is motionless or vomiting. Patients with real pain but with an over-reaction to their pain are likely to brighten up with increasing response to the clinician's questions during examination. The behavioral response to severe pain can prove a major interference in obtaining a history and performing an examination, thus causing great concern to the clinician because this very factor accentuates the need for careful and rapid diagnosis. One further tip concerning the behavioral response to pain is that although most patients with head pain usually lie still, patients who have meningeal irritation, either due to subarachnoid hemorrhage or infection, consistently exhibit extreme restlessness, the bedclothes being found awry with the patient sprawled across the bed.

The General Habitus

The general habitus of the patient can frequently indicate a degree of social and economic deprivation. The clinician might find it useful to consider that patients emerging from sections of the community where such deprivation is significant are less likely to afford themselves the luxury and cost of a physician consultation for headache of minor nature. Obviously other features of habitus may become of record. For example, if the appearance suggests participation in a brawl, then head trauma could be the cause of headache.

Appropriate and thorough examination of the head and neck may reveal a cause for headache due to abnormality of pericranial structures. Key structures likely to be involved in the differential diagnosis of headache are the tempromandibular joint, sinuses, teeth and muscles of the head and neck. Trapezius muscle spasm may be either a direct cause of head pain or secondary to intracranial mischief. Nuchal rigidity should always be tested for.

Arteries

Never fail to examine the arterial pulses of the head and neck and particularly that of the temporal arteries in the elderly. Tenderness of the extracranial arteries is the hallmark of arteritis in the case of the temporal artery or carotidynia in the case of the internal carotid.

Acute Red Eye

The examiner should be satisfied that no acute red eye exists, particularly since acute glaucoma may present with headache and be a cause of rapidly progressive blindness (see Chapter 14).

Lymph Nodes

The presence of enlarged tender lymph nodes on examination of the head and neck occasionally may be relevant to the presenting symptom of headache. Such finding in the region of the occipital canal can be associated with severe ipsilateral hemicranial pain of vascular or lancinating type. This pain is probably caused by entrapment of the occipital nerve as it passes, together with the occipital artery, through the occipital canal. Enlargement of lymph nodes in this canal may compress the occipital nerve and produce a pulsatile headache. Infection in the bone or scalp causing localized headache is usually accompanied by enlargement of regional nodes. Remember to look for tubercular nodes (Scrofula) when dealing with a case of painful ophthalmoplegia or Tolosa-Hunt syndrome.

External Acoustic Meatus

Blood in the *external acoustic meatus* may indicate an intracranial hematoma secondary to head injury. While examining the ear also ascertain that there are no signs of infection or the cholesteatoma which, although rarely, may erode into the intracranial cavity. In a patient with trauma do not miss the boggy mass in the region of the temporalis muscle under which lurks a ruptured middle meningeal artery and an intracranial, extradural hematoma! Be sure that the fluid leaking from the nose is related to lacrimation and not to a CSF leak!

Always listen with a stethescope for the bruit of atherosclerotic origin in the extracranial arteries, as well as over the eyes for the bruit of a cavernous sinus fistula and over the head for the bruit of an arteriovenous malformation.

Dermatological Exam

A dermatological exam sometimes may be helpful in the diagnosis of headache. Look in particular for rashes on the head and neck, such as herpes zoster or simplex. Remember also, that the skin of patients with migraine may be pale, cold and clammy in a hemifacial distribution. This is thought to result from the shunting of blood from the skin to the deep vasculature. The dermatological exam has to extend to a search for puncture sites for narcotic injection. Body rashes in general may indicate a systemic disease causing the headache.

Temperature

An elevated temperature may indicate a systemic cause for headache, but note that patients with acute migraine may have a temperature elevation on rare occasions.

Blood Pressure

The measurement of blood pressure is vital to the differential diagnosis of headache and should be recorded from both arms as well as erect and supine since postural hypotension may produce a characteristic low pressure headache.

Otherwise, a general exam of the chest, cardiovascular system and abdomen should be performed with a view to identifying systemic diseases, many of which have headache as a part of the presenting symptomatology.

KEY POINTS IN THE NEUROLOGICAL EXAM

A complete neurological exam is important, particularly when the history suggests involvement of the central nervous system and particularly if full examination of other systems has been unrevealing. Only the key points of the examination will be emphasized.

Higher Cortical Functions And Conscious State

The assessment of the higher cortical functions and conscious state is essential. The presence of confusion or depression of consciousness indicates a high probability of a serious neurologic lesion.

Fundoscopic Exam

Fundoscopic exam should never be passed over in the patient with acute headache. Time should be taken to ensure that the optic disc is clearly seen. Never dilate the pupils to do this, because in so doing, the important sign of unilateral pupillary dilation consequent upon brain herniation may be missed.

Visual Fields

Check the visual fields closely. Remember that a bitemporal field deficit in a patient with severe fronto-temporal headache can be caused by an expanding pituitary adenoma. Scotomas or hemianopic field defect may indicate less common causes of headache, such as a brain tumor or AVM.

Ophthalmoplegia

Ophthalmoplegia should always be treated with gravity, although in the long run it may prove due to complicated migraine. Unilateral third nerve palsies and unilateral or bilateral sixth nerve palsies are frequently related to aneurysms of the cerebral vasculature or raised intracranial pressure and brain herniation (see Chapters 4 and 14). Unilateral ophthalmoplegia plus sensory loss in the first division of the fifth cranial nerve in association with unilateral retroorbital headache may be due to a superior orbital fissure syndrome, painful ophthalmoplegia or Tolosa-Hunt syndrome. Miosis together with excessive sweating may indicate post-traumatic dysautonomic cephalalgia.[9]

As symptoms and signs emerge that indicate structural lesions within the central nervous system, further neurological exam should be intensified to localize lesions and identify a cause.

DIFFERENTIAL DIAGNOSIS

When the history and the physical examination are complete, the clinician is left with three broad diagnostic categories into which the headache may fall:

1. Headache with symptoms and signs of a systemic disorder;

2. Headache with symptoms and signs of a CNS disorder;

3. Headache alone.

Headache With Symptoms And Signs Of A Systemic Disorder

In this first category, the cause of headache can frequently be found on the basis of clinical examination and can be supported by appropriate clinico-pathological investigation. The varieties of headache in this category include non-vascular headache of intracranial origin produced by such systemic conditions as acute pressor reactions. Also, extracranial non-vascular headache (e.g., sinusitis and temporo-mandibular joint problems) and non-migrainous vascular headache (e.g., simple intracranial vasodilation secondary to toxic or metabolic factors). The diagnoses are listed in greater length in Table 18.2.

Headache With Symptoms And Signs Of CNS Disorder

The category of patients with headache and associated neurological deficit can be placed in three broad diagnostic subcategories, intracranial non-vascular headache and non-migrainous vascular headache and vascular headache of migrainous type. The diagnostic conditions in the first two categories include some of the potentially more serious and life-threatening causes of headache as well as some of the most challenging diagnoses in terms of differentiation from the vascular headache associated with complicated migraine. In view of this, some time will be spent in reviewing the problem.

Complicated Migraine

The syndrome of migraine has a number of dramatic symptoms and signs which make the term complicated migraine well-earned. These include field defects, ophthalmoplegia, hemiplegia, dysphasia, ataxia and meningeal signs, among others. The major diagnostic concern surrounding this pattern of symptoms and signs is the relationship between complicated migraine and structural lesions of the cranial vasculature and brain. Another major clinical concern in complicated migraine, which complicates diagnosis, is the occasional irreversibility of neuronal function, presumably secondary to severe ischemia. Uncommonly, frequent attacks of severe and complicated migraine can lead to cumulative neurological deficit possibly caused by repeated episodes of cerebral ischemia and infarction. Evidence for this can be found in clinical, angiographic, biochemical, blood flow and CT studies.[11]

Descriptions of complicated migraine have been in the literature since the mid 19th century. Two articles of note are listed in the references.[1,5] In the view of this author, the classification of complicated migraine includes all episodes termed migraine headache which have associated neurological deficit. The syndrome incorporates classical migraine because experience shows that the neurological complications of the classic prodrome frequently continue into the headache phase and even for a period of time after the headache has subsided. A list of the varieties of complicated migraine is included in Table 18.2. The major category of headache to be considered in the differential diagnosis is that of the vascular non-migrainous type. Non-migraine conditions causing this type of headache are listed in Table 18.3.

Classical Migraine

The clinical description of classical migraine may encompass symptoms and signs of hemiplegic, basilar, meningeal, ophthalmic or retinal origin, presenting as a prodrome and followed by headache, usually hemicranial in distribution.

Table 18.3 Non-migraine Causes of Symptoms and Signs Mimicking a Complicated Migraine Headache

I. Vascular causes
   A. Arteriovenous malformation
   B. Cerebral infarction or hemorrhage
   C. Transient ischemic attack
   D. Expanding cerebral aneurysm
   E. Subarachnoid hemorrhage

II. Non-vascular causes
   A. Tumor of brain or pituitary
   B. Cavernous sinus inflammation
   C. Brain abscess

Hemiplegic Migraine

The syndrome of hemiplegic migraine includes both motor and sensory symptoms occurring in a unilateral distribution as part of an attack of migraine. Approximately 50 percent of patients will also suffer from dysphasia. Tables 18.4 and 18.5 are modified from the paper by Bradshaw and Parsons and describe the distribution, frequency and duration of symptoms in hemiplegic migraine. From even a brief perusal of these tables one can see how difficult complicated migraine can be to differentiate from conditions such as occlusive cerebral vascular disease. One of the factors that can be helpful is the number of neurological episodes that the patient has suffered prior to assessment. In 46 percent of migraine patients, multiple attacks will have occurred and in 37 percent, 2–6 attacks. In only 17 percent of cases, will patients be seen for the first time with a single attack. Therefore, a history of prior events is important in the differential diagnosis.

In hemiplegic migraine the weakness usually occurs on the same side in each attack, lasts hours or days and can outlast the headache. In some cases the conscious state is impaired. Uncommonly, hemiplegic migraine

Table 18.4 The Distribution of Symptoms in Complicated Migraine

	Per Cent	Per Cent
Headache		100
Generalized	29	
Contralateral	47	
Homolateral	22	
Inconspicuous	2	
Paraesthesiae		100
Hand, face and leg	39	
Hand and face	36	
Hand and leg	12	
Hand only	13	
Speech disturbance		47
Dysphasia	44	
Dysarthria	3	
Impaired consciousness		23
Syncope	12	
Diminished awareness	8	
Stupor	3	
Visual disturbance		88
Teichopsia	54	
Hemianopia	39	
Diplopia	12	
Blindness	6	
Central scotoma	6	

(from Bradshaw, P., Parsons, M.: Hemiplegic migraine, a clinical study. Quart. J. Med., 34:65, 1965; reprinted with permission.)

Table 18.5 The Duration of Limb Symptoms in the Average Attack of Complicated Migraine

Duration	Per Cent
< 1 hour	58
1–3 hours	14
3–24 hours	12
1–14 days	16

(from Bradshaw, P., Parsons, M.: Hemiplegic migraine, a clinical study. Quart. J. Med., 34:65, 1965; reprinted with permission.)

exists in families. The hemiplegic migraine frequently occurs on the same side in each family member.

The major differential diagnoses in cases of classical and hemiplegic migraine includes arteriovenous malformations, transient ischemic attacks and neoplasia. Subarachnoid hemorrhage with vasospasm is also, though rarely, a consideration. The most likely structural lesion presenting as classical or hemiplegic migraine in younger age groups is, in the experience of this author, an arteriovenous malformation. Although attacks are usually stereotyped as to the side of hemicrania and distribution of neurological deficit, this cannot be relied upon because an arteriovenous malformation can steal blood flow from either cerebral hemisphere.

There are some pointers to the differential diagnosis of hemiplegic migraine which can be summarized at this stage. The diagnosis is more likely to be complicated migraine, (1) when the patient is comparatively young, (2) when the patient is female, (3) if there have been previous episodes, (4) if there is a familial history, and (5) if there is a relation to humoral factors such as menses, contraceptive pill use or estrogen therapy.

Basilar Artery Migraine

Basilar artery migraine occurs mainly in young people, particularly adolescent girls. The symptoms are vertigo, double vision, teichopsia, visual field defects, bilateral paresthesiae, dysarthria and ataxia. The most common symptoms are bilateral visual scintillating phenomena and bilateral numbness and dysesthesiae of the mouth, tongue and hands. Headache and vomiting are frequent occurrences. Rarely basilar migraine may be associated with loss of consciousness.

The major differential diagnosis of this condition is, of course, a transient ischemic attack in the vertebro-basilar circulation. The age of presentation is usually the most helpful feature, but when, as sometimes occurs, basilar migraine presents for the first time around middle age, the differential diagnosis can be a major dilemma and can be resolved only by intensive evaluation of the patient, frequently with limited confidence in the conclusions.

Ophthalmoplegic Migraine

An attack of migraine headache can be accompanied by third, fourth or sixth cranial nerve paresis, either as a prodrome or during the headache phase. In 80 percent of cases the ocular palsy involves the third nerve, in 12 percent the sixth. The ophthalmoplegia is at first transient but after repeated episodes can become permanent. The mechanisms involved in the production of ophthalmoplegic migraine remain speculative. To account for the third nerve paresis, it has been suggested that the occulomotor nerve becomes compressed between edematous and engorged posterior cerebral and superior cerebellar arteries.

The major differential diagnosis is aneurysmal dilation, either developmental or atherosclerotic, of the cerebral arteries, particularly the internal carotid artery or the posterior communicating artery. All cases should be promptly evaluated with spinal tap, CT scans and arteriography.

Ophthalmic Migraine

Although the familiar prodrome of homonymous hemianopia, flashing lights, zig-zags, color spectra, teichopsia and spreading scotoma are considered occipital in origin, visual field defects can be produced by retinal changes. This is extremely rare but field defects that present during migraine occasionally become permanent. The differential diagnosis includes extracranial cerebral vascular disease. Rarely occipital tumors may masquerade in this fashion.

Migraine Equivalents or Variants

All forms of neurological deficit described in association with the headache phase of migraine may be seen in the absence of the headache. This is usually regarded as a migraine equivalent or migraine variant. More rarely, epilepsy may cause a migraine-like neurological deficit, but the headache phase which normally would follow that prodrome is absent. Migraine equivalents are always a diagnostic dilemma, lessened somewhat when they occur in the young. All of the structural lesions mentioned above can present in this way.

In the opinion of this author, all patients presenting with neurological deficit associated with suspected migraine should be studied thoroughly. The performance of an EEG, CT scan with contrast infusion and, if indicated, digital subtraction angiography would now be the appropriate approach. Cerebral arteriography is rarely needed, and is a decision to be taken seriously during the acute phase of the migraine, in view of the possibility of accentuating vasospasm.

Headache Alone

Vascular Headache of Migraine Type

The majority of patients in the category of headache alone will suffer from vascular headache of migraine type. Hallmarks of this condition are found in the history. It is a paroxysmal headache, unilateral or bilateral in its cranial distribution, frequently being fronto-temporal or occipital, radiating to the frontal or retro-orbital regions. The headache may be pulsatile but it is often described as a continuous pain with a severe aching quality. Frequently there are superimposed icepick-like pains.[7] Associated symptoms of nausea, photophobia and hyperacusis aid in the diagnosis as does a history of past attacks occurring with neurological deficit. A strong family history will support the diagnosis. A diagnosis of headache can be supported by subtle findings on examination such as cooling of skin temperature, pallor of the skin and asymmetry of pulses in the extracranial arteries.

A major difficulty in the differential diagnosis of migraine is caused when it presents for the first time in older age groups. This author has found it a good rule of thumb that, when a headache of this nature presents for the first time at age 40 and upwards, particularly in the elderly, the patient should be intensively investigated. A list of non-migraine causes of migraine-like headache is provided in Tables 18.3 and 18.6.

Muscle Contraction Headache

This category may also include patients who suffer from a severe exacerbation of muscle contraction headache. In these instances, stress may play an important role in initiating the attack. For example, Professor W.B. Mathews in his textbook describes the onset of severe head pain in a man who found in his wife's pocket a brand of cigarettes that neither of them smoked. This type of headache, frequently called psychogenic headache, raises the problem of differentiation from headache presenting as a conversion symptom (see below).

The features of muscle contraction headache are well known. The pain is usually situated in a hatband-like distribution, over the vertex or localized to the occipital area and neck area. Pain is described as a tight constricting

Table 18.6 Additional Causes of Migraine-like Headaches (See Table 18.3)

Acute glaucoma
Cranial (Temporal) arteritis
Acute sinusitis
Sphenoid sinus mucocele
Masseter muscle spasm due to dental malocclusion

chronic ache. Associated features on examination are variably present and include spasm or increased tension and tenderness of the muscles of the head and neck.

Organic Non-migrainous Headache

The most anxiety-provoking patients who present solely with headache are those with headache of organic origin which is non-vascular or vascular in character but non-migrainous. In these patients, the clinician must search obsessively for clinical features that imply serious intracranial mischief and are potentially life threatening (see Tables 18.3 and 18.6). When such a headache presents for the first time, particularly in old age groups, intensive investigation is in order.

Psychogenic Headache

The final type of headache that presents without signs or symptoms of systemic or CNS disorder is psychogenic headache. However, the term psychogenic is used inappropriately when it is meant to imply conversion headache. For example, muscle contraction headache which does involve organic pain mechanisms can be precipitated by psychological factors. Use of the term conversion headache is preferred. The condition can be defined best as a headache in which the clinical disorder is a conversion reaction in the absence of central or peripheral pain mechanisms. Conversion headache is one of the most difficult forms of headache to diagnose, indeed it is almost a diagnostic feature of this disorder that there is a delay in diagnosis.

Most cases have an abrupt onset with exacerbations and remissions. The sex incidence is nearly the same. It occurs predominantly in younger adults of age range 18 to 30 but can be observed in all ages. The character of conversion headache frequently cannot be differentiated from other types of headache. In addition, major abnormalities in the mental status are seldom found in patients with conversion reaction. Furthermore, laboratory, electrophysiological and radiological studies are normal. The usual duration of this problem is from months to years, but in the majority of cases, diagnosis is made within 1 year of its initial presentation. Another marker of the diagnosis is that the disorder is rarely relieved by medication.

Key points in history and examination that will aid in making this diagnosis are as follows: Firstly, it must be stressed that a thorough history is essential and this must include psychiatric history. The response to the question, "How long have you had the headache?" may reveal that the patient has seen several doctors, received multiple medications without symptomatic relief and currently is suffering an exacerbation of a headache problem that has been going on for a number of months.

When patients are asked to what they attribute their headache, they may have responses which reveal secondary gain. For example, they may state that it always occurs when they perform a particular job at their place of work, a job which on further questioning may be revealed as onerous. Thus, the headache complaint may be the patients' attempt to remove themselves from this adverse situation. The headache presentation may also be time-locked with emotional conflicts or precipitating social events such as the death of a close relative or friend. Remember, however, that in cases of conversion headache, the patients frequently deny any disturbing emotional relationships or conflicts in their life. Therefore, relatives or close friends should be questioned as to any disturbing psychological or social events in the patients' lives at the time of headache presentation.

Some patients may give an unusual account of the character of the head pain which does not resemble any of the usual headache syndromes. Patients may also identify the character of the headache with the headaches suffered by a person with whom there may be some unrevealed emotional conflict. Alternatively, patients may not be able to describe appropriate character-ological features of any type of headache. For example, although the pain may have a description similar to intracranial pressure headache, the patient may not be able to support this with other expected historical features (e.g., accentuation by bending, stooping, coughing, etc.).

The major abnormalities on exam will be of behavioral nature. The patients may have a total indifference to their symptomatology despite bitter complaints of pain. Also symptoms may be overdramatized, particularly when they are of an unusual description. There may be either extreme passivity or hostile denial when questions are asked about emotional problems. The psychiatric examination is rarely revealing of serious psychiatric disease but the personality profile may reveal an immature dependent person.

In the management of the patient with conversion headache, psychological testing, including the Minnesota Multiphasic Personality Inventory, can be done to confirm clinical impressions. Psychiatric intervention, particularly the employment of psychoanalytical or psychotherapeutic techniques may be successful in treating the complaint. This in itself points to conversion headache.

THERAPEUTIC MANAGEMENT

This section concentrates on the therapy of acute headache due to muscle contraction and migraine. The management of acute headache associated with other neurological diseases is discussed in other chapters as part of the management of the specific CNS disorders. The headache associated with the types of systemic disease that have been discussed in this chapter are usually best managed with simple analgesics and most importantly by treating the disease itself.

Muscle Contraction Headache

An acute exacerbation of muscle contraction headache is best treated by bed rest and complete relaxation. The identity of any precipitating factors should be noted during the interview and, if at all possible, these can be discussed with the patient and reassurance and psychological support provided.

Gentle massage of the head and neck area together with hot packs applied to these areas are physical maneuvers that may be helpful in alleviating some of the pain.

Only minor analgesics should be used in view of the risk of analgesic addiction in patients with chronic headache. However, if the patient has consistently used scheduled analgesics such as codeine, the pain of an acute exacerbation of severe muscle contraction headache may not respond to anything other than parenteral narcotics. Instead of pursuing this line of treatment, it is preferable to treat the patient with those tranquilizers which are also neuromuscular relaxants such as diazepam (Valium) and which may have the added beneficial effect of causing drowsiness and sleep. Other muscle relaxants such as carisoprodal are only occasionally effective in the acute exacerbation. The recent development of non-steroidal anti-inflammatory agents such as naproxene (Anaprox), ibuprofen (Motrin) and other has provided a useful alternative analgesic, effective in some patients. In the view of this author, Fiorinal, one of the most popular medications for muscle contraction headache, should not be used because of its barbiturate content and polypharmaceutical nature.

In terms of future management of the muscle contraction headache it is wise to make another appointment with the patient to discuss further therapy rather than discuss this during the headache, when most likely the patient will be unable to concentrate on the advice given.

Migraine

There are any number of therapeutic approaches recommended for the problem of acute migraine. Because of the variable effectiveness of therapy for the acute attack of migraine in the hands of different practitioners, and because the precise cause of migraine is unknown, no absolute drug indications can be recommended. The following therapeutic approach represents the preference of this author.

1. When patients with acute or complicated migraine are seen during the acute headache phase, metoclopramide (Reglan), 10 mg is given by slow IV push over a 2 to 5 minute period. This therapy has been accepted by some as the treatment of choice not only for combating the nausea and vomiting of migraine but for improving gastric motility and intestinal

absorption of analgesic.[10] One of the problems of treating migraine overcome by metoclopramide has been the delay in gastric emptying during the attack and therefore the consequent delay in absorption of oral analgesic. Metaclopramide tablets, 10 mg, can also be given by mouth but are less rapid and effective in action. Oral medication is, however, the treatment of choice for acute migraine attacks that are not attended by a physician.

The analgesic used with metaclopramide in this clinic is naproxene sodium (Anaprox) 275 mg tablets; two at the time of attack. This therapy is chosen because in the opinion of this author there is much evidence that suggests a role for prostaglandin involvement in the platelet dysfunction, cerebral hemodynamic response and genesis of pain in the migraine attack. There have been a number of studies using prostaglandin inhibitors which have proven to be effective during acute headache.[4,8] Aspirin 600 mg together with metaclopramide is an alternative popular in certain British clinics. (Wilkinson, M., Personal Communication)

2. If this form of therapy is ineffective, the ergot derivitives may be tried next. However, if the migraine attack is complicated by neurological deficit, in the opinion of this author, the ergot derivatives are contraindicated because of their potentially vasospastic effect. Dihydroergotamine, 1 mg, intramuscularly is the mode of choice. However, some authorities have safely and effectively given this dosage intravenously.[6] This treatment can be repeated every 8 hours but no more than three doses should be given. Patients occasionally have nausea and vomiting from the use of ergot. Metaclopramide is the antinauseant of choice for both the nausea and vomiting of migraine and ergot therapy. For those few patients in which metaclopramide is ineffective promethazine (Phenergan) suppositories, 25 mg every 8 hours is used as an alternative.

3. For those patients who have a severe and prolonged attack of migraine and who qualify for the description status migrainosus, hydrocortisone 100 mg IV *stat,* and then 6 or 8 hourly for 24 hours if needed, is often effective in breaking the headache cycle.

4. The use of intramuscular narcotics such as meperidine (Demerol) is an easy way out for the treatment of acute headache. The shot, called in to the emergency room for the migraineur with another severe attack is convenient and usually effective. However, this will build up an adverse behavioral pattern in the migraine patient and possibly lead to addiction. There are occasions when in the judgement of the clinician, the pain and distress of severe migraine is so great, the intramuscular narcotics are indicated. The oft-time quoted aphorism "Keep the needle out of the butt of the patient with migraine!" carries with it an element of rigid intolerance to the patient who is seriously afflicted with this disorder. However, there should only be exceptional use of this treatment in the

individual patient and only after examination by a physician who has considered it warranted.

These above therapies should be used in combination with supportive measures such as bed rest in a darkened, quiet, if possible, sound proof room. Some patients feel comfort from the application of cold compresses.

Complicated Migraine

This is the most difficult of the acute headaches to manage. The same therapeutic approach as described above for non-complicated migraine can be used with the exception of ergot derivatives. The question frequently arises, if the complicated features of the migraine are due to vasospasm, what is the place of cerebral vasodilators? Unfortunately, cerebral vasodilators may seriously intensify the headache. Furthermore, some authors believe that the neurological deficit associated with complicated migraine may be due to steal of blood flow from the intracranial to extracranial vasculature.[12] Cerebral vasodilators, particularly papaverine (Pavabid) which has a marked extracranial vasodilator influence, may enhance steal from the intracranial circulation and worsen both the neurological deficit and the extracranial headache. Nevertheless, although infrequently, the clinician can be faced with a migraine patient who has prolonged neurological deficit after the headache phase is resolved. Furthermore, there is evidence that severe and repeated episodes of complicated migraine can lead to permanent structural change in the brain. The therapeutic strategy for this type of case is a matter of great concern for which there is no definitive answer at this time.

REFERENCES

1. Bradshaw, P., Parsons, M.: Hemiplegic migraine, a clinical study. Quart. J. Med., 34:65, 1965.
2. Dalessio, D.J., ed.: Wolff's Headache and Other Head Pain. 4th Ed. Oxford U. Press, New York, 1980.
3. Friedman, A.P.: Headache. Ch. 13. In Baker, A.B., Baker, L.H., eds.: Clinical Neurology. Vol. 2. Harper & Row, Philadelphia, 1981.
4. Hakkarainen, H., Vapaatolo, H., Gothoni, G., et al.: Tolfenamic acid is as effective as ergotamine during migraine attacks. Lancet, 2:326, 1979.
5. Pearce, J., Ed.: Modern Topics in Migraine. William Heinemann Medical Books, London, 1975.
6. Raskin, N.H., Appenzeller, O.: Headache. W. B. Saunders, Philadelphia, 1980.
7. Raskin, N.H., Schwartz, R.K.: Icepick-like pain. Neurology, 30:203, 1980.
8. Vardi, Y., Rabey, I.M., Streifler, M., et al.: Migraine attacks: alleviation by an inhibitor of prostaglandin synthesis and action. Neurology, 26:447, 1976.

9. Vijayan, N., Dreyfus, P.M.: Post-traumatic dysautonomic cephalalgia. Arch. Neurol., 32:649, 1975.
10. Volans, G.N.: The effect of metoclopramide on the absorption of effervescent aspirin in migraine. Clin. Pharmacol., 2:57, 1975.
11. Welch, K.M.A., Chabi, E., Nell, J., et al.: Similarities in biochemical effects of cerebral ischemia in patients with cerebrovascular disease and migraine. In Greene, R., ed.: Current Concepts in Migraine Research. Raven Press, New York, 1978.
12. Welch, K.M.A., Spira, P.J., Knowles, L., et al.: Effects of prostaglandins on the internal and external carotid blood flow in the monkey. Neurology 24:705, 1974.

19

Early Diagnosis and Management of Acute Infections of the Nervous System

Larry E. Davis, M.D.
Russell D. Snyder, M.D.

INTRODUCTION

Patients with acute infections of the central nervous system (CNS), often present to the emergency room. These patients may have a diffuse infection of the membranes covering the brain (meningitis), a diffuse infection of the brain parenchyma (encephalitis) or localized infection of the brain parenchyma (brain abscess). Viruses and bacteria are the organisms most commonly responsible for these infections. The emergency room physician should be especially alert for CNS infections because these patients may not always present with the usual signs of an infection. They may lack a fever, signs of systemic illness, or elevated blood white cell count. Examination of the cerebrospinal fluid (CSF) is frequently the most helpful diagnostic test in CNS infections and the LP should be considered in the emergency room. However this test should not be performed indiscrimately. It will not help, and may be contraindicated, in patients with a brain abscess. The prompt recognition, diagnosis, and appropriate treatment of these infections is important since a delay in starting treatment may result in death or serious injury to the nervous system.

VIRAL MENINGITIS

> ***PRINCIPLE 1:*** The rapid onset of fever, headache, and stiff neck without other neurological signs or depressed mental status suggests viral meningitis or bacterial meningitis.

Viral meningitis occurs primarily in children and young adults. The illness usually begins with the abrupt onset of fever, headache, nuchal rigidity and occasional vomiting.[1,18] The patient may be irritable and drowsy but confusion or severe depression of consciousness is rare. Other systemic signs may be present depending upon the infecting virus. Mumps meningitis is frequently preceded by parotitis but not always. Coxsackie and echovirus meningitis may be accompanied by rashes, myalgias, diarrhea, or herpangina.

> **PRINCIPLE 2:** Most cases of viral meningitis occur during the summer and early fall.

Although several viruses can cause meningitis (Table 19.1), the majority of cases are due to enteroviruses (echovirus and coxsackie virus).[18] During the summer and early fall, epidemics of strains of enteroviruses commonly spread across the United States infecting children and adults. Over 90 percent of the infections are asymptomatic or result in mild gastroenteritis or an upper respiratory tract infection. In occasional patients viral meningitis also develops.

> **PRINCIPLE 3:** The CSF in viral meningitis has a lymphocytic pleocytosis and normal glucose.

The clinical diagnosis of viral meningitis is made on the basis of typical signs and symptoms plus a characteristic CSF. The lumbar CSF usually has a normal or slightly elevated opening pressure. The spinal fluid contains a moderate pleocytosis with 20–1,000 WBC/mm.[3] Characteristically these white cells are predominately lymphocytes (Table 19.2). Very early in the illness, however, polymorphonuclear neutrophils may transiently predominate.[24] The CSF protein level is normal or slightly elevated. The CSF glucose level is characteristically normal. Although occasional patients with proven viral meningitis (especially mumps) have had depressed CSF glucose levels, this finding should be cause for concern. Bacterial and fungal cultures of the CSF should be sterile.

Patients should not have signs or X-rays suggestive of a parameningeal

Table 19.1 Causes of Viral Meningitis

I. Common
  A. Echovirus
  B. Coxsackie virus
  C. Mumps
II. Uncommon
  A. Arboviruses such as Western equine and St. Louis
  B. Lymphocytic choriomeningitis
  C. Herpes simplex, type 2
  D. Poliovirus
  E. Adenovirus

Table 19.2 Spinal Fluid Profiles in CNS Infections*

	O.P. Pressure	White Blood Cells	Protein	Glucose	Bacterial Culture
Viral meningitis	N or sl↑	20–1,000 mainly lymphs	sl↑	N	Negative
Bacterial meningitis	↑	50–10,000 mainly PMNs	↑	↓	Positive
Brain abscess	↑	0–40 lymphs & PMNs	N	N	Negative
Viral encephalitis	sl↑	10–200 mainly lymphs	N or sl↑	N	Negative
Epidural abscess	N or sl↑	0–40 mainly lymphs	N or sl↑	N	Negative
Subdural empyema	↑	10–1,000 mainly PMNs	sl↑	N	Negative

*N = Normal
 sl = slight
 ↑ = increased
 ↓ = decreased

focus such as sinusitis, otitis media, or skull fractures. If these are present, the possibility of a subdural empyema or brain abscess should be considered.

To establish the specific etiology of viral meningitis, one must isolate a virus from the CSF or demonstrate a significant rise in serum antibody titers to a likely viral pathogen between the acute and convalescent sera. However, in practice it is seldom necessary to establish the specific viral cause.

> *PRINCIPLE 4:* The clinical course is usually benign.

The majority of patients completely recover within one to two weeks without hospitalization.[1] Occasional patients will require hospitalization because of severe vomiting, headache, or an atypical CSF. At times, it may be difficult to distinguish viral meningitis from bacterial meningitis particularly if the CSF contains a low glucose level or a predominance of polymorphonuclear neutrophils. In this situation it is prudent to hospitalize the patient and treat with broad spectrum antibiotics until the CSF and blood cultures are known to be sterile.

Most patients with viral meningitis are treated symptomatically with drugs aimed to reduce the headache, nausea, and vomiting.

BACTERIAL MENINGITIS IN CHILDREN AND ADULTS

Bacterial meningitis is a major problem in diagnosis and management for physicians providing emergency care. Delay in the diagnosis or institution of intensive therapy may result in permanent brain damage and even death.[25] Approximately 30 percent of cases have significant neurologic handicaps following recovery[22] and 5 to 10 percent die during the acute illness. Appropriate diagnosis and rapid institution of therapy improve the outlook in most cases. A high level of physician awareness of the clinical presentation of bacterial meningitis is imperative to achieve appropriate emergency management.

> **PRINCIPLE 1:** The classical signs and symptoms of acute bacterial meningitis are fever, headache, and stiff neck.

The onset of bacterial meningitis may be abrupt or develop over a few days. Initial manifestations include chills, malaise, fever, vomiting, and headache. These symptoms may remit briefly and then return with increased severity. Headache is characteristically severe, diffuse in nature, and may radiate down the neck and back. The infection often causes meningeal inflammation resulting in pain and rigidity in the cervical region (stiff neck or nuchal rigidity). Characteristically, the patient complains of pain and discomfort when the neck is flexed either passively or actively. Brudzinski's sign (flexion of the legs when the neck is flexed) and Kernig's sign (inability to extend the knee when the hip is flexed) are also frequently present. Meningeal signs are less reliable in meningitis during the first year of life. In the elderly, cervical osteoarthritis may be difficult to distinguish from the stiff neck of meningitis. Patients with arthritis usually have resistance to both neck flexion and lateral rotation while patients with meningitis mainly have resistance to neck flexion. As the infection progresses, the development of cortical inflammation and cerebral edema may cause irritability, lethargy, confusion, depressed consciousness, hypertonia, hypotonia, seizures, posturing, papilledema, sixth nerve palsies, and, in small children, a full fontanel. A skin rash may be present, especially if the patient has bacteremia. The rash is usually petechial or hemorrhagic with meningococcal infections, but similar rashes occur in other bacterial and viral diseases. Meningitis occurs more frequently in patients with a history of alcoholism or immunosuppression.

The differential diagnosis encountered in bacterial meningitis is presented in Table 19.3.

> **PRINCIPLE 2:** A febrile infant or child with a full fontanel or neurologic signs has bacterial meningitis until proven otherwise.

Bacterial meningitis occurring during the first year of life may not present with the classical signs and symptoms. In infants, the signs and symptoms of meningitis may be relatively non-specific. In fact, poor feeding may be the only initial manifestation. Fever may not be present. Often, infants are lethargic, irritable, and may have mild diarrhea. A bulging fontanel usually develops, but may not be an early manifestation. Seizures commonly

Table 19.3 Differential Diagnosis of Bacterial Meningitis

Viral meningitis
Encephalitis
Febrile seizure
Subdural hematoma or empyema
Subarachnoid hemorrhage
Septicemia
Brain abscess
Leukemia or carcinomatous meningitis
Pharyngeal abscess
Lead poisoning
"Viral" myositis
Toxic-metabolic encephalopathy
Reye's syndrome

occur. Likewise, throughout the first year of life, children may have only subtle signs. Headache and papilledema are rare signs in this group. In a child who has fever and seizures and who is not known to have febrile convulsions or epilepsy, strong consideration should be given to the diagnosis of meningitis. If there is any suggestion of neurologic involvement in a febrile child, a lumbar puncture is imperative. Children with idiopathic febrile seizures should have normal CSF.

PRINCIPLE 3: When bacterial meningitis is suspected, a lumbar puncture becomes an emergency measure.

The only definitive way to establish the diagnosis of bacterial meningitis is by examination and culture of the cerebrospinal fluid. Since delay in the diagnosis of bacterial meningitis has an adverse effect on outcome, a lumbar puncture should be performed immediately in the emergency room. The CSF should be examined and cultured immediately after withdrawal. Appropriate laboratory tests usually performed on the CSF are listed in Table 19.4. If the CSF pressure is not markedly elevated, 10–15 ml of fluid should be obtained in four consecutive tubes. Protein and glucose should be determined from the first tube, culture from the second, cell count from the third, with the fourth used for special tests or saved in a frozen state. The CSF findings in central nervous system infections are shown in Table 19.2. A CSF white cell count greater than 10 is very suggestive of disease of the central nervous system or meninges. Usually in bacterial meningitis the CSF glucose is below 35 mg/dL and is also less than 40 percent of a simultaneously obtained blood glucose. Confusion in interpretation of the CSF-blood glucose ratio may occur when intravenous glucose has been given to the patient. The blood glucose may not equilibrate with CSF for 2 hours or more, thus producing an artifactually low CSF to blood glucose ratio.

**Table 19.4 Laboratory Tests on CSF in Suspected
Bacterial Meningitis**

I. Essential tests
   A. Total and differential cell count
   B. Glucose
   C. Protein
   D. Gram stain of CSF sediment
   E. Bacterial culture of CSF sediment

II. May be indicated
   A. India ink preparation of CSF sediment
   B. Tuberculosis culture
   C. Fungus culture
   D. Countercurrent immunoelectrophoresis
   E. Latex agglutination for *H. influenzae*, etc.
   F. Limulus assay for Gram-negative endo-
      toxin
   G. Cryptococcus antigen
   H. Coccidioidomycosis antibody
   I. Viral culture
   J. VDRL

However, the absolute value of CSF glucose is usually below 35 mg/dL in bacterial meningitis even when serum levels are high.

The lumbar puncture should be performed even in the presence of suspected increased intracranial pressure if meningitis is strongly suspected. The risk of complication from a lumbar puncture in a patient with bacterial meningitis is small. If lateralizing signs such as a hemiparesis are present, the possibility of other diagnoses, such as a brain abscess should be considered. If a CT scan can be obtained quickly (i.e., in less than 30 minutes) it should be done first. However, if brain swelling is suspected and a CT cannot be done, emergency measures directed toward correcting intracranial pressure are indicated while the patient is being prepared for lumbar puncture. Mannitol, 0.5–1.5 gm/kg can be infused intravenously over a period of 20 minutes, followed by the cautious withdrawal of 2–5 cc of CSF (see Chapter 3).

Although most patients with bacterial meningitis have classical changes in their CSF, occasional patients may have one or more CSF parameters which vary from the rule. Prior treatment with antibiotics, a common occurrence in meningitis, may cause the CSF findings to be more nearly normal, but such prior treatment rarely produces CSF which is completely normal.

PRINCIPLE 4: Always obtain a blood culture.

Blood cultures drawn prior to the administration of antibiotics will grow bacteria in about 75 percent of the patients with bacterial meningitis. Commonly, sensitivities will become available on the blood isolate before the CSF isolate allowing for rapid adjustment of appropriate antibiotics. Occasionally, a blood culture will be positive when no organism is grown from the CSF.

> ***PRINCIPLE 5:*** Appropriate antibiotic therapy should be immediately instituted after all cultures have been obtained.

If the clinical picture and CSF suggest bacterial meningitis, immediate institution of antibiotic therapy is appropriate.[3] The type of antibiotic selected will depend on the results of the Gram stain, the most common organisms seen in that age group or patient population, and local experience with various bacterial sensitivities (Table 19.5). To be effective, the antibiotic must reach the CSF and central nervous system in sufficient concentrations to be bacteriocidal or inhibit bacterial growth. To accomplish this, the antibiotic must cross the blood-brain barrier. Therefore, agents should be preferentially selected which cross the blood-brain barrier (Table 19.6). Allergy to drugs must be ruled out before they are administered.

Antibiotic therapy should be divided into two phases. The first phase covers the period of treatment prior to identification of the organism and determination of sensitivities. During this phase, broad spectrum antibiotics, such as chloramphenicol and ampicillin, are frequently given. These drugs cross the blood-brain barrier well, especially when the meninges are inflamed. However, if the Gram stain or clinical situation suggests an unusual Gram-negative organism, the addition of new cephalosporins[5A,8] or an aminoglycoside such as gentamicin, should be considered.

In the second phase, after the organism has been isolated and antibiotic

Table 19.5 Likely Etiologic Agents in Various Settings as Causes of Bacterial Meningitis

Setting	Likely Etiologic Agent
Newborn	Gram negative bacilli (esp. *E. coli*) Group B streptococcus, *H. influenzae, S. pneumonia, S. aureus*
Childhood	*H. influenzae, S. pneumonia, N. meningitis*
Young adult	*N. meningitis, S. pneumonia*
Hyposplenism	*S. pneumonia, H. influenzae*
CSF rhinorrhea	*S. pneumonia*
Alcoholic	*S. pneumonia, L. monocytogenes* and uncommon organisms
Epidemic or cluster	*N. meningitis*
Endocarditis	*S. pneumonia* or *S. aureus*
Penetrating trauma and post-operative	*S. aureus,* Gram negative bacilli
Immunosuppressed	Gram negative bacilli, unusual bacteria and fungi
Ventriculo-atrial shunt	*S. epidermidis*

Table 19.6 Penetration of Antibiotics into CSF

Antibiotic	Normal Meninges	Meningitis
Penicillins		
Penicillin G	Poor	Good
Ampicillin	Poor	Good
Carbenicillin	Poor	?
Methicillin	Poor	?
Nafcillin	Poor	Fair
Cephalosporins		
Cephalothin	Poor	Poor-fair
Cefazolin	Poor	Fair
Cephaloridine	Fair	Fair
Moxalactam	Fair-good	Fair-good
Cefotaxime	Poor-fair	Fair-good
Aminoglycosides		
Gentamicin	Poor	Fair
Kanamycin	Poor	Fair
Amikacin	Poor	Poor
Tetracyclines		
Tetracycline	Poor-fair	Fair
Oxytetracycline	Poor	Poor
Chlortetracycline	Poor	Poor
Doxycycline	Fair-good	Fair-good
Miscellaneous antibacterial		
Chloramphenicol	Good	Good
Clindamycin	Poor	Fair
Metronidazole	Fair-good	Good
Trimethoprim	Good	Good
Sulfonamides	Fair-good	Good
Rifampin	Fair	Good
Polymyxin B	Poor	Poor
Vancomycin	Poor	Good
Erythromycin	Poor	Poor-fair

sensitivities are known, treatment should be as specific as possible. If *Staphylococcus aureus* is isolated, penicillinase-resistant penicillins should be used. If Gram-negative bacilli are isolated, it may be necessary to deliver appropriate amino-glycoside antibiotics intrathecally in the lumbar space, or intraventricularly through a surgically inserted reservoir. Because meningeal inflammation may be associated with intrathecal administration of gentamicin which contains preservatives, a preservative-free preparation is available for intrathecal use. The only currently available cephalosporin which may achieve bacteriocidal levels in CSF following parental administration is moxalactam. Moxalactam appears effective in Gram-negative bacillary meningitis. It is customary to treat patients for 10 to 14 days with an effective antimicrobial agent in therapeutic dosages. At present, there is no evidence that the addition of corticosteroids is beneficial.

In children under the age of five, *Hemophilus influenza* is the most common cause of bacterial meningitis with *Streptococcus pneumonia* and *Neisseria meningitis* being second and third. In these children, a combination of ampicillin and chloramphenicol is usually delivered during the first phase of treatment as some strains of *H. influenza* are now ampicillin-resistant.

Dosages are suggested in Table 19.7. However, recommendations change frequently; check for current recommendations in recent medical journals or recent issues of the Medical Letter.

PRINCIPLE 6: When in doubt, treat for meningitis.

The incidence of neurological residua from bacterial meningitis is significant and may, in part, be related to delay in treatment. Thus, in individuals in whom the clinical suspicion of bacterial meningitis is high and the cerebrospinal fluid is somewhat atypical, it appears prudent to treat with appropriate antibiotics until culture of the CSF and blood are available and the clinical course has been determined. Viral meningitis, early in the clinical course, may resemble bacterial meningitis and have a predominance of polymorphonuclear cells in CSF. Antibiotic treatment may be stopped 2 to 3 days after CSF and blood cultures are negative. If the patient has had prior inadequate treatment with antibiotics, cultures may be sterile, CSF may resemble viral meningitis, and a full course of appropriate antibiot-

Table 19.7 Antibiotic Dosage for Bacterial Meningitis

Drug	Adult Dose	Child Dose	Route
Penicillins			
Penicillin G	20–24 million units/day divided q2–3h	100,000 to 500,000 u/kg/day divided q2h to q6h	IV
Ampicillin	12–14 gm/day divided q4h	300–400 mg/kg/day divided q4h	IV
Carbenicillin	25–35 gm/day divided q4h	400–600 mg/kg/day divided q4h to q6h	IV
Methicillin	8–12 gm/day divided q4–6h	250–300 mg/kg/day divided q6h	IV
Nafcillin	8–12 gm/day divided q4–6h	150–250 mg/kg/day divided q6h	IV
Cloxacillin	1.5–2 gm/day divided q6h	100–200 mg/kg/day divided q6h to q8h	IV
Aminoglycosides			
Kanamycin	15 mg/kg/day divided q12h	15–20 mg/kg/day divided q12h	IV
Gentamicin	3–5 mg/kg/day divided q8h	2–6 mg/kg/day divided q8h	IV
	5–10 mg/day	1–5 mg/day	INTRATHECAL
Others			
Chloramphenicol	50–100 mg/kg/day divided q6h	75–100 mg/kg/day divided q6h	IV
Moxalactam	6–12 gm divided q8h (?)	75–150 mg/kg/day divided q8h (?)	IV
Cefotaxime	50–150 mg/kg/day divided q4h (?)	100–200 mg/kg/day divided q4h (?)	IV

ics may be indicated. If the clinical picture resembles tuberculous or fungal meningitis, alterations in treatment may be made.

Isolation of patients with bacterial meningitis is not necessary, with the exceptions of *N. meningitis* infection or tuberculous meningitis with associated active pulmonary tuberculous.

> ***PRINCIPLE 7:*** Reduce maintenance fluids to minimize cerebral edema.

Individuals with bacterial meningitis may develop inappropriate hypothalamic release of antidiuretic hormone (ADH) and fluid retention. Overhydration with intravenous fluids may exacerbate the situation and possibly predispose to cerebral edema. If the blood pressure is not low, it is customary to administer one-half to two-thirds of the calculated daily maintenance fluid intravenously during the first several days of illness. Usually, the fluid is given as one-quarter to one-third normal saline in 5 percent dextrose. Blood pressure should be followed carefully. Frequent serum sodium levels should be obtained, looking for hyponatremia. Urinary output should also be followed for signs of inappropriate ADH secretion. Cerebral edema can occur in meningitis even with fluid restriction. Steroids do not appear to be beneficial in the cerebral edema occurring during meningitis.[12]

> ***PRINCIPLE 8:*** Watch for complications of bacterial meningitis and treat early.

Patients with bacterial meningitis have frequent neurologic complications (Table 19.8).

In the presence of clinical deterioration, the following studies should be obtained: electrolytes, coagulation parameters, computed tomography of the head, EEG, and repeat lumbar puncture and examination of CSF. Other studies may be indicated, depending upon the clinical setting. Appropriate measures should be taken for any abnormalities discovered.

Table 19.8 Complications of Bacterial Meningitis

I. Common
  A. Cerebral edema
  B. Shock
  C. Subdural effusion
  D. Seizure
  E. Brain infarction or necrosis
  F. Inappropriate ADH secretion

II. Uncommon
  A. Obstructive hydrocephalus
  B. Subdural empyema
  C. Brain abscess
  D. Disseminated intravascular coagulation

Seizures are a relatively common complication of meningitis, especially in children. They usually occur early in the course of the illness. Identifiable causes for seizures are listed in Table 19.9, although the precise cause often cannot be discovered. Treatment with phenytoin, phenobarbital, or diazepam should be instituted if seizures develop.

> **PRINCIPLE 9:** Household contacts should be treated prophylactically when infection is caused by *N. meningitis.*

Household contacts of patients infected with *N. meningitis* and others including ER and hospital personnel who have had close contact with the patient should receive chemoprophylaxis. Rifampin is the appropriate drug. Adults should receive rifampin, 600 mg, once daily for 4 consecutive days. The dose for children 1–12 years of age is 20 mg/kg/day for 4 days in a single daily dose and for children under 1 year, 10 mg/kg given in the same schedule.

Contacts of *S. pneumonia* do not need prophylactic treatment. Recommendations regarding prophylactic treatment following exposure to *H. influenza* meningitis are not well defined. Treatment of household contacts under four years of age with rifampin may be indicated,[23] utilizing the same dosage and schedule used for prophylaxis of *N. meningitis.*

BRAIN ABSCESSES

Brain abscesses are notoriously difficult to recognize early because of their subacute onset and non-specific symptoms.[21] If unrecognized and untreated they are fatal. However, if detected early and treated appropriately, cure is often possible.

> **PRINCIPLE 1:** The subacute development of headaches, focal neurological signs, seizures, papilledema, and intermittent fevers should suggest a brain abscess.

Table 19.9 Causes for Seizures in Bacterial Meningitis

Hyponatremia
Brain irritation
Brain infarction or necrosis
Subdural effusion
Subdural empyema
Brain abscess
High fever

Table 19.10 Presenting Signs and Symptoms of Brain Abscesses

I. Common
  A. Headache
  B. Confusion
  C. Hemiparesis
  D. Seizures
  E. Intermittent fever
II. Less common
  A. Nuchal rigidity
  B. Stupor
  C. Coma

Brain abscesses occur in males twice as often as in females and are slightly more common in children and young adults. The patient usually presents with a subacute progressive course characterized by increasing headaches, lethargy, confusion, focal neurological signs and generalized or focal seizures (Table 19.10). The focal neurological signs commonly include hemiparesis, aphasia, hemianopsia, or ataxia. Intermittent fevers occur in about half the patients.

As the abscess progresses, signs of increased intracranial pressure occur with the patient developing stupor or coma, papilledema, and third nerve palsies. (Warning—do not dilate pupils to look for papilledema as it may mask the ability to detect the development of a third nerve palsy.) If untreated, death often occurs following herniation. Because of the subacute onset and varying clinical characteristics, the diagnosis of brain abscess is often not made until the second week of symptoms.[21]

The differential diagnosis includes brain tumors (metastatic or primary), subdural hematoma, subdural empyema, lateral venous sinus thrombosis, encephalitis (especially herpes simplex encephalitis), and cerebral cysticercosis. Rarely an arteriovenous malformation that has bled or an acute focal hemorrhagic stroke may present like an acute brain abscess.

> **PRINCIPLE 2:** The CT or radionuclide brain scan are the diagnostic tests of choice.

The CT scan is an excellent diagnostic test especially after the abscess is well-formed or encapsulated.[16] At that time the abscess shows a center of mixed low density changes with a peripheral enhancing rim reflecting the development of the capsule (Fig. 19.1). Occasionally, brain tumors or infarcts with necrotic centers also have this appearance. If the CT scan is performed when only a cerebritis is present, the scan may appear as only a low density area, possibly with mass effect, with variable surrounding enhancement. The CT scan also identifies multiple abscesses.

The radionuclide brain scan is sensitive and accurate and may show abnormalities in the cerebritis stage before the CT scan shows specific changes.

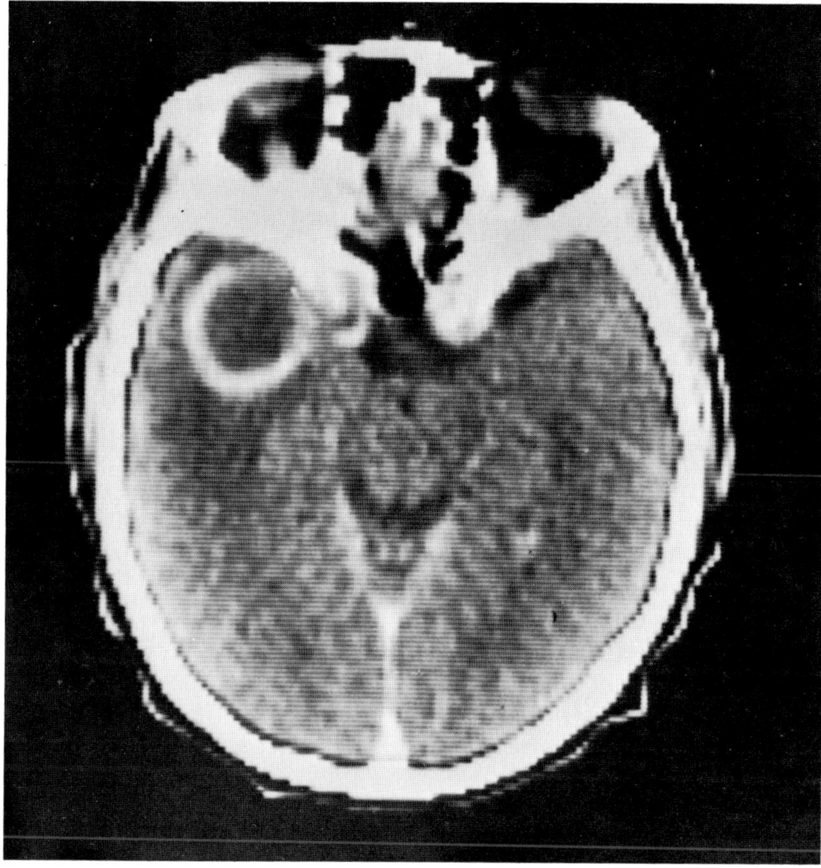

Fig. 19.1 CT scan of patient with left temporal lobe brain abscess. Note well encapsulated contrast enhancing rim, the central low density and surrounding cerebral edema.

However, the radionuclide brain scan may not distinguish between abscesses, necrotic foci from herpetic encephalitis, cerebral infarcts, or brain tumors.

A careful search should also be made for the primary focus from which the abscess developed (see Principle 3 below). Skull and sinus X-rays should be obtained looking for evidence of sinusitis, mastoiditis, skull fractures, or other parameningeal abnormalities. A chest X-ray should be obtained looking for evidence of lung abscesses, pneumonia, bronchiectasis, or empyema. A urinalysis may show evidence of pyelonephritis.

If the diagnosis of brain abscess is suspected, a lumbar puncture is not indicated and may be hazardous because of the risk of herniation. If, however, a lumbar puncture is inadvertently performed, the CSF is usually under increased pressure and has a mild pleocytosis of polymorphonuclear leukocytes and lymphocytes, mildly elevated protein, and normal glucose (Table 19.2). Bacterial and fungal cultures are usually sterile even when the agents are subsequently cultured from the abscess pus.

The electroencephalogram is usually abnormal with focal delta waves localizing cerebral but not cerebellar abscesses. However, the EEG changes suggest only space occupying lesions and are not specific for a brain abscess.

> ***PRINCIPLE 3:*** Brain abscesses develop by hematogenous spread or from direct extension of otic or sinus infections.

Most series report up to 40 percent of brain abscesses occur as a direct extension from otic or mastoid infection. In developing countries these figures may be higher. Typically, patients have a chronic low-grade sinusitis, orbital infection, or mastoiditis by which bacteria or fungi directly spread across bone, dura, arachnoid, and into the adjacent brain. Thus, patients with frontal sinus infections have abscesses in the frontal lobes while patients with otic infections have abscesses either in the temporal lobes (upward extension) or cerebellum (posterior extension). If a brain abscess is due to adjacent sinus or otic infections, both the abscess and the adjacent infection should be treated.

Brain abscesses also occasionally occur following head trauma or neurosurgical operations. The presence of a skull fracture should be cause for concern.

Abscesses occurring as a result of hematogenous spread are seen most often in patients with lung infections (lung abscess, pneumonia, empyema, or bronchiectasis), right to left cardiovascular shunts (cyanotic congenital heart disease), and chronic foci of infection such as osteomyelitis or chronic pyelonephritis. Additional sources include septic abortions and tooth or facial infections. Subacute bacterial endocarditis seldom causes brain abscesses but acute bacterial endocarditis may cause multiple abscesses. Occasionally no systemic focus is identified.

Experimental studies show that normal brain is relatively resistant to hematogenous spread of bacteria. Thus bacteremias rarely cause brain abscesses. However, the presence of bacterial stasis in vessels (infected emboli) or ischemic brain (cyanotic congenital heart disease) predispose to brain abscesses. Hematogenous brain abscesses usually begin at the border of the gray and white matter and rapidly develop into the white matter. Occasionally they rupture into ventricles causing a disastrous and often fatal ventriculitis. Abscesses involving the brainstem or spinal cord are rare.

> ***PRINCIPLE 4:*** Anaerobic bacteria are common causes of brain abscesses.

Bacteria causing brain abscesses differ from those that commonly cause meningitis. Anaerobic bacteria rarely cause meningitis but are found in up to 50 percent of brain abscesses.[6] Common causes of brain abscess include *Bacteroides fragilis, Streptococcus viridens, Streptococcus pyogenes, S. aureus* and *Peptostreptococcus.* Less common causes include *Klebsiella species, Proteus species, Escherichia coli, Nocardia asteroides, Mycobacterium tuberculosis, S. pneumonia, Actinomyces,* and *Entamoeba histolytica.* Often, several bacterial strains are cultured from a brain abscess.

It is impossible to accurately predict which organisms will be found in a brain abscess. However, abscesses originating from the sinuses are more likely to contain streptococci, either alone or with other organisms. Abscesses arising from an otic focus are more likely to contain anaerobic organisms including *Bacteroides fragilis* as well as other aerobic organisms. Post traumatic abscesses, including those following neurosurgery, often contain *S. aureus.*

If the abscess is surgically drained, it is important that the pus be cultured for both anaerobic and aerobic organisms as well as fungi. Mycobacterial cultures should be started if clinically indicated.

> **PRINCIPLE 5:** Current treatment is antibiotics plus surgery or antibiotics alone.

As soon as the diagnosis of brain abscess is made, wide spectrum antibiotic therapy should be instituted. The antibiotics must be selected for their effectiveness against all likely pathogens (anaerobic and aerobic) and their ability to penetrate the brain abscess and surrounding brain parenchyma.[7] Table 19.11 gives a listing of the ability of antibiotics to penetrate the brain parenchyma and abscess. In general, chloramphenicol and penicillin are commonly used unless fungi or unusual bacteria like *S. aureus* are suspected. Chloramphenicol is effective against a wide variety of organisms including

Table 19.11 Penetration of Antibiotics Into Brain Abscesses and Brain Tissue

Antibiotic	Penetration
Penicillin G	Poor-good
Ampicillin	Poor-good
Methicillin	Fair-good
Nafcillin	Poor
Cephalothin	Poor-fair
Gentamicin	Poor
Amikacin	Poor
Oxytetracycline	Poor
Chloramphenicol	Fair-good
Clindamycin	Fair-good
Metronidazole	Good
Trimethoprim	Good
Sulfamethoxazole	Good

most anaerobic bacteria and many aerobic gram-positive and gram-negative organisms. The drug penetrates well into the brain tissue but somewhat erratically into the pus of brain abscesses. Penicillin is effective against most Gram-positive organisms, both anaerobic and aerobic, with the exception of most strains of *S. aureus.* Penicillin penetrates erratically into brain abscesses.

Chloramphenicol (50–100 mg/kg/day in divided doses) and penicillin (200–300 mg or 320,000–480,000 units/kg/day in divided doses) are generally given parenterally. If *Nocardia* infections are suspected, sulfamethoxazole penetrates well into brain abscesses and is effective against most anaerobic bacteria. Metronidazole may be particularly useful in abscesses with anaerobic bacteria.[15]

Most brain abscesses have considerable surrounding brain edema that contributes to the "mass effect" of the abscess. If the patient is in danger of herniation, mannitol at 0.25 gm/kg (low dose) to 1.5 gm/kg should be given intravenously over 20 minutes. Dexamethasone (in adults, 16–24 mg/ 24 hr in 4 to 6 divided doses) may be necessary preoperatively and then tapered postoperatively.

In addition to antibiotics, surgical excision of the abscess is commonly recommended to: (1) culture the organism, (2) prevent herniation, and (3) promote rapid healing. Optimally, the abscess should be near the cortical surface and have a necrotic center and well-formed capsule allowing easy surgical removal. Unfortunately, if the abscess is multi-lobulated, total excision of the abscess may be impossible and surgical drainage of the pus is then indicated. If the abscess is detected at the early cerebritis stage (i.e., localized brain inflammation without a surrounding capsule) surgical intervention is seldom helpful, and it is often necessary to wait until a capsule is formed. Some medical centers have, on occasion, elected not to operate upon brain abscesses but treat them only with antibiotics.[4] This is commonly considered when the abscess is at the cerebritis stage, is deep or near critical areas (motor cortex or speech areas), or when multiple abscesses are present. In these situations, broad spectrum antibiotics (metronidazole, penicillin, chloramphenicol) followed by serial CT scans to ensure the abscess is not expanding have met with considerable success.

Mortality rates for brain abscesses have been reported to be 30 to 65 percent with the lower rates reported for those patients who have received optimal therapy following the early diagnosis. About one-half the survivors have neurologic sequelae, especially seizures and mild focal neurological signs. In many centers, patients are routinely placed on phenytoin or phenobarbital for 1 to 2 years to prevent seizures.

ACUTE ENCEPHALITIS

Acute encephalitis results from a widely disseminated viral infection of the brain parenchyma with destruction of neurons and glial cells. Table 19.12 lists the major causes of acute encephalitis in the United States. This section,

Table 19.12 Major Causes of Encephalitis in the United States

Virus	Vector	Geographic Distribution
Western equine	Mosquito	West of Mississippi river
St. Louis	Mosquito	Nationwide esp. along Mississippi river
Eastern equine	Mosquito	Atlantic coast
Venezuelan equine	Mosquito	Southwest and Florida
California	Mosquito	Northern midwest and Northeastern states
Colorado tick fever	Tick	Rocky mountain and Pacific coast states
Mumps	—	Nationwide
Herpes simplex	—	Nationwide
Rabies	Dog, skunk, fox, bat, raccoon	Nationwide

however, will deal primarily with the two most important causes of encephalitis: arboviruses and herpes simplex virus. Most other infectious causes of encephalitis, except rabies, follow a clinical course similar to that of arbovirus encephalitis.

> ***PRINCIPLE 1:*** Acute encephalitis is characterized by fever and the abrupt onset of headache and depression of consciousness.

Encephalitis differs from meningitis primarily in that patients present with prominent depressed consciousness and minimal or absent stiff neck.[17] The presence of fever, headache, and obtundation are the hallmarks of this disease. Inappropriate or bizarre behavior may be noted. Patients may develop one or more signs and symptoms presented in Table 19.13. The severity of these signs will depend upon the infecting organism. For example, mumps usually causes a mild meningoencephalitis while rabies encephalitis is almost always fatal. Also, the very young and the very old usually experience a more severe encephalitis.

Depending upon the infecting agent, a prodrome, involving another organ

Table 19.13 Signs and Symptoms of Encephalitis

I. Common
  A. Fever
  B. Headaches
  C. Confusion, delirium
  D. Depression of consciousness
  E. Seizures
  F. Mild stiff neck

II. Less common
  A. Nausea and vomiting
  B. Hemiparesis
  C. Cranial nerve palsies
  D. Aphasia
  E. Ataxia
  F. Blindness

system, may precede the encephalitis. In mumps, parotitis is common while malaise and myalgias frequently precede arbovirus encephalitis.

> **PRINCIPLE 2:** The most useful diagnostic tests are an EEG and lumbar puncture.

The EEG is almost always abnormal in encephalitis and usually shows diffuse bilateral slowing with occasional seizure activity.[19] This is in contrast to viral meningitis which usually has a normal EEG. The lumbar puncture has an opening pressure that is normal or elevated (Table 19.2). The CSF is clear and colorless and contains 10 to several hundred WBC/mm³, predominately lymphocytes. CSF glucose is normal while the protein may be normal to mildly elevated (40–200 mg/dl). Virus is seldom isolated from the CSF except in the case of mumps. Radionuclide brain scans and CT scans are not very helpful and may be normal or show non-specific abnormalities.

There is usually a moderate leukocytosis in the peripheral blood.

> **PRINCIPLE 3:** Most patients with viral encephalitis do not require isolation procedures.

Patients with arbovirus infections do not transmit the infection person-to-person; a vector is required. However blood and needle precautions should be taken. Likewise, patients with herpes encephalitis are not contagious. Patients with mumps encephalitis should be considered contagious to non-immune individuals as the virus is present in the patient's saliva. If rabies is suspected, isolation is required as rabies virus is present in several body secretions including saliva.

ARBOVIRUS ENCEPHALITIS

> **PRINCIPLE 1:** Clustering of encephalitis cases in the summer suggests an arbovirus.

Arboviruses, or togaviruses, comprise over 250 strains that are found mainly in the tropics. These viruses are transmitted by hematophagous arthropods such as mosquitos or ticks. In the United States the most important viruses of this group include Western equine, Eastern equine, Venezuelan, St. Louis, California, and Colorado tick fever. Of these, St. Louis and Western equine encephalitis are the most common and are transmitted to man by mosquitos.[19] Arbovirus encephalitis, therefore, occurs during the late spring, summer and early fall when mosquitos and ticks are prominent. This often results in a clustering of cases within specific areas of the country.

Most infections with arboviruses are asymptomatic or mild. Fortunately, only a small percent of non-immune patients infected with arboviruses will develop encephalitis. The majority will develop fevers and myalgias and occasionally a picture of viral meningitis. If arbovirus encephalitis is suspected clinically, health authorities should be immediately notified as an epidemic could be developing.

> **PRINCIPLE 2:** The treatment of arbovirus encephalitis is symptomatic.

No effective antiviral agent has been developed for arbovirus encephalitis or any viral encephalitis except herpes simplex encephalitis. Therefore, attention and care should be directed to the airway, bladder, fluid and electrolyte balance, fever, and seizures if they occur.[19] In comatose patients intubation and artificial ventilation along with urinary catheterization are usually required. The presence of seizures may necessitate the use of intravenous phenytoin (see Chapter 6).

In viral encephalitis cerebral edema and localized hemorrhages may result in increased intracranial pressure and possible herniation. Treatment of the increased intracranial pressure should include reduction of intravenous fluids to 2/3 maintenance, hyperventilation to achieve arterial PCO_2 of 25–35 torr, and intermittent use of Mannitol 0.25–1.5 g/kg by IV over 20 minutes. Since there is experimental evidence that corticosteroids may potentiate spread of the viral encephalitis, use of corticosteroids remains controversial. Use of an intracranial pressure monitor may also be considered.

The acute encephalitis lasts 1 to 3 weeks. Recovery may occur over weeks to months. The prognosis of encephalitis varies with the viral cause. Encephalitis from mumps, lymphocytic choriomeningitis, Colorado tick fever, and Venezuelan equine results in only rare deaths and few sequelae. Encephalitis from Western equine, St. Louis, and California results in 2 to 10 percent mortality and occasional sequelae.[10] Encephalitis from Eastern equine has a 20 percent mortality and 50 percent of the survivors have neurological sequelae. Rabies is almost always fatal.

> **PRINCIPLE 3:** The diagnosis of arbovirus encephalitis is best made by serology.

In most patients with encephalitis, a virus is rarely isolated from the CSF, blood, throat, urine or stool. Therefore, the diagnosis of arbovirus encephalitis is usually confirmed by demonstrating a titer rise to a given arbovirus between acute and convalescent serum specimens. Since most individuals lack arbovirus antibodies, a single convalescent serum with an elevated arbovirus titer will allow a presumptive diagnosis.

HERPES SIMPLEX ENCEPHALITIS

Herpes simplex (HSV) encephalitis has been separated from the other viral encephalitides because specific treatment is now available.[27] Therefore, clinical distinction of HSV encephalitis from the other forms of encephalitis is important. Most cases of herpes simplex encephalitis occur from a type 1 herpes simplex viral infection in previously healthy individuals.[20] Present evidence suggests that most cases are not a primary infection but result following reactivation of a latent virus probably present in the trigeminal ganglia.[30]

> ***PRINCIPLE 1:*** There are no pathognomonic signs and symptoms of herpes simplex encephalitis.

Herpes encephalitis can occur in patients of any age, sex, or socioeconomic status at any time of the year. There are no specific signs or symptoms although most patients present with the classic signs of fever, headache, and altered mental status.[27] Patients with herpes encephalitis are slightly more likely to have focal seizures than generalized seizures but this is not specific enough to be helpful in an individual case.

The presence of a cold sore at the time of admission or a history or recurrent cold sores does not have any diagnostic significance.[30]

The clinical course rapidly progresses over the first several days, often leading to a profound coma and death. The acute encephalitis usually lasts 1 to 2 weeks with a prolonged convalescence occurring over weeks to months.

> ***PRINCIPLE 2:*** There are no specific laboratory tests to establish the diagnosis but periodic lateralized epileptiform discharges on the EEG and temporal lobe abnormalities on the CT or radionuclide brain scan suggest the diagnosis.

All patients with HSV encephalitis will have a diffusely abnormal EEG.[29] In addition, about 80 percent of patients will develop high voltage complexes originating from one or both temporal lobes characterized as periodic lateralized epileptiform discharges (PLEDs).[30] PLEDs occur more commonly in patients with herpes encephalitis than in other forms of encephalitis.

The radionuclide brain scan often shows abnormalities demonstrating damage to the blood-brain barrier in one or both hemispheres early in the clinical course.[29] When the abnormalities localize to one temporal lobe, the possibility of herpes simplex encephalitis is increased. The CT scan typically becomes abnormal later in the clinical course than the radionuclide brain scan. CT abnormalities include low density lesions in one or both temporal lobes and areas of hemorrhagic necrosis. While this finding may suggest herpes encephalitis, it is not specific and may be confused with early brain abscesses, arteriovenous malformations, traumatic contusions, and brain tumors.

The CSF is under increased pressure and typically has a mononuclear pleocytosis with 5–500 WBC/mm.[3] Occasionally, the CSF may contain many red cells suggesting brain necrosis and hemorrhage. The CSF protein is mildly elevated (50–200 mg/dl) while the glucose is usually normal. Herpes simplex virus is seldom isolated from the CSF.

As yet no serological test for herpes simplex virus in blood or CSF has been found to be useful in the diagnosis of herpes simplex encephalitis. This occurs because most adults and many children have been previously infected with herpes simplex virus and have pre-existing antibodies. Likewise, the isolation of herpes simplex virus from the lip or throat has no diagnostic significance.[30]

> ***PRINCIPLE 3:*** A brain biopsy is currently the only method of acutely diagnosing herpes encephalitis.

As previously mentioned, there are no clinical symptoms, signs, or laboratory tests that are specific for this diagnosis. Therefore, at the present time, the diagnosis can be only established by brain biopsy.[28,29] A cerebral cortex biopsy should be seriously entertained in any patient with unknown encephalitis in whom antiviral treatment with adenine arabinoside is being seriously considered. Experience from the NIH Cooperative Encephalitis Study has shown that of patients clinically suspected of having herpes encephalitis, 50 percent will be subsequently shown to have other diagnoses [28] (Table 19.14).

The cerebral cortex biopsy is best obtained by an open biopsy taken near the area of maximal pathology, usually from the posterior frontal or temporal lobes. An open biopsy allows a better histological diagnosis and has fewer complications than a needle biopsy. If properly performed, surgical biopsies of the cerebral cortex have few complications. The major complication is subsequent seizures in approximately 5 percent, that are easily controlled with phenytoin.

Once the biopsy is obtained, several studies on the tissue should be performed to establish the diagnosis. A suspension of the brain tissue should be inoculated onto susceptible tissue culture cell lines for viral isolation. If herpes simplex virus is present, viral cytopathic effects usually develop

Table 19.14 Diseases That May Mimic HSV Encephalitis

Cryptococcal meningitis
Tuberculous meningitis
Arbovirus encephalitis
Other viral encephalitis
Toxoplasma encephalitis
Brain abscess
Brain tumor
Arteriovenous malformation
Cerebral hemorrhage
Bacterial endocarditis

in 1 to 4 days. However, occasionally up to 2 weeks may be required. Frozen sections of the brain biopsy may be stained for herpes simplex viral antigens by immunofluorescence. This method can establish the diagnosis within hours. Experienced laboratories will demonstrate specific fluorescence in up to 80 percent of the virus-proven cases. However, 5 to 10 percent of false positives occur. The remainder of the tissue should be fixed for conventional histologic examination. This may be helpful if the diagnosis is not herpes simplex encephalitis.

PRINCIPLE 4: Early treatment with antiviral agents is important.

Patients with herpes simplex encephalitis who are untreated have a mortality rate as high as 70 percent. The NIH Collaborative Anti-viral Study has shown that the use of adenine arabinoside (Vidarabine or ARA-A) can reduce mortality to 30 percent.[27] ARA-A is diluted and given by slow, continuous intravenous infusion in a dose of 15 mg/kg/day for 10 days. This drug is most effective when given early in the clinical course before coma develops. The drug can be given as much as 12 hours before the brain biopsy is obtained without interfering in the ability to isolate virus from the biopsy specimen.

Following the brain biopsy adenine arabinoside should be continued for 5 days. At that time the patient and laboratory tests should be reevaluated. If the culture is negative for herpes virus and histologic sections of the brain biopsy suggest other diagnoses, adenine arabinoside can be discontinued.

Adenine arabinoside has side effects and should not be used indiscriminately. It has no antiviral effect on RNA viruses such as arboviruses, mumps, or rabies. Large amounts of fluid are necessary to dissolve the drug and administration of high fluid volumes aggravate cerebral edema. The drug also has recognized neurologic, oncogenic, and some immunosuppressive properties. Nevertheless, in herpes encephalitis the drug is clearly beneficial. The NIH Anti-viral Cooperative Study found patients less than 30 years of age had a better outcome than those who were older.[27] In the younger patients, 77 percent survived and 50 percent of those surviving returned to normal. In the older patient group, 65 percent survived and 38 percent of those surviving returned to normal.

A new drug, acyclovir, may also prove beneficial in the treatment of herpes simplex encephalitis. The drug appears to possess potent anti-herpes simplex viral activity with considerably less drug toxicity. Studies evaluating this drug are now underway.

HERPES ZOSTER (SHINGLES)

Herpes zoster (shingles) is due to the exacerbation of a latent varicella-zoster (VZ) virus. Following a primary infection of chickenpox, the VZ virus becomes latent in the dorsal root ganglia for years. Exacerbation of this latency rarely occurs in children and young adults. However, over the age of 50 the incidence of herpes zoster slowly climbs reaching an incidence of 1 percent per year by age 90.[14] In addition, patients of any age who have defects in their cellular immune system are at increased risk for developing herpes zoster. Patients with cancer have a risk of approximately 2 percent while patients with Hodgkin's disease have a risk of almost 50 percent of developing herpes zoster.

> **PRINCIPLE 1:** Herpes zoster causes a characteristic vesicular eruption in the distribution of a dermatome.

Typically, the patient develops a sharp, burning, uncomfortable sensation in a dermatomal distribution 1 to 4 days before the appearance of the rash.[5] The rash then develops in the same dermatome and consists of papules evolving into vesicles. Freely moveable, non-painful, local adenopathy is usually present in the lymph nodes draining the effected area. Over the next several weeks, the vesicles evolve into pustules, crust, and skin ulceration (Fig. 19.2). Generally the zoster appears in only one dermatome.[14] However, occasional patients may have several consecutive dermatomes or sporadic dermatomes involved and rare patients may develop pain in a dermatomal distribution without a rash (*zoster sine herpete*). The rash occurs on the trunk in 50 percent of cases, on the head in 20 percent, and in the extremities in 30 percent.

If a lumbar puncture is performed, the CSF, in about one-third of patients, will show a mild lymphocytic pleocytosis, normal to mildly elevated protein, and normal glucose. Varicella-zoster virus is seldom isolated from the CSF although it can be isolated from skin vesicles.

The diagnosis is easily made when the vesicular rash is in a dermatomal distribution. In the pre-eruptive stage, however, the pain may be confused with the pain of angina pectoris, biliary or renal colic, or other chest or abdominal problems.

Herpes Zoster Opthalmicus

When herpes zoster occurs over the first division of the trigeminal nerve, vesicles typically develop over one side of the forehead and around the eye.[11] About one-third of these patients will also have a viral infection of the cornea and uvea producing severe pain and occasionally blindness. Clinically, patients with corneal involvement often have vesicles over the tip of the nose since both areas are innervated by the nasociliary branch of the first division of the fifth cranial nerve.

> **PRINCIPLE 2:** Treatment of uncomplicated herpes zoster is primarily symptomatic.

Most patients with uncomplicated herpes zoster do not require hospitalization. If complications develop (see Principle 3 below) or the pain is severe,

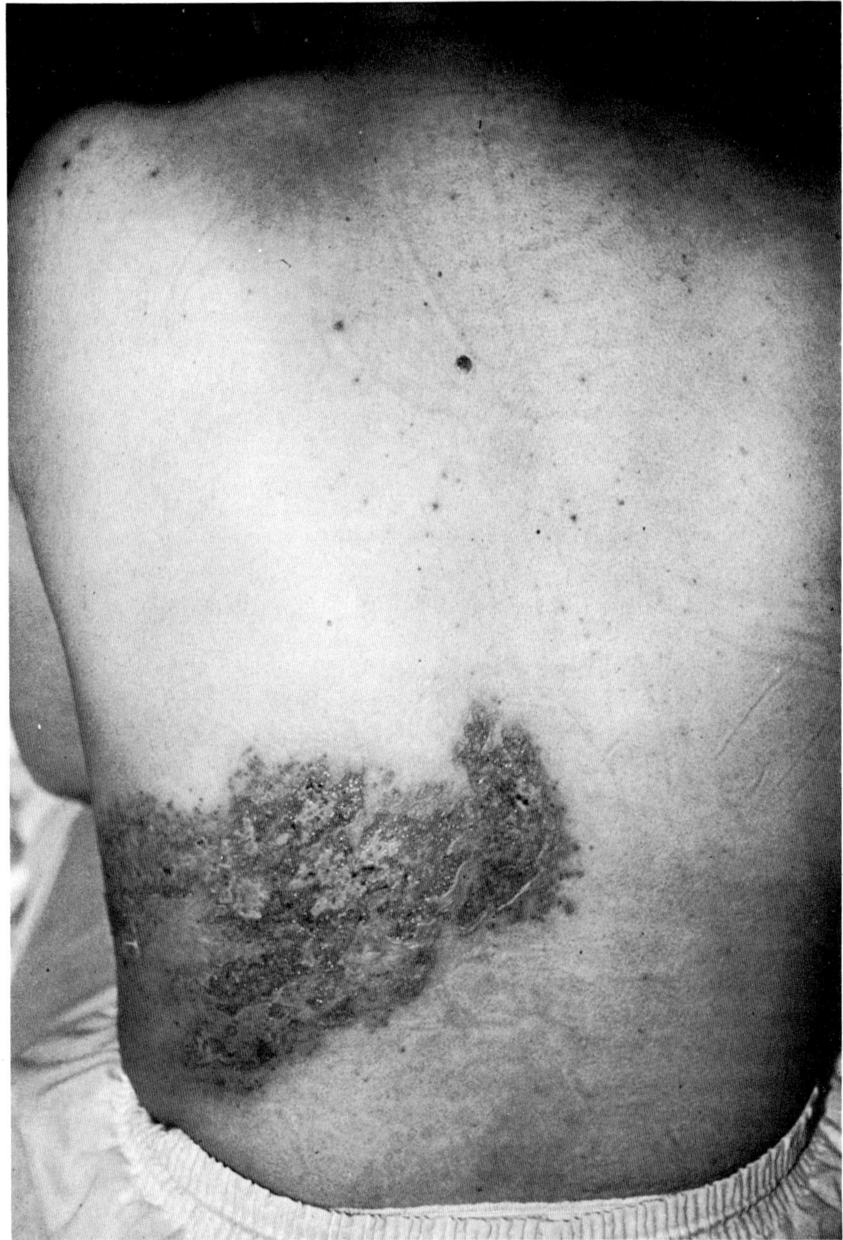

Fig. 19.2 Herpes zoster involving left lower thoracic dermatome.

hospitalization may be indicated. The acute disease is often treated by the application of cool, wet compresses applied to the skin vesicles to aid in healing.[14] The vesicles should be kept clean and not allowed to become bacterially infected. If a secondary bacterial infection develops, bacitracin ointment applied to the rash may be useful. If the infection progresses, bacterial cultures should be taken and systemic antibiotics should be administered. Analgesics may be required for the acute pain. Occasionally, antihistamines may be required for itching. If the patients are not hospitalized, they should be followed carefully as some complications develop days after primary vesicular rash occurs.

Use of systemic corticosteroids during the acute phase is thought by some to reduce the incidence of post-herpetic neuralgia, especially in the elderly. Regimens commonly employed consist of prednisone 60 mg/day in divided doses for 1 week and then tapering over the next 2 weeks. Consideration must be given to the risk of suppressing the immune response with the prednisone, resulting in viral dissemination.

In the majority of patients symptomatically treated, the dermatomal pain slowly subsides over a month leaving a residual mild hypo or hyperesthesia.[5,14] Occasional patients, however, will develop a residual post herpetic neuralgia (see Principle 3 below).

> **PRINCIPLE 3:** Complications of herpes zoster include dissemination of the rash, motor paralysis, encephalomyelitis, and post-herpetic neuralgia.

Dissemination Of Varicella Zoster

In patients with cellular immune defects, herpes zoster poses a greater risk to spread from the original dermatome distribution.[9] Typically, 1 to 2 weeks after the original dermatomal eruption, secondary vesicles develop over the skin resembling chickenpox. The progression may terminate at this time or progress to a severe, widespread skin rash, viral pneumonia, and visceral involvement which may be fatal. Because of this possibility, treatment of herpes zoster in these patients is often more aggressive. Experimental use of adenine arabinoside (ARA-A) has been shown to be effective in accelerating the healing and virus clearance from the rash.[26] This drug must be given intravenously at 15 mg/kg/day over 10 days in a hospital setting. The drug appears to be somewhat more effective if given prophylactically at the time of the initial dermatomal rash. However, the drug can be given after dissemination has started. There is some feeling that the drug may also reduce the risk of subsequent post-herpetic neuralgia.

Intramuscular human leukocyte interferon, when given to immunosuppressed patients with herpes zoster, has also resulted in a shorter clinical course with reduced incidence of post herpetic neuralgia. Interferon is an endogenous protein with potent, wide spectrum, antiviral activity. Unfortunately, the drug is in limited supply and expensive. Until production is increased and costs are reduced, interferon is not a practical form of therapy.

Zoster immune globulin has not been found to be beneficial in the treatment of uncomplicated herpes zoster and it appears that the immune globulin has no value in preventing dissemination of the virus.

Motor Paresis

Occasionally, patients with herpes zoster may also develop segmental motor weakness. Although any muscle may be involved, facial muscles (Ramsay Hunt syndrome), diaphragmatic paralysis and acute urinary retention are the most common. Patients with the Ramsay Hunt syndrome will usually have vesicles over the ear pinna or skin behind the pinna as well as ipsilateral peripheral facial weakness and possibly dizziness, tinnitus, or hearing loss.[2] The prognosis is generally favorable with recovery of motor function occurring in over 85 percent of patients.

Encephalomyelitis

This is a rare but serious complication of herpes zoster.[13] These patients may develop acute back pain corresponding to the dermatome of the rash followed by sensory loss below the spinal cord level and possibly weakness below that level giving the clinical appearance of transverse myelitis. It is thought that the virus has spread proximally from the involved sensory ganglia to the spinal cord. Upon reaching the spinal cord the virus may cause a localized infection (transverse myelitis) or disseminate to produce a widespread encephalomyelitis (see section on viral encephalitis). These patients are acutely ill and require hospitalization usually in an intensive care unit. The CSF of these patients typically shows a moderate lymphocytic pleocytosis and elevated protein with a normal glucose. Cultures of the CSF should be bacterially sterile and occasionally may contain varicella zoster virus. These patients should receive adenine arabinoside (15 mg/kg/day intravenously over ten days) or other antiviral drugs (acyclovir) because this complication is potentially life-threatening.

Post-Herpetic Neuralgia

This is an uncommon, but greatly feared complication of herpes zoster.[14] It rarely occurs in younger patients but occurs to some degree in about half the patients over the age of 60. In these patients the pain involving the dermatomal distribution persists long after the rash has completely healed. Typically, these patients experience a steady, uncomfortable burning or aching pain involving the dermatome. Superimposed, excruciating lancinating pains may occur upon cutaneous stimulation of the dermatome.

Treatment of post-herpetic neuralgia is difficult and often results in only partial relief. Patients may benefit from the use of a transcutaneous electrical stimulator with the stimulating electrode placed on the back near the midline over the involved dermatome. Other patients benefit from the use of tricyclic antidepressants such as amitriptyline. Doses of this drug between 50 and 200 mg/day are frequently beneficial. Occasionally, Prolixin 1 mg/day may also be added for pain relief. In patients with lancinating pains, carbamazepine in the dose used to treat tic doulourex (600 mg to 1,000/ day) may be tried. Recently tried treatments that have had some success include sympathetic ganglion block with lidocaine, sympathectomy, and Sinemet (25/100, 3 times per day). Non-narcotic analgesics may bring some, but seldom total, relief. However, the use of narcotic analgesics should be carefully monitored as the pain in these patients is often chronic allowing them to become tolerant or addicted to narcotics.

PRINCIPLE 4: Acute herpes zoster is contagious.

Non-immune individuals exposed to patients with herpes zoster can develop chickenpox as the varicella-zoster virus causes both conditions. Patients should be considered infectious until the vesicles have completely crusted over. However, unlike patients with chickenpox, there is no risk of respiratory spread of the virus.

REFERENCES

1. Adair, C.V., Gauld, R.L., Smadel, J.E.: Aseptic meningitis, a disease of diverse etiology: clinical and etiologic studies on 854 cases. Ann. Int. Med., 39:675, 1953.
2. Aleksic, S.N., Budzilovich, G.N., Lieberman, A.N.: Herpes zoster oticus and facial paralysis (Ramsay Hunt syndrome). J. Neurol. Sci., 20:149, 1973.
3. Bell, W.E.: Treatment of bacterial infections of the central nervous system. Ann. Neurol., 9:313, 1981.
4. Berg, B., Franklin, G., Cuneo, R., et al: Non-surgical cure of brain abscess: early diagnosis and follow-up with computerized tomography. Ann. Neurol., 3:474, 1978.
5. Burgoon, C.F., Burgoon, J.S., Baldridge, G.D.: The natural history of herpes zoster. JAMA, 164:265, 1957.
5A. Cherubin, C.E., Corrado, M.L., Nair, S.R., et. al.: Treatment of Gram negative bacillary meningitis: role of the new cephalosporin antibiotics. Rev. Infect. Dis., 4 (Suppl.): S453, 1982.
6. De Louvois, J., Gortvai, P., Hurley, R.: Bacteriology of abscesses of the central nervous system: a multicenter prospective study. Br. Med. J., 2:981, 1977.
7. De Louvois, J., Gortvai, P., Hurley, R.: Antibiotic treatment of abscesses of the central nervous system. Br. Med. J., 2:985, 1977.
8. Dillon, H.C.: Studies of moxalactam for Gram-negative and Haemophilus influenzae meningitis: an appraisal. J. Pediatr., 99:907, 1981.
9. Dolin, R., Reichman, R. C., Mazur, M.H., et al: Herpes zoster-varicella infections in immunosuppressed patients. Ann. Int. Med., 89:375, 1978.
10. Earnest, M.P., Goolishian, H.A., Calverley, J.R., et al: Neurologic, intellectual and psychologic sequelae following western encephalitis. Neurology, 21:969, 1971.
11. Edgerton, A.E.: Herpes zoster ophthalmicus. Arch. Ophthalmol., 34:40, 1945.
12. Fishman, R.A.: Steroids in the treatment of brain edema. N. Engl. J. Med., 306:359, 1982.

13. Hogan, E.L., Krigman, M.R.: Herpes zoster myelitis. Arch. Neurol., 29:309, 1973.
14. Hope-Simpson, R.E.: The nature of herpes zoster: a long term study and new hypothesis. Proc. Roy. Soc. Med., 58:9, 1965.
15. Ingham, H.R., Selkon, J.B., Roxby, C.M.: Bacteriological study of otogenic cerebral abscesses: chemotherapeutic role of metronidazole. Br. Med. J., 2:991, 1977.
16. Kaufman, D.M., Leeds, N.E.: Computed tomography (CT) in the diagnosis of intracranial abscesses. Neurology, 27:1069, 1977.
17. Kennard, C., Swash, M.: Acute viral encephalitis: its diagnosis and outcome. Brain, 104:129, 1981.
18. Lepow, M.L., Carver, D.H., Wright, H.T., et al: A clinical, epidemiologic and laboratory investigation of aseptic meningitis during the four-year period, 1955–1958. N. Engl. J. Med., 266:1181, 1962.
19. Monath, T.P.: St. Louis encephalitis. Am. Publ. Health Asoc., Washington, DC, 1980.
20. Nahmias, A.J., Norrild, B.: Herpes simplex viruses 1 and 2—basic and clinical aspects. Disease-A-Month 25:10, 1979.
21. Samson, D.S., Clark, K.: A current review of brain abscess. Am. J. Med., 54:201, 1973.
22. Sell, S.H.W., Merrill, R.E., Doyne, E.O., et al: Long-term sequelae of Hemophilus influenzae meningitis. Pediatr., 49:206, 1972.
23. Smith, A.L.: Is Haemophilus influenzae meningitis contagious? N. Engl. J. Med., 301:155, 1979.
24. Sullivan, R.J., Davis, L.E., Jones, V.A., et al: Viral aseptic meningitis: 12 years experience. Missour. Med., Sept. 11–15, 1971.
25. Swartz, M.N., Dodge, P.R.: Bacterial meningitis—a review of selected aspects. N. Engl. J. Med., 272:725–731, 779–787, 842–902, 954–960, 1003–1010, 1965.
26. Whitley, R.J., Ch'ien, L.T., Dolin, R., et al: Adenine arabinoside therapy of herpes zoster in the immunosuppressed. N. Engl. J. Med., 294:1193, 1976.
27. Whitley, R.J., Soong, S.J., Dolin, R., et al: Adenine arabinoside therapy of biopsy-proved herpes simplex encephalitis. N. Engl. J. Med., 297:289, 1977.
28. Whitley, R.J., Soong, S.J., Hirsch, M.S., et al: Herpes simplex encephalitis. Vidarabine therapy and diagnostic problems. N. Engl. J. Med., 304:313, 1981.
29. Whitley, R.J., Soong, S.J., Linneman, C., et al: Herpes simplex encephalitis—clinical assessment. JAMA, 247:317, 1982.
30. Wolinsky, J.S.: Herpes simplex encephalitis. Johns Hopkins Med. J., 147:157, 1980.

20

Legal Aspects of Neurological Emergency Care

H. Richard Beresford, M.D., J.D.

INTRODUCTION

Physicians need no reminding that law affects their professional activities. Not only is there a pervasive concern about malpractice suits, but issues relating to confidentiality, informed consent, care of the hopelessly ill, and the growing impact of hospital or governmental regulations regularly confront the practitioner. Accordingly, the physician may see law as overly intrusive or at best as a mixed blessing. Yet no matter what the physician's attitude, having some understanding of what the law requires and why the rules are what they are should be of some practical value.

The purpose of this chapter is to discuss how law functions with respect to physicians caring for patients with neurological disorders who need immediate treatment. The focus will be on general concepts, using as examples cases involving emergency neurological care, and no systematic effort will be made to advise physicians how to handle the legal aspects of specific situations. In this chapter the term "emergency" indicates a condition which may result in severe disability or death, and for which any delay in providing treatment increases the risk to the patient.

LEGAL DUTIES OF THE PHYSICIAN IN EMERGENCIES

General Considerations

Underlying the law of medical practice is the notion of professional responsibility. Society views physicians as persons who possess knowledge and skills which they apply to the care of patients in accordance with certain norms.

Physicians themselves have defined with variable precision standards of competence and ethical behavior, and law has largely adopted its conception of what constitutes acceptable performance from these. Thus, in most medical malpractice litigation the central question is whether the defendant physician met reasonable or accepted standards of medical practice, and the answer turns on the testimony of other physicians as to what these standards are. It is exceptional for a court to impose standards that differ from professional ones.

Another aspect of the law of medical practice is the problem of how to encourage physicians to meet professional standards. In this area social goals are important determinants. If the goal is deterring future injuries to patients, a variety of approaches might be tried, ranging from mandatory continuing education or consultation to suspension or revocation of licensure. If the goal is primarily to compensate injured patients, the physician's status is like that of any other unsuccessful defendant in a personal injury action who must pay the costs his or her negligence has imposed on an injured person (e.g., medical expenses, loss of income, pain and suffering). If the goal is punishment, the "guilty" physician becomes analogous to the white-collar criminal whose penalty is measured in part by the extent to which the wrongful conduct offends prevailing mores. In fact, most litigation involving physicians is malpractice, and in this form of action the usual remedy is the payment of money damages. On occasion, awards, although labelled as compensatory, may include an unspecified element of punishment if judge or jury are particularly outraged by a physician's conduct. The deterring effect of a money award on future misconduct is speculative, particularly where insurance covers all or most of a judgement, but it may be that a physician who pays for a negligent act will be more careful in the future.

Whatever its value in promoting observance of accepted standards of care, a malpractice liability system may have the undesirable consequence of inducing defensive medicine. Critics of the current system see this as one of its major failings,[1] and any meaningful reform of the current system should address the problem posed by the legitimate self-protective concerns of physicians. The aggregate economic, social and personal costs of a system which causes physicians to think they must conduct tests or procedures primarily to thwart lawsuits appear unacceptably high.

Patient-Oriented Duties

Professional Standards

The physician's legal duty in an emergency is identical to that in other contexts: to provide care that is reasonable under the circumstances.[2] If the patient is facing imminent death or severe disability, the physician must do what other similarly qualified physicians would do in a like situation.

To illustrate, consider the following example: A young man is brought to a hospital emergency room at 2 AM following a motor vehicle crash. He is comatose and has slow irregular respirations, a widely dilated and unreactive right pupil, decerebrate posturing and bilateral extensor plantar responses. Here the severity of the head injury is obvious, as is the need to provide respiratory support, reduce intracranial pressure, and consider prompt neurosurgical treatment. A physician who fails to recognize the nature of the problem, or who fails to take immediate therapeutic and diagnostic steps or to obtain consultative assistance would not meet professional norms for a physician at almost any level of training or experience.

However, suppose the patient is drowsy but oriented and coherent, the respirations are normal, the pupils equal, only the left plantar response is extensor, and no abnormal posturing is observed. Suppose further that the on-call physician is a board certified internist, that he orders skull X-rays which are reported to him as normal, that he places the patient in a bed-holding area to be observed by a nurse every ½ hour, and that he does not seek a neurological or neurosurgical consultation. Suppose, finally, that 2 hours later the patient is found comatose and apneic with a fixed dilated right pupil and, despite prompt neurosurgery, dies of the effects of a right epidural hematoma.

Here the question whether the physician behaved reasonably or not is open to debate. He examined the patient, found little in the way of focal neurological signs, apparently excluded a skull fracture, and kept the patient for observation. He can be criticized for failing to attach enough significance to the patient's drowsiness and to the left extensor plantar response and for not seeking prompt neurological or neurosurgical consultation. If the hospital had available 24-hour computerized tomography, he could also be faulted for failing to order this test. But a legal conclusion that he violated relevant professional standards must rest on testimony from another comparably experienced internist that he failed to meet reasonable or accepted standards for an internist by not seeking consultation or failing to perform more testing. In other words, the physician's conduct is measured by what he could reasonably be expected to know or do, not by what a hypothetical expert in the management of neurological disorders would have done in a similar situation.

The law's message here is that a physician must meet society's expectations for a certain level of performance, *but* that this level is to be defined by what professional peers deem reasonable. Some have criticized this reliance on professional standards as overly protective of physicians. But much about medical practice is either too complex or too dependent on accumulated knowledge and experience to permit a determination of what is reasonable or acceptable practice to be made by non-physicians. This seems especially true where the effect of the determination may be to penalize an individual physician.

Other Standards

While the law tends to defer to professional standards in judging competence, it still insists that physicians behave as fiduciaries of their patients' interests. The notion is that there is more to the physician's duty than acting competently. He or she must also be faithful and respectful. This means that privacy and confidentiality must be protected and that patients must be informed participants in decisions which may have a major impact on their well-being. Although the outer limits of the doctrines of confidentiality and informed consent are often unclear, both legal rules and professional ethics recognize that these doctrines provide indispensable protections for patients. In a medical emergency, however, the need for immediate treatment may eclipse concerns about whether a patient's personal autonomy is being adequately respected. Here the physician's capacity to perform with technical competence becomes the dominant factor in deciding whether the physician has met the legal duty to a patient.

Aside from principles established by court decisions or professional standards, a growing body of regulations enacted by hospitals, accrediting bodies (e.g., JCAH), and administrative agencies cover aspects of physicians' conduct towards patients. Most do not specifically deal with the treatment of medical emergencies, but some do. For example, hospitals or accrediting agencies may require that all hospital staff physicians attain competence in cardiopulmonary rescucitation, regardless of specialty. Hospitals may limit the privileges of some physicians with respect to treatment of some types of emergencies (e.g., acute head or spinal injuries). Accrediting or governmental agencies or hospital by-laws may require certain staffing patterns for emergency rooms or intensive care units, or governmental agencies may establish or support centers for the treatment of acute head injuries or other forms of neurological trauma. These and other forms of regulation thus determine who is permitted to treat some emergencies or affect the distribution of patients suffering some types of life-threatening illnesses.

Society-Oriented Duties

In most medical emergencies the interests of patients and society are congruent. Preventing death or severe disability in an injured or sick person is a goal to which society attaches the highest priority, and many resources are devoted to it. But occasionally a physician may be asked to compromise personal interests of patients to promote other societal goals. For example, while treating an injured but apparently intoxicated patient, a physician may be asked by a police officer to obtain a blood sample for the sole purpose of measuring alcohol or drug levels. Obviously information derived from such a test may be used in a criminal prosecution of the patient. Or a physician may be required by state or local law to report certain types of injuries (e.g., knife or gunshot wounds) to governmental authorities, and such reports may be a link in a chain of incriminating evidence.

Requiring physicians to breach confidentiality in these circumstances is justifiable in the sense that all citizens have a general social duty to aid the enforcement of the criminal law. While some physicians may recoil at this mingling of law enforcement concerns with the altruistic act of providing care in an emergency, assisting law enforcement is not incompatible with providing adequate care. What the physician most owes a patient in an emergency is speedy, appropriate and well-administered treatment.

Rarely the physician may encounter a patient who rejects (or whose family rejects) medical care for a life-threatening disorder. The usual example is the Jehovah's Witness who refuses blood transfusions that are essential to preserve life, but other situations may arise when a patient declines vitally needed treatment. So long as the patient is legally competent, a physician may not lawfully compel treatment. But if the patient is legally incompetent, either by reason of illness or age, it is generally lawful to administer treatment over the objections of the patient or family where the alternative is death or severe disability. Here the societal interest in preserving life or health overcomes the presumptively unreasoning objections of the patient, or the objections of family members who may reject treatment on religious or other grounds unrelated to the health of the patient.

LIABILITY FOR BREACH OF LEGAL DUTIES

Malpractice

Negligence

In the typical medical malpractice suit a physician is charged with negligently harming a patient. To establish negligence a claimant must show that the physician's conduct was not consistent with reasonable or accepted standard of medical practice. To meet this burden the claimant must present testimony from other professionals describing what are reasonable or accepted standards of practice and stating how the defendant breached these standards.[3]

Testifying physicians must be qualified to offer an opinion, and it is grounds for excluding a physician's testimony that he or she lacks expertise in the subject matter of a suit. Accordingly, a general practitioner would not be permitted to testify in a suit against a neurologist or a specialist in emergency care. The exceptions are when the generalist either has special training or experience with the problem at issue or the problem itself can be analyzed in the context of non-specialized medical knowledge.[4] For example, a court would probably reject a generalist's testimony in a suit against a neurologist for failure to diagnose a spinal disorder unless the generalist provides evidence of special competence or the medical facts justify a finding that any reasonably competent physician should have made the diagnosis (as in a case where a patient complains of numbness and weakness in the legs after sustaining back trauma).

While the general rules about qualifications of physicians to testify are as stated, it is probably also fair to say that some courts will allow marginally qualified medical witnesses to testify. One reason for this may be that a particular court is unwilling or unable to make discriminating judgements about medical competence. It is easier to allow the matter of what weight to attach to medical testimony to be resolved by a jury than to endure lengthy arguments of counsel about whether a particular physician is expert enough to offer an opinion.[5] Also, a court may be reluctant to undercut a claimant's case at the outset by rejecting an offer of medical testimony, even if there are questions about its potential weight, because of the law's requirement that a case be dismissed if the claimant does not prove the relevant standards of care.[6]

Once a claimant presents evidence that a physician has failed to meet reasonable or accepted standards of care, the defendant has two avenues of attack. One is to demonstrate by artful cross-examination that the opinions of the claimant's medical witnesses are not well-founded. If it can be shown that the claimant's witnesses have not carefully analyzed the medical data, have reached conclusions that are not supported by facts, or have had little or no personal experience in handling cases similar to the one at issue, a court may conclude that the claimant's medical evidence is too uncertain to establish liability.[7] The other avenue is for the defendant to produce medical witnesses who testify that the defendant in fact met reasonable or accepted standards of care. Then it falls to the court to decide which testimony is the more persuasive. Since the burden is on the claimant to establish with a reasonable degree of certainty that the defendant was negligent, a stand-off in the medical testimony works to the benefit of the defendant.

To win a malpractice case it is not enough for a claimant to show that a physician breached reasonable or accepted standards of care. There must also be proof that the sub-standard care caused harm. This is illustrated by two court decisions in New York and California, both involving neurological emergencies.

In the New York case,[8] the issue was whether an inadequate evaluation of a patient with subarachnoid hemorrhage injured the patient. The patient lost consciousness at work and was brought to a hospital emergency room where, after a cursory examination, an intern diagnosed him as drunk and released him. Shortly after leaving he again lost consciousness and was then hospitalized for "cerebral dysfunction." He died a few hours later and at autopsy was found to have sustained subarachnoid hemorrhage from a ruptured aneurysm. In a suit against the hospital the claimant's medical witness testified that the intern's evaluation was substandard and that, had the patient been promptly admitted and placed at bed rest, he would have had an even chance of survival. A jury verdict for the claimant was reversed on appeal. The appellate court reasoned that, even though the intern may have been negligent, the medical testimony was insufficient to establish that non-negligent care would have prevented death from the intracranial hemorrhage.

In the California case,[9] the issue was whether a general practitioner's careless handling of a patient with a head injury caused the patient's death. The patient was brought to a hospital emergency room after an auto crash, "semiconscious," smelling of alcohol, and having a scalp laceration. On neurological examination he had "dilated and divergent" pupils and unassessable plantar responses. Because no neurosurgeon was available, the physician ordered that the patient be sent by ambulance to another hospital. He did not call the other hospital to advise it of the transfer nor did he try to ascertain if a neurosurgeon would be available there. While enroute the patient died. At autopsy he had many brain contusions and acute pulmonary edema. In a suit against the general practitioner, a neurosurgeon testified that the patient would probably have died no matter how he was treated. The court condemned the defendant's conduct, but agreed that the medical evidence did not support a finding that it caused the patient's death.

These cases illustrate the rule that, before liability is imposed on a physician, the claimant must prove that the physician's misconduct caused injury, not the disease or disorder itself. This rule protects a physician from penalty for not averting what is impossible to prevent. But if it is known that a patient would have had a reasonable chance of cure or survival if non-negligent care had been provided, no such protection exists. Indeed it is probable that courts will be increasingly disposed to finding a causal connection between sub-standard conduct and injury in any case where there is credible evidence that proper medical intervention might have been successful.

The issue of causation is often the determining factor in litigation involving emergency care. A physician responds to a life-threatening event and the patient dies or is left severely impaired. It is then asserted that the physician's response was not reasonable or acceptable under the circumstances, and the whole question of who or what caused what quantum of injury emerges.

In broad terms the legal concept of causation can be stated in one of two ways: A causal relationship between conduct and harm exists either (1) if *but for* the physician's conduct no permanent harm would have ensued, or (2) if the physician's conduct was a *substantial factor* in producing the harm. Thus, if a patient has a predictably lethal head injury, it would be unreasonable to attribute death to the physician's conduct, no matter how outrageous. But if a patient has a diagnosable and treatable head injury and the physician's response is careless, the physician's conduct decisively affects the outcome. Determining causation therefore involves asking what the physician could have done to change the outcome. If the answer is nothing, or if the answer is that the physician did what other similarly qualified physicians would have done, the physician is not legally responsible for a patient's death or disability.

Only in the exceptional case will a court find that a physician caused harm in the absence of unequivocal medical testimony to that effect. One example is where a layman could reasonably conclude that a causal relationship exists between medical misconduct and outcome, as where a physician at a suitably equipped hospital fails to order diagnostic X-rays for a traumatically-injured unconscious patient and the patient dies of a resectable subdural or epidural hematoma. In this hypothetical situation, a court might invoke the "common knowledge" doctrine to allow a claimant to prevail without expert medical testimony on the issue of causation.[10] A variation on the "common knowledge" doctrine is the concept of *res ipsa loquitor* ("the matter speaks for itself"). Under this doctrine, the burden of proving a lack of causal relationship between conduct and injury is placed on the defendant physician if the claimant shows (1) that the claimant's injury was not one which ordinarily occurs in the absence of negligence, (2) that the defendant was in control of the situation in which the injury occured, and (3) and the claimant did not act carelessly.[11] *Res ipsa loquitor* is sparingly applied by courts, and even then a court is likely to insist that there be medical testimony to the effect that the injury was improbable without negligence.

Lack of Informed Consent

In an unequivocal medical emergency the issue of informed consent is less significant than in other contexts. The physician is legally justified in doing what is medically appropriate to prevent death or disability, even if the patient resists or fails to cooperate.[12] Only if a claimant establishes that the physician acted unreasonably in concluding that an emergency existed would the issue of informed consent be seriously entertained by a court. Moreover, the claimant must also show that the non-consensual treatment was injurious before liability can be imposed.[13]

As an example of how an informed consent question might arise out of emergency care, consider the following case. Suppose that a patient is brought to a hospital emergency room after sustaining head trauma and is observed to have a single generalized seizure, following which he gradually becomes alert. In this circumstance there is no apparent threat to life. The intravenous administration of large dosages of anticonvulsants over the patient's objections is probably inappropriate—but not primarily because of the patient's objections. The central issue here is whether such treatment is reasonable after only one seizure. If as a consequence of the treatment the patient sustained cardiorespiratory arrest and permanent brain damage, the legal focus would be on the indications for the particular form of treatment, rather than on the fact that the patient did not consent to it. Nevertheless, a claimant's lawyer might also allege that, in addition to the negligent use of anti-convulsants, the physician also injured the patient by not obtaining consent to a potentially hazardous treatment.

The concept of informed consent has tortured physicians, lawyers and philosophers. There seems little disagreement in principle that doctors should tell patients enough to allow them to make some sort of informed choice before they agree to potentially harmful care. But how much to tell and by whose standards the adequacy of telling is evaluated are questions that have evoked a variety of answers. Also, even if one assumes a patient has been adequately informed, uncertainties may arise about whether agreeing to a particular treatment in the context of an acute illness is a free exercise of choice. Weighty as these concerns are, they may miss the point. What ordinarily determines the outcome of treatment of an immediately life-threatening disorder is the physician's skill, not the dialogue which antedates the treatment.

When the issue of informed consent is central to a suit against a physician, differing legal standards may apply depending on where the suit arises. In some states, a failure to obtain informed consent (however defined) may be deemed a battery,[14] and a physician is then subject to liability even if the patient suffers no harm. In most states, however, the issue of informed consent is considered analogously to negligence.[15] That is, liability turns on whether the physician's failure to disclose what reasonable medical practitioner would disclose harmed the patient. Without harm there is no liability. Thus, if a physician fails to obtain an informed consent to angiography for a patient with clinical evidence of subdural hematoma, the physician is not liable if the angiogram is both normal and uneventful. Whatever the rationale for liability, a suit based on lack of informed consent to an uncomplicated procedure is unlikely since there is scant basis for computing money damages.

In determining whether a physician acted reasonably in obtaining informed consent, one of two general standards applies. In some states, the focus is on what other physicians would have communicated in similar circumstances.[15] In other states, the adequacy of the informing process is assessed according to what a hypothetical reasonable person in the patient's position would need to know.[16,17]

These differing criteria have been referred to as "reasonable doctor" and "reasonable patient" standards, respectively. For example, if the conventional practice in state A which has adopted the "reasonable doctor" standard is that neurosurgeons do not tell patients that a risk of laminectomy for a herniated lumbar disc is loss of normal bladder function, a patient who sustained this complication could not recover solely on the basis of a lack of informed consent. But in state B which follows a "reasonable patient" standard, a different result is possible if the patient can establish that he would have rejected surgery had he known of this particular risk. Note, however, that even if a physician fails to meet a "reasonable patient" standard of disclosure, the claimant must still prove that the non-disclosure affected his or her decision. This may be a difficult task, particularly if the indication for the treatment was compelling (as where the patient had intractable pain and progressive loss of motor function).

There is no magic formula for achieving a lawful informed consent. The duty to inform clearly includes communication of the indications for test or treatment, alternative courses of action and the known hazards. But the manner in which information is communicated will obviously affect how well it is understood. An exhaustive, jargon-laden explanation may only confuse, although it may at least make the point that a particular test or treatment is not to be taken lightly. Similarly, a hurried last-minute explanation while the patient is being transported to surgery or X-ray does little to enhance the patient's understanding and would not constitute an adequate disclosure.

Where no emergency exists, physician and patient usually have enough time to discuss pros and cons of a particular test or treatment. But if the clinical situation does not permit extensive dialogue, the physician may be unable to assess whether patient or family truly perceive what is at stake. Here the physician must do the best he or she can, recognizing that the law will judge conduct by what is reasonable under the circumstances and not by what would have been optimal in the light of hindsight. As already indicated, where the need for prompt treatment is urgent, the issue of informed consent is a secondary legal consideration.

Signed consent forms, no matter how elaborate, do not fully resolve the issue of informed consent. They are, however, evidence that there was an attempt to explain and secure consent to a test or treatment, and together with other evidence may be very helpful to the physician who is accused of not obtaining a lawful consent. Thus, the combination of a signed consent form, witnessed by one who overheard the physician's explanation as well as the patient's assent, and a note by the physician in the patient's hospital record describing the attempt to inform should effectively counter any assertion that the physician ignored the duty to inform. The following notation in a patient's chart should be useful in this respect:

"(Insert date and time) I explained to (Mr., Mrs., Ms.) _____________ the indications and the risks of (test, treatment), including the risks of (indicate major known complications), and the available alternatives, and (he/she) then agreed to undergo it.

_____________(signature)_____________

Many patients who present as neurological emergencies are legally incompetent. One who is comatose, grossly demented, or in the throes of an agitated delirium can neither comprehend a physician's disclosure nor exercise a right of choice. If the notion of informed consent is to have any meaning in this circumstance, there must be someone to speak for the patient. In some emergencies, the physician must fill this role since awaiting the arrival of a family member or the appointment of a legal representative would be unthinkable if treatment is to have any chance of success.

Where a major treatment can be deferred without further harm to the patient, as in some cases of surgery for primary intraparenchymal brain hemorrhage, it is feasible and legally desirable to have the participation of a family member of other legal representative in the decision to employ risky and perhaps debatably useful treatments. But whatever are the physician's concerns about the patient's competence to consent to treatment in an emergency, the overriding legal consideration is the medical appropriateness of the treatment that is actually given. Law does not require the physician to make fine judgements about a patient's decision-making competence where to delay indicated treatment clearly risks further harm to the patient.[12] Indeed delaying treatment because of a preoccupation with the issue of the patient's competence or autonomy may open the physician to a claim of negligence.

Breach of Confidentiality

While most suits against physicians allege some form of malpractice, most often negligence and sometimes a failure to obtain informed consent, other claims may be pressed. One of the more significant is the claim that a physician has harmed a patient by an unauthorized disclosure of confidential matters.[18]

By legislation in many states a physician is barred from disclosing to others or to the general public information acquired in the course of providing medical care. Also, courts have fashioned a legal cause of action based on the notion of invasion of a personal right of privacy which is broad enough to include unauthorized disclosure by a physician of confidential medical information.[19,20]

While not a major legal risk, physicians providing emergency neurological care might become enmeshed in suits alleging breach of confidentiality. For example, suppose a prominent rock musician is brought to a hospital emergency room in coma from overdosage of an illicit drug. Because of the patient's stature the attending physician receives several phone calls from reporters and during the course of a conversation with one of them he discloses the cause of the coma. In this circumstance, he may be liable to the patient for whatever provable harm results from publication of this information.[18] That the physician was telling the truth is no defense here.

Or suppose that, in the absence of a law requiring that he report use of the particular intoxicant to state authorities, the physician nevertheless informs the police of the patient's drug usage. Although the physician might believe he is serving societal goals by such a disclosure, he has no firm legal basis for violating the patient's privacy. Other examples are readily conceivable, but the above examples emphasize the general rule that disclosure of medical data by a physician is legally impermissible unless the patient authorizes it, regardless of who the patient is or why he is ill.

There are important exceptions to the confidentiality rules. One is where a physician is required by legislation or administrative regulation to disclose specific medical data. The laws of many states require physicians to report to public health agencies certain infectious diseases (including neurosyphillis), epilepsy, drug addiction, or certain traumatic injuries (i.e., gunshot or knife wounds), and as part of the reporting process patients are identified by name.[21] Failure to comply with a reporting law is usually punishable by a fine or other penalty, but the physician who complies with a particular statute or regulation is immune from civil liability for breach of confidentiality. If it were otherwise, the social goals of the reporting laws would be thwarted and the physician would be placed in an intolerable position.

Even if a physician is not required by law to disclose confidential information, it may be permissible to do so to protect a patient or those whom the patient might injure. Although it would seldom arise in the circumstances of emergency neurological care, an important issue for physicians treating patients with epilepsy is how to handle reporting to motor vehicle agencies.[22] A brief discussion of this issue will illustrate the tension that may arise between the physician's duty to a patient and a more general social duty, and will apply to other situations where a patient's neurological condition makes driving dangerous (e.g., visual field loss, severe dementia, limb weakness that interferes with braking or steering).

Some states make epilepsy a reportable disease and leave the physician no choice about disclosure. Other states require patients to report their own epilepsy to motor vehicle agencies and the agencies then seek medical data from physicians after the patient has reported. Compliance with these laws by epileptics is clearly less than complete, but the extent of non-compliance is unclear. The physician may perceive a legal dilemma when caring for a patient whose epilepsy is poorly controlled yet who continues to drive. If a physician is not required by statute to report epilepsy but is unable to convince a patient not to drive, the physician faces a choice between making an unauthorized disclosure of confidential information or tolerating the risks the patient poses to self or others. In either case, the physician may feel legally vulnerable. Disclosure may evoke an invasion of privacy suit, while non-disclosure may open the physician to suit by a person whom the patient has injured.[23]

The physician's dilemma may be more apparent than real, however. If it is medically certain that the patient's epilepsy is poorly controlled or is otherwise apparent that driving is risky, it is improbable that a court would sustain an invasion of privacy suit if the physician reports the patient to a state agency. Courts in other situations have held that physicians may lawfully breach confidentiality where a patient's conduct threatens the interests of third persons,[19,24,25] and reporting the patient with uncontrolled epilepsy seems to fall within the rules of these cases. Further support for reporting can be found in codes of medical ethics which allow breaches of confidentiality to protect third persons.[26]

Divulging of confidential medical information by a physician is likely to disrupt the physician-patient relationship. No matter what the legal justifications, therefore, the physician should consider both the alternatives to disclosure (including repeated admonitions to the patient) and how to tell the patient that disclosure is forthcoming. A patient who understands that a physician is sensitive to privacy interests and yet is determined to protect the patient and others from harm, even if it means violating privacy, may be more willing to comply with medical instructions than one who sees the physician as essentially disloyal.[27] But if the physician cannot secure a patient's cooperation and the doctor/patient relationship is severed, the physician should still assist the patient to obtain another physician who is competent to treat epilepsy. The same principle holds for other disclosures, the result of which is to end a professional relationship.

Criminal Liability

Conceptual Basis

At first sight criminal law would seem irrelevant to the care of neurological disorders. Yet decisions about withholding or withdrawing care from patients with severe permanent neurological impairment raise the question of what constitutes homicide. Is the act of turning off a respirator in a permanently comatose patient with intact cardiovascular function murder, manslaughter, or an otherwise wrongful act? What of a refusal to attempt to rescucitate a profoundly demented patient? If not, what is the basis for excepting these acts from the law's prohibitions against conduct which causes or contributes to the death of a person?

These questions have surfaced in recent legislation and judicial decisions. Before discussing specific cases, however, certain themes of criminal law should be noted. One is that, before conduct is classified as criminal, there should be a societal consensus that it is morally culpable. Another is that defining certain forms of conduct as criminal should either promote socially desirable behavior or at least deter socially undesirable behavior. And, for those who engage in criminal conduct, there should be proportionate punishment, one feature of which is to deter future wrongful behavior. These themes underlie consideration of legal issues relating to brain death and withholding care from those with severe and permanent neurological impairment. While such issues seldom arise during treatment of a medical emergency, they concern any physician who must choose how vigorously to treat a comatose patient.

Brain Death

Since publication of the report of the Harvard ad hoc committee in 1968,[28] a consensus has developed among physicians that patients who meet certain criteria for irreversible loss of brain function are dead. Recognizing this consensus, a majority of state legislatures have enacted laws which authorize physicians to declare death on the basis of loss of brain functions. In a few other states the brain death concept has been adopted by judicial decision.[29-31] Moreover, commissioners of uniform state laws and representatives of the American Bar and Medical Associations have recently agreed on a Uniform Determination of Death Act (UDDA). This proposed legislation would allow death to be determined on the basis of "irreversible cessation" of either cardiorespiratory or brain functions, provided the determination is made "in accordance with accepted medical standards." The UDDA has been endorsed, among others, by the American Academy of Neurology and a presidential commission for the study of ethical problems in medicine, with the recommendation that it be adopted by all states.[32]

Given the broad agreement between medicine and law that irreversible cessation of brain function constitutes death, it is highly improbable that a physician in a state without brain death legislation would be found to have violated homicide laws by withdrawing care from a patient who met prevailing criteria for brain death. The only significant legal question in such a case would be the factual basis for the determination of brain death. Several sets of criteria for brain death have been published and, despite differences in some details, they agree on major principles. The essential elements of brain death are irreversible cessation of all cerebral and brainstem functions (including respiratory reflexes), and proof that the cause of coma is a disease or injury of the structure of the brain.[33] Methods of clinical testing for cerebral and brainstem function are well-described in standard texts. Table 20.1 summarizes the elements of a determination of death based on irreversible cessation of brain functions. From a medico-legal viewpoint, the physician making the determination of brain death must know the criteria and be competent to perform the appropriate clinical tests (including the assessment of oculovestibular reflexes and respiratory functions). If a physician is uncertain about either the criteria or how to test for loss of

Table 20.1 Determination of Death Based on Irreversible Cessation of Brain Functions

I. Cessation of brain functions
    A. Cerebral
        1. Unreceptivity and unresponsiveness to external stimuli
        2. Confirmable by electroencephalography or blood flow studies
    B. Brainstem
        1. Absence of pupillary, corneal, oculocephalic, oculovestibular and pharyngeal reflexes
        2. Absence of reflex ventilatory effort in presence of hypercarbia

II. Irreversibility of functional loss
    A. Etiology of coma known and accounts for clinical signs
    B. Adequate period of evaluation and treatment
    C. No basis for predicting recovery

III. Exclusion of factors that may interfere with determination
    A. Drug or metabolic intoxications
    B. Hypothermia
    C. Age less than 5 years
    D. Hypovolemic shock

brain functions, consulting with a knowledgeable physician is a self-evident legal and ethical requirement.

Once brain death has been determined, the physician must record in the patient's chart the findings which support the determination (e.g., cause of coma, absence of responses to noxious stimuli, absence of pupillary and oculovestibular responses, absence of respiratory effort in response to hypercarbia, electrocerebral silence on a technically adequate EEG, etc.). At present, the failure to prepare a suitably detailed note is one of the more certain ways to invite embroilment in a legal proceeding. For example, the brain death issue has most often reached the courtroom through an assertion by a defendant in a murder trial that the physician who turned off the respirator killed the patient, not the defendant who inflicted the head injury.[29-31] While courts have uniformly rejected this argument where there was adequate medical evidence of brain death, it should be apparent that an incomplete or illegible record of how brain death was determined will at the very least open the physician to uncomfortable questions about the validity of the determination.

Permanent Severe Neurological Impairment

The consensus about brain death does not extend to decisions about withdrawing or withholding care from those who are profoundly demented or malformed. A few courts have considered decisions of this nature, but there is little pertinent legislation. In the realm of emergency care of the neurologically impaired, the question is likely to be whether or not to initiate resuscitation. Decisions about withdrawing care are usually more deliberative. From the viewpoint of legal analysis, the difference between withdrawing and withholding life-support may not be significant. The important factors are the accuracy of the medical prognosis and by whom and how the decisions about care are reached. Prognosis is a technical question, but other aspects of the decisions call for participation by family (or legal representative) and consultants, and perhaps even by knowledgeable non physicians (e.g., ethicists, theologians, lawyers, judges).

Since "right" answers in this area are elusive, discussion will center on contrasting judicial approaches. Whether any one will gain wide adherence is speculative, but the physician who is confronted with writing or acting on an order not to rescucitate or who must otherwise make a therapeutic choice for a neurologically-impaired patient should be aware of the differing viewpoints. In states where the highest court has ruled on these matters (e.g., New Jersey, Massachusetts, New York), some rather specific legal guidance exists. Elsewhere the choice lies between acting on a carefully thought out agreement with a patient's family or relying on the advice of an experienced health care lawyer.

Much has been written about orders not to rescucitate (ONTR), but there is little law on the subject.[34] A Massachusetts appellate court recently considered the lawfulness on an ONTR for a woman with advanced Alzheimer Disease.[35] She was profoundly demented, incontinent, incapable of self-care, and had generalized vascular disease. Her physician predicted she would die within a year and foresaw the possibility of cardiac arrest at any time. He and her family (including a physician-son) agreed that an ONTR was appropriate, but the hospital administrators believed that an authorizing court order should be obtained. When asked to decide, however, the court ruled that advance judicial approval of an ONTR is unnecessary where the effect of rescucitation is a "mere suspension of the act of dying." The court observed that this particular case "presents a question peculiarly within the competence of the medical profession of what measures are appropriate to ease the imminent passing of an irreversibly, terminally ill patient." In Massachusetts it would now appear that, where the medical prognosis is reasonably certain and the attending physician and the patient's legal representatives are in agreement, an ONTR is lawful.

What is lawful in Massachusetts may not be elsewhere; thus, in developing a policy about ONTR, medical institutions in other states should consult their attorneys about what guidelines will best comply with local laws. It is probable that, in most states, guidelines will be found acceptable if they require a high degree of certainty about a prognosis that the patient is dying of an irreversible disease process and require participation by a patient's family or legal representative in the decision-making process. Once institutional guidelines are developed, physicians and nurses can implement ONTR with less uncertainty and anxiety than many now seem to experience.

Those who formulate guidelines for an ONTR or for any other decision to withhold or withdraw care will find in three recent state supreme court cases contrasting models of decision making. These cases are not the last word on the subject and as more litigation occurs a trend may develop. At the moment, however, no clear trend is discernible.

In the well-known case of Karen Quinlan,[36] the high court of New Jersey authorized the guardian of one in a persistent vegetative state to direct removal of a respirator and thereby exercise her constitutional right of "privacy," provided that the attending physician and a hospital "ethics committee" agreed she had no reasonable possibility of regaining "cognition or sapience." The court did not clarify what it meant by an "ethics committee," but the tenor of its opinion suggests that it viewed the committee as a means of validating the prognosis.

In the *Saikewicz* case,[37] the Massachusetts supreme court ruled that a judicial hearing is required before the doctrine of substituted judgement can be used to empower a guardian to authorize withholding of palliative treatment from an incompetent patient with an incurable disease. At issue was the propriety of withholding chemotherapy for an acute leukemia. The medical evidence indicated that treatment had a limited chance of producing a remission and no chance of cure. In stressing the need for a judicial order, the court expressed disdain for the role of medical or multidisciplinary committees in the decision-making process.

In the *Storar* decision,[38] which involved two companion cases, the New

York high court considered the issue of substituting judgement for incompetent patients. In one case it held that it is lawful to withdraw treatment from a patient in a chronic vegetative state without prior judicial approval if there is "clear and convincing" evidence that the patient had during competency indicated a desire not to have life-support in such a circumstance. In the other case, it refused to authorize discontinuance of palliative blood transfusions for a severely retarded adult male with terminal cancer who had never been competent to indicate a preference, even though his mother had asked that the transfusions be stopped. In other words, the New York court would permit withdrawal of life-sustaining treatment only where it is shown that this accords with the patient's wishes, *as expressed by the patient,* not by others acting on the patient's behalf.

These cases have provoked extensive comment, both critical and approving. While they involve differing factual situations and propose different methods of arriving at decisions to withhold or withdraw care, they hold that under certain circumstances it is legally acceptable to shorten a person's life by omission of some forms of treatment. *Quinlan* would keep the locus of decision-making within the medical institution, while *Saikewicz* would require judicial authorization. *Storar* would permit a private agreement between physicians and family (or legal representative) to withdraw care, but only if the patient's preference for this course of action is clearly evident. The court in *Storar* did suggest, however, that the state legislature should consider the problem, and the decision itself implies that a "living will" is one means by which a person can prevent the administration of purposeless care.

Several state legislatures have wrestled with proposed "living will" and "right to die" laws, but few laws have been enacted. Where they have, as in California,[39] the terminology is confusing and the coverage is uncertain.[40] Nevertheless, such legislation does suggest an emerging societal consensus about the "rightness" of stopping treatment.

One seeming advantage of legislation is to reassure participants in decisions about hopelessly ill or dying patients that stopping care is neither immoral nor, under specified circumstances, unlawful. A potential disadvantage is the difficulty of drafting a law which will cover the many different situations which may arise. There is also the deeper, less technical concern that society should be wary about granting advance legal immunity to those who would shorten other people's lives. The "best" decisions about terminal care are arguably those in which physicians and families retain a degree of uncertainty about the legal and moral consequences of their conduct, and are cautious, compassionate and thorough in their deliberations.[40]

The Problem Of Child Abuse

In response to data about the considerable extent of child abuse, the laws of all states now authorize or require physicians to report to public agencies instances of suspected child abuse.[41] Where reporting is mandatory, as it is in most states, non-reporting may be punishable by a fine or other penalty, and the physician is protected from liability for "good faith" reporting. Details of reporting requirements vary considerably from state to state and any physician who cares for traumatically-injured children should become familiar with relevant state reporting laws. No attempt will be made here to discuss the different type of reporting statutes.

A physician who treats a child with a neurological disorder that may be due to trauma inflicted by a parent or other adult has two forms of legal duty. Both derive from an obligation to the child. One is to provide appropriate medical care, and the other is to try to protect the child from future harm. The physician has no duty to protect the parents or other caretakers of the child from an investigation by the state. Indeed, the physician who carelessly fails to identify a case of child abuse may be liable to the child for injuries which the child later sustains at the hands of the abusing parents. This legal risk is exemplified in a recent California case.[41] There a physician did not appreciate that a child's injuries might be the result of parental abuse and thus did not report the case to the state. The child was later severely injured by one of the parents and the court held the physician liable to the child because he had negligently breached his duty to the child by failing to identify and report possible parental abuse. While this decision has drawn much criticism, it emphasizes that the social goal of protecting children from abuse places a major responsibility on the physician to be both aware of the problem of child abuse and an active participant in trying to control it.

LEGAL RISKS IN EMERGENCY MEDICINE (Table 20.2)

Providing medical care in an emergency undoubtedly carries with it a risk of later legal inquiry. This is true no matter how expert the care is. Of those who require emergency care, some will die or be left severely impaired. While improvements in physicians' abilities to treat life-threatening disorders have been dramatic, poor or fatal outcomes are inevitable and will be a source of lawsuits. The reflective emergency care physician will appreciate that no highly reliable prescription for avoiding lawsuits exists, and that medico-legal concerns are secondary in importance to the goal of practicing emergency medicine of the highest quality.

The notion that litigation is an inescapable accompaniment of emergency medical care is not particularly reassuring. So it is still proper to think in terms of reducing legal risks. But what reduces legal exposure most effectively is practicing in accord with professional norms. The legalistic premises of defensive medicine, which emphasize liberal use of diagnostic technology, may obscure the importance of careful clinical assessments. The following examples are illustrative.

One potential pitfall of emergency care is the failure to appreciate the significance of behavioral or emotional symptoms. Faced with a patient

Table 20.2 Legal Risks in Emergency Care

I. Preventable—high probability of civil liability
   A. Misdiagnosis because of:
      1. Careless examination or history taking
      2. Careless failure to perform indicated diagnostic tests
      3. Careless failure to obtain consultation
   B. Careless treatment

II. Preventable—possibility of civil liability
   A. Failure to obtain "informed consent" where it is feasible to do so
   B. Breach of confidentiality
   C. Failure to arrange or conduct adequate follow-up care
   D. Failure to document otherwise acceptable care

III. Preventable—civil liability improbable
   A. Careless failure to diagnose untreatable condition
   B. Careless treatment of predictably fatal or disabling disorder
   C. Failure to obtain informed consent to procedure which causes no harm

IV. Unpreventable—suit possible; liability improbable
   A. Unsuccessful treatment of predictability fatal or disabling disorder
   B. Misdiagnosis despite observing accepted medical standards
   C. Erroneous choice of treatment where choice not careless
   D. Failure to inform of unlikely complication of procedure and complication occurs

whose neurological status is normal but for agitation, irritability, inattentiveness, or a "peculiar" affect, the physician may dismiss the symptoms as responses to stress or as elements of the patient's pre-existing personality. Yet what these symptoms call for is further inquiry into their significance, be it careful re-examination, neurologic consultation, or more laboratory testing and X-rays. Depending on the clinical context, they may be due to hypoxia, other metabolic disturbances (e.g., hyponatremia), CNS infection or an early stage of increased intracranial pressure secondary to an epidural or subdural hematoma.

Earlier chapters have covered the approach to evaluating these symptoms. Suffice it to say here, many a malpractice suit arising from emergency care has rested on a physician's failure to evaluate emotional or behavioral symptoms by performing a careful examination of mental status. It is probably no longer defensible for any physician to claim that he or she can not be expected to know that such symptoms may reflect a neurological disorder. The symptoms must be evaluated, not because this will protect the physician from a lawsuit but because it may lead to diagnosis of a treatable disorder.

Similar considerations apply to other not readily explicable symptoms. One who complains of tingling extremities after a "whiplash" may have a compressive lesion of the cervical spinal cord, despite an unremarkable neurological examination and normal spine X-rays. One who is persistently nauseated after a seemingly minor concussion may have an epidural hematoma, despite otherwise normal findings. And so forth. The physician who quickly concludes that such relatively minor symptoms are of no account incurs a legal risk to be sure. More importantly, the physician fails to meet professional norms which call for careful re-evaluation and/or consultation.

The term "defensive medicine" implies testing that cannot be justified in terms of potential benefit to a patient. It may well be that routinely performing skull X-rays on all patients who have sustained head trauma, no matter how trivial, is censurable as defensive medicine. But it is also censurable as dubious medical judgement. The legal standard of care is determined by what is medically reasonable under the circumstances. There is no compelling medical indication to order skull X-rays for a patient who was briefly stunned, is now asymptomatic, has a completely normal neurological examination (including mental status), and can readily be followed as an outpatient. If the patient nevertheless turns out to have an epidural hematoma, it is the totality of the physician's conduct which will determine civil liability, not the mere failure to order an X-ray for which there was no clinical indication.

Another potential medico-legal hazard arises when appraisal in an emergency unit (including X-rays) leads to hospitalization for observation, and the observation itself is inadequate. As an example, consider again the patient with tingling in the extremities after a "whiplash." Suppose the patient is hospitalized, placed at bedrest, and is examined with decreasing frequency. Suppose, further, that on the second day the patient complains of difficulty moving his legs or difficulty urinating, but an incomplete bedside examination (which doesn't include an attempt to have the patient stand or walk) reveals no definite new findings. Finally, on the third day the patient becomes paraplegic from the effects of a spinal epidural hematoma at the cervicothoracic junction.

The point here is that early negative test results and clinical stability may lull clinicians into performing inadequate follow-up appraisals. All resources of emergency care, including consultants and X-rays, are marshalled for the initial appraisal and seldom are tests omitted which later assume medico-legal significance. But when the patient either seems to be stable or follows an atypical course, signs of deterioration are not promptly identified and an opportunity to intervene for the patient's benefit is missed. In this situation, the legal focus would be on the question of whether the follow-up care met professional standards. That initial appraisal was complete and medico-legally impeccable would not defeat a claim of negligence, although it might support an argument that there was no particular reason why physicians should have anticipated neurologic deterioration.

Another recurring issue in litigation arising from emergency care is the adequacy of the follow-up of patients who are treated and released. The assumption here is that the initial decision to release is compatible with professional standards, and that the only legal question is whether the patient was properly advised or proper arrangements were made for later care. For example, consider patients who are treated and released after seemingly minor head injuries. Many emergency units provide printed material describing what symptoms might herald clinical deterioration (e.g., increasing headache or lethargy, nausea and vomiting) and instructing the patient promptly to seek medical care if such symptoms appear. While these "head sheets" are probably useful from a medico-legal viewpoint, their primary purpose should be to alert patients (and families) to the potential seriousness of a head injury.

The releasing physician should also be satisfied that the patient or a competent family member comprehends the instructions, he should determine whether it is in fact feasible for the patient to return promptly to medical care if clinical worsening occurs, and should inquire if there is someone readily available to assist the patient in this circumstance. Where a patient expresses a preference for follow-up care by a physician other than the original examiner, it is necessary to ascertain who will follow the patient and communicate relevant medical information.

While it may seem simplistic to stress the medico-legal importance of adequate medical records in emergency care, poor record-keeping still plagues physicians and hospitals in their defense of malpractice suits. Despite harping on the subject by medical school professors and hospital administrators, lawyers and risk managers, too many medical records are fragmentary, uninformative or illegible. The result may be difficulty proving that a physician actually performed a complete neurological examination or considered differential diagnostic possibilities for a patient with neurological symptoms. Or, harkening back to the informed consent issue, a failure to record the fact of a discussion with a patient and/or family about the risks of an angiogram, myelogram or other potentially hazardous procedure complicates defense of a claim based on lack of informed consent.

A note which describes positive findings and pertinent negatives, summarizes results of laboratory and radiological tests, and indicates the management plan and its rationale is medically valuable and will more often than not be helpful in defending a lawsuit. This would seem particularly true in the context of emergency room care because the emergency room physician seldom has the opportunity to write follow-up notes which fill in details that were omitted during the first contact with a patient. Some notes may be turned against a physician in a legal proceeding, particularly when they describe facts to which the physician incorrectly responded. An example is a note which describes the appearance of pupillary asymmetry in a head-injured patient, but which also reflects that the physician did not perceive the clinical significance of the finding. On balance, however, descriptive and thoughtful notes will provide the physician far more benefit than harm in the medico-legal sense.

As a final cautionary note on record-keeping, a failure to maintain adequate medical records may be grounds for disciplinary action under state medical licensure laws. For example, regulations issued under the disciplinary sections of Maryland's licensure law[42] require the following with respect to medical records:"The records should be up to date, legible and should contain all pertinent patient information including history and physical examination, follow-up notes, laboratory work and notes from consultants.

The medical problems should be clearly stated . . ." (Guidelines-Peer Review–Title 10 section 1 (f))

CONCLUSION

In most respects the law of medical practice is straightforward (see Table 20.3). The basic rule is that the physician must meet reasonable or accepted standards of practice for his or her specialty or type of practice. This is as true for emergency care as for any other form of practice. However, law takes into account that the circumstances of emergency care are often such that some errors are unavoidable, errors that might be classified as negligence in circumstances where more deliberate care is feasible. Generally speaking, it would seem that the best way for the physician to cope with the threat of lawsuits arising out of emergency care is to maintain knowledge and skills that meet professional norms for emergency care. In other words, practice medicine that will satisfy one's peers and let the legal chips fall where they may. The central legal question in nearly every case reaching litigation will be the extent to which the physician's conduct deviated from professional standards as defined by physicians.

In those few cases where the issue of informed consent is dominant, the rules are not so straightforward. Where the "reasonable doctor" standard applies, the approach is similar to that in negligence actions. What other physicians do sets the standard. But in those several jurisdictions which apply a layman-oriented approach to what a physician ought to communicate, the physician may be uncertain about how much and in what form to communicate information relevant to a patient's choice. Even here, a disclosure which coherently describes risks, potential benefits and alternatives should not be a difficult exercise for most physicians and should provide adequate legal protection. Moreover, the number of cases which turn on the informed consent issue is small, far smaller than the amount of writing on the subject would indicate.

Until recently, cases involving withdrawal or withholding of care from hopelessly ill or dying persons had been handled informally by physicians and families without legal scrutiny. A few recent, highly publicized judicial decisions have proposed a more formal role for law in resolving these issues, and there is now considerable debate over the degree to which legal institu-

Table 20.3 Legal Duties of Physicians in Emergencies

   I. Conform to accepted or prevailing medical standards for managing particular problem

  II. Obtain "informed" consent of patient (or family member) for invasive procedures, but do not delay urgently needed procedures because of uncertainty about adequacy of consent

 III. Protect confidentiality of doctor-patient communications

 IV. Conform to state or local laws or regulations on reporting or on assisting law-enforcement

---

tions should participate. At this writing it is unclear what general principles will emerge, although there does seem to be a consensus that it is lawful either to allow or to some extent hasten the deaths of some hopelessly ill persons. As to questions about when death is diagnosable, the medical consensus that irreversible cessation of all functions of the brain indicates death has been largely adopted by legal institutions. The failure of some state legislatures to enact brain death legislation and the lack of uniform draftsmanship of existing laws have troubled some commentators, but there is little doubt about the general legal validity of the brain death concept.

REFERENCES

1. Calabresi, G.: The problem of malpractice. Trying to round out the circle. Toronto Law J 27:131, 1977.
2. Waltz, J.R. and Inbau, F.E.: *Medical Jurisprudence,* Macmillan, New York, 1971, pp. 38–58.
3. *Phillips v Stillwell,* 99 P 2d 104 (Sup Ct Ariz 1940).
4. *Frost v Mayo Clinic,* 304 Fed Supp 285 (DC Minn 1969).
5. *State v Carter,* 46 So 2d 897 (Sup Ct La 1950).
6. Curran, W.L., Shapiro, E.D.: Law Medicine and Forensic Science. 2d Ed., Little Brown & Co, Boston, 1970, pp. 329–330.
7. *Lawlor v Kolarsick,* 223 A 2d 281 (Super Ct NJ 1966).
8. *Myers v County of Nassau,* 319 NY Supp 2d 268 (Sup Ct NY 1971).
9. *Black v Caruso,* 9 Cal Rptr 67 (Cal App 1969).
10. *Corn v French,* 289 P 2d 173 (Sup Ct Nev 1955).
11. *Mayor v Dowsett,* 400 P 2d 234 (Sup Ct Ore 1965).
12. Waltz, J.R., Inbau, F.E.: Medical Jurisprudence. Macmillan, New York, 1971, p. 168.
13. *Rogers v Lumbermen's Mutual Casualty Co,* 119 So 2d 649 (La App 1960).
14. *Schloendorff v Soc of New York Hosp,* 105 NE 92 (Ct App NY 1914).
15. *Williams v Menahan,* 379 P 2d 292 (Sup Ct Kans 1963).
16. *Canterbury v Spence,* 464 Fed 2d 793 (DC Cir 1972).
17. *Cobbs v Grant,* 502 P 2d 1 (Sup Ct Calif 1972).
18. *Simonsen v Swenson,* 117 SW 831 (Sup Ct Neb 1920).
19. *Berry v Moench,* 331 P 2d 814 (Sup Ct Utah 1958).
20. *Hammonds v Aetna Casualty & Surety Co,* 237 Fed Supp 96 (ND Ohio 1965).
21. Waltz, J.R., Inbau, F.E.: Medical Jurisprudence. Macmillan, New York, 1971, Ch. 21, pp. 309–326.
22. Masland, R.L.: The physician's responsibility for epileptic drivers. Ann. Neurol., 4:485, 1978.
23. *Freese v Lemmon,* 210 NW 2d 576 (Sup Ct Iowa 1973).
24. *Tarasoff v Regents,* 17 Cal 2d 425 (Sup Ct Calif 1976).
25. *McIntosh v Milano* (L–44368–76 Calendar No 77–3811, Super Ct NJ 6/12/74).
26. Judicial Council Opinions and Reports. Amer Med Assn, Chicago, 1977, p. 5.
27. Stone, A.: The Tarasoff decision: suing psychotherapists to safeguard society. Harvard Law Rev. 90:358, 1976.
28. Beecher, H.K.: A definition of irreversible coma. JAMA, 205: 337, 1968.

29. *Commonwealth v Golston,* 366 NE 2d 744 (Sup Jud Ct Mass 1977).
30. *Lovato v Dist Ct,* 601 P 2d 1072 (Sup Ct Colo 1979).
31. *State v Shaffer,* 574 P 2d 205 (Sup Ct Kans 1977).
32. President's Commission for the Study of Ethical Problems in Medicine and Biomedical and Behavioral Research: Defining Death—Medical, Legal and Ethical Issues in the Determination of Death. US Gov Printing Off, Washington, 1981.
33. Guidelines for the determination of death. JAMA 246:2184–2186, 1981.
34. Allan, S.M.: No code orders vs rescucitation: the decision to withhold life-prolonging treatment from the terminally ill. Wayne Law Rev 26:139–172, 1979.
35. *In the Matter of Shirley Dinnerstein,* 380 NE 2d 134 (Mass App 1978).
36. *In re Quinlan,* 355 A 2d 647 (Sup Ct NJ 1976).
37. *Supertindent of Belchertown State School v Saikewicz,* 370 NE 2d 417 (Sup Jud Ct Mass 1977).
38. *Matter of Storar,* 52 NY 2d 363 (Ct App NY 1981).
39. Redleaf, D.L., Schmitt, S.B., Thompson, W.C.: The California Natural Death Act: an empirical study of physicians' practices. Stanford Law Rev 31:913–945, 1979.
40. Burt, R.A.: Taking Care of Strangers: The Rule of Law in Doctor-Patient Relations. The Free Press, New York, 1979.
41. *Landeros v Flood,* 551 P 2d 389 (Sup Ct Calif 1976).
42. Annotated Code of Maryland, Health Occupations, Section 14–404, 1981.

Index

Page number followed by t represent tables.

Abdominal aortic by-pass surgery, neurologic
    complications, 326
Abducens nerves in intracranial hypertension, 69
Abscess
    brain, 475–480
        antibiotic regimens, 479–480
        causative agents, 478–479
        diagnostic tests, 39–40, 134t, 476–477
        differential diagnosis, 476
        hematogenous, 478
        in children, 405
        incidence, 476
        intracranial hypertension in, 65
        mortality, 480
        signs and symptoms, 476, 476t
        surgery for, 480
        treatment, 479–480
    spinal epidural, 318–320
Absence seizures, 107, 109–110, 119
Acetazolamide (Diamox), in acute glaucoma, 333
Acetylcholine, 220–221
Acetylcholinesterase, 220–221, 266
Acid maltase deficiency, 242
ACTH, 119, 371
Acyclovir, 486
Adenine arabinoside (ARA-A; Vidarabine)
    in herpes simplex encephalitis, 333, 486
    in herpes zoster, 489, 490
Affective disorders, vs delirium, 280
Air myelography, 29
Airway management, in neurologic emergencies,
    4–5, 100, 177, 253–255, 253t
Akinetic mutism, 99
Akinetic seizures, 107, 108
Alcoholism
    coma diagnosis in, 83
    dementia and, 306
    myopathies in, 242
    neuropathy in, 265, 268
    seizures and, 110–111
Alternating hemiplegia, 139
Alzheimer's disease, 304
Aminoglycosides, in bacterial meningitis, 473t
Amipaque myelography, 29
Amitriptyline (Elavil), 263, 490

Amnesia. *See also* Amnesic syndromes
    anterograde, 293
    psychogenic, 297
    retrograde, 294, 298–299
    transient global, 295
Amnesic syndromes, 293–299. *See also* Amnesia
    chronic, 299
    clinical evaluation, 297–299
    differential diagnosis, 297
    diffuse causes, 296–297
    etiology, 295–296, 295t
    focal causes, 295, 297
    in dissociative reactions, 281
    symptoms, 265, 294, 296t
Amphetamine abuse, 367
Ampicillin, 473t
Amyotrophic lateral sclerosis (ALS), 227–230,
    250, 366
Amyotrophy
    diabetic, 232–233
    neuralgic, 250
Amytal interview, 283
Analgesics in head injury, 179
Anemia
    blackouts due to, 166
    causing anoxia, 415–416
Anesthesia
    and metabolic coma, 82
    in patients with neuromuscular disease, 243,
        225
    paraplegia due to, 327
Aneurysm
    aortic, spinal cord complications of, 326
    intracranial. *See also* Hemorrhage, intracranial
        etiology, 130
        third nerve palsy and, 351–352
        vision loss and, 342
Angiography, cerebral
    in central nervous system infections, 40
    in intracranial hemorrhage, 152, 153–154,
        155
    in ischemic disease, 136, 139–141
    in TIA evaluation, 31, 173
    in trauma assessment, 38
    intravenous digital subtraction (IVDSA), 45

Angiography—*continued*
  value, risks and costs, 28–29, 30t
  vs computed tomography, 29
Anomic aphasia, 290
Anoxia, brain
  amnesia and, 296
  anaerobic metabolism, 413
  anemic, 415–416
  anoxic, 414–415
  cerebral syndromes following, 420–421, 421t
  coma and, 425–427
    management, 434–435
  compensatory mechanisms, 413, 415
  edema due to, 64
  effects on consciousness, 413
  histotoxic, 416–417
  ischemic, 417
    clinical neurologic syndromes following, 420,
      422, 421t
    neuropathological features, 417–420
  post-cardiac arrest, 434–435
  primary vs secondary events, 435–436
  radiologic evaluation, 43
  spinal cord syndrome following, 421–422, 421t
  treatment, 432–436
  types of, 414–417, 414t
Antidepressants, toxicity, 263. *See also* under
  individual drug names
Anterior cord syndrome, 198
Antibiotics, penetration of brain parenchyma,
  479t
See also under individual drug names
Anticoagulants
  in cerebral infarction, 143
  in TIAs, 174–175
Anticonvulsants
  in neonates, 399–400, 400t
  overdose, 263
Antiepileptic drugs
  characteristics of, 122t
  general principles, 119–121
  in chronic epilepsy, 115
  volume of distribution, 116t
Antifibrinolytic agents, 153
Antiplatelet drugs, in TIAs, 175
Anxiety, and transient neurologic symptoms, 163,
  167–168
Aphasia. *See also* Aphasic syndromes
  anomic, 290
  Broca's, 288–289
  conduction, 289
  expressive, 288–289
  fluent, 290–291, 291t
  global, 290
  non-fluent, 287
  transcortical motor, 289
  transcortical sensory, 289
  Wernicke's, 289
Aphasic syndromes, 284–285. *See also* Aphasia
  classic lesions, 289t
  classification, 288–290

differential diagnosis, 288t
  evaluation, 287–288, 291–293
Apnea, criteria for brain death, 424
Apoplexy, pituitary, 342
Apraxia(s), 300–303
  anatomic lesions causing, 302
  buccofacial, 301, 302
  clinical features, 301t, 301–302
  differential diagnosis, 303
  evaluation, 303
  ideational, 301
  ideomotor, 301
  unilateral limb, 301, 302
Arachnoid villi, 60
Arousal. *See* Consciousness, level of
Arrhythmias, cardiac
  in neuromuscular disease, 255–256
  transient neurologic symptoms due to, 163
  with cerebral infarction, 137
Arsenic poisoning, neurologic effects, 263, 265,
  268, 329
Arteriography, in TIAs, 173
Arteriosclerosis, transient visual loss and, 342
Arteriovenous malformations (AVM)
  cerebral hemorrhage and, 158, 443
  in children, 403
  vision loss due to, 344
Arteritis
  giant cell (GCA) and vision loss, 336, 337–338
  presentation, 449
  temporal, 241
Aspirin therapy in TIAs, 175
Ataxia, acute
  in cerebellar hemorrhage, 74
  in childhood, 408–410, 409t
  in migraine, 447
  in multiple sclerosis, 377
Atrophy
  cerebral neuronal, 304–305
  localized, vs subdural hematoma, 42
Atropine, 267, 271
Auditory comprehension in aphasia, 292
Aura
  in classical migraine, 164, 366, 453
  in seizure disorders, 103, 104
Axonal neuropathies, 231t, 233–235

Babinski sign, 15, 87, 92
Back pain, non-traumatic, 312
Baclofen (Lioresal), for multiple sclerosis, 373
Barbiturates. *See also* under individual drug
  names and intracranial hypertension, 101–102,
  192
    post-cardiac arrest, 436
    toxicity, 88, 91–92, 264, 265
Basilar artery
  migraine, 455
  thrombosis, 100, 344
Becker's dystrophy, 240
Behavioral disorders, drug and toxin induced,
  264–265

Bell's phenomenon, 92
Biopsy
  brain, 485–486
  muscle, 225
Blackouts, 104, 104t, 165–167
Black widow spider bites, 251
Bladder dysfunction
  in multiple sclerosis, 377–378
  in spinal injury, 211, 312
Bleeding disorders, lumbar puncture in, 49, 50, 49t
Blepharitis and visual loss, 331
Blood flow, cerebral
  in anoxia, 413
  in blackouts, 165, 166
  management in cerebral infarction, 136–137
  post-ischemic vasoconstriction, 436
Botulism
  electromyography, 225
  infantile, 407
  presentation and diagnosis, 237, 245t, 355
  treatment, 238
Bowel dysfunction, in multiple sclerosis, 377–378
Brachial neuritis, 233–250
Brachial plexus injuries, 213, 233
Brain
  abscess. *See* Abscess, brain
  anatomy and physiology, 59–61
  antibiotic penetration, 479t
  anoxia. *See* Anoxia, brain
  biopsy, in herpes encephalitis, 485–486
  cell death, common causes, 3t
  compressive lesions, 70, 73. *See also*
    Intracranial pressure, increased
  edema. *See* Edema, brain
  hemorrhage. *See* Hemorrhage, intracranial
  herniation. *See* Herniation, brain
  ischemic lesions. *See* Infarction, intracranial
  mass lesions. *See* Mass lesions, intracranial
  pain pathways, 440–441, 440t
  post-cardiac arrest syndromes, 418–420, 434–435
  post-electric shock syndromes, 429–430
  structural vs non-structural lesions, 5–7, 13t, 14t, 16t, 16–17
  tumors. *See* Mass lesions, intracranial
  vascular lesions. *See* Cerebrovascular disease
  vasculature, 128–130
Brain death
  clinical criteria, 22, 422–425, 423t, 506t, 506–507
    in children, 389, 410
    supplementory tests, 425
  emergency room determination, 95
  legal issues, 505–507
  vs cerebral death, 422
Brainstem
  anatomy and physiology, 59
  compressive lesions, 69, 70. *See also*
    Intracranial pressure, increased
  hemorrhagic lesions, 178

  in coma, 80
  infarction, 138–139. *See also* Infarction, intracranial
  multiple sclerosis lesions, 375–377
  reflexes
    in brain death, 424–425
    in coma diagnosis, 87, 97t
    in increased intracranial pressure, 68–74
  tumors, 65
Brain syndrome, organic, drug-induced, 264–265
Breath holding spells, pediatric, 104, 401–402
Breath odor, in coma diagnosis, 94
Brown-Séquard syndrome, 197
Bruit, carotid, 147
Bulbar palsy, 227
Burr hole, cranial, 189–190
Butyrophenones (Haldol) poisoning, 264
Bypass surgery
  abdominal aortic, neurologic complications, 326
  extracranial-intracranial, 146, 174

Caffeine toxicity, 263, 265
Caloric stimulation, 90–91
Carbamate toxicity, 266
Carbamazepine (Tegretol)
  in multiple sclerosis, 375–378
  in post-herpetic neuralgia, 491
  in status epilepticus, 124
  toxicity, 263, 264
Carbenicillin, 473t
Carbohydrate metabolism, disorders of, 413–414, 435
  in infants, 408
Carbon disulfide toxicity, 268
Carbon monoxide toxicity
  neuropathology, 264, 265, 268, 416
  treatment, 271
Cardiac arrest
  anoxic coma following, 425–427
    management, 434–435
  clinical neurologic syndromes following, 420–422, 421t
  following electric shock, 428, 430
  neuropathology, 415, 417–420, 418t
Cardiopulmonary resuscitation (CPR)
  techniques, 432–434
Cardiovascular dysfunction in neurologic disease, 5, 255–256
Carnitine palmityltransferase (CPT) deficiency, 242
Carotid artery
  anatomy, 128–130
  aneurysm
    and third nerve palsy, 352
    and vision loss, 342
  bruit, 147
  occlusion
    etiology, 140
    symptoms, 169–170, 170t
    TIAs associated with, 31t, 170, 170t, 172, 173

Carotid artery—*continued*
   traumatic, 188
   vision loss due to, 342
Carotid-cavernous fistula, 188, 353–354
Carpel tunnel syndrome, 231
Catatonia, vs coma, 98–99
Cauda equina injuries, 198–199
Causalgia, 214
Cavernous sinus lesion, 353
Cefotaxime, 473t
Central cord syndrome, 197
Cephalosporin, 472
Cerebellar incoordination. *See* Ataxia
Cerebellar lesions
   hematoma, 156–157
   hemorrhage, 70, 74, 80–81, 100
   infarctions, 146
   presentation, 80, 100
Cerebral aneurysms. *See* Aneurysms, intracranial
Cerebral angiography. *See* Angiography,
  cerebral
Cerebral blood flow. *See* Blood flow, cerebral
Cerebral hemorrhage. *See* Hemorrhage,
  intracranial
Cerebral infarction. *See* Infarction, intracranial
Cerebrospinal fluid (CSF)
   analysis. *See* Lumbar puncture
   antibiotic penetration, 472t
   circulation, 60
     abnormal, 66–68
   excess, 68
   in acute encephalitis, 482
   in bacterial meningitis, 18–19, 469–470, 470t
   in brain abscess, 477–478
   in brain infarction, 143–144
   in central nervous system infections, 467t
   in coma diagnosis, 96
   in herpes encephalitis, 484–485
   in increased intracranial pressure, 54–55
   in intracranial hemorrhage, 152
   in multiple sclerosis, 381
   in obstructive cord lesions, 315
   in seizure disorders, 109, 117
   in viral meningitis, 466–467
Cerebrovascular disease. *See also* Hemorrhage,
  intracranial; Stroke; Thrombosis; TIA
   anatomy and pathophysiology, 128–136
   incidence, 127
   in infants and children, 402–404
   ischemic. *See* Infarction, intracranial; Stroke
Cervical collars, 194
Cervical lesions. *See* Spinal cord injuries
Cervical osteoarthritis, vs meningitis, 468
Charcot-Marie-Tooth disease, 235
Cheyne-stokes respirations, 70, 92
Chiasmal compression, 342
Chickenpox, 491
Child abuse
   legal aspects, 509–510
   neurologic signs, 404

Children
   acute ataxia in, 403–410
   bacterial meningitis, 467–475
   brain death criteria, 389, 410
   cerebrovascular disease, 402–404
   complex headaches in, 404–405
   drowning, 430, 431–432
   increased intracranial pressure, 393–394, 395t
   metabolic diseases, 407–408, 408t
   neurologic diseases, incidence and etiologies,
    387, 388t
   neurologic exam in, 388–389, 391–392
   seizures, 119, 397–402, 399t
   spinal muscular atrophies, 226–227
   use and interpretation of lab tests, 392–393
Chloramphenicol
   in bacterial meningitis, 473t
   in brain abscess, 479–480
Chlordane toxicity, 268
Choroid plexus papilloma, 68
Chvostek's sign, 250
Ciliary flush, 333
Cimetidine, 191
Circle of Willis, 129–130
Clonazepam, 119
Cloxacillin, 473t
Cocaine abuse, 264, 265
Codeine, 179
Coma, 79–102
   anatomical, 82
   anoxic post-cardiac arrest, 410, 421, 425–427
    management, 434–435
   attempted arousal, 86
   causes, 97t, 99–100
   criteria for brain death in, 422–423
   definition, 80
   differential diagnosis, 98–100
   drug-induced, 263, 264
   emergency room assessment, 82–102
   eye reflexes, 68–69, 87–92
   history, 82–83, 83t
   in children, 396, 403
   incidence, 79
   laboratory tests, 43, 95–98
   lumbar puncture, 96
   metabolic, 82, 86
   neurologic exam, 83–92
   pathoanatomy, 80–82
   pathophysiology, 80–82
   physical exam, 93–94
   posturing, diagnostic significance, 84–87
   prognosis, 94–95, 427
   radiologic patterns, 79, 95–96, 97t
   respiratory patterns in, 92
   structural causes, 84t
   subacute onset, 99
   sudden, 99
   toxicologic analysis, 96–98, 261–263
   treatment in ER, 100–102, 271
Coma scales, 94–95
Command testing in aphasia, 292

Commission on Classification and Terminology
of the International League Against Epilepsy,
106
Compression. *See also* Intracranial pressure,
increased
brain, 70, 73
peripheral nerve, 212
spinal cord. *See* Spinal cord compression
syndromes
Computed tomography (CT)
cerebral toxins and, 43
in acute disorders of mental status, 42
in anoxia, 43
in bacterial meningitis, 470
in brain abscess, 476
in cerebellar hematoma, 157
in children, 393, 404
in coma diagnosis, 43, 79, 95–96, 97t
in encephalitis, 40, 134–136, 484
in headache, 404
in infections of the CNS, 39–40, 134–136, 470,
489
in intracranial hemorrhage, 48, 150–152
in intracranial hypertension, 38, 75
in multiple sclerosis, 43, 381
in seizure management, 40–41, 117–118
in spinal lesions, 317
in stroke management, 31, 33, 134–136
in TIA, 171
in trauma assessment, 37–38, 37t
limitations, 21
risks, 27–28, 30t
vs cerebral angiography, 29
vs nuclide brain scan, 28
Concussion
cerebral, 180
spinal, 196
Conduction aphasia, 289–290
Confabulation phenomena, 297–298
Confidentiality, breach of, 503–505
Confrontation naming in aphasia, 291–292
Confusion. *See* Dementia; Memory disorders;
Orientation disorders
Conjunctivitis and vision loss, 331
Consciousness
content of, acute disorders, 42, 275–309, 275t
level of
diagnostic significance, 8–9, 9t
in children, 392
in head injury, 178
in stroke patient, 132
posturing, diagnostic significance, 84–87
terminology, 80
Constipation, in multiple sclerosis, 377–378
Contusion, cerebral, 4, 181
in children, 403
Conus medullaris lesions, 198
Conversational speech in aphasia, 291
Conversion headache, 458–459
Conversion reactions, 281–282

Cornea
inflammation of, 332–333
reflexes, in coma diagnosis, 92
ulcerated, 333
Corpus callosum lesions, 302
Corticosteroids
adverse reactions, 371
in acute myelopathy, 318, 320, 323, 324, 327
in herpes zoster, 489
in intracranial hypertension, 76
in multiple sclerosis, 371–372
in optic neuropathy, 341, 374, 375
Cranial nerve signs, 138–139
in children, 391
in trauma, 184, 188
Craniectomy, 190–191
Craniopharyngioma, cystic, 342
Craniotomy, fronto-temporo-parietal, 191
CRAO. *See* Retinal artery occlusion, central
Cresyldiphenyl phosphate toxicity, 268
Criminal liability in emergency care, 505–509
Crutchfield tongs, 204–205
CT. *See* Computed tomography
Current, electric, effects on human body, 428
Cyanide kit, 271
Cyanide poisoning, 271, 417
Cyst, cerebellar, 366

Dacryoadenitis, 331
Dacryocystitis, 331
Dantrolene sodium (Dantrium), 373
DDT, neurologic syndromes, 268
Death
brain. *See* Brain death
cerebral, 422
Delirium
agitated, 277
causes, 277, 278t
drug-induced, 264–265
post-operative, 279
presentation, 276–277
withdrawal, 276–277
Delirium tremens, 277
Dementia, 303–308
alcoholic, 306
differential diagnosis, 304–305
evaluation, 306–307
multi-infarct, 305
terminology, 303–304
tumor-induced, 306
vs pseudodementia, 307–308, 307t
Depression
in multiple sclerosis, 378–379
vs dementia, 307, 307t
Dermatological exam, 450
Dermatomyositis, 241
Desipramine (Norpramine) toxicity, 263
Devic's disease, 324–325
Dexamethasone (Decadron)
in brain abscess, 480
in cerebral edema, 76, 143

522 *Index*

Dexamethasone—*continued*
  in head injuries, 179, 191
  in intracranial hemorrhage, 150
  in metastatic epidural neoplasm, 318
  in spinal cord injury, 195
Diabetes insipidus, and head injury, 93, 193
Diabetes mellitus, neuromuscular complications, 232–234
Diabetic dysequilibrium syndromes, 65
Diaphragm, in neuromuscular disease, 254
Diazepam (Valium)
  in multiple sclerosis, 373
  in pediatric seizures, 400, 401
  in status epilepticus, 109, 123
2,4-dichlorophenoxyacetic (2,4-D) toxicity, 268
Diet, in multiple sclerosis, 370
Digitalis, 277
Dihydroergotamine, in migraine, 461
Diphtheria, neuromuscular complications, 235
Diplopia, 348–360
  comitant, 356
  crossed, 357
  emergent, 69, 351–359
  in multiple sclerosis, 376
  monocular, 356
  non-diplopia, 356
  non-emeregent, 356
  restrictive, 356
  uncrossed, 357
Diplopia fields, 357–358
Diplopia syndromes
  diagnosis, 360
  examination, 357–360
  ocular ductions in, 357
  ocular versions in, 357
Dislocations, spinal, 205–207
Disordered repetition, 287–288
Dissociative reactions, 281–282
Dizziness
  causes, 167
  clinical and laboratory tests, 168–169
Doll's eyes, 69, 90
Double simultaneous stimulation (DSS), 300
Double vision. *See* Diplopia
Doxepin (Sinequan) toxicity, 263
"Drop attacks", 107, 108, 170
Drowning
  clinical features, 431
  dry vs wet, 430
  freshwater, 430–431
  incidence, 430
  neuropathology, 431–432
  saltwater, 431
  treatment and prognosis, 431–432
Drug-induced neurologic syndromes, 259–272, 269t
  behavioral disorders, 264–265
  clinical evaluation, principles of, 260–261
  diagnosis, 259–260
  laboratory evaluations, 261–263
  management, 270–272

  metabolic changes, 82, 264
  movement disorders, 264
  neuromuscular problems, 266–268
  orientation disorders, 264–265, 275t, 278t
  physical examination, 260
  physiologic antagonists, 271
  reflex changes, 87, 88, 92, 260
  seizures, 263–264
Duchenne muscular dystrophy (DUD), 239–240, 256
Dural sinuses, 60
Dysarthric disorders, 285–288
Dyskinesia, orofacial, 264
Dysphagia, in neuromuscular diseases, 246–247, 253, 254–255
Dysphasias, 114
Dysphonia, 246–247, 253, 254–255
Dystrophies
  Becker's, 240
  Duchenne muscular, 239–240, 256
  facioscapulohumeral, 240
  limb girdle, 240
  myotonic muscular, 240, 250, 251
    neonatal, 406–407
  scapuloperoneal, 240

Eaton-Lambert syndrome, 225, 238
Eclampsia, vs intracranial hemorrhage, 157
Edema, brain
  computed tomography in, 38, 75
  cytotoxic, 62
  hydrocephalic, 64
  in brain abscess, 480
  in brain infarction, 143
  in meningitis, 474
  vasogenic, 63
EEG. *See* Electroencephalogram
Elderly patients, seizures in, 111
Electrocution injuries, 427–430
  acute syndromes following, 429–430
  incidence, 427–428
  resuscitation, 430
Electroencephalogram (EEG)
  as criterion for brain death, 410
  during brain anoxia, 413
  in acute encephalitis, 482
  in brain abscences, 478
  in children, 393, 394t, 402
  in coma diagnosis, 95
  in disorientation disorders, 282–283
  in seizures, 107–108, 118–119
Electromyography (EMG), in neuromuscular disorders, 223–224
Elderly patients, seizures in, 111
Embolus, with brain infarction, 130, 131t, 140–141
Emesis, induced, 271
EMG. *See* Electromyography
Encephalitis, acute, 480–482
  arbovirus, 482–483
  causes, 481t

diagnostic tests, 40, 134–136, 482, 484
herpes simplex, 483–486
increased intracranial pressure in, 64–65
signs and symptoms, 481–482, 481t
Encephalomyelitis, 325, 490
Encephalopathy
anoxic, 430–432
hepatic, 94
hypertensive, 187
lead, 65
metabolic, 82
Endophthalmitis, 345
Endrin toxicity, 268
Epidural pressure monitoring, 188
Epidural tumor, metastatic, and spinal
syndromes, 317–318
Epiglottitis, 389
Epileptic seizures
akinetic, 107
differential diagnosis, 166
definition, 104
generalized, 106, 107–108, 119
in children, 397–402
international classification of, 106–108, 106t
intractable, 115
partial, 106–107
post-traumatic, 193
psychomotor, 106
secondary corticoreticular, 107
temporal lobe, 106
unclassified, 108
vs hypotensive episode, 85
Episcleritis and visual loss, 331
Epsilon aminocaoroic acid (Amicar), 153
Erb's paralysis, 213
Ethanol abuse, 265, 268
Ethosuximide (Zarontin), in seizures, 114, 119,
123–124
Ethylene glycol toxicity, 264
Euphoria, in multiple sclerosis, 378–379
Evoked potentials testing, 379–381
Exercise
in multiple sclerosis, 370
rhabdomyolysis due to, 252
Extracranial-intracranial (EC-IC) bypass, 146, 174
Eye. *See also* Vision loss
herpes zoster infections, 487
myopathies affecting, 240
reflexes, 68–69, 87–92, 260

Facial nerve lesions, 188
Facilitating myasthenic syndrome, 238
Facioscapulohumeral dystrophy, 240
Factitious disorders, 280–281
Falx cerebri, 59
Febrile seizures, 401
Femoral nerve, 213
Fever, with neurologic signs, 18, 93. *See also*
Abscess, brain; Encephalitis, acute; Meningitis
Fisher syndrome, 354
Fistula, carotid-cavernous, 188, 353–354

Flashlight ophthalamic exam, 347–348
Fluid management
in comatose patient, 101
in head injuries, 191–192
in meningitis, 474
in pediatric neurologic disease, 389
Foramen magnum tumors, vs multiple sclerosis,
366
Foramen of Magendie, 60
Foramina of Lushka, 60
Forced duction tests, 356
Fourth nerve palsy, 353
Fractures
cranial
basilar, 38, 91, 180–181
depressed, 38, 181
linear, 180
radiologic assessment, 37–38
spinal, 199–203
management, 204–208
Frontal lobe lesions, cognitive disorders of, 283–
284
Furosimide (Lasix)
in brain edema, 76
in intracranial hemorrhage, 150

Ganser state, 294, 297
Gasoline vapor inhalation, 268
Gentamicin, 472, 473t
Giant cell arteritis, 336, 337–338
Glasgow Coma Scale, 94, 95t, 178, 178t
Glaucoma, acute, 333–334, 447, 449
Gliomas, 65, 112
Glucose, cerebrospinal fluid levels, 55, 56–57

Glucose metabolism, cerebral
in anoxia, 413–414, 435
in infants, 408
Glue-footed gait, 284
Gower's sign, 239
Grand mal seizures, 107–108
Graves' disease, 341, 356
Guillain-Barré syndrome
cardiac complications, 256
diplopia and, 354
signs and symptoms, 234, 244, 245t, 250
treatment, 234–235
Gunshot wounds
analgesics in, 211
head injuries, 184
nerve lacerations, 213
spinal lesions, 199

Hallucinations, 276, 277, 280
Halo brace, 200, 205–206
Hangman's fractures, 200
Harrington distraction rods, 203, 208
Headache
character and severity, 445–446
classification, 441–442
clinical exam, 448–451

Headache—*continued*
  conversion, 458–459
  diagnostic approach, 439–443
  differential diagnosis, 69, 452–459
  duration, 444
  etiology, 55, 441–442t
  in children, 404–405
  migraine. *See* Migraine headaches
  motor disturbances, 447
  muscle contraction, 457–458, 460
  nerve pathways, 440
  neurologic exam in, 451–452
  organic non-migrainous, 458
  pain location, 440–441, 445
  patient history, 443–448, 448
  psychogenic, 458–459
  signs and symptoms, 450, 447
  therapy, 459–462
  vascular, 457
    vs non-vascular, 442–443
  visual symptoms, 446
  vomiting, 446–447
  with central nervous system disorder, 69, 452–456
  with systemic disorder, 452
Head injuries, 177–193
  complications, 192–193
  cranial nerve lesions, 184, 188
  edema, 64
  fractures. *See* Fractures, cranial
  gunshot wounds, 184
  increased intracranial pressure in, 64
  in infants and children, 402–403
  initial evaluation and treatment, 177–179, 191
  intracranial hemorrhage. *See* Hemorrhage, intracranial
  radiologic tests, 179
  sedation and pain relief, 179
  signs and symptoms, 449, 450
  surgical management, 188–191
  vascular injuries, 188
Heat stroke, 93
Heavy metal toxicity
  laboratory analysis, 262
  neurologic effects, 264, 265, 267
  treatment, 268
Hematoma
  cerebellar, 66, 156–157
  epidural, 65, 65t, 181
  in children, 404
  increased intracranial pressure and, 65, 65t, 66
  radiologic testing, 34–35, 38, 42, 134t
  spinal epidural, 320–321
  subdural, 42, 65, 134t, 181–182
Hematomyelia, 196, 328
Hemi-inattention syndromes, 299–300, 300t, 303
Hemiparesis
  diagnostic significance, 179
  signs and symptoms, 84
Hemispheric dominance and language disorders, 285

Hemorrhage, intracranial
  angiogram in, 152, 153–154, 155
  basal ganglionic, 99
  causative mechanisms, 130–131, 131t, 147–150, 154
  cerebellar, 70, 74, 80–81, 100
  computed tomography in, 134t, 146, 150–152
  increased intracranial pressure in, 65, 150
  infratentorial, 184
  lumbar puncture in, 47–48, 152
  management, 147–158, 151t
    early measures, 150
    medical, 64, 154–155
    surgical, 154, 155–156
  neonatal intraventricular, 403–404
  pontine, 100
  signs and symptoms, 64, 70, 99, 149–150, 178–179
  subarachnoid, and acute spinal cord syndrome, 328
  supratentorial, 181–183
  thalamic, 89, 99
  transient neurological symptoms with, 163
  traumatic, 182, 184
  vs hypertensive encephalopathy, 157
  vs infarction, 132, 133t, 133, 146
Hemorrhage, spinal cord, 199, 328
Heparin
  in brain infarction, 143
  in coma, 101
  in spinal cord injury, 209
  in TIA, 174–175
Herniated disc syndromes, 321–322
Herniation, brain. *See also* Intracranial pressure, increased
  and third nerve palsy, 352
  central, 59, 70
  early symptoms, 70
  lumbar pucture and, 47, 49
  uncal, 59, 71–72, 352
Herpes simplex encephalitis, 483–486
  antiviral treatment, 486
  diagnostic tests, 484–485
  differential diagnosis, 485t
  mortality, 486
  signs and symptoms, 484
Herpes simplex keratitis, 332–333
Herpes zoster, 486–491
  complications, 489–491
  incidence, 486–487
  management, 487–489
  myelitis, 327
  opthalmicus, 487–489
  signs and symptoms, 487
High altitude anoxia, 414
Hip fractures, vs hemiparesis, 84–85
Hippus, 88
Horner's syndrome, 88, 213–214
Hydrocephalus
  acute, 70
  communicating, 66

in children, 409
intracranial hypertension and, 64
mechanisms of, 66–68
normal pressure, 305–306
obstructive, 66
signs and symptoms, 69
Hydrocortisone, in migraine, 461
Hyperadrenalism, myopathies in, 242
Hyperkalemia, and periodic paralysis, 243
Hyperosmolar agents, in intracranial
hypertension, 76
Hyperpathia, in multiple sclerosis, 375
Hypertension, intracranial. *See* Intracranial
pressure, increased
systemic
in brain infarction, 137
in coma diagnosis, 93
in intracranial hemorrhage, 150
Hyperthermia, malignant, 243, 252
Hyperthyroidism, myopathies and, 241
Hyperventilation, 76, 163
Hypoadrenalism, myopathies in, 242
Hypocalcemia, myopathies, 250
Hypoglycemia
and transient neurologic symptoms, 163–166
vs brain infarction, 147
Hypokalemia, and periodic paralysis, 242
Hypomagnesemia, 250
Hyponatremia, complicating head injury, 192–
193
Hypotension
following spinal injury, 196, 210
in coma diagnosis, 93
orthostatic, 163, 166
postural, 168
secondary to drug and toxin poisoning, 270
vs epilepsy, 85
Hypothermia, in coma patient, 93
Hypothyroidism, myopathy and, 241, 251
Hypoxia, cerebral. *See* Anoxia, cerebral
Hysteria, vs organic neurologic disease, 19–20
Hysterical paralysis, 199
Hysterical seizure disorders, 104t, 116, 119
Hysterical unresponsiveness, vs coma, 98

Ice pick pains, 169, 446
ICP. *See* Intracranial pressure, increased
Increased intracranial pressure. *See* Intracranial
pressure, increased
Idoxuridine (Stoxil), 333
Infants. *See also* Children
bacterial meningitis in, 468–469
botulism, 237, 407
myasthenia gravis in, 236
neurologic exam in, 388–389, 391–392
spinal muscular atropies, 226–227
Infarction, brain. *See also* Stroke
anticoagulant therapy, 143
border zone, 419
central retinal artery, 334–335
cerebellar, 146
cerebral angiography, 139–141
ciliary artery, 336–339
computed tomography in, 134t
dementia in, 305
early management, 4, 136–147
end zone, 419–420
following global anoxic ischemia, 418–420, 419t
hemi-inattention syndromes and, 299–300
increased intracranial pressure and, 65
in pediatric patient, 403
in young adults, 145, 145t
localizing the lesion, 138–139, 138t
lumbar puncture in, 143–144
mechanisms, 130, 133
preservation of brain tissue, 136–138
progressing, 141–143
surgery in, 145–146
systemic hypertension and, 137
transient neurologic symptoms and, 163
vs hypoglycemia, 147
vs intracranial hemorrhage, 132–133, 33t
Infarction, spinal cord, 325–327
Infections, central nervous system
early diagnosis and management, 465–491
delerium in, 278t
in children, 405–406
radiologic techniques in assessment, 39–40
Infectious diseases, complicating neuromuscular
disease, 257
Influenza, myalgias in, 250
Informed consent in neurologic emergency care,
500–503
Innervation ratio, 220
Insecticides, toxic effects, 266
Intensive care unit delirium, 279
Interferon, human leukocyte, in herpes zoster,
489
Intervertebral disc, herniated, 321–322
Intracranial pressure, increased, 59–77
abnormalities of cerebrospinal fluid flow and,
66–67
acute encephalitis, and, 483
anatomy and physiology, 59–61
benign, 68
brain abscess, and, 476
diffuse, 64–65, 64t
etiologies, 64–68
evaluation, 74–75, 74t
following head injury, 191–192
in children, 393–394, 395t
in intracranial hemorrhage, 150
lumbar puncture in, 54–55, 75
mass lesions, and, 65–66
mechanisms of, 62–64
radiologic evaluation, 42
rapid onset, 69, 70
signs and symptoms, 68–74
slowly developing, 69
transient vision loss, 69, 343
treatment, 75–77, 101
vomiting, 446–447

Intrathecal infections, acute spinal cord
  syndrome and, 327
Intubation, 5, 101
  in children, 389
Iridectomy, 333–334
Ischemia, cerebral. *See* Infarction, intracranial;
  Transient ischemic attack
Isoniazid toxicity, 264, 268

Jefferson fractures, 200

Kanamycin, 473t
Keratitis, 331, 332–333
Ketamine toxicity, 265
Ketogenic diet, 119
Korsakoff's syndrome, 294, 297–298
Kugelberg-Welander disease, 227
Kussmaul respirations, in coma diagnosis, 92

Labrynthine disease
  transient neurologic symptoms, 163, 167
  vs multiple sclerosis, 376–377
Lacerations
  nerve, 213
  scalp, 177, 180, 188
Language disorders
  aphasic. *See* Aphasia
  disordered expression, 287
  dysarthric, 285–288
  hemispheric dominance, 285
  schizophrenic, 290–291, 291t
  signs and symptoms, 265, 367–368
Legal aspects of neurologic emergency care, 493–
  497
  child abuse, 509–510
  criminal liability, 505–509
  patient-oriented duties
  professional standards, 494–496
  reducing legal risks, 510–514, 511t
  society-oriented duties, 496–497
Lennox-Gastaut syndrome, 402
Leukoencephalopathy
  anoxic, 418–419
  progressive multifocal, 367
Lhermitte's sign, 324, 375
Lightning strikes, 427–430
Limb girdle dystrophy, 240
Limb movement in coma diagnosis, 84–87
Lindane toxicity, 268
Literal paraphasias, 287
Lithium toxicity, 264, 265
Locked-in syndrome, 98
Lumbar puncture, 47–57
  artifacts, 21, 56
  acute spinal cord syndromes following, 327
  complications, 52–54, 55, 53t, 320–321
  contraindications, 6, 48–50, 49t
  in acute encephalitis, 482, 484–485
  in bacterial meningitis, 18–19, 469–470,
    470t
  in brain abscess, 477–478

  in brain infarction, 143–144
  in children, 392
  in coma diagnosis, 96
  indications, 47–48, 48t, 75
  in increased intracranial pressure, 54–55
  in intracranial hemorrhage, 152
  in mass lesions of the brain, 49
  in multiple sclerosis, 381
  in seizure disorders, 109, 117
  in spinal cord lesions, 315
  in status epilepticus, 109
  in viral meningitis, 466–467
  interpreting results, 54–57
  technique, 51–52
  traumatic tap, 54–55
Lumbosacral plexopathy, 233
Lupus erythematosis, disseminated, 326–327

Malingering, voluntary, 280–281
Malpractice, 497–505
Mannitol
  contraindications, 192
  in brain abscess, 480
  in brain edema, 76
  in coma, 101
  in head injured patient, 192
  in intracranial hemorrhage, 150
Marcus-Gunn pupil, 334, 347
Mass lesions, intracranial
  abscess. *See* Abscess, brain
  brain herniation and, 70–72
  coma and, 81
  dementia and, 306
  delirium and, 277, 278t
  hematoma. *See* Hematoma, intracranial
  hemorrhage. *See* Hemorrhage, intracranial
  intracranial hypertension and, 65–66, 65t
  lumbar puncture in, 49t, 49–50
  posterior fossa subdurals, 409
  radiologic tests, 134t
  sixth nerve palsy and, 352
  subtentorial, 65, 66t, 70, 73–74
  supratentorial, 65, 65t
  vs multiple sclerosis, 366
McArdles disease, 242
Meclizine HCL (Antivert), 377
Median nerve injuries, 213
Memory disorders, 293–299
  chronic, 293–299
  clinical evaluation, 297–299
  differential diagnosis, 297
  etiology, 295–296, 295t
  modality specific, 298
  short-term, 294
  symptoms, 294, 295t
Meningioma, 65
Meningitis
  bacterial, 467–475
    antibiotic therapy, 471–474, 472t
    blood cultures, 470–471

cerebrospinal fluid analysis, 18–19, 47, 48, 469
  common etiologic agents, 471t
  complications, 405
  differential diagnosis, 109, 469t
  neurologic complications, 474–475
  prognosis, 468
  signs and symptoms, 468
  treatment, 475
  hemophilus influenza, 405, 472, 475
  increased intracranial pressure in, 64–65
  radiologic tests, 40
  viral, 465–467, 466t
    diagnostic tests, 47, 48, 466–467
Mental status, acute changes in, 275–308
Meperidine (Demerol), in migraine, 461–462
Meralgia paresthetica, 213
Mercury neuropathy, 265, 267
Metabolic disease, in infancy, 407–408, 408t
Metabolic imbalance
  in anoxic anoxia, 415
  delirium due to, 278t
  drug-induced, 264
Metastatic disease, spinal, 43
Methadone toxicity, 264, 271
Methaqualone (Quaaludes), 263
Methicillin, 473t
Methohexital, 101
Methemoglobinemia, 271
Methylene Blue, 271
Metoclopramide (Reglan), 460–461
Metrizamide myelography, 29
Migraine headaches
  basilar artery, 455
  classical, 453
    underlying lesions, 443
  complicated, 453, 454t
    lesions mimicking, 453t, 457t
    management, 462
  cutaneous signs, 450
  differential diagnosis, 366–367, 452–456
  familial history, 448
  hemiplegic, 454–455, 455t
  narcotic therapy for, 461–462
  ophthalmic, 456
  ophthalmoplegic, 456
  pediatric, 404–405
  prodromal period, 164, 366, 453
  therapy, 460–462
  transient neurologic symptoms and, 104, 163
  variants, 456
  visual symptomatology, 344, 446
Moneuritis multiplex, 232–233
Mononeuropathy, 231–232
Morphine, in head injured patient, 179
Motor neuron
  normal anatomy, 220
  pathology, 226–230, 226t, 244, 245t, 250
  signs in spinal lesions, 198, 313
Movement disorders, drug-induced, 264

Moxalactam, 472, 473t
Moya-Moya disease, 403
Mucocoele, sinus, 342
Mucormycosis, 353
Multiple sclerosis
  age of onset, 363
  ataxia and tremor in, 377
  benign form, 363
  bowel and bladder dysfunction, 377–378
  brainstem dysfunction, 375–377
  classification criteria, 361–363
  complicating infections, 367
  course, 361–363
  demyelination mechanisms, 365
  diagnostic tests, 43, 379–384
  diet, 370
  differential diagnosis, 365–369, 368t, 369t
  epidemiology, 364
  etiology, 364–365
  exacerbation, 363, 370
    incidence, 363, 364
  exercise in, 370
  malignant, 363
  management
    general principles, 370–371
    steroid, 371–372
  mental and psychological symptoms, 378–379
  nausea and vertigo, 376, 377
  paroxysmal symptoms, 378
  placebo response, 371
  prognosis, 363–364
  remission, 363–364, 365
  sensory dysfunction, 375
  signs and symptoms, 162, 168, 369–370
  stress in, 370, 379
  transverse myelopathy, 324–325
  weakness and spasticity, 372–373
Mumps meningitis, 466
Muscle(s)
  aches, 249–251, 249t
  biopsy, 225
  cell destruction. *See* Rhabdomyolysis
  contraction, 221–222
  cramps, 250–251, 249t
  diseases of, 238–243, 239t. *See also* Myopathies;
    Neuromuscular diseases
  fibers, 222
  weakness
    associated problems, 247–248, 454–455
    complicating herpes zoster, 490
    differential diagnosis, 245t
    distal, 244
    drug and toxin induced, 266–268
    facial, 244–246
    in multiple sclerosis, 372–373
    laboratory investigations, 248
    management, 248–249
    pharyngeal, 246–247
    proximal, 244
    ptosis, 244
Muscle tension headaches, 457–458, 460

Muscular atrophy, progressive, 227
Muscular dystrophies, 239–240
Mutism, akinetic, 99
Myalgias, 249–251, 249t
Myasthenia gravis, 225, 235–237, 244, 245t
  diplopia in, 354
  laryngeal muscle function, 246
  myalgia, 250–251
  transient neonatal, 236, 406
Myelin, anatomy and physiology, 220
Myelinating neuropathies, 231t, 233–235
Myelinolysis, central pontine, 367
Myelitis
  acute transverse, 322–323, 323t
  in multiple sclerosis, 324–325
  herpes zoster, 327
  spinal cord, 322–325, 327
Myelography
  contraindications, 322
  in spinal cord disease, 315
  risks and costs, 29–31, 30t
Myelopathy. *See* Spinal cord, disorders of
  acute necrotic, 328
  lupus, 327
  radiation, 323–324
  transverse, 322–323, 323t
  toxic, 329
  vs recurrent neoplasm, 324t
Myoclonus, drug-induced, 264
Myoglobinuria, 251–252
Myopathies. *See also* Neuromuscular disorders
  alcoholic, 242
    endocrine, 241–243, 244
    inflammatory, 240–241, 245, 250
    metabolic, 241–243, 244
    ocular, 240
    toxic, 241–243, 2
Myophosphorylase deficiency, 242
Myosin, 221–222
Myositis, 241
Myotonia, 251
Myotonic muscular dystrophy, 240, 251

Nafcillin, 473t
Naloxone toxicity, 271
Naproxene sodium, in migraine therapy, 461
Narcolepsy, 104
Narcotic antagonists, 100, 271
Narcotics, pupillary reactions, 88
Nasal symptoms in acute headache, 447
N-butyl-ketone toxicity, 268
Neck stiffness, 447
Necrosis, spinal cord, 328
Negligence, professional, 497–500
Neologism, in aphasia, 287
Neonate. *See also* Children; Infants
  intracranial hemorrhage in, 403–404
  myotonic dystrophy in, 406–407
  seizures in, 398–401, 399t, 400t
  transient myasthenia gravis, 406–407

Neostigmine (Prostigmine), in myasthenia gravis, 236
Nerve(s), peripheral
  anatomy and physiology, 220
  biopsy, 226
  compression, 212
  conduction velocity (NCV), 222–223
  diseases of, 230–235, 231t, 245t
  injuries, 212–217
    initial evaluation and management, 212
  irritability, 250
  lacerations, 213
  pathways, 440
  rehabilitation, 216–217
  root avulsions, 213
  stretching, 212
  surgical management, 215–216
Neuralgia, post herpetic, 489, 490–491
Neuralgic amyotrophy, 250
Neurinoma, acoustic, 25
Neuritis, optic, 373–374
Neurologic examination, 14–16, 14t
  in cerebrovascular disease, 132
  in comatose patients, 83–92
  in drug and toxin-induced neuropathy, 263–264
  in headache, 451–452
  in increased intracranial pressure, 75
  in infants and children, 388–389, 391–392
  in spinal cord lesions, 312–315
Neurologic impairment, severe, legal aspects of care in, 507–509
Neurologic syndromes
  diagnostic methods in, 8–10
  diagnostic pitfalls in, 17–22
  differential diagnosis, 11t
Neuroma, following nerve injury, 214
Neuromuscular anatomy and physiology, 220–222
Neuromuscular disorders, 219–257
  cardiac complications, 255–256
  clinical presentation, 243–249
  diagnostic techniques, 222–226, 248
  drug-induced, 266–268
  dysphagia and dysphonia, 246–247, 253, 254–255
  electrodiagnostic studies, 222–225
  infectious complications, 257
  lower motor neuron diseases, 226–230, 226t, 244, 245t, 250
  mechanical ventilatory support, 253–255, 253t
  muscle aches and cramps, 249–251
  muscle biopsy, 225
  muscle disease, 238–243, 239t. *See also* Muscle; Myopathies
  muscle weakness, 244–249, 245t
  nerve biopsy, 226
  neuromuscular junction, 235–238, 245t
  pediatric, 406–407
  peripheral nerve diseases, 230–235, 231t, 245t
  respiratory complications, 253–255, 253t

Neuromuscular junction
  normal anatomy and physiology, 220, 235t
  diseases of, 235–238, 235t, 244, 245t
Neuromyelitis optica, 324–325
Neurons
  anoxic sensitivity, 418, 420
  motor
    normal anatomy and physiology, 220
    pathology, 226–230, 226t, 245t
Neuropathy
  diabetic proximal, 232–233
  diphtheric, 235
  drug and toxin-induced, 266–268
  optic. *See also* Diplopia; Vision loss
    compressive, 341
    in multiple sclerosis, 373–375
    ischemic, 336–339, 343
    pressure, 162–163
N-hexane toxicity, 268
Nitroprusside, in hypertensive stroke patient,
  137, 150
Nodes of Ranvier, 220
Normal pressure hydrocephalus, 305–306
Nuclear Magnetic Resonance (NMR), 45
Nuclide brain scan
  for brain abscess, 476–477
  in stroke diagnosis, 33, 136
  value and limitations, 28, 30t
Nutritional causes of orientation disorders, 278t
Nystagmus, in multiple sclerosis, 375–376

Occlusion, vascular. *See* Infarction, intracranial;
  Thrombosis
Ocular bobbing, 89
Ocular dipping, 89
Oculocephalic maneuver, 90
Odontoid fractures, 201
Olfactory nerve lesions, 184, 188
Ophthalmoparesis, 91–92
Ophthalmopathy. *See* Vision loss
Ophthalmoplegia, 240, 256
  bilateral, 354
  inernuclear, 355, 376
  unilateral, 353–354, 451–452
Ophthalmoscopy, 348
Organic brain syndrome, toxic, 164–165
Organophosphates, neuromuscular effects, 238,
  245t, 266–267
  treatment, 267, 271
Orientation disorders, 275–284. *See also*
  Dementia
  defective cognitive control, 283–284
  differential diagnosis, 277–282, 278t
  drug and toxin induced, 264–265, 275t, 278t
  evaluation, 282–283
  in multiple sclerosis, 378
  schizophrenia, 279–280
  symptoms, 276–277
Orthoisoprophenyldiphenyl phosphate toxicity,
  268
Orthostatic hypotension, 163

Otic infections and brain abscess, 478
Otorrhea, in head injuries, 180–181
Overdose, drug. *See* Drug overdose
Over-the-counter (OTC) agents and organic brain
  syndrome, 265
Oxygen therapy, in carbon-monoxide poisoning,
  271

Pain
  behavioral response to, 449
  pathways in head and neck, 440–441
Pain sensitive intracranial structures, 440t
Palsy
  brachial, 233
  bulbar, 227
  fourth nerve, 353
  ocular, 456
  peroneal, 232
  radial nerve, 232
  sixth nerve, 69, 88, 91, 352
  third nerve, 87–88, 91, 351–352
  upgaze, 355
Pantopaque myelography, 29
Papaverine (Pavabid), in migraine therapy, 462
Papilledema
  in intracranial hypertension, 69, 344
  vs optic neuritis, 374
Paraldehyde, in status epilepticus, 123, 123t
Paralysis
  drug and toxin induced, 266–268
  hysterical, 199
  periodic, 242–243, 245t
Paraphasias, evaluation, 287
Parasympathetic nervous system, and increased
  intracranial pressure, 69
Paresthesia, drug and toxin induced, 266–268
Parietal lobe lesion, and hemi-inattention
  syndrome, 300
Patient follow-up, legal aspects, 19, 512–513
Patient history in neurologic emergency care,
  10–13, 12t
Pediatric neurologic disease. *See* Infants;
  Children
Penicillin
  in bacterial meningitis, 473
  in brain abscess, 480
Pentobarbital, in intracranial hypertension, 101–
  102
Periarteritis nodosa, myelopathy and, 327
Periodic paralysis, 251
Peroneal palsy, 232
Personal identity, loss of in amnesia, 294, 297
Petit mal, 107
Phenastix testing, in phenothiazine toxicity, 98
Phencyclidine (PCP, angel dust) toxicity, 262, 265
Phenobarbital
  in neonatal seizures, 400t, 400
  in subarachnoid hemorrhage, 153
  toxicity, 263
Phenothiazines toxicity, 263, 264

Phenytoin (Dilantin)
  in multiple sclerosis, 375, 378
  in neonatal seizures, 400
  in status epilepticus, 123, 124
  toxicity, 263, 264, 265
Philadelphia collar, 206–207
Phosphofructokinase deficiency, 242
Physical exam in neurologic emergencies, 13–14, 13t
Physostigmine, in coma, 87–88, 101
Pilocarpine, 3, 333
Pinprick testing in spinal cord injuries, 196, 313
Pins and needles, in multiple sclerosis, 375
Pituitary apoplexy, 354
Plain film diagnostic techniques, 26–27, 30t
Plexopathy, 233
Pneumoencephalography (PEG), 28–29
Pneumonia, complicating neuromuscular disease, 257
Poison. *See* Toxin
Poison control center, 262
Poliomyelitis, 230, 245t
Polymyalgia rheumatica (PMR), 241, 250, 337, 338
Polymyositis, primary, 241
Polyneuropathy, 233–235
Pontine lesions, 80, 86, 88, 100
Porphyria, 235, 245t
Positron emission tomography (PET), 45
4-poster brace, 206–207
Posterior communicating artery aneurysm, 348–352
Posterior fossa. *See* Subtentorial compartment
Post-operative delirium, 279
Posturing
  decerebrate, 68, 85–86
  decorticate, 68, 85–86
Pott's disease, 320
Prednisone
  in Graves' ophthalmopathy, 341
  in multiple sclerosis, 372
Pregnancy, eclampsia vs intracranial hemorrhage, 157
Pressure, intracranial
  increased. *See* Intracranial pressure, increased
  monitoring techniques, 188–189
Pressure neuropathy, 162–163
Pressure sores, and spinal injury, 211
Primary lateral sclerosis, 227
Primidone, 121
Principles of neurologic emergency management, 3–22
Prochlorperazine (Compazine), in multiple sclerosis, 377
Promethazine (Phenergan), in migraine therapy, 461
Propoxyphene (Darvon) toxicity, 271
Prostaglandin inhibitors, in acute migraine, 461
Protein
  cerebrospinal fluid, 56
  metabolism disorders, 408

Pseudocholinesterase deficiency, 243
Pseudocoma, 98
Pseudodementia, 307–308, 307t
Pseudo-seizures, 116
Pseudotumor
  cerebri, 42, 68, 69
  orbital, 356
Pulmonary function in neuromuscular disease, 253–255, 253t
Pupillary reactions
  in brainstem herniation, 70, 71
  in coma, 87–88
  in head injuries, 178
  innervation, 68–69
Pyridostigmine (Mestinon), in myasthenia gravis, 236

Quadriplegia, 179, 195, 196, 210–211

Radial nerve lesions, 213, 232
Radiation myelopathy, 323–324, 324t
Radiologic tests in neurologic emergencies, 25–45
  acute disorders of mental status, 42
  anoxia, 43
  cerebrovascular disease, 31–35
  coma, 43
  computed tomography. *See* Computed tomography
  in children, 393
  increased intracranial pressure, 42
  infections, 39–40
  effectiveness, 21, 25–31, 30t
  multiple sclerosis, 43
  nuclide brain scan. *See* Nuclide brain scan
  plain film. *See* Plain film
  seizures, 40, 117
  spinal cord disorders, 315–317, 319
  spinal injuries, 43–45, 195
  stroke patients, 31, 33, 134–136
  toxins, 43
  trauma, 36–38
Radionuclide brain scan. *See* Nuclide brain scan
Ramsay Hunt syndrome, 490
Reading assessment in aphasia, 292–293
Reasonable doctor standard of disclosure, 501
Record-keeping, medico-legal aspects, 513
Red blood cells in cerebrospinal fluid, 54, 55, 56
Red eye, and glaucoma, 449
Reduction methods, in spinal dislocations, 205–207
Reflex responses
  criteria for brain death, 423t, 423–424
  drug-induced changes, 263–264
  in children and infants, 391
  in coma, 83–92
  pupillary. *See* Pupillary reactivity
Renal failure, acute
  due to myoglobin challenge, 252
  in coma, 93
Repetition testing in aphasia, 292

Repetitive stimulation, in neuromuscular
 disorders, 224–225, 248
Res ipsa loquitor, 500
Respirator disconnection procedures in brain
 death, 424–425
Respiratory arrest, in electric shock, 428, 429
Respiratory complications
 in children, 389
 in coma, 92, 100
 in intracranial hypertension, 68, 70–71
 in neuromuscular disorders, 253–255, 253t
 in trauma, 177
Responsive naming, in aphasia, 292
Resuscitation
 cardiopulmonary techniques (CPR), 432–434
 in electrical trauma, 430
Resuscitation orders, legal aspects, 507–509
Reticular activating system, (RAS)
 and coma, 80–82
 in intracranial hypertension, 68
 pathoanatomy, 59, 80
Retinal artery occlusion, central, (CRAO), 334–
 336, 344
Retinal detachments, 340
Retinal holes, 340
Retrobulbar neuritis, 374
Reye's syndrome, 394–395, 398t
Rhabdomyolysis, 245t, 247, 251–252, 251t
 drug and toxin induced, 252, 264
Rhegmatogenous detachments, 340
Rhinorrhea, 180
Rifampin, in meningitis, 475
Rum fits, 110–111

Salicylates toxicity, 264
Scalp lacerations, 177, 180, 188
Scapuloperoneal dystrophy, 240
Schizophrenia, 279–280
 vs fluent aphasia, 290–291, 291t
Sciatic nerve injuries, 213
Sclerosis
 amyotrophic lateral (ALS), 277–230, 250, 366
 multiple. *See* Multiple sclerosis
 primary lateral, 227
Scoliosis, 255
Sedimentation rates, in optic neuropathy, 337
Seizure disorders, 103–125
 alcohol related, 110–111
 atypical presentation, 110
 biochemical tests for, 117
 case studies, 103, 109–110, 111–112
 classification, 106–108, 108t
 clinical examination, 112–114
 clinical presentation, 103–112
 definitions, 104
 differential diagnosis, 104–105t
 drug differentials associated with, 263–264
 history, 112–113
 hysterical, 104t, 116, 119
 indications for hospital admission, 114–116
 in meningitis, 475, 475t

 in children, 397–402, 399t
 in post-arrest coma, 434
 in the elderly, 111
 laboratory investigations, 40, 116–119
 management, 119–124
  general principles, 120, 121t
 multiple sclerosis and, 367, 378
 physical examination, 113–114
 post traumatic, 111, 162, 168
 psychosocial aspects, 116, 124
 radiological tests, 117–118
 reflex anoxic, 401–402
 status epilepticus. *See* Status epilepticus
 symptomatic seizures, 111–112, 115
 structural etiologies, 113t, 113–114
 tonic, 378
Sensory dysfunction
 in multiple sclerosis, 375
 in severe headache, 447
Sexual dysfunction, in spinal cord disorders, 312
Shingles, 486–491. *See also* Herpes zoster
Sinemet, in post herpetic neuralgia, 491
Sinusitis, and brain abscesses, 478
Sixth nerve lesions, 69, 88, 91, 352
Skew deviation, 355
Skin infections, and lumbar puncture, 49, 50
Skull films
 in coma diagnosis, 96
 in seizure disorders, 117
 in trauma assessment, 36–37, 37t
 efficacy, 26, 30t
Skull fractures
 basilar, 38, 91, 180–181
 depressed, 38, 181
 linear, 180
 radiologic assessment, 37–38
Skull percussion, in coma diagnosis, 93
Sodium amobarbital, 283
Soft cervical collar, 194, 207
Spasticity
 following spinal injury, 211
 in multiple sclerosis, 372–373
Speech disorders, 285–288
 evaluation, 286–288
 motor aspects, 286–288
 symptoms, 285
Spike-wave stupor, 95
Spinal cord anatomy, 311
Spinal cord compression syndromes
 epidural abscess, 318–319
 epidural hematoma, 320–321
 metastatic epidural, 317–318, 319t
 symptoms, 11t, 17–18, 312, 317, 319
Spinal cord disorders, 196–199, 197t, 311–329
 acute non-compressive syndromes, 322–328
 and cervical spondylosis, 328
 anoxic, 421
 complicating lumbar puncture, 327
 compression syndromes. *See* Spinal cord
  compression syndromes
 diagnostic approach, 311–317

Spinal cord disorders—*continued*
  diagnostic tests, 43, 195, 313, 315–317
  hematomyelia, 196, 328
  hemisection, 197, 313
  hemorrhage, 199
  infarction, 325–327
  in subarachnoid hemorrhage, 328
  motor signs, 198, 313
  necrosis, 328
  partial injury syndromes, 197–198
  patient history, 311–312
  physical examination, 312–315, 312t
  post-infectious encephalomyelitis, 325
  radiation myelopathy, 323–324, 324t
  respiratory management, 196, 211
  sensory examination, 196, 313
  surgery in, 207–208
  transections, 196–197
  traumatic lesions. *See* Spinal cord trauma
Spinal shock, 313
Spinal cord injuries, 193–211
  cauda equina lesions, 198–199
  cervical lesions, 195, 196, 197t
  complications, 209–211
  conus medullaris lesions, 198
  gunshot wounds, 199
  initial evaluation, 50, 193–196
  management, 204–208
  neurologic examination, 194–195
  radiologic tests, 43, 195
  rehabilitation, 211
  surgery in, 207–208
  syndromes, 196–199, 197t
  traction, 204–208
Spinal cord tumors
  metastatic epidural, 317–318, 318t, 319t
  primary, 322
Spinal films, role in neurologic emergencies, 26, 30t
Spinal fluid myelin basic protein assay (MBP), 383–384
Spinal fluid oligoclonal banding, 381
Spinal fractures, 199–203. *See also* Vertebrae
  evaluation, 43, 199–203
  neurologic examination, 194–195
  management, 204–208
  radiologic tests, 43, 195
  reduction, 205–207
  thoracic, 202
Spinal fusion, 50, 201, 208, 255
Spinal injuries, 193–211
Spinal muscular atrophies (SMA), 226–227
Spinal shock, 197, 211
Spinal stenosis, 45
Spondylitis, tuberculous, 320
Spondylosis, cervical
  vs multiple sclerosis, 366
  symmetrical central cord syndrome in, 328
Status epilepticus, 108–110
  case study, 109–110
  classification, 108, 109t

  convulsive, 108–109
  indications for hospital admission, 115–116
  management, 121–124, 123t
  mortality, 108
  non-convulsive, 109–110
Status migrainosus, 461
Stenosis, spinal, 45
Stress, in multiple sclerosis, 370, 379
Stroke. *See also* Hemorrhage, intracranial; Infarction, intracranial
  definitions, 131–132
  differential diagnosis, 132
  early management, 131–132, 131t
  embolic, 140–141
  focal neurologic signs, 132
  history, 132
  impending, 344
  incidence, 127
  infarction vs hemorrhage, 133t
  mechanisms, 130–131, 131t, 133
  neurologic exam, 132
  physical findings, 132
  radiologic tests, 31, 33, 134–136
  vision loss, 336, 344
Strychnine poisoning, 251
Stye, 331
Subarachnoid hemorrhage. *See* Hemorrhage, subarachnoid
Subarachnoid pressure monitoring, 188
Subtentorial compartment
  anatomy, 59
  mass lesions, 65–66, 66t
Succinylcholine, 238
Sulfinpyrazone (Anturane), in TIAs, 175
Supratentorial compartment
  anatomy, 59
  mass lesions, 65t, 65
Swallowing dysfunction, 246–247, 253, 254–255
Symmetrical central cord syndrome in, 328
Sympathetic nervous system, in intracranial hypertension, 69
Syncope, 104, 166
Syndrome(s)
  Brown-sequard, 197
  carpal tunnel, 231
  central cord, 97
  diabetic dysequilibrium, 65
  diplopic, 348, 360
  Eaton-Lambert, 225, 238
  facilitating myasthenic, 238
  Fisher, 353
  hemi-inattention, 299–300, 300t, 303
  herniated disc, 321–322
  Horner's, 88, 213–214
  Lennox-Gastaut, 402
  locked-in, 98
  Ramsay Hunt, 490
  Reye's, 394–395, 398t
  toxic organic brain, 264–265
  Uhthoff's, 363, 374

Tentorial notch, 59
Tentorium cerebelli, 59
Tetanus, 251
Tetany, 250
Thalamic lesions, 89, 99
Thallium poisoning, 268
Theophylline toxicity, 263, 265
Thiamine, in coma management, 100
Third nerve lesions, 87–88, 351–352
Thoracic spine fractures, 202
Thrombosis
    basilar artery, 100
    carotid, 140
    cavernous sinus, 353
    venous sinus, in children, 405–406
Thymectomy, 237
Thymomas, 236
TIA's. *See* Transient ischemic attacks
Tic douloureux, 376
Tick paralysis, 235, 245t
Toe reflexes, 15, 87, 92
    in infants, 391
Toluene toxicity, 264, 265
Tomography, computerized. *See* Computerized
    tomography
Toxicologic analysis, 96–98, 261–262
Toxin-induced neurologic syndromes, 252, 259–
    272, 269t
    and multiple sclerosis, 366, 367
    behavioral disorders, 264–265
    clinical evaluation, 260–261
    diagnosis, 259–260
    management, basic principles, 270–272
    metabolic changes, 264
    neuromuscular effects, 252, 266–268
    orientation disorders, 278t
    physical examination, 260
    physiologic antagonists, 271
    radiologic evaluation, 43
Trance, vs coma, 98–99
Transcortical aphasia, 289
Transient ischemic attacks, 169–175
    anterior circulation, 169–170
    clinical anatomy, 169
    clinical management, 171–175
    criteria for hospital admission, 173
    differential diagnosis, 172t
    embolic, 173
    history, 170–171
    pathophysiology, 169
    posterior circulation, 170
    radiologic workup, 31–33, 31t
    surgical workup, 173–174
    symptoms, 169–170
Transient neurologic symptoms, 161–175
    blackouts, 104t, 104, 165–167
    causes, 161–164, 162t
    dizziness, 168–169
    history, 164–165, 164t
    TIA. *See* Transient ischemic attacks
Transverse myelopathy, 322–323, 323t

Trauma
    head. *See* Head injuries
    orbital, 356
    post-traumatic seizures, 111
    radiologic techniques in assessment, 36–38
Tremor, in multiple sclerosis, 377
2,4,5-trichlorophenoxyacetic acid (2,4-D),
    toxicity, 268
Tricyclic antidepressants, overdose, 262, 264, 265
Trifluorothymidine (Viroptic), 333
Trimethobenzamide HCl (Tigan), in multiple
    sclerosis, 377
Triorthocresyl phosphate (TOCP), 268
Tropomyosin, 222
Trousseau's sign, 250
Tumor
    intracranial. *See* Mass lesions, intracranial
    spinal, 43, 317–318, 318t, 319t, 322
Tunnel vision, 345

Uhthoff's syndrome, 363, 374
Ulcers, corneal, 333
Ulnar neuropathy, 231–232
Uniform Determination of Death Act (UDDA),
    506
Upgaze palsy, 355
Urine tests, in coma diagnosis, 98
Uveitis, anterior, 332

Valproate, in seizure management, 119, 121
Valproic acid (Depakene), toxicity, 263
Varicella zoster, 395, 489
Vascular disease
    hypertensive. *See* Hypertension, systemic;
        Intracranial pressure, increased
    occlusive. *See* Infarction, intracranial
Vascular headache. *See* Headache
Vegetative state, 99, 422
Ventricular pressure monitoring, 189
Ventricular puncture, 102
Verbal paraphasias, 287
Vertebrae, injuries of, 199–203
    Hangman's fractures, 200
    Jefferson fractures, 200
    lower lumbar fractures, 203
    management, 204–208
    odontoid fractures, 201
    thoracic spine fractures, 202
    thoracolumbar junction, 202–203
    unilateral facet damage, 201–202
    whiplash, 199
Vertebral-basilar vascular system
    anatomy, 128–130
    occlusion, 169–170, 170t, 341
Vertigo
    in multiple sclerosis, 376–377
    vs cerebellar ataxia, 409–410
Vision loss, non-traumatic, 331–348
    anterior segment, 331–334
    binocular, 346
    common causes, 332t

Vision loss—*continued*
  examination, 346–348
  feigned, 344
  hemi-inattention syndromes, 300
  monocular, 346
  patient history, 345
  posterior segment, 334–339
  retrobulbar, 341–342
  scotomatous, 346
  transient, 342–344
Visual acuity testing, 345
Visual evoked potentials (VEP), 379–381
Visual symptoms, in acute headache, 446
Voluntary movement disorders. *See* Apraxias
Vomiting
  in acute headache, 446–447
  in intracranial hypertension, 69, 70

Warfarin, in TIA, 175
Werdnig-Hoffmann disease, 226
Wernicke's aphasia, 289
West's syndrome, 108
Whiplash injury, 199
White blood cells in cerebrospinal fluid, 56
Word finding difficulty in aphasia, 288
Writing assessment, in aphasia testing, 293
Wrong way eyes, 90

Xanthochromia, cerebrospinal fluid, 55, 56

Zoster immune globulin, 489